AF581207

Emergency Asthma

CLINICAL ALLERGY AND IMMUNOLOGY

Series Editor

MICHAEL A. KALINER, M.D.

Medical Director
Institute for Asthma and Allergy
Washington, D.C.

1. Sinusitis: Pathophysiology and Treatment, *edited by Howard M. Druce*
2. Eosinophils in Allergy and Inflammation, *edited by Gerald J. Gleich and A. Barry Kay*
3. Molecular and Cellular Biology of the Allergic Response, *edited by Arnold I. Levinson and Yvonne Paterson*
4. Neuropeptides in Respiratory Medicine, *edited by Michael A. Kaliner, Peter J. Barnes, Gert H. H. Kunkel, and James N. Baraniuk*
5. Provocation Testing in Clinical Practice, *edited by Sheldon L. Spector*
6. Mast Cell Proteases in Immunology and Biology, *edited by George H. Caughey*
7. Histamine and H_1-Receptor Antagonists in Allergic Disease, *edited by F. Estelle R. Simons*
8. Immunopharmacology of Allergic Diseases, *edited by Robert G. Townley and Devendra K. Agrawal*
9. Indoor Air Pollution and Health, *edited by Emil J. Bardana, Jr., and Anthony Montanaro*
10. Genetics of Allergy and Asthma: Methods for Investigative Studies, *edited by Malcolm N. Blumenthal and Bengt Björkstén*
11. Allergic and Respiratory Disease in Sports Medicine, *edited by John M. Weiler*
12. Allergens and Allergen Immunotherapy: Second Edition, Revised and Expanded, *edited by Richard F. Lockey and Samuel C. Bukantz*
13. Emergency Asthma, *edited by Barry E. Brenner*

ADDITIONAL VOLUMES IN PREPARATION

Food Hypersensitivity and Adverse Reactions, *edited by Marianne Frieri and Brett Kettelhut*

Emergency Asthma

edited by

Barry E. Brenner

The Brooklyn Hospital Center
member of New York–Presbyterian Hospitals
Weill Medical College of Cornell University
Brooklyn, New York

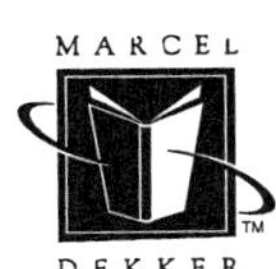

MARCEL DEKKER, INC. NEW YORK • BASEL

Library of Congress Cataloging-in-Publication Data

Emergency asthma / edited by Barry E. Brenner
p. cm. -- (Clinical allergy and immunology ; 13)
Includes bibliographical references and index.
ISBN 0-8247-1945-X (alk. paper)
1. Asthma. 2. Respiratory emergencies. I. Brenner, Barry E.
II. Series.
[DNLM: 1. Asthma. 2. Emergencies. W1 CL652 v. 13 1999 / WF 553
E53 1999]
RC591.E46 1999
616.2'38--dc21
DNLM/DLC
for Library of Congress 98-56653
CIP

This book is printed on acid-free paper.

Headquarters
Marcel Dekker, Inc.
270 Madison Avenue, New York, NY 10016
tel: 212-696-9000; fax: 212-685-4540

Eastern Hemisphere Distribution
Marcel Dekker AG
Hutgasse 4, Postfach 812, CH-4001 Basel, Switzerland
tel: 41-61-261-8482; fax: 41-61-261-8896

World Wide Web
http://www.dekker.com

The publisher offers discounts on this book when ordered in bulk quantities. For more information, write to Special Sales/Professional Marketing at the headquarters address above.

Current printing (last digit):
10 9 8 7 6 5 4 3 2 1

PRINTED IN THE UNITED STATES OF AMERICA

Series Introduction

There are about 14–17 million asthmatics in the United States today. On average, one of 10 will make an emergency visit this year for acute asthma management. Proper management will result in resolution of asthma in most of the patients, although about 500,000 will need to be admitted for inpatient management. With such an important disease, and so much emergency room intervention, one would expect asthma and its management to be major topics in the educational programs of emergency room physicians. However, most emergency room physicians and their assistants learn about asthma primarily from experience. Medical students do not rotate through an asthma specialist's office in order to see outpatient asthma management. There is little formal education offered on pathophysiology, allergy, psychology, and the myriad factors that exacerbate asthma. Moreover, no focused text is available to assist in this educational process.

Emergency Asthma, edited by Barry E. Brenner, is designed to provide a concise, focused, yet comprehensive text on asthma designed specifically for the emergency physician. It covers asthma completely, although the focus is on emergency cases. Each component of underlying causes, examination, treatment, and follow-up is addressed. The chapters are relatively brief and focused but, in total, very comprehensive. This book should be required reading for all emergency physicians, and the information presented here should prove invaluable to all medical practitioners in their battle against asthma.

Michael A. Kaliner, M.D.

To my family,
Cheryl, my wife, Rachel, Dovi, Hudi, Avi, Ari, and grandchildren

May this work serve to improve the care
for the acute asthmatic in the emergency department.

Foreword

On my initial reflection, it seemed that an entire book devoted to the emergency medicine considerations of asthma would be excessive, but when I thought about how much of every emergency department (ED) workload is devoted to asthma, the increasing numbers of patients who present with that disease, the fluctuating—but real—mortality from the disease, and the limitations of my own knowledge concerning this significant problem, it was with great interest and gratitude that I read this book.

Osler thought that asthma never caused mortality, but we currently seem to be in the rise of the sine curve of asthma mortality. Death usually occurs in a middle-aged person with a history of moderate asthma. It often comes quickly from an attack that initially seems no different from previous, less severe attacks. Everyone is surprised—neither the medical professional nor the layperson expects there to be a death. Naturally, there are recriminations, hard feelings, and sometimes litigation. This book will hopefully help to minimize these tragic occurrences, not only by teaching us how to respond to asthma in an efficient and educated fashion, but also by the stimulation of new research and, even more importantly, new thoughts on how to deal with the evaluation of the asthmatic.

For a disease that is as ancient as asthma, it is remarkable how little we understand of its origins and its pathophysiology, and how limited are our treatment options. A succinct definition of the disease applicable to the ED remains obscure. The first chapter, on the history of asthma, is not only fascinating, it reminds us how long patients and physicians have been trying to cope with this terrible affliction. Although we have made enormous improvements in our approach to this disease—especially compared to what was available even a few decades ago—there is still much frustration in finding the right combination of agents that will have reliable and lasting effects without tachyphylaxis.

In my medical lifetime, we have seen the development of selective β-agonists; inhaled, ingested, and parenteral steroids; some prophylactic agents; and more effective delivery technologies. Nevertheless, asthma still remains a tremendous challenge. For example, the airway management of asthma remains highly difficult. As emergency physicians have developed a comfortable expertise with rapid-sequence intubation techniques, they often forget that the airway obstruction in the asthmatic patient is not at the level of the vocal cords. When facing the gasping, failing asthmatic patient, it is tempting to believe that all will be solved by ''taking over the airway,'' but because endotracheal intubation does not relieve bronchospasm—and may in fact worsen it—the job of ventilating the patient merely starts with endotracheal intubation. Even if one can manually overcome the high airway pressures required for inhalation, we have at present no technology that will assist the patient in exhalation, and until the bronchospasm can be relieved, ventilation will remain enormously difficult.

The origins of the reactive airway overreaction are thoroughly discussed in this book, but in many patients they remain obscure. It is rare that we can find a specific etiology that triggers an attack, and even more unlikely that we will find a specific allergen that could be avoided in the future. The fact that we have an increase in environmental factors seems almost self-evident to anyone who has ever witnessed the visible smog conditions of our major cities, and it is probable that our love for the automobile has been gratified at the expense of a harsh increase in reactive airway disease. There are other problems that may also be environmental but are not caused by anything within our obvious control. For example, we have seen an increase in asthma following an apparently mild case of mycoplasma bronchitis or pneumonia in many patients who have never before suffered from asthma, only to be left with an increasingly serious case of reactive airway disease. This form of asthma may initially present with persistent cough rather than wheezing. It also might be true that if we could recognize asthma sooner, then we, by aggressive treatment with inhaled steroids and bronchodilatators, might well be able to prevent the descent into long-term chronic serious disease.

Many aspects of asthma require special consideration, and these are also discussed in this book. For example, asthma during pregnancy is often exacerbated. It is not only that two lives are at risk from the severe forms of the disease, but often that the asthma is exacerbating an underlying pregnancy comorbidity, such as hyperemesis gravidarum in the first trimester or preeclampsia in the third. Moreover, although many asthmatic medications are safe to use in pregnancy, others may have undesirable side effects.

The pediatric patient with asthma is always a special challenge. In addition to the difficulty of achieving adequate delivery of medications, the sight of ventilatory difficulty is psychologically very stressful not only to the parents but also to medical personnel who have dealt mostly with adults and are not accustomed to seeing children in distress. It would also appear that our noxious environments are producing more pediatric asthmatics, and I found the discussions of pediatric management in this book to be very informative.

We often overlook the importance of an effective prehospital management strategy, but there is every reason to believe that if aggressive care can commence in the field, it would make our job easier in the ED and, in fact, may well prevent mortality. This book reviews some special field considerations, and I found it a useful stimulus to review my own relationship with the paramedics with whom I interact. For example, in San Diego, California, it is possible—and often very helpful—to have the paramedics deliver the first respiratory inhalation treatment. But in Jackson Hole, Wyoming, paramedics are not yet permitted to do this, and the number of agents that can be given is very limited (essentially epinephrine and atropine). As every physician knows, trying to change field protocols is often time-consuming, difficult, and frustrating. It is, however, worthwhile to try to institute these changes to make field management aggressive and efficient.

As our society and the way we practice medicine evolve, there are ever-increasing challenges to the management of the asthmatic patient. It does not matter how effective a therapeutic regimen is if the patient has no access to that regimen. For far too many patients in our population, the ED remains the only source of care for acute asthma. Although the emergency physician does an admirable job of caring for acute asthma and status asthmaticus patients, disposition from the ED and long-term care are not as good. I do not say this as an indictment of the emergency physician. Our society has not provided the structure in which to place the nonfunded asthmatic patient. The ED is effective for several visits but not for long-term follow-up. Even for a series of asthmatic visits, it is often impossible to have the same physician and nurse see the patient, and starting all over again on each return visit is unlikely to lead to intelligent management of the patient. Moreover, the various administrative concerns of the managed-care system often lead to limitations in drug formularies, pulmonary testing, and diagnostic procedures that do not serve the best interests of the episodic patient. Even if there were adequate primary care, it is often impossible to obtain a timely visit to the primary physician, and the patient must again resort to the ED for a mild exacerbation. However, what is most worrisome is the severe attack in the indigent patient that is properly but only partially relieved in the ED. The patient has nowhere to go for follow-up. Even if the patient is capable of returning to the ED, the long-term management of this patient will remain suboptimal despite the best efforts of the emergency physician.

The discussions of many of these concerns, which are found in this book, will be of great help to the practicing emergency physician as well as to the residents in training who are in the process of learning that medical knowledge is not sufficient to care for many ED patients. The diagnosis of asthma usually is not subtle, but the effective disposition and optimal long-term management strategy often are. Decisions for admission are progressively being driven by sociological necessities that do not belong in medicine but have become the pressure points for medical decision making. For example, it should not be the responsibility of the hospital staff to obtain shelter for the homeless, but when confronted with a homeless patient with a moderate asthmatic attack, how is it possible to avoid admission when the alternative is the patient's return to a bush or bench in the park in the middle of a rainstorm?

I believe that the emergency physician who reads this book will find answers to many of the common, and some not-so-common, questions about the management of this disease. Acute asthma is omnipresent; it is difficult to define, to manage effectively, and to prevent. Early relapse and return visits to the ED are common. I believe that this book provides an important discussion of the present state of knowledge about this serious disease, especially in the context of the ED. It should also be useful to other physicians who are responsible for asthmatic patients, whether in their offices or on inpatient services after the patients have been treated in the ED. This book will help to provide some insight into the decisions the emergency physician has to make and may ameliorate some of the second-guessing that inevitably occurs after a patient's initial management.

Having read this book, I now approach the asthmatic patient with a greater sense of confidence about how to manage this problem. I believe the book will provide for all readers a stimulus to curiosity about the future management of this disease, as well as an improved daily performance.

Peter Rosen, M.D.
Professor and Residency Director
Department of Emergency Medicine
University of California, San Diego

Preface

Acute asthma is one of the most common specific illnesses that present to an emergency department (ED). Over the last 20 years, many changes have occurred in the management of asthma in the ED. Intravenous aminophylline and subcutaneous epinephrine used to be the mainstays of acute asthma treatment in adults. In children, serial injections of subcutaneous epinephrine followed by a "chaser" of aqueous suspension epinephrine, Susphrine®, were routine. Patients were discharged from the ED when they were asymptomatic and "wheeze-free." Concomitantly, emergency medicine has come of age as a specialty to care for many patients with acute asthma from a unique perspective. There are now practice guidelines, noninvasive measures of oxygenation, and monitors of airway flow rates for acute asthmatics in the ED. However, in the last 20 years there has also been a worldwide increase in asthma morbidity and mortality. Each year there are over one million visits to the ED for acute asthma, with asthma representing 10% of ED visits in certain regions. The total direct economic cost has been estimated at $6.2 billion.

This book is intended to serve as a concise but thorough, clinically useful compendium dedicated to both the clinician and patient with acute asthma in the ED. Each chapter is a short but well-referenced state-of-the-art review of the subject. Where appropriate, the chapters discuss asthma in children as well as adults. The aim of this book is to provide scholarly information applicable at the bedside or "asthma chair." To this end, I have sought chapter authors from a cross section of fields—including epidemiology, allergy and immunology, pulmonary, and critical care medicine—who have achieved prominence in asthma. Most of the chapter authors are academic emergency physicians and clinicians involved with both pediatric and adult emergency medicine.

The book covers a wide range of topics, including an introduction to past and future directions in asthma, i.e., the history of asthma and trends in future asthma research; pathophysiology; epidemiology of acute asthma, especially in urban centers; factors that result in the visit to the ED; clinical manifestations; evaluations such as pulse oximetry, spirometry, laboratory work, electrocardiograms, and X-rays; management of acute asthma involving the National Institutes of Health (NIH) protocol, among others, and specific treatments; management of the airway and endotracheal intubation; special situations, such as the pregnant asthmatic or intractable severe asthma; disposition from the ED and the role of the observation unit; and how to prevent relapse.

Emergency Asthma reviews the current thinking about asthma, especially as it presents to the ED. The definition and diagnosis of acute asthma are covered in several chapters in this book (see Chapters 5, 13, and 14 on epidemiology, differential diagnosis, and spirometry, respectively). Of particular note is that there is no overall diagnostic or treatment plan covering the entire subject of acute asthma. For this purpose, I suggest the reader refer to Chapter 18 for guidelines for the management of adult asthma, which lists the 1997 National Asthma Education and Prevention Program (NAEPP) guidelines. The impact of algorithmic treatment guidelines for acute asthma in the ED remains an area of investigation.

It is my hope that this book will be a starting point to stimulate new interventions; develop effective management protocols; and forge partnerships between emergency physicians, private practitioners, and researchers. It is also my goal that this collaboration will work to reverse the tide of increasing ED visits, admissions, and mortality due to asthma. This effort is dedicated to the patients, the best justification for the academic excellence of the clinician.

Barry E. Brenner

Acknowledgments

I would like to thank Lilli Sentz of the Rare Book Room of the N.Y. Academy of Medicine for invaluable assistance; Fred Rosner, M.D., and the library of the Jewish Theologic Seminary for information on Maimonides; the Phillip Reichert family; Ron Cunningham from the American College of Emergency Physicians; and Henning Ruben, M.D., and Ole Koehnke from Ambu Inc. for all their help. I would like to give a special thanks to Carlos Camargo, M.D., and Robert Silverman, M.D., for their special help with this project, as well as to all of the chapter contributors who worked so exhaustively to produce this landmark work.

I would like to thank Drs. Bjorn Ibsen and Erik Jacobsen for the extraordinary accounts of their medical experiences, as well as Dorte Askgaard, Ph.D., Lotte Mortensen, head nurse, and Neil Frandsen for information about Vivi Ebert and the 1952 epidemic of polio in Copenhagen. I would also like to thank the patients that I met, Mr. Olsen and Mr. Knulson, for taking the time to describe their experiences.

I would like to express my gratitude to Audrey Ellis, whose effort to keep me organized in this task were nearly exhausted, and to the publishing assistance of Sandra Beberman, Linda Schonberg, and Sebastian Thaler. A special thanks to Michael Kaliner, M.D., for initiating this project with me and for his careful advice.

Finally, I thank Scott Inkley, M.D., F.C.C.P., whose patients with acute asthma gave me the drive and determination to improve the care for all asthmatics.

Barry E. Brenner

Contents

Part Four PROVOCATIVE FACTORS FOR EMERGENCY DEPARTMENT VISITS

Part Five CLINICAL MANIFESTATIONS

Part Six MANAGEMENT

Contributors

Jill M. Baren, M.D. Assistant Professor, Departments of Emergency Medicine and Pediatrics, University of Pennsylvania School of Medicine, Philadelphia, Pennsylvania

Barry E. Brenner, M.D., Ph.D. Vice-Chairman and Research Director, Department of Emergency Medicine, The Brooklyn Hospital Center, member of New York–Presbyterian Hospitals, Weill Medical College of Cornell University, Brooklyn, New York

Robert Bristow, M.D. Clinical Instructor, Department of Emergency Medicine, Columbia-Presbyterian Hospital, Columbia University School of Medicine, New York, New York

Susan M. Brugman, M.D. Associate Professor of Pediatrics, University of Colorado Health Sciences Center, Denver, Colorado

Charles B. Cairns, M.D. Associate Professor of Medicine, University of Colorado Health Sciences Center, and Director, Colorado Emergency Medicine Research Center, Denver, Colorado

Carlos A. Camargo Jr., M.D., Dr.P.H. Attending Physician, Department of Emergency Medicine, Massachusetts General Hospital and Harvard Medical School, Boston, Massachusetts

Ellen F. Crain, M.D., Ph.D. Professor of Pediatrics, Albert Einstein College of Medicine, and Director of Pediatric Emergency Medicine, Jacobi Medical Center, Bronx, New York

Rita Kay Cydulka, M.D. Associate Professor and Residency Director, Department of Emergency Medicine, MetroHealth Medical Center/Case Western Reserve University, Cleveland, Ohio

Charles L. Emerman, M.D. Chairman, Department of Emergency Medicine, MetroHealth Medical Center/Cleveland Clinic Foundation, Cleveland, Ohio

Susan Fuchs, M.D. Associate Professor, Department of Pediatrics, Northwestern University Medical School, Chicago, Illinois

Theodore J. Gaeta, D.O. Assistant Professor and Program Director, Department of Emergency Medicine, New York Methodist Hospital, member of New York–Presbyterian Hospitals, Weill Medical College of Cornell University, Brooklyn, New York

Louis G. Graff, M.D. Associate Professor, Department of Traumatology and Emergency Medicine, University of Connecticut School of Medicine, Farmington, Connecticut

Kim Guishard, M.D. Clinical Director, Department of Emergency Medicine, The Brooklyn Hospital Center, member of New York–Presbyterian Hospitals, Weill Medical College of Cornell University, Brooklyn, and Assistant Professor of Clinical Surgery/ Emergency Medicine, New York University School of Medicine, New York, New York

Jin H. Han, M.D. Department of Emergency Medicine, State University of New York Health Science Center at Brooklyn Kings County Hospital Center, Brooklyn, New York

Michael A. Kaliner, M.D. Medical Director, Institute for Asthma and Allergy, Washington Hospital Center, Washington, D.C.

Jill P. Karpel, M.D. Professor of Medicine, Albert Einstein College of Medicine, and Department of Medicine, Montefiore Medical Center, Bronx, New York

Martin S. Kohn, M.D., M.S. Chairman, Department of Emergency Medicine, The Brooklyn Hospital Center, member of New York–Presbyterian Hospitals, Weill Medical College of Cornell University, Brooklyn, and Assistant Professor of Clinical Surgery/ Emergency Medicine, New York University School of Medicine, New York, New York

Monica Kraft, M.D. Director, Carl and Hazel Felt Laboratory for Asthma Research, National Jewish Medical and Research Center, and Assistant Professor of Medicine, Division of Pulmonary and Critical Care Medicine, University of Colorado Health Sciences Center, Denver, Colorado

David M. Lang, M.D. Chief, Division of Allergy/Immunology, and Associate Professor, Department of Medicine, Allegheny University of the Health Sciences, Philadelphia, Pennsylvania

Mark J. Leber, M.D. Attending Physician and Faculty Member, Emergency Medicine Residency Program, Department of Emergency Medicine, The Brooklyn Hospital Center, member of New York–Presbyterian Hospitals, Weill Medical College of Cornell University, Brooklyn, New York

Richard J. Martin, M.D. Head, Pulmonary Division, and Vice Chair, Department of Medicine, National Jewish Medical and Research Center, and Professor of Medicine, University of Colorado Health Sciences Center, Denver, Colorado

Paul Mayo, M.D. Associate Professor of Medicine, Albert Einstein College of Medicine, Bronx, and Co-Director, Medical Intensive Care Unit, Beth Israel Medical Center, New York, New York

Michael F. McDermott, M.D. Director of Observation Medicine, Department of Emergency Medicine, Cook County Hospital, Chicago, Illinois

Eric S. Nadel, M.D. Instructor of Medicine, Harvard Medical School, and Department of Emergency Medicine, Brigham and Women's Hospital, Boston, Massachusetts

Richard M. Nowak, M.D., M.B.A. Associate Professor and Vice-Chairman, Department of Emergency Medicine, Henry Ford Health Systems, Detroit, Michigan

Harold H. Osborn, M.D. Chairman, Department of Emergency Medicine, Long Island College Hospital, Brooklyn, New York

Edward A. Panacek, M.D. Professor of Medicine, Division of Emergency Medicine, University of California, Davis, Sacramento, California

Charles V. Pollack Jr., M. A., M.D. Clinical Associate Professor and Chairman, Department of Emergency Medicine, Maricopa Medical Center, Phoenix, Arizona

Kerry Alexander Powell, M.D., Ch.B. Instructor, Department of Emergency Medicine, Johns Hopkins Bayview Medical Center, Baltimore, Maryland

Michael Stavros Radeos, M.D. Assistant Professor of Medicine, New York Medical College, and Director of Research, Department of Emergency Medicine, Lincoln Medical and Mental Health Center, Bronx, New York

Donald G. Raible, M.D. Associate Professor of Medicine, Division of Pulmonary/Critical Care Medicine, Allegheny University of the Health Sciences, Philadelphia, Pennsylvania

Phillip L. Rice Jr., M.D. Director and Assistant Professor, Department of Emergency Medicine, Kings County Hospital Center, Brooklyn, New York

Lynne D. Richardson, M.D. Vice-Chairman and Residency Director, Department of Emergency Medicine, Mount Sinai School of Medicine, New York, New York

Richard J. Scarfone, M.D. Associate Professor of Pediatrics, MCP-Hahnemann School of Medicine, and Medical Director, Section of Pediatric Emergency Medicine, St. Christopher's Hospital for Children, Philadelphia, Pennsylvania

Steven M. Scharf, M.D., Ph.D. Professor, Department of Medicine, Albert Einstein College of Medicine, Bronx, and Long Island Jewish Medical Center, New Hyde Park, New York

Mona Shah, M.D. Clinical Assistant Professor, Department of Emergency Medicine, Oregon Health Sciences University, Portland, Oregon

Robert Silverman, M.D. Assistant Professor of Emergency Medicine and Epidemiology and Social Medicine, Albert Einstein College of Medicine, Bronx, and Department of Emergency Medicine, Long Island Jewish Medical Center, New Hyde Park, New York

Richard Sinert, D.O. Assistant Professor and Research Director, Department of Emergency Medicine, State University of New York Health Science Center at Brooklyn Kings County Hospital Center, Brooklyn, New York

Emil M. Skobeloff, M.D. Clinical Associate Professor, Department of Emergency Medicine, MCP-Hahnemann Medical College, Crozer-Chester Medical Center, Philadelphia, Pennsylvania

Karen L. Stavile, M.D. Assistant Professor and Associate Director, Department of Emergency Medicine, State University of New York Health Science Center at Brooklyn Kings County Hospital Center, Brooklyn, New York

Mary H. Stewart, M.D. Senior Instructor, Department of Emergency Medicine, MetroHealth Medical Center, Cleveland, and Director, Emergency Department, Allen Memorial Hospital, Oberlin, Ohio

Samuel J. Stratton, M.D. Medical Director, Los Angeles County EMS Agency, Los Angeles, and Associate Professor, Department of Emergency Medicine, Harbor–UCLA Medical Center, Torrance, California

George D. Thurston, Sc.D. Associate Professor, Department of Environmental Medicine, New York University School of Medicine, New York, New York

Joseph Adrian Tyndall, M.D. Attending Physician, Department of Emergency Medicine, The Brooklyn Hospital Center, member of New York–Presbyterian Hospitals, Weill Medical College of Cornell University, Brooklyn, New York

Brian T. Williams, M.D. Research Fellow, Department of Emergency Medicine, University of Colorado Health Sciences Center, and Colorado Emergency Medicine Research Center, Denver, Colorado

1

Where Have We Been?

The History of Acute Asthma

Barry E. Brenner

The Brooklyn Hospital Center, member of New York–Presbyterian Hospitals, Weill Medical College of Cornell University, Brooklyn, New York

Almost all the serious consequences of bronchial asthma occur during acute asthmatic episodes. Emergency asthma, the subject of this book, is the type of acute asthma that is seen in emergency departments (EDs). There are 1.5 million emergency department visits for acute asthma in the United States per year. (see Chapter 5, ''Epidemiology of Asthma''). According to the Multi-Center Asthma Research Collaboration (MARC), 40% of adults with an episode of acute asthma have not seen a primary care provider (PCP) in the last year. For an asthma problem, 95% of the population studied go to the ED if they have no PCP, and even 65% come to the ED even if they have a PCP (1). Thus the ED is the main resource for patients with acute asthma. Emergency physicians prevent much of the morbidity and mortality associated with bronchial asthma and also serve as the only source of care for many asthmatic patients.

Asthma is a frequent, serious, and chronic disease with acute exacerbations commonly seen in all EDs. Many recurrent presentations of other illnesses are for symptoms, e.g., headache, chest pain, or abdominal pain. Acute asthma seems to present in a similar fashion in most patients. For experienced clinicians the signs, symptoms, and response to therapy for most cases of acute asthma seem quite predictable. Such a specific disease should have been well recognized by clinicians hundreds of years ago and for the most part diagnosed correctly based on this repetitive clinical presentation. Therefore, a review of the history of acute asthma is achievable. As the introduction to this book on emergency asthma, the history of the concepts and treatments in patients with acute asthma before the advent of EDs, emergency medicine, or even before pharmaceutical companies will be reviewed. Developments in asthma did not happen in isolation from the major changes in medicine in general; many of these advances impacted profoundly on the diagnosis and therapy of acute asthma. Some of the most relevant and interesting of these will be reviewed as well.

I. ANTIQUITY

The Ebers papyrus in Egypt from 1500 B.C. refers to a condition whose description is consistent with acute asthma and was treated with enemas and animal excreta, including crocodile and camel, together with herbs such as squill and henbane. Henbane, whose active ingredient is scopolamine, was placed on a heated brick rock and the vapors were inhaled (2,3). Scopolamine has strong anticholinergic properties, and anticholinergic agents have been useful in patients with acute asthma even in today's EDs. Asthma was described in the oldest medical book, the Chinese *Nei Ching*, written by Huang-Ti in approximately 1000 B.C. In this connection the author mentions the Ma Huang plant, from which the sympathomimetic ephedrine was extracted in the early 1900s (4).

Ayurvedic medicine from ancient India termed a condition Tamaka Swasa that is consistent with asthma. It was described in the Caraka Samhita, a two-volume medical book written in Sanskrit from at least the first century A.D. It was noted that Tamaka Swasa often started with a ''cold'' leading to shortness of breath, wheezing, and much coughing. In more severe cases the patient may not be able to speak or lie down. He may be wide-eyed and sweating. The treatment consisted of steam, inhaled cinnamon, castor bean oil, an insect resin (lac), tumeric, arsenics, *Datura* (see section later on belladonna alkaloids), and herbal ointments (5).

Asthma is a Greek word meaning *panting*. It was first used in Homer's Iliad and also found in the works of the poet Pindar, the playwright Aeschylus, and the philosopher Plato. The term was used by Hippocrates and implied a certain sound. Hippocrates (460–370 B.C.) (Fig. 1) separated medicine from superstition and infused scientific spirit and ethical principles into medicine. The condition of asthma was regarded as paroxysmal and more severe than simple dyspnea. Its spasmodic nature was compared to an epileptic convulsion, and it was considered a divine visitation.

With the destruction of ancient Greece by the Romans, Greek medicine was incorporated into Roman practices. Initially hindered by Pliny the elder, who stated that Rome had been successful for over 600 years without physicians, Asclepiades established Greek medicine in Rome, and the Greek physician Galen (131–201 A.D.) became Rome's greatest medical practitioner. Seneca, the Roman philosopher, suffered with asthma (6). Galen and other Roman physicians, notably Aretaeus, noted that acute asthma was more frequent during the winter than the summer and during the night compared to the day. ''There was a wheezing noise heard in the chest. The voice may be weak and the neck stretched. The asthmatic appears anxious'' (7–9). Roman physicians and the practitioners of Ayurvedic medicine had given asthma a remarkably accurate descriptions before the start of the Middle Ages.

II. MIDDLE AGES AND BYZANTINE PERIOD

After centuries of the ''Dark'' Middle Ages came the Moslems, who in their conquests acquired Greek manuscripts and brought the ancient medical wisdom of Greece and Rome to Arabia and Spain. Treatments of asthma involved mixtures of licorice, cotton, melon, Mohameddan cucumber, and gum arabic (10). Moses Maimonides (1138*–1204), an ex-

* Many books list Maimonides' year of birth as 1135. The best source of the year of his birth is Maimonides' Commentary to the Mishnah written in 1168, where he states in his own handwriting that he was thirty years old when he finished writing this work.

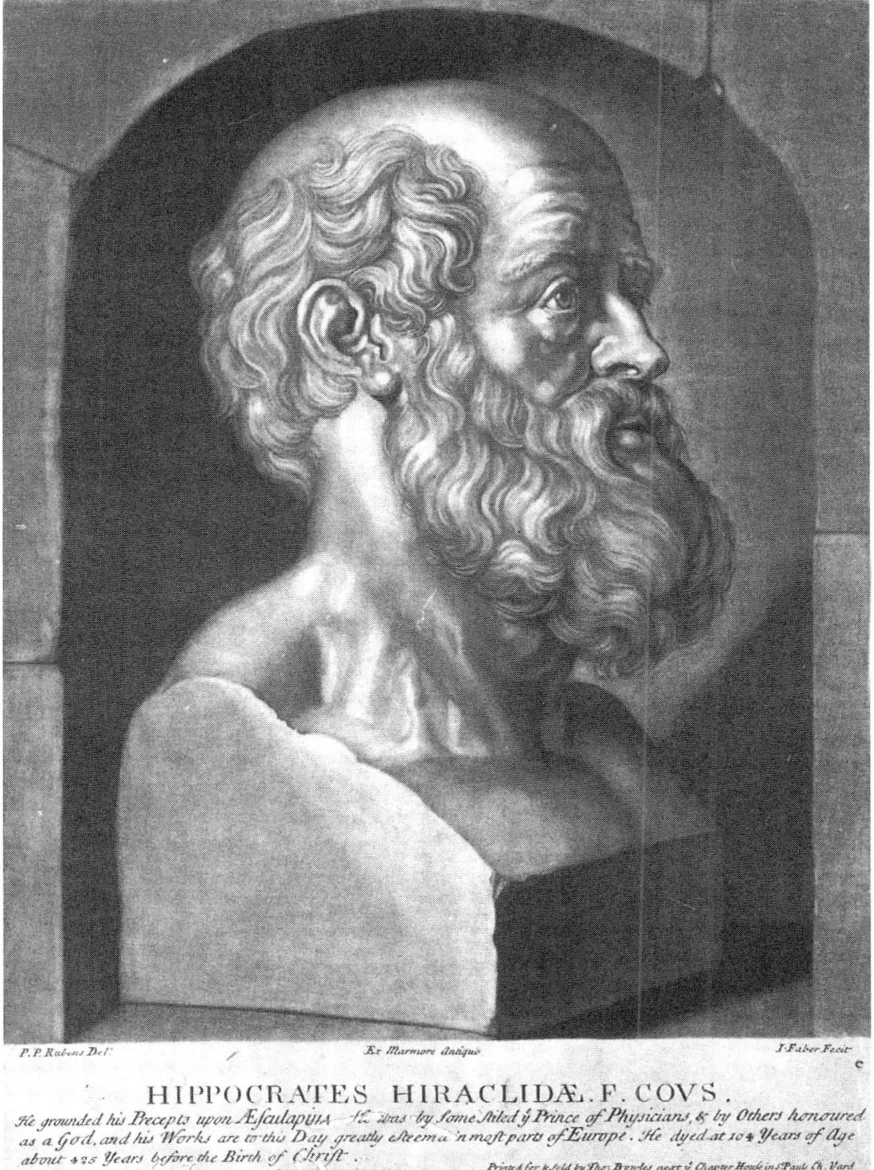

Figure 1 Mezzotint by J. Faber after Peter Paul Reubens (1577–1640). Reubens painted this picture from an ancient statue of Hippocrates from the Greek island of Kos, where the famous physician resided. The bottom of the mezzotint reads, "He grounded his Precepts upon Aesculapius. He was by some styled as Prince of Physicians, and by others honoured as a God, and his Works are to this Day greatly esteemed in most parts of Europe. He died at 104 years of Age about 425 Years before the Birth of Christ." (Courtesy of the Wellcome Institute Library, London, England.)

traordinary talmudic scholar, philosopher, and physician, lived in Cordova, Spain (Fig. 2). To escape Islamic persecution in Spain the family fled, wandering for 10 years in Spain to arrive in Fez, Morocco, where Maimonides devoted himself to the study of medicine and Judaism. The family finally settled in Egypt, where his reputation as a physician grew. He became appointed as the physician to the great Saladin and then became physician to the Saladin's son, Prince Al Afdal Nur ad Din Ali, when the Prince assumed the throne at age 40 in 1193.†

Maimonides was requested to write dietary advice on asthma for the Prince. This resulted in a Treatise on Asthma (11) written in the latter 14 years of Maimonides' life. He states that he has no magic cure for asthma and that he will cite as many sources as he can remember "to give greater force to any discourse."† He noted that he relied heavily on Galen. Maimonides wrote that asthma often starts with a common cold during the rainy season, noted that the "air pollution" of Cairo may in part be responsible for the asthma, and recommended a change in climate for the Prince. His description of the city seems amazingly modern: "Town air is stagnant, turbid, and thick; it is the natural result of its big buildings, narrow streets, and garbage. . . . Air winds carry stealthily inside the houses and many become ill with asthma without noticing it. Concern for clean air is a foremost rule in preserving the health of one's body and soul." He proceeded to recommend various diets and therapeutic herbs. Some were to be inhaled as vapors. He also recommended old chicken soup to thin the phlegm and serve as an expectorant. In the modern era chicken soup was reported to have similar effects (12,13). Many dietary recommendations were provided by Maimonides to the Prince (14,15). He emphasized that medical conditions should be taken care of by scientifically based physicians and urged the Prince not to chase after magic cures. Maimonides stated in this treatise that:

> he who puts his life in the hands of a physician skilled in art but lacking in science is like a mariner who trusts his luck, relying only on the sea winds. Sometimes they blow in the direction you want with good luck; other times not and this may lead to doom.

III. THE RENAISSANCE

For the next 400 years the scientific study of asthma and other diseases was suppressed by feudalism and the repressive interests of established religions. At the end of this time period, man again began to contemplate himself and the universe, and the Renaissance began. Just preceding this time (1400 A.D.) the Greek word for asthma was brought into the English language as two different words: asmy and asma. Around 1600 A.D. the word asthma came into usage (7).

Van Helmont (1577–1644) in France, who suffered with asthma, noted that the bronchi were the origin of asthma and that inhaling dust or eating fish in certain individuals brought on attacks. He noted that the bronchi would react with spasm to dust, especially from the demolition of houses and temples (16). He described a monk who, while eating

† There in Egypt he wrote his prodigious compilation of Jewish law, Mishneh Torah (finished in 1168), and the philosophic treatise, Guide for the Perplexed. The former work was highly criticized for not being referenced well enough to its source, the Talmud.

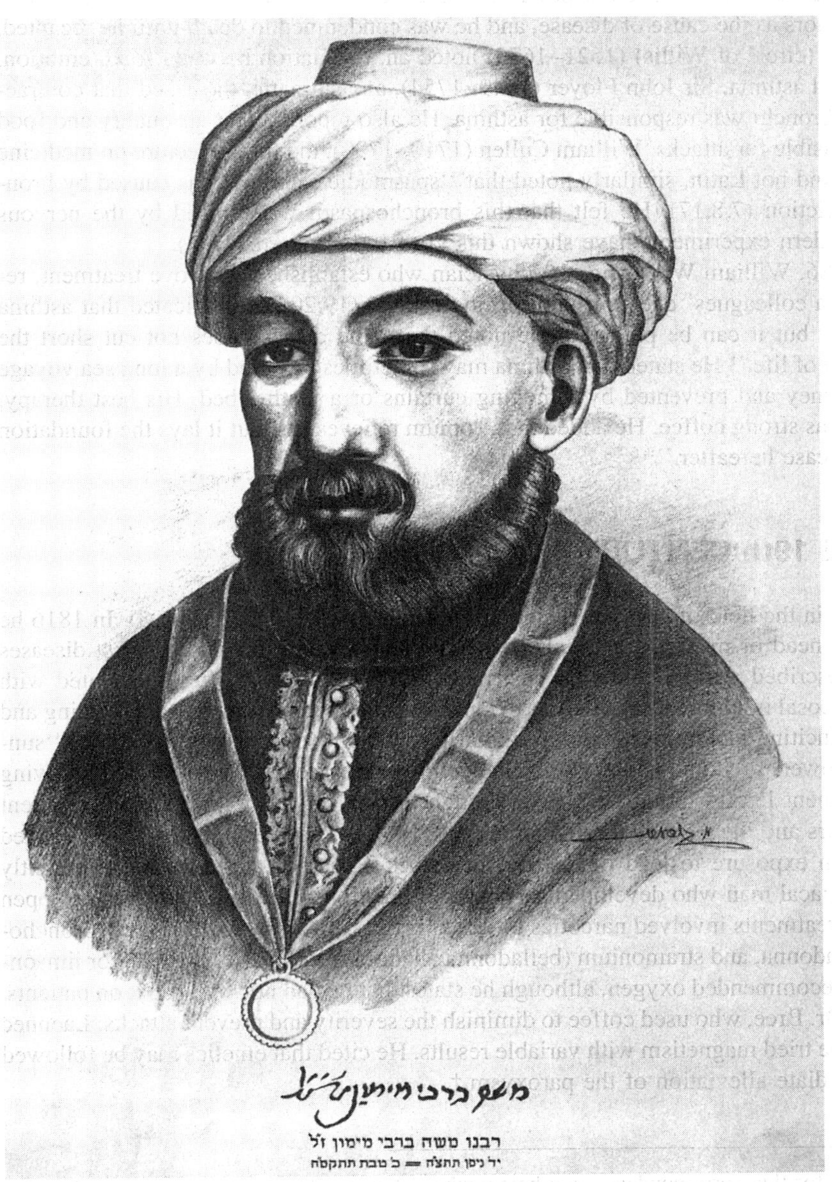

Figure 2 Top: Moses Maimonides photogravure. (Courtesy of the Wellcome Institute Library, London, England.) Bottom: Signature from letter by Maimonides pleading for funds to ransom Jewish captives taken prisoner in 1168 by the Crusader, Almaric of Jerusalem, after his attack. From the Cairo Genizah of the Ben Ezra synagogue in Fostat, Egypt, 1897. (Courtesy of the Jewish Theological Seminary of America.)

fish fried in oil, fell down, deprived of breathing, "so that he was scarce distinguished from a strangled man." This concept put him in conflict with the official Church view of internal humors as the cause of disease, and he was condemned to death until he recanted.

Willis (circle of Willis) (1621–1675) noted an association between food, emotion, heredity, and asthma. Sir John Floyer (1649–1754), an asthmatic, theorized that contraction of the bronchi was responsible for asthma. He also reported that air quality and food were responsible for attacks. William Cullen (1710–1790), the first to lecture on medicine in English and not Latin, similarly noted that "spasmodic asthma" was caused by bronchial constriction (7,8,17). He felt that this bronchospasm was caused by the nervous system. Modern experiments have shown this view to be incorrect (18).

In 1786, William Withering, the physician who established foxglove treatment, responded to a colleagues' questions concerning asthma (19,20). He indicated that asthma is incurable, but it can be palliated. He noted that "the disease does not cut short the usual period of life." He stated that asthma may sometimes be cured by a long sea voyage or land journey and prevented by removing curtains or a feather bed. His best therapy, he stated, was strong coffee. He added that "opium relieves fits, but it lays the foundation of more disease hereafter."*

IV. THE 19th CENTURY

A luminary in the field of chest medicine was Laennec (1781–1826) (Fig. 3). In 1816 he became the head of medicine at Necker Hospital and wrote a treatise on chest diseases (21). He described asthma as due to spasms of the bronchi most often associated with catarrh (mucosal inflammation). Asthma symptoms were increased during the evening and nighttime. Inciting factors were emotions, marital relations, odors (bulb flowers or "sun-seeking" flowers or stored apples), or a change in the weather. It was produced by living in an apartment low to the ground, even though the air was changed by the movement through doors and the passage through chimneys. He also reported occupationally related asthma from exposure to lead oxides. He describes a case of an agoraphobic, slightly hypochondriacal man who developed shortness of breath repeatedly on exposure to open areas. His treatments involved narcotics to lessen respiratory drive and decrease bronchospasm, belladonna, and stramonium (belladonna alkaloid from the *Datura* plant or jimsonweed). He recommended oxygen, although he states that he had not yet used it on patients. He cited a Dr. Bree, who used coffee to diminish the severity and prevent attacks. Laennec stated that he tried magnetism with variable results. He cited that emetics may be followed by an immediate alleviation of the paroxysm.†

* The source for this correspondence is a holographic letter, written in English, and displayed at the Royal Society of Medicine, London, England.

† Leannec's treatise is famous for the description of the use of the stethoscope. He described his auscultation through the stethoscope as *mediate auscultation* (Laennec's term) as opposed to listening with one's own ear, termed *immediate auscultation*. He coined the terms we use today for the different types of rhonchi, râles, egophony, bronchophony, and pectoriloquy. His colleagues argued strongly against this mediate auscultation in which one would have to carry an instrument. It seemed unnecessary to depend on another instrument when you always would have your ear. Laennec countered by arguing that the stethoscope was good for listening in areas in which it

Charles B. Williams (1805–1889) in 1840 demonstrated that smooth muscle contraction was a probable cause of airway obstruction in asthma. He demonstrated in animals that the airways contracted to electrical stimuli and that contractions were abolished by belladonna, stramonium, or morphine (22).

Salter (1823–1871), an asthma sufferer, provided vivid accounts of acute asthma, emphasizing the hereditary aspects of the disease and distinguishing bronchial from cardiac asthma. He also considered asthma to be both related to inflammation of the bronchi as well as bronchospasm. His work on asthma was considered the standard during the late 1800s (17,23).

Ramadge (1793–1867) wrote a review of the subject of asthma about 15 years after Laennec. He described the onset of asthma to be associated with food, weather, menstruation, or emotions. He stated that asthma occurred mostly at night. In the summertime it was associated with periods of excessive heat and in the winter it occurred with the early frost or a ''close, foggy'' state. On physical examination he described accessory muscle use and hyperinflation of the chest (24): ''The patient may sit up, lean forward, breathing as if to suck in his air. The patient may not be able to speak.'' He reported on the auscultation with a stethoscope of wheezing and spasm of the bronchi. As for therapy, he noted that what works for some patients does not work for others. He stated that narcotics should be discredited as these agents make matters worse, but early in the attack they may be useful if judiciously used. He notes that Laennec used narcotics to relax the respiratory drive, which caused an effect similar to that of hibernation in animals. He cited Willis, who noted that opiates impede respiration that was already ''oppressed'' and that opiates endanger life. Ramadge, who seems very forward thinking, recommended stramonium, which ''produces a grateful forgetfulness and a balmy oblivion like opiates.'' He also recommended a change from city to country living (24).

Trousseau, the French physician famous for his sign of hypocalcemia, describes a personal worst attack, which came on in minutes with intense profuse rhinorrhea and watery discharge from his eyes, dyspnea, and oppression, and was relieved in 10 minutes by smoking a cigar! At the time of the asthma attack, Trousseau was in the hayloft watching a coachman, who he suspected of dishonesty, measuring oats (25). He notes that with some asthmatics, the mere presence of a cat or rabbit in a room causes bronchospasm. Trousseau urged treatment with stramonium, ether, chloroform, or potassium nitrate fumes.

---

was difficult for the ear to maneuver: the axilla, bony prominences, and the space occupied by the breast. Listening with the ear was too fatiguing on the posture and head itself. In addition the physician could not assess egophony, bronchophony, or pectoriloquy. He described the sounds of asthma as wheezing. In this chapter of his textbook he discusses the construction of his stethoscope. His prototype was paper, but he found wood more durable. He tried metal, but it was too cold for the patient. The stethoscope recommended by Laennec was made out of wood or Indian cane, 1 ft long (to avoid exposure to the patient's breath), 0.5–1.5 inches in diameter, and perforated longitudinally by a bore three lines wide. The part to go on the chest wall was a 1.5 inch funnel for the lung exam. The funnel was to be plugged to examine the heart. The stethoscope came into two parts to allow for portability, and the physician could listen with only one ear at a time. Initially Laennec's idea was ridiculed, and he retired to the countryside. During his lifetime, however, the book and the stethoscope grew in acceptance eventually to become the standard in internal and chest medicine. Dr. George Camman introduced the binaural stethoscope in 1855 with flexible tubing. The tubing was covered with tight coils dipped covered with silk and dipped in a gum elastic. This stethoscope looks quite similar to those in use today (Figures 4A-D).

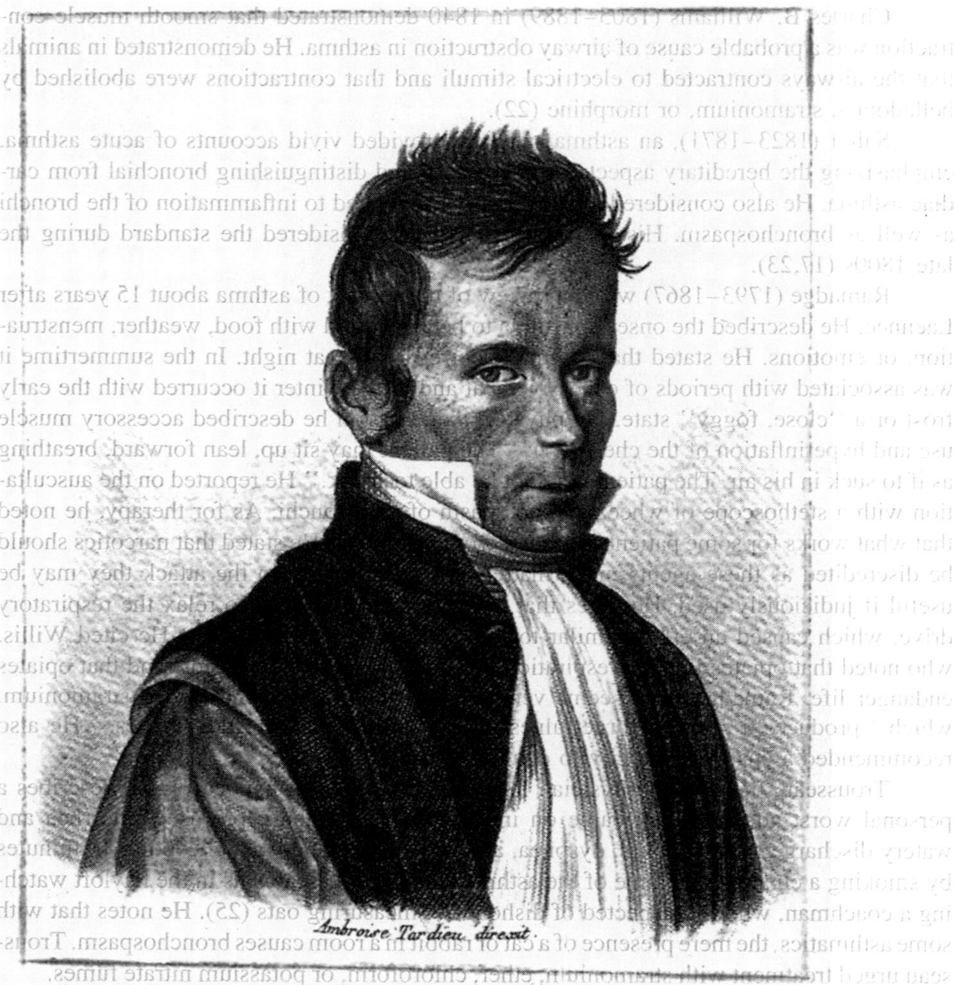

Figure 3 Engraving of Rene Theophile Hyacinthe Laennec by Ambroise Thadieu. (Courtesy of Wellcome Institute Library, London, England.)

Thorowgood published many works on asthma from 1870 until 1900 based on his clinical experience with 160 patients with asthma. He described the use of ozone paper (see Fig. 9 on page 16) which was smoked and contained potash (potassium hydroxide) or potassium iodide. He indicates that at earlier times *Datura* (jimsonweed) was chopped and smoked in a pipe, but in his more modern times it had been placed into the paper of

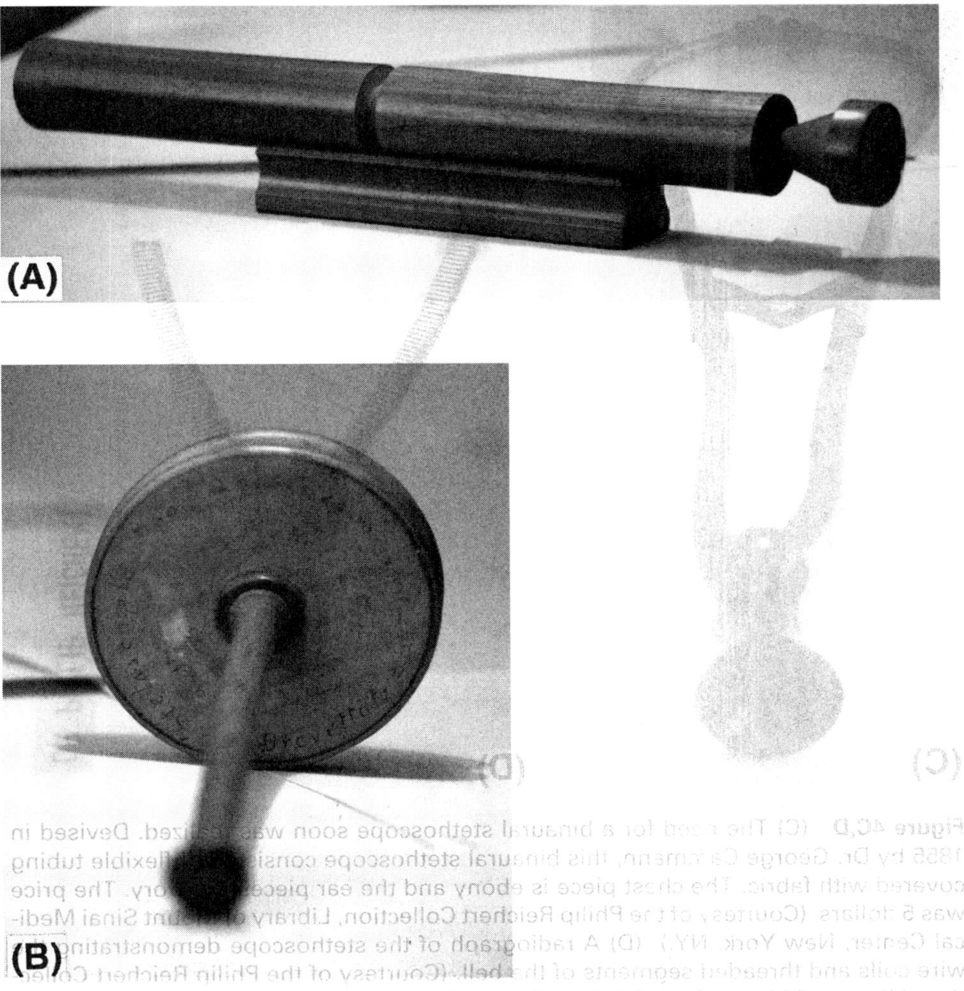

Figure 4A,B (A) A reconstructed model of Laennec's original stethoscope, 1819. It was separable for portability. (Courtesy of the Philip Reichert Collection, Library of Mount Sinai Medical Center, New York, NY.) (B) The earpiece of the stethoscope may be unscrewed for ease in carrying, as in all monoaurals. This specimen is inscribed in ink: "Stethoscope tipo Laennec megafonico. Brevettato. Doctt Corradino Malloli Faligno Bevagna. (Courtesy of the Philip Reichert Collection, Library of Mount Sinai Medical Center, New York, NY.)

a cigarette. Other therapies recommended were chloroform, ether, amyl nitrite, nitre paper (paper suffused with potassium nitrate), and sprays made from a solution of lobelia and belladonna alkaloids. He noted the highly effective use of chloroform for a severe asthmatic in 1847. Chloroform, if used early in very small amounts, he stated, would abort an attack, but larger amounts are needed for an established episode. His standard treatment was 5–10 drops in a handkerchief or an inhaling pipe. He reported tachyphylaxis to the

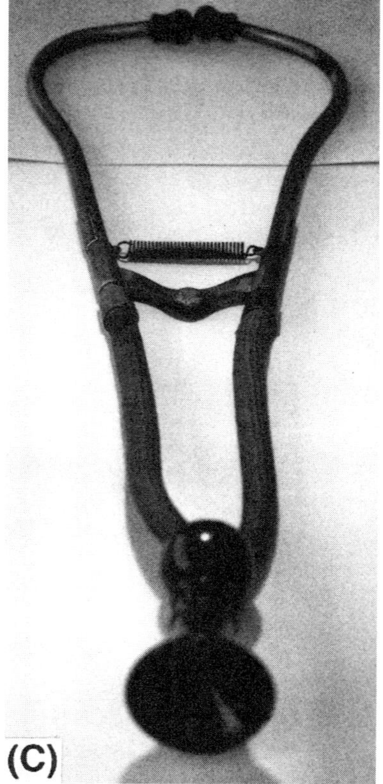

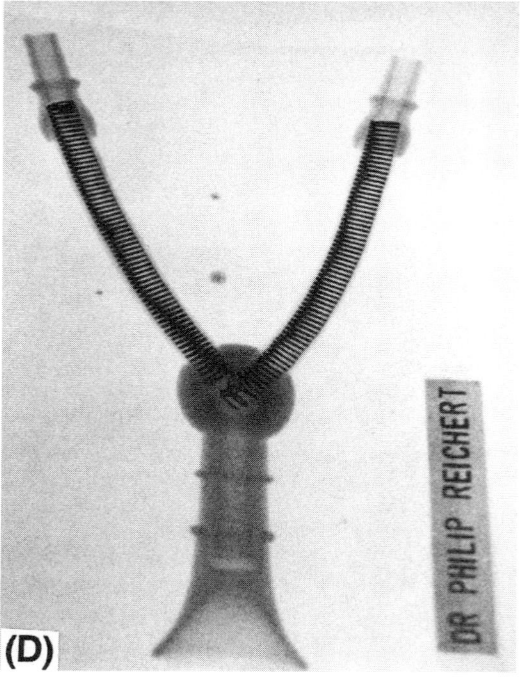

Figure 4C,D (C) The need for a binaural stethoscope soon was realized. Devised in 1855 by Dr. George Cammann, this binaural stethoscope consisted of flexible tubing covered with fabric. The chest piece is ebony and the ear pieces are ivory. The price was 5 dollars. (Courtesy of the Philip Reichert Collection, Library of Mount Sinai Medical Center, New York, NY.) (D) A radiograph of the stethoscope demonstrating the wire coils and threaded segments of the bell. (Courtesy of the Philip Reichert Collection, Library of Mount Sinai Medical Center, New York, NY.)

effects of chloroform and stated ''the doses (of chloroform) may need to be increased as the system becomes less susceptible during repeat episodes.'' (26)

Einthoven (1860–1927), the inventor of the electrocardiograph (EKG), evaluated three theories of pathogenesis of asthma popular at his time: bronchospasm vs. spasm of the diaphragm vs. capillary-leak. He demonstrated experimentally that spasm of the bronchi was the etiology (27).

This was a time period of great observation by physicians and scientists, and the sputum did not escape their notice. Leyden (1832–1910) (Fig. 5) in 1871 found octohedral crystals in the sputum of asthmatics and believed that these caused bronchospasm (28). Actually, they were first found in sputum by Charcot (1825–1893) (the famous neurologist) in 1853, but he did not associate these crystals with asthma at that time. Curshmann (1846–1910) (Fig. 6) in 1882 found spirals in the sputum and felt that they must cause the bronchospasm, since Leyden crystals were not always found in sputum (29,30). Ehrlich, then a young physician in Leipzig experimenting with aniline dyes, stained blood

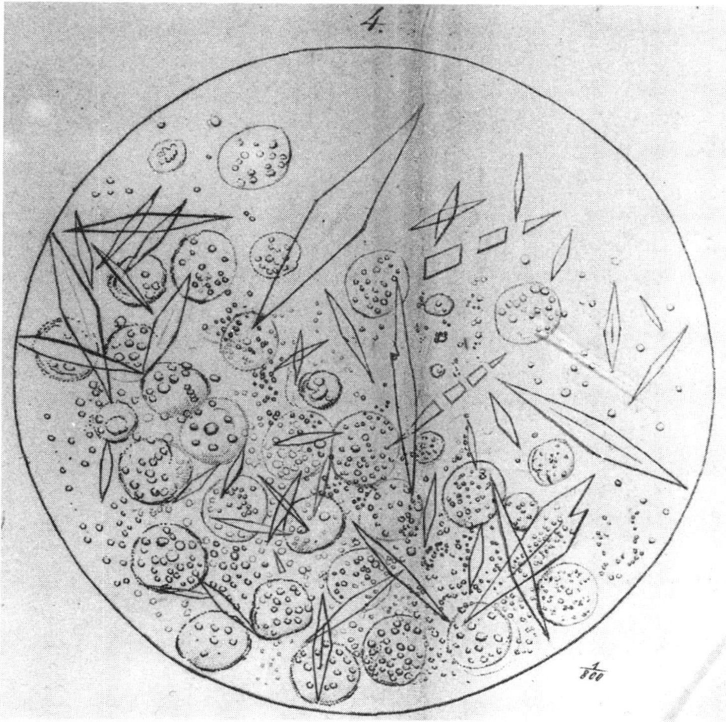

Figure 5 Leyden crystals formed from eosinophilic debris. (From Ref. 28.)

and essentially discovered the eosinophil (31). Gollasch, reporting on his own work and unpublished works of Müller in 1889, noted eosinophilia in sputum (32). Fink (33) as well as Gabritschewsky (34) demonstrated eosinophilia in the blood of asthmatics in 1890. Concomitantly it was demonstrated that during exacerbations, blood eosinophilia was increased as compared with ''wheeze-free'' intervals (35). The eosinophil, Charcot-Leyden crystals, and Curshmann spirals had captured much interest concerning their role in the pathogenesis of acute asthma at this time period (36). The eosinophilia in acute asthma, however, could not explain the myriad clinical manifestations of acute asthma.

V. THE TURN OF THE 20th CENTURY

In 1902, Richet (1850–1935) found that injection of a foreign protein from Portuguese men-of-war or sea anemones into dogs was followed by a condition of greater susceptibility to the protein. He termed this phenomenon *anaphylaxis* to express its antithesis to prophylaxis or protection afforded by injection of certain proteins (37). With the injection of diphtheria antitoxin in 1894, there was ample opportunity to observe the effect of injections of foreign proteins. In 1910 Meltzer noted a similarity between anaphylaxis and asthma in which a person became sensitized to a definite substance, and an attack occurred every time the substance entered the circulation. Minute quantities of the substance, if inhaled, would bring on an attack of asthma (38). In 1906 Von Pirquet, an Austrian pedia-

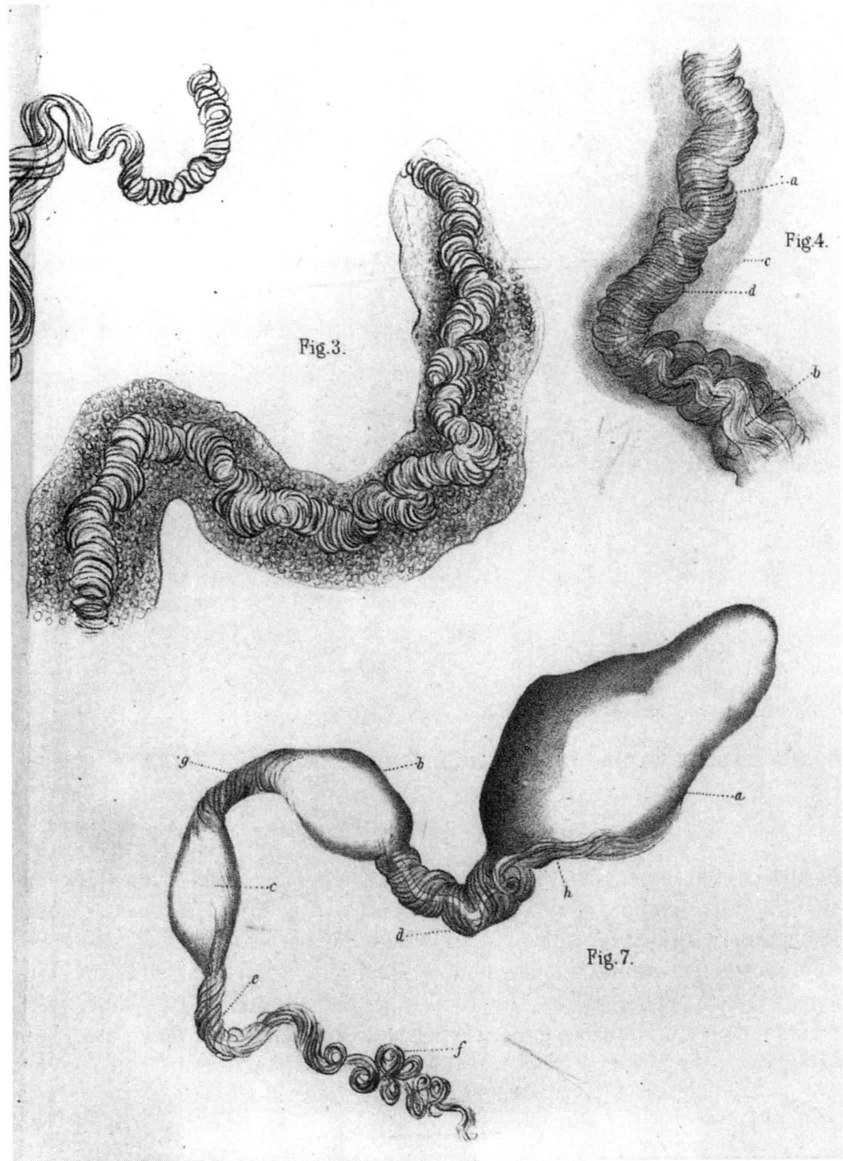

Figure 6 Curschmann spirals formed from mucus and eosinophilic debris. (From Ref. 29.)

trician, introduced the term *allergy*, from the Greek word *allos* (meaning other) based on their studies of serum sickness (39). Asthma now was felt to be an allergic phenomenon and a cure would be effected by injecting these foreign proteins.

Just before the turn of the century (1892), standards in internal medicine were being established. Sir William Osler wrote a single authored textbook, *The Principles and Practice of Medicine* (Figs. 7A, B, and 8). Textbooks give us a view into the standard of practice at that time period. He notes that in the pathogenesis of asthma there is a contribution of both inflammation and spasm of the bronchi. His description of acute asthma outlined a typical acute episode and recognized the urgency of the problem. He stated that "immediate and prompt relief is demanded" (26). He noted the following therapies, similar to Thorowgood mentioned earlier (26). Osler noted that chloroform, a few whiffs, provided prompt but temporary relief. Although somewhat contradictory to the adult with acute asthma, Osler stated "in a child with very severe asthma, immediate and permanent relief can be achieved with chloroform." Amyl nitrite was useful with 2–5 drops supplied in a handkerchief. Morphine and cocaine combined were good for obstinate attacks. Belladonna, henbane, lobeline, and stramonium could be used in solution or in cigarettes. Nitre

THE PRINCIPLES AND

PRACTICE OF MEDICINE

DESIGNED FOR THE USE OF
PRACTITIONERS AND STUDENTS OF MEDICINE

BY
WILLIAM OSLER, M. D.
FELLOW OF THE ROYAL COLLEGE OF PHYSICIANS, LONDON
PROFESSOR OF MEDICINE IN THE JOHNS HOPKINS UNIVERSITY AND
PHYSICIAN-IN-CHIEF TO THE JOHNS HOPKINS HOSPITAL, BALTIMORE
FORMERLY PROFESSOR OF THE INSTITUTES OF MEDICINE, MC GILL UNIVERSITY, MONTREAL
AND PROFESSOR OF CLINICAL MEDICINE
IN THE UNIVERSITY OF PENNSYLVANIA, PHILADELPHIA

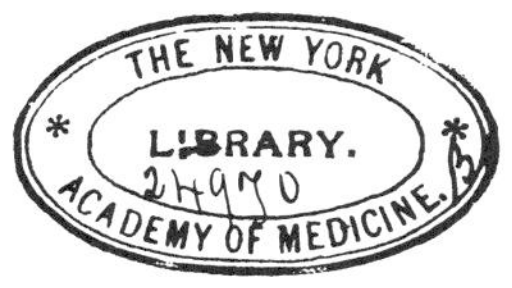

(A)

NEW YORK
D. APPLETON AND COMPANY
1892

Figure 7A Title page from Osler's textbook, *The Principles and Practice of Medicine*, 1892.

paper with nitrate of potash burned to provide fumes seemed to help at night (Fig. 9) (see page 8). He stated that oxygen may also be tried. To prevent recurrence, potassium iodide was important. The asthmatic was better living in the city than the country. Most notably, Osler stated that ''we have no knowledge of the morbid anatomy. Death during the attack is unknown'' (40). This statement seems so surprising now, since at that time period there was no epinephrine, beta-agonists, or glucocorticoids. Furthermore Osler encouraged the use of a respiratory depressant, morphine. Both the sixth edition published in 1905 and the eighth edition [the last edition published while the author was alive (Osler died in 1919)] published in 1917 were unchanged in the entire therapy of asthma from the original 1892 textbook.

At the turn of the century the aspects of allergy and asthma were beginning to become clarified. The therapeutic agent, belladonna alkaloids, e.g., lobeline, and stramonium, repeatedly appeared in many physicians' therapeutic armamentarium of asthma. A common source for these parasympatholytic agents, as mentioned before was the *Datura* plant. In India, the *Datura* plant was smoked since at least the 1600s for asthma and was introduced into England from India in the early 1800s. As mentioned in many sources above, these medicines formed the mainstay of asthma therapy in the 1800s (41). With optimal use a patient could inhale 0.5 mg of belladonna alkaloid per cigarette; with more casual use, 0.15 mg could be readily inhaled (42). Physicians making house calls even in the early 1920s experienced a noisome odor in the homes of asthmatics that reeked of smells and fumes of burnt niter paper, stramonium, and lobeline (43).

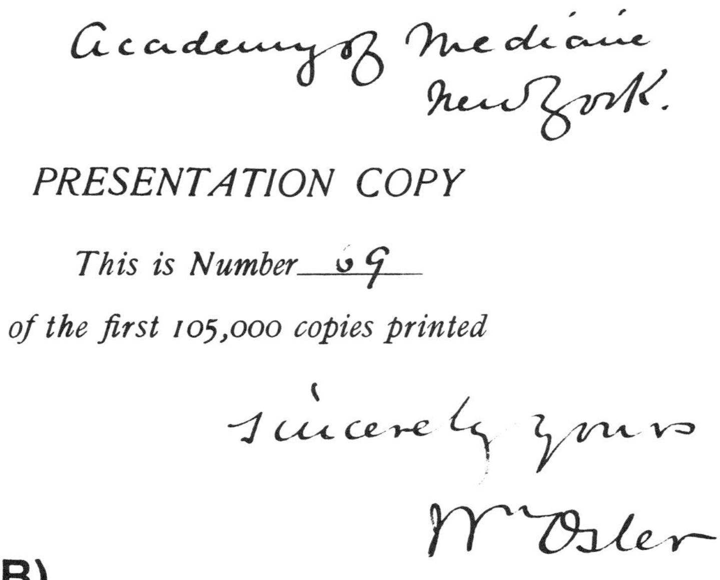

Figure 7B Osler's signature on a signed copy of his textbook. (Courtesy of the NY Academy of Medicine Library, New York, NY.)

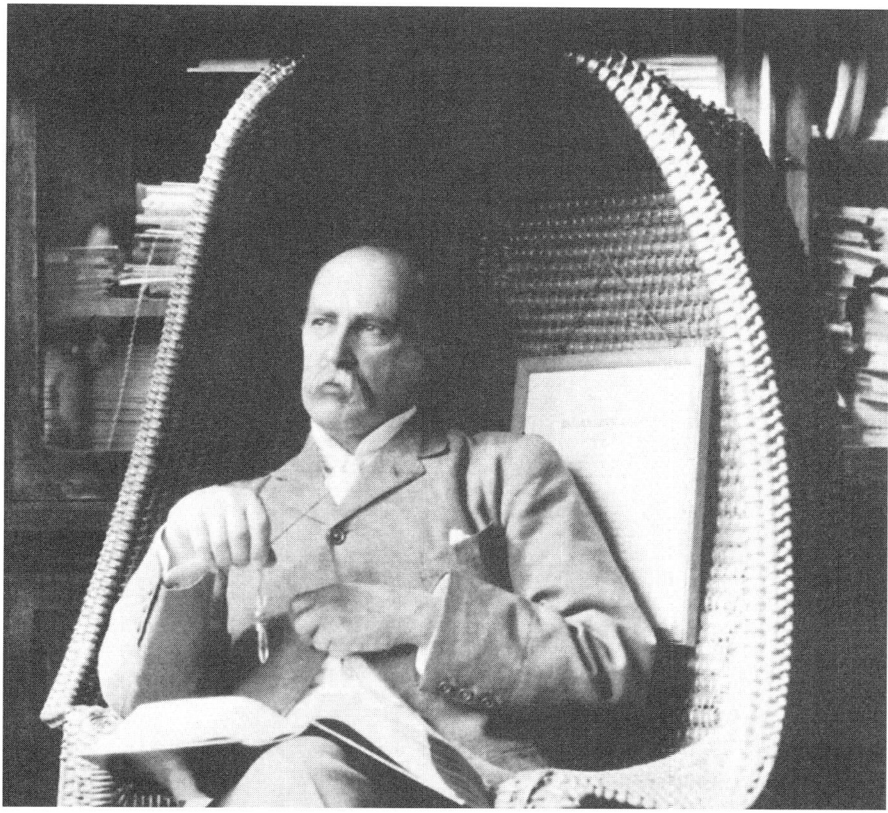

Figure 8 Osler sitting in Sir Edward Jenner's chair in the room of the Regius Professor at the Oxford University Museum, Oxford, England. (Courtesy of the Wellcome Institute Library, London, England.)

VI. THE 20th CENTURY

Highly effective "modern" therapy of acute asthma began with the development of epinephrine. The first parenteral use of epinephrine for acute asthma was in 1903, reported from Montefiore Home for Chronic Invalids (44). In the introduction, authors remark that opium and morphine, by mouth, rectum, or subcutaneously, are effective only while the patient is stuporous, but the asthma attack returns when the patient awakens. Only temporary beneficial effects were observed with chloroform. They reported a new, highly effective agent, adrenaline, administered subcutaneously at doses from 0.15 to 0.3 mg (1:1000 epinephrine). Administration by the inhaled route (atomizer), however, waited until 1929 (45). The Ma Huang plant, as mentioned at the beginning of this chapter, was used for thousands of years in China for treating what was apparently asthma. Its active ingredient, ephedrine, was isolated in 1884 in Japan but introduced into the western hemisphere in 1924 (46).

In the early 1900s, Rackemann evaluated 150 patients with asthma at the Massachusetts General Hospital, mostly outpatients and ward patients. They all had blood, sputum,

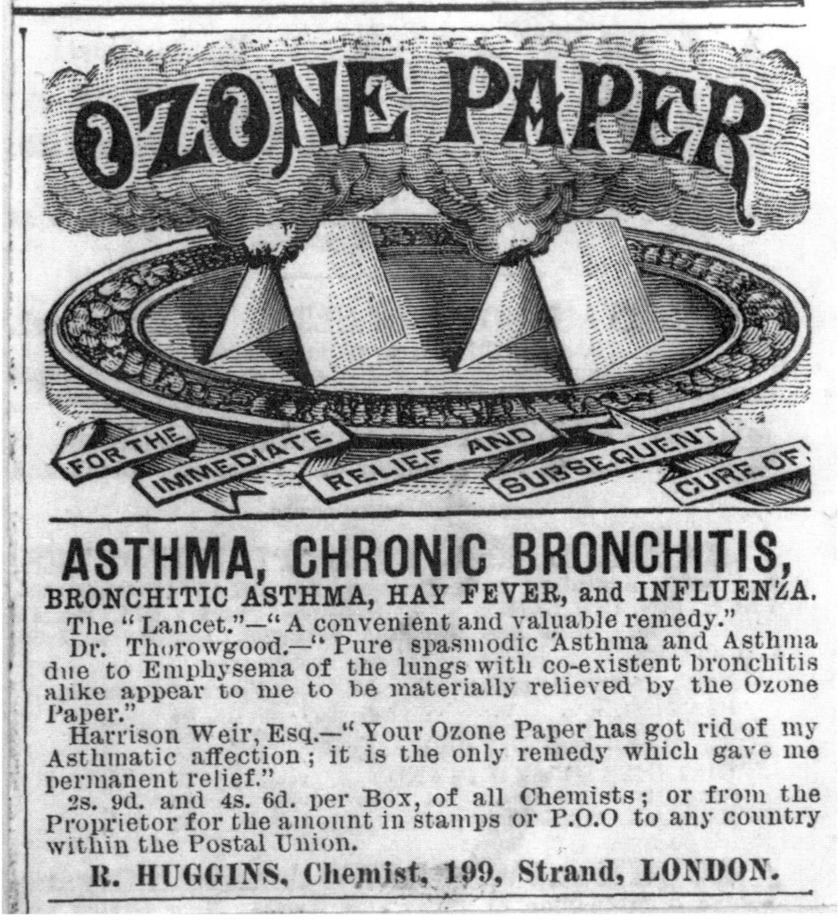

Figure 9 Advertisement for an antiasthmatic paper in the Illustrated London News, November 26, 1892. "Ozone paper" was paper suffused with potash (potassium hydroxide) or potassium iodide (see page 8). (Courtesy of the Mary Evans Picture Library, London, England.)

and roentgenographic evaluations to exclude organic cardiac, blood, or other pulmonary disease. All patients presented as having episodic dyspnea with wheezing and no other etiology could be found. He classified the cases into extrinsic asthma, i.e., related to allergy to proteins that are extrinsic to the body (28% of cases), such as allergens (horse hair was classic), as opposed to intrinsic asthma (53%), where the "allergen" was inside the body, such as acute bronchitis. The remaining 20% of cases were unclassified. The age of onset of extrinsic asthma was typically 12 years while intrinsic asthma was 26 years of age. In the treatment section, this article states, "adrenalin is a very important drug in the treatment of asthma; a subcutaneous injection of adrenalin chlorid solution (Parke Davis) will control the attack in almost every case" (47).

To obtain a clearer picture of asthma in the early 1900s, the time of discovery of a drug or case reports of its use are helpful to demonstrate what agents were available. But classification, clinical manifestations, and treatments as recommended in standard textbooks of that time period indicate more of the contemporary general practice and thinking about asthma. The sixth edition of Stedman's Medical Dictionary published in 1920 listed 16 different types of asthma and provided the nosology and terminology of that time period (48). Under asthma was included: *alveolar asthma* due to emphysema, *amygdaline asthma* due to enlarged tonsils or adenoids; *asthma nocturnum* due to a nightmare; *bronchial asthma*, the common form, due to either bronchospasm or bronchial edema; *bronchitic asthma* due to bronchitis; *cardiac asthma* due to cardiosclerosis, often occuring at night; *catarrhal asthma*, the same as bronchitic asthma; *essential asthma*, nervous asthma associated with no bronchial edema; *grinders asthma* due to siderosis or silicosis; *hay* asthma, asthma associated with hayfever; *Heberden's asthma*, angina pectoris; *horse asthma* due to proximity to horses; *miner's asthma* from anthracosis; *nasal asthma* from intranasal causes such as a deviated septum; *potter's asthma* due to pneumoconiosis; *reflex* asthma, which is symptomatic asthma; *renal asthma* due to renal disease; *sexual asthma* due to either venereal disease or excessive sexual excitement; *stone asthma* associated with pressure and burning of the chest due to a bronchial calculus, relieved when coughing dislodges the calculus; *thymic asthma* a spasmodic closure of the larynx in children due to an enlarged thymus gland, also known as *Kopp's asthma.*

Rackemann wrote the chapter on bronchial asthma as part of the Allergy section in the first edition of *Cecil, a Textbook of Medicine by American Authors* (49). Rackemann noted that asthma affected all ages and races. Some asthma clinics were seeing 100 patients per week. Under extrinsic asthma, Rackemann lists many well-known allergens that cause bronchospasm. Under intrinsic he included acute bacterial bronchitis, occurring quite regularly in the spring and fall, often following colds, especially in children. He noted other causes of intrinsic asthma such as reflex asthma, due to disturbances in the nose or throat or pregnancy or menses (47,50) or toxic asthma, due to sinusitis, tonsillitis, or teeth decay. He noted that asthma may occur with a positive syphilis test or with diabetes and resolved with treatment of both, as well as cardiac and renal asthma, which resolved with treatment of the underlying condition. Curiously, like Osler (40), he wrote that death from acute asthma was rare, with only 21 reported cases in which pathology was available. He noted that eosinophilia of blood and sputum as well as Charcot-Leyden crystals were characteristic of asthma. Clinical manifestations were described in a fashion common to present day textbooks, including a description of wheezing, defined as musical or sonorous râles. He describes in detail an asthma attack with the onset due to horse dander. He noted that asthma may occur with dust, fumes, or exercise or idiopathically. Occupational asthma was well described along with sensitivities to many agents, foods, specific dusts, and animal dander. In a glimpse into those times, he stated (49),

> Individuals subject to these attacks are never without their pet remedy which may be a powder containing stramonium leaves, the smoke of which is inhaled, or some nasal spray containing cocaine, or adrenalin. Such patients are uncomfortable at night. It is common for them to wake up three to four times per night to burn their powder or take their adrenalin.

He noted that the patients could not eat during the attack and weight loss often was common and marked. Musical or sonorous râles might be heard. Cyanosis was not present unless there was a coexistent pulmonary infection. He noted that there was a sharp systolic fall in blood pressure with inspiration, i.e., pulsus paradoxus. His recommended treatment was 0.25 ml of adrenalin chloride (epinephrine) repeated at half-hour intervals as needed.

One and a half milligrams of dry powder under the tongue in children, he stated, was frequently efficacious. Stramonium in asthma powders and cigarettes were helpful. He stated that morphine was not specific and rarely indicated. Ephedrine, which works like adrenalin, can be given parenterally or orally (25–50 mg three times per day). He stated that adrenalin was much more effective than ephedrine. Among the general recommendations he provided are allergen avoidance, moving to a dry climate such as Arizona, potassium iodide, and ipecac.

Aminophylline was first used clinically after demonstration of its bronchodilating effect on bronchial smooth muscle in the laboratory This finding was made in 1922 in Frankfurt, Germany, by Samson Raphael Hirsch* (51,52). After a 14-year hiatus, aminophylline was used for acute asthma, especially cases that did not respond to epinephrine (adrenaline-fast). During their investigations of diuretics and treatments for pulmonary edema, Hermann et al. in 1937 reported on the efficacy of intravenous aminophylline in 41 cases of severe asthma. In these cases 480 mg was "pushed slowly" intravenously with few side effects and all but two cases had prompt, complete, and persistent relief of dyspnea (53).

The study that was way ahead of its time was published in 1900. At that time Solis–Cohen prepared a crude extract of the adrenal gland and used it in the treatment of acute asthma (54). In the late 1930s, cortisone was finally isolated, and it was used successfully in the late 1940s for the treatment of rheumatoid arthritis. After this time period, the development of the use of steroids for asthma followed a traditional pathway of case reports, then clinical series, from small to larger, than double-blind clinical trials. In the time period from 1949 to 1950 the use of ACTH for acute and chronic asthma was found to be highly effective in many several small clinical series with the first report from Johns Hopkins Hospital (55,56). In the early 1950s, Carryer et al. gave 100 mg of cortisone intramuscularly every day to a very small series of patients in a double-blind placebo controlled trial and established corticosteroids as a highly effective treatment of asthma (57). Other studies came out shortly afterwards corroborating these effects of both cortisone and ACTH (58–61). By 1955, the agent with which present-day physicians are most familiar, namely prednisone (initially called metacortandracin), was developed and also found effective in acute asthma (62,63). In one study in 1955 on 10 patients concerning the effect of ACTH in refractory acute asthma, a glimpse of the times and medical care for acute asthma can be perceived. In one typical case they report (64):

> An intelligent and sensible housewife aged 53 was seen at home as an emergency in status asthmaticus so severe that two hour previously her own practitioner had thought her to be on the point of death. In spite of intravenous aminophylline she was still extremely shocked and distressed in her breathing. She was at once admitted to the hospital and given ACTH 30 mg intramuscularly six-hourly. Within 12 hours she was comfortable, and within forty-eight hours she was completely free from wheezing. The total dosage was 730 mg in nine days.

---

* Dr. Hirsch was the great grandson of the famous German rabbi by the same name. Since Dr. Hirsch lived in Frankfurt, Germany, some authors expressed concern about Dr. Hirsch's welfare since there was no academic productivity from 1933 onward. However, Dr. Hirsch went underground in 1933 and escaped to Belgium in 1938 where he remained underground. After the war, he opened up a private practice in internal medicine in Belgium. He died in 1960.

An extraordinarily progressive study adumbrating modern practices with chronic asthma was published in 1951. In this study 30 patients were directed to self-inject ACTH and determine their own daily doses based on symptoms. The self-injection was not problematic, since the patients were already well-experienced in self-injecting epinephrine. The study was successful in that all patients improved over the 10 month study period with doses varying from 20 mg every day to 12 mg every other day. Relapse occurred soon after discontinuing the drug.

In a multicenter study with 13 sites (but only 32 patients), patients who did not improve after 24 hr of acute therapy (subcutaneous epinephrine, intravenous aminophylline, inhaled isoproterenol, oxygen, antibiotics, and sedatives) received either placebo or 1.25 g of cortisone orally over 9 days in a tapering regimen (starting with 350 mg on day 1). The major findings were that by the fourth day of the study fewer patients in the cortisone group had disabling symptoms as compared with the placebo group [66% (n=15) vs. 24% (n=17)] (65).

In the early 1950s, modifications of epinephrine were made resulting in isoproterenol (isoprenaline), a pure β-agonist without any α activity like epinephrine; isoproterenol was used by inhalation to treat acute asthma. In the 1940s the spray atomizer, like that used for perfume, was a common inhalant route used for bronchodilating drugs, such as epinephrine. In 1956 Maison, a medical consultant at Riker Laboratory (now 3M Pharmaceuticals), developed a canister with a one-way valve, resulting in a spray containing approximately the same amount of drug per spray (a metered dose). The potential of this product was soon realized by the pharmaceutical industry and "reliable" metered dose inhalers (MDIs), Medihalers®, became available (66). In 1948 Ahlquist developed the concept of α- and β-receptors to explain the different effects of sympathomimetics on different organs (67). In 1967 Lands et al. suggested that there were two forms of the β-receptor, β_1 and β_2. When stimulated the β_1- receptors cause lipolysis and a chronotropic and inotropic effect on the heart. β_2-receptors cause vasodilation, bronchodilation, skeletal muscle tremor, and muscle glycogenolysis (68). Pharmaceutical companies endeavored to make MDIs and aerosolized solutions with as much β_2 and as little β_1 properties as possible.

The state of knowledge about acute asthma was exhaustively reviewed by Brenner in the early 1980s (69,70). By this time, comparative trials of different therapeutic agents had been reported, and sedatives were widely condemned during acute asthma episodes as their use was associated with increased risks for intubation and fatality (71,72). Intermittent positive pressure breathing (IPPB) devices, to decrease the work of breathing of the acute asthmatic, was the primary means to administer inhaled β agonists. IPPB was the standard method in the 1960s and 1970s to deliver these agents, but was found to be associated with increased risks of barotrauma and was replaced by the equally effective method of nebulizing the β agonists in a "well," through which air or oxygen was introduced; the resulting "steam" was inhaled by the patient (73,74).

In 1998 patients that present to the ED with near-fatal asthma receive oxygen, endotracheal intubation, and mechanical ventilation. This was not always the case. Oxygen was discovered by Priestly (1733–1804) in 1774 by heating mercuric oxide over mercury in a closed vessel. He stated that "dephlogisticated air" was released. This air made a candle burn brighter and supported the life of mice. Priestly came to dinner at the home of Lavoisier (1743–1794), in 1775, at which time Priestley described his findings (Fig. 10). Lavoisier, along with his colleague LaPlace, studied oxygen and showed that respiration was like combustion, and oxygen was inhaled and carbon dioxide and water were exhaled. He termed the gas *oxygen* because it caused or generated combustion. The unhappy ending of this great scientific career occurred when Lavoisier was condemned as an enemy of the people of France and guillotined on May 8, 1794 (75,76).

For the treatment of diphtheria, O'Dwyer in 1882 developed endotracheal tubes that would be placed by a blind digital intubation. Endotracheal intubation was developed to avoid tracheotomy in these patients with diphtheria. Cuffed tracheal tubes were developed around 1890. The laryngoscope and placement of the tube under direct visualization was pioneered in 1895. For surgery, patients were intubated and then ventilated with a bellows-like device (77–79).

Mechanical ventilation was accomplished in 1927, after Drinker made a negative pressure ventilation device that was termed the *iron lung*. Due to the "iron shell" surrounding the patient, access for nursing care was difficult. However, for patients with respiratory depression secondary to polio, this device was inadequate and the mortality rate was approximately 90%. In 1952 there was an epidemic of polio in Copenhagen, Denmark, where there were almost 3000 admissions with acute poliomyelitis and several hundred patients in respiratory failure; most of the patients were children between 1 and 14 years of age. The referral center for Copenhagen and eastern Denmark was the 500-bed Blegdams Hospital; this facility had only seven negative pressure ventilators. At this time anesthesiology was a new specialty, officially recognized in Denmark in 1950. Anesthesiologists only worked in the operating room under the auspices of the surgeon, who even chose the anesthetic. At the start of the epidemic in the beginning of August 1952, 31 patients had been admitted to this hospital with polio and respiratory depression. Despite treatment with negative pressure ventilators, 27 died within three days of admission. Dr. Bjørn Ibsen, an anesthesiologist, was consulted. He urged a boldly different treatment with tracheostomy to allow for easy removal of secretions, insertion of a cuffed tracheal tube to prevent aspiration, and a connection of a bag to the tracheal tube to allow for manual positive pressure ventilation. His plan was met with skepticism. On August 27, 1952, he was assigned just one patient on which to try this new therapeutic plan, a 12-year old girl paralyzed in all four extremities, "gasping for breath, drowning in her own secretions, cyanotic, sweating, and a temperature of 40.2 C" (80). Under local anesthesia a tracheostomy was successfully performed, but the patient still could not be ventilated through the tracheal tube. The patient was "dying in his hands." Intravenous pentothal was given, and the patient relaxed and was now able to be ventilated. Cyanosis was gone and the patient stabilized (Fig. 11). This positive pressure, however, required someone to manually ventilate the patients by "squeezing the bag" until they could spontaneously and adequately breathe.* Most patients required three months to reach this level of improvement. This manual ventilation was provided initially by 200 medical students who worked in shifts of 24 hr per day seven days per week "bagging" patients with poliomyelitis and respiratory failure. The death rate was dramatically reduced from 90 to 25% (80). In the week from August 28 to September 3, 1952, 335 polio patients were admitted to Blegdams Hospital, and at the height of the epidemic 70 patients were manually ventilated on the same day. By November 1952 approximately 1500 medical and dental students had put in 165,000 hours of manual ventilation, intermittently even monitoring the P_{CO_2} and oxygen saturation (81,82) (Figs. 12–14).† The need for positive pres-

* Dr. Ibsen and two other colleagues manually "bagged" this patient for another 18 hr. She survived the hospitalization, succumbing 19 years later to an unrelated condition.

† The students had the advantages of early technology with a continuous P_{CO_2} monitoring. Bromthy-

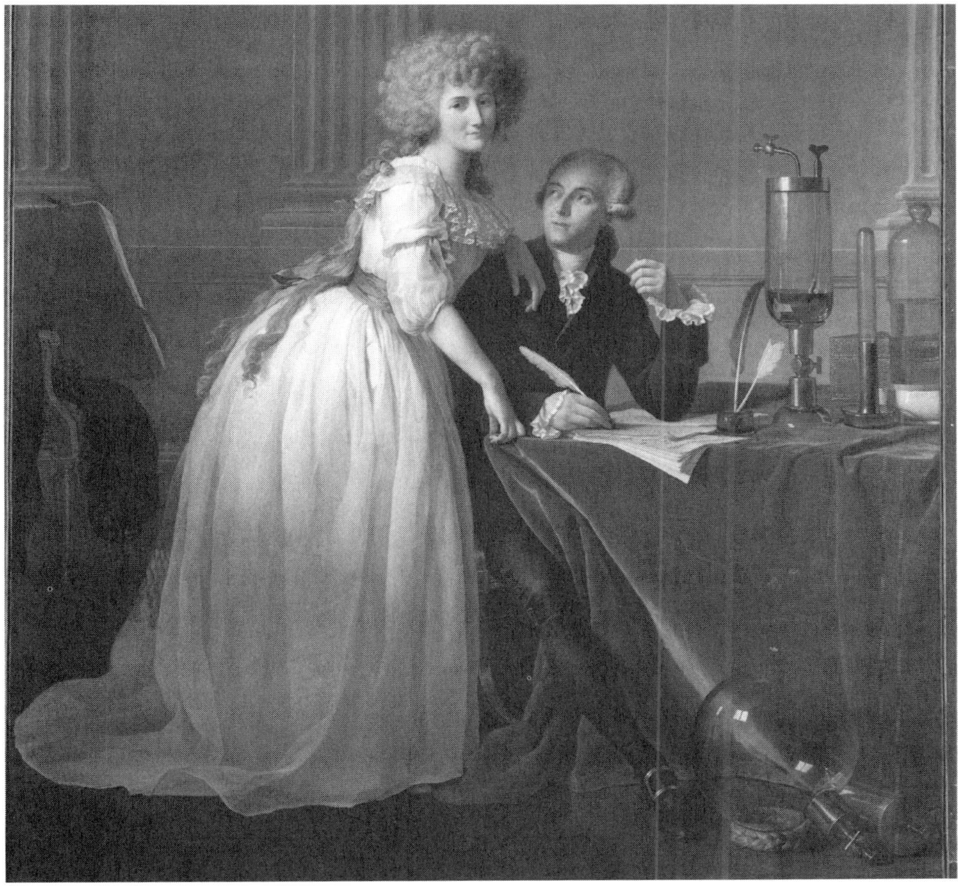

Figure 10 Antoine Lavoisier and his wife, Marie Anne Pierette Paulze, 1788, by Jacques Louis David. (Courtesy of the Metropolitan Museum of Art, New York, NY, all rights reserved.)

mol blue was used as an indicator, where the color varied with the P_{CO_2}. The color changes were recorded by a photelectric cell connected to a galvanometer. This device was termed a Carbovisor. In addition they had an oximeter, which was a noninvasive monitor of oxygen saturation developed for combat airplane pilots in order that the pilots could adjust their oxygen supply. It worked using differences between oxygen rich and poor blood. The oximeter was applied to the ear lobe. At this time, arterial blood gases were not available, but serum bicarbonate measurements did exist. Since some of the patients had a chronic respiratory acidosis, the physicians felt that the problem with these patients was a high bicarbonate, since an elevated arterial P_{CO_2} was unknown and not able to be measured. They misinterpreted the findings of respiratory failure as manifestations of poliomyelitis.

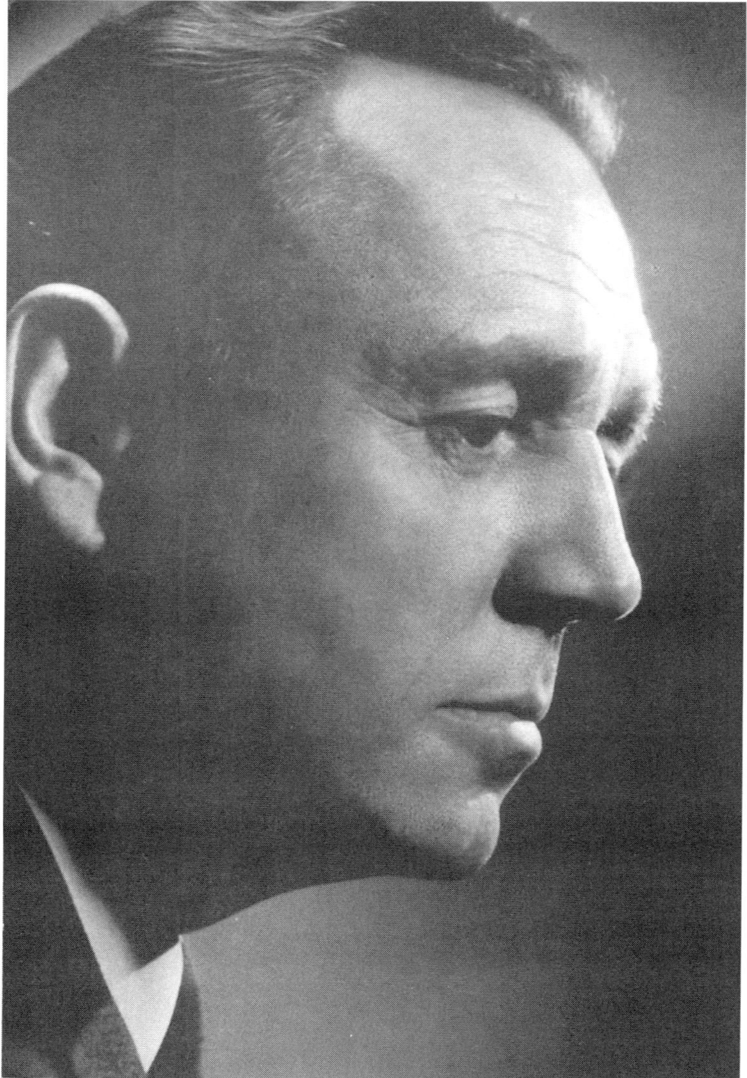

Figure 11 Dr. Bjorn Ibsen, the first intensivist. On Friday, August 24, 1952, there was a chiefs of services meeting in which the problem of poliomyelitis was discussed. On rounds that day, Dr. Ibsen observed the lungs of two deceased boys that had had poliomyelitis. He noted that the lungs were entirely normal. He concluded that the problem of ventilation in polio could be solved by manually ventilating the patients. The Danish physicians at that time "were desperate for an effective therapy." On Monday, August 27, he was given a 12-year-old patient, Vivi Ebert, on whom he would attempt his new procedure. Twelve to fourteen physicians observed, and all but one or two left when the patient took a downhill course (see text) (personal communication with Dr. Ibsen, June 1998).

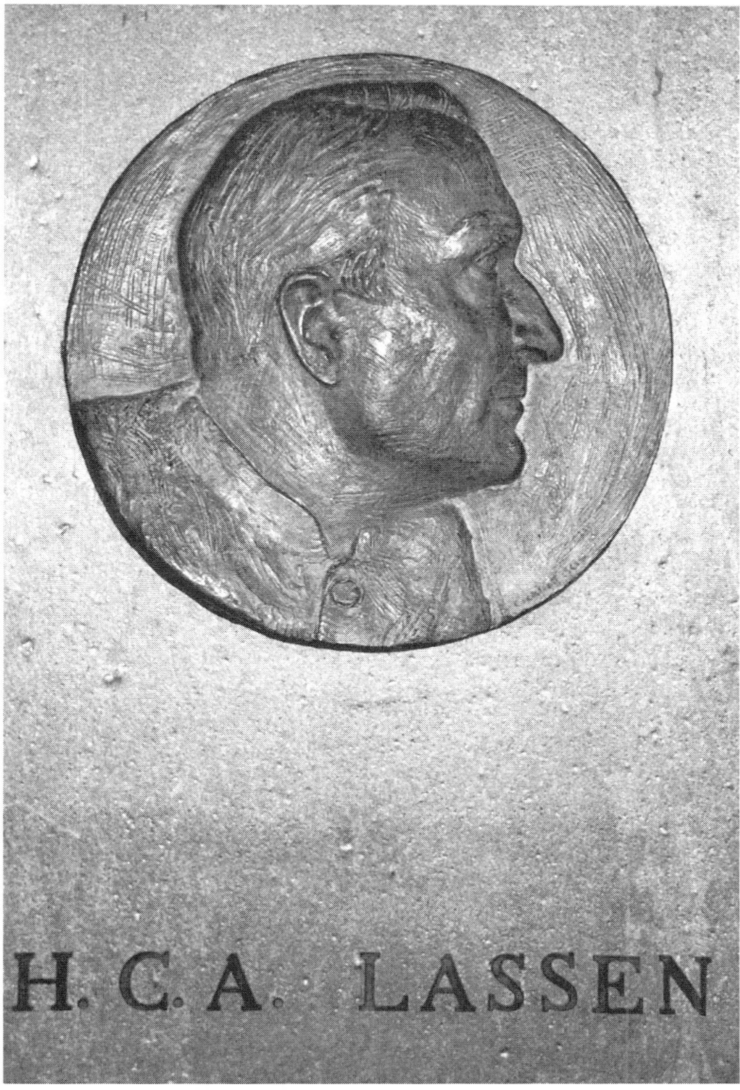

Figure 12 Dr. H.C.A. Lassen, chief of infectious disease and head of medicine during the polio epidemic in 1952 and subsequent years. From relief sculpture at Rigs Hospital, Copenhagen, Denmark.

sure mechanical ventilation to replace manual ventilation arose, since clearly 1500 students were not the permanent answer to respiratory failure. The answer would come from machines.

The first Bennett pressure cycled ventilator was developed in approximately 1946 (75,83). Volume cycle respirators were developed in the early 1960s and popularized about ten years later. The first intensive care unit in the United States was in the early

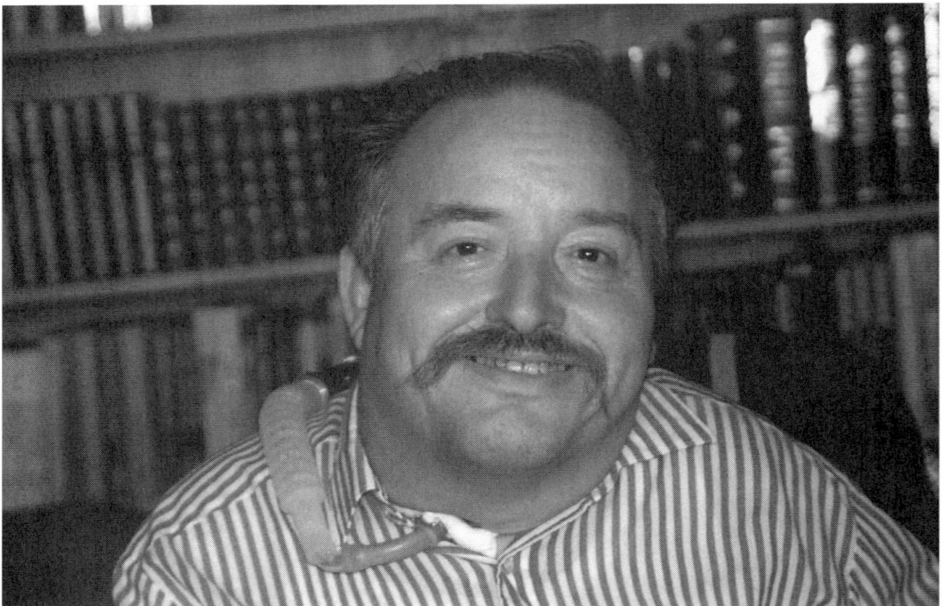

Figure 13 Torben Olsen, patient manually ventilated at age 2 during the 1952 polio epidemic. By the end of the epidemic, 20 patients could not survive without mechanical ventilation. Mr. Olsen has been continuously ventilated from 1952 to the present. He has a bachelor's degree in language and literature. (June, 1998.)

1950s at Peter Bent Brigham Hospital (75). In the early and mid-1960s the two therapies of endotracheal intubation and mechanical ventilation for acute asthma were combined and successful results were reported (84–89).

As mentioned earlier, the death rate from asthma was very rarely recorded in the medical literature before 1930 (90). In fact, Rackemann reported on 2000 consecutive cases of extrinsic asthma without a single death (91). This near absence of death may be due to mis-classification of asthma, inaccuracy of death certificates, and infrequency in which one physician would encounter death in an acute asthmatic (92). In the recently completed Multicenter Asthma Research Collaboration, there was only one death out of 1896 consecutive adults with acute asthma (personal communication, C. Camargo, M.D., for MARC investigators). Speizer and Doll, reporting on the death rate from acute asthma, note that it had been stable in the last century (1867–1961), at 4.6 per million in males and 4.3 per million in females (93). Since 1952, when corticosteroids were introduced, a decrease in the death rate from acute asthma was *not* noted. These data were based on death certificates in the age range of 5–34 years when death from acute asthma would be less confused with diagnoses such as bronchiolitis in infants or cardiac disease and emphysema in the older populations. With the advent of β-agonist therapy, corticosteroids, oxygen administration, antibiotics, endotracheal intubation, and mechanical ventilation in the 20th century, it is still astonishing that we could not demonstrate a lower mortality rate than that in the 19th century, especially considering the dangerous therapies

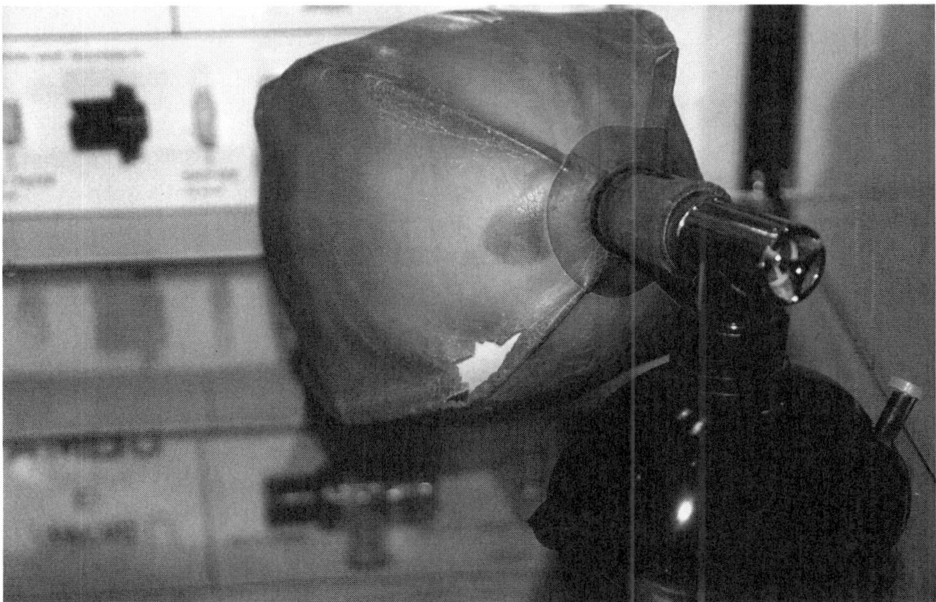

Figure 14 The first Ambu bag. The first bag-masks were "to and fro" systems where the exhaled air of the patient was washed out by hooking the bag up to oxygen. The medical students in Denmark were replaced by mechanical ventilators, the earliest of which were termed "the Student from Skive" and designed by Bang and Olufsen (presently famous for high-fidelity sound systems). A truckers' strike occurred in Denmark in around 1954, threatening the supply of oxygen to the polio patients on mechanical ventilation. Although the shortage in oxygen never became critical, Dr. Henning Ruben was concerned about what would have occurred. He adapted his one-way valve, which was in use in anesthesia, to a self-expanding bag. This bag was portable (ambulant from where Ambu Inc. derives its name) and was not dependent on an external oxygen source. This bag-valve-mask was introduced in Europe in 1956, and Dr. Ruben brought a sample with him when he went to work with Dr. James Elam (developer of mouth-to-mouth resuscitation) in 1958. Dr. Elam was instrumental in bringing the Ambu bag to the United States (personal communication Dr. Henning Ruben, Ole Koehnke, Ambu Inc.).

of the time, such as morphine, and less effective therapies, such as inhaled belladonna alkaloids.

VII. EMERGENCY MEDICINE

In the 1950s and earlier, acute asthmatics would go to the physician's office or the physician would make a house call if the patient were too ill to leave the house. Subsequently, with the baby boom era, the increased population, and spread of urban areas, house calls became more time consuming for practitioners. There was a concomitant decline in the

In commemoration of the
successful negotiations and
efforts of those
who persevered in the long
effort to achieve
recognition of the specialty
of emergency medicine.
September 21, 1979
American College of
Emergency Physicians

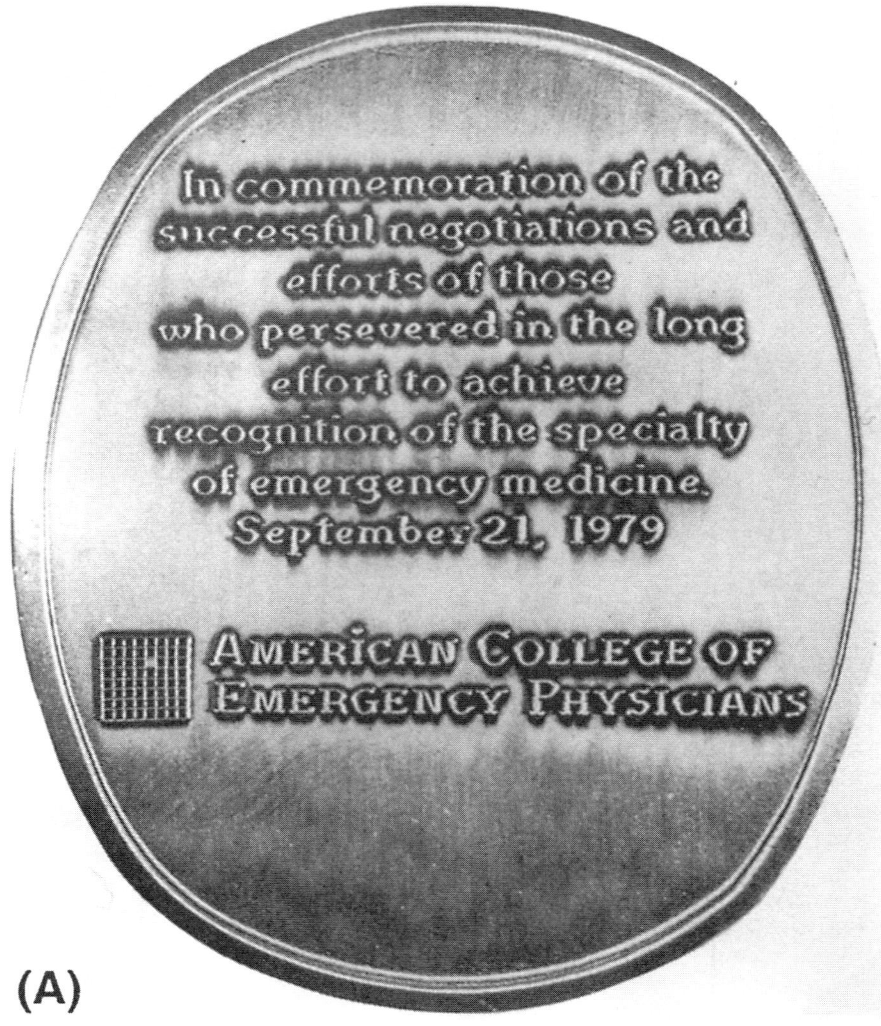

(A)

Figure 15 Coins commemorating the recognition of specialty status for emergency medicine by the American Board of Medical Specialties, September 21, 1979. A is the front and B is the obverse side. (Courtesy of the American College of Emergency Physicians.)

number of general practitioners as specialists became more numerous. Lastly, emergency care was more completely paid for by the individual's health insurance carrier while a house call was not. Patients would then go to the hospital for their emergencies and the "emergency room" was born. Public ambulance systems reappeared in the mid-1960s for the transport of emergencies, such as acute asthma (94). The first emergency medicine residency program was started in 1969 at the University of Cincinnati and by that time national ED visits had increased over 365% from 1955. The first board examination and

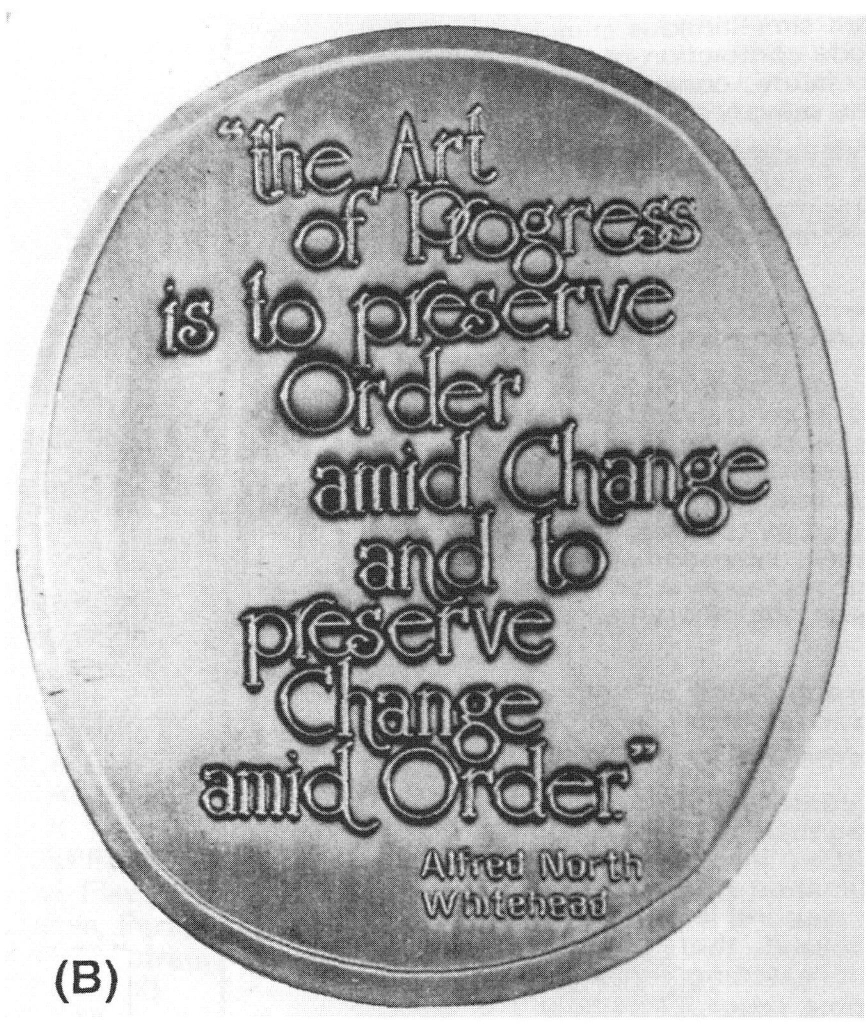

(B)

certification was in 1979 (Figs. 15A and B), and by 1998 119 accredited emergency medicine residencies had emerged (95, 96). By 1996 there were 100 million ED visits per year, 5000 EDs, and 1.5 million ED visits for acute asthma.

REFERENCES

1. Woodruff PG, Singk AK, Camargo CA Jr. Role of the emergency department in chronic asthma care. Am J Respir Crit Care Med 1998;157 (3, Part 2): A611.
2. Cohen SG. Asthma in antiquity: the Ebers papyrus. Allergy Proc 1992; 13:147–154.

3. Sakula A. A history of asthma. J Royal Coll Phys 1988; 22:36–44.
4. Saavedra-Delgado AM, Cohen SG. Huang-Ti, the yellow emperor and the Nei ching: antiquity's earliest reference to asthma. Allergy Proc 1991; 12:197–198.
5. Viswanathan R. Historical aspects of bronchial asthma. Ind J Chest Dis. 1964; 6:165–169.
6. Panzani RC. Seneca and his asthma: the illness, life, and death of a Roman stoic philosopher. J Asthma 1988; 25:163–174.
7. Keeney EL. The history of asthma from Hippocrates to Meltzer. J. Allergy. 1964; 35:215–226.
8. Stolkind E. History of bronchial asthma. Proc Roy Soc Med 1933; 26:1120–1126.
9. Marketos SG, Ballas CN. Bronchial asthma in the medical literature of Greek antiquity. J Asthma 1982; 19:263–269.
10. Marketos SG, Eftychiades AC. Bronchial asthma according to Byzantine medicine. J Asthma 1986; 23:149–155.
11. Maimonides, M. Treatise on asthma. Translated by S. Muntner, In Medical Writings of Moses Maimonides, Vol 1. Lippincott, Philadelphia, PA, 1963, pp. 2, 57, 61–74.
12. Saketkhoo K, Januszkiewicz A, Sackner MA. Effects of drinking hot water, cold water, and chicken soup on nasal mucus velocity and nasal airflow resistance. Chest 1978; 74:408–410.
13. Rosner F. Hot chicken soup for asthma. Lancet 1979; 2:1079.
14. Cosman MP. A feast for Aesculapius: historical diets for asthma and sexual pleasure. Annu Rev Nutr 1983; 1–33.
15. Rosner F. Moses Maimonides' Treatise on Asthma. J Asthma 1984; 21:119–129.
16. Van Helmont JB. Oriatrike or Physick Refined. Lodowick, Lloyd, London, England, 1662, pp. 356-373.
17. Kahn MA. Historical survey of our knowledge of bronchial asthma. Medical Life 1928; 35: 109–162.
18. Corris PA, Dark JH. Aetiology of asthma: lesson from lung transplant. Lancet 1993; 341: 1369–1371.
19. Persson CGA. Glucocorticoids for asthma: early contributions. Pulm Pharmacol 1989; 2:163–166.
20. Mann RD. Modern Drug Use:an Enquiry on Historical Principles. MTP, Lancaster, PA, 1984; 355–362.
21. Laennec RTH. A treatise on the Diseases of the Chest and on Mediate Auscultation, (originally published in 1818; translated by J. Forbes) Wood, Collins, Hannay, Grigg, Avner, New York, NY, pp. 7-56, 413–425.
22. Williams CJB. Pathology and diagnosis of diseases of the chest comprising a rational exposition of the physical signs. J Churchill, London, England, 1840, pp. 320–331.
23. Salter HH. On asthma: its pathology and treatment. J. Churchill, London, England, 1860.
24. Ramadge FH. Asthma, its species and complications, or researches into the pathology of disordered respiration; with remarks on the remedial treatment applicable to each variety, being a practical and theoretical review of this malady, considered in its simple form, and in connection with disease of the heart, catarrh, indigestion, etc. Longman, Rees, Orme, Brown, Green, Longman, London, England, 1835, pp. 41–102.
25. Cohen SG. Asthma among the famous. Armand Trousseau (1801–1867), French physician. Allergy Proc 1997; 18:40–42.
26. Thorowgood JC. Notes on asthma: its nature, forms, and treatment. J. Churchill, London, England, 1870, pp. 41–56.
27. Tammeling GJ. Willem Einthoven as a pioneer in bronchial function. Eur J Cardiol 1978; 8: 299–302.
28. Leyden E. Zur Kenntniss des Bronchial-Asthma. Archiv Pathol Anat Physiol 1872; 54: 324–352 [in German].
29. Curschmann H. Bronchiolitis exsudativa und ihr Verhältniss zum Asthma nervosum. Deutsches Archiv Klin Med 1882; 32:1–34 [in German].

30. Sakula A. Charcot-Leyden crystals and Curshmann spirals in asthmatic sputum. Thorax 1986; 41:503–507.
31. Ehrlich P. Ueber die specifischen Granulationen des Blutes. Archiv für Physiologie. Physiologische Abtheilung des Archives für Anatomie und Physiologie. 1879; 571–579 [in German].
32. Gollasch. Zur Klenntniss der asthmatischen Sputums. Fortschritte der Medizin 1889; 7:361–365 [in German].
33. Fink. Beitrage zur kenntnis des eiters und des sputums, Martiri und Gruttefren, Elberfeld, 1890, pp. 1–33 [in German].
34. Gabritschewsky G. Klinische hämatologische Notizen. Archiv Exp Pathol Pharmakol 1890; 28:83–96 [in German].
35. Von Noorden C. Beiträge zur pathologie des Asthma bronchiale. Zeit Klin Med 1892; 20: 98–106 [in German].
36. Müller HF. Zur Lehre vom Asthma bronchiale. Zentralblatt für Allgemeine Pathologie 1893; 4:529–541.
37. Portier MM, Richet Ch. De l'action anaphylactique de certains venins. Comptes Rendu des Seances de la Societie de Biologie 1902; 54:170–172 [in French].
38. Meltzer SJ. Bronchial asthma as a phenomenon of anaphylaxis. JAMA 1910; 55:1021–1024.
39. von Pirquet C. Allergie. Muenchener Medizinische Wochenschrift 1906; 53:1457–1458 [in German].
40. Osler W. The Principles and Practice of Medicine: designed for the use of practitioners and students of medicine. First edition. D. Appleton, New York, 1892, pp. 497–501.
41. Gandevia B. Historical review of the use of parasympatholytic agents in the treatment of respiratry disorders. Postgrad Med J 1975; 51(suppl 7):13–20.
42. Hertz CW. Historical aspects of anticholinergic treatment of obstructive airways disease. Scand J Respir Dis Suppl 1979; 103:105–109.
43. Waldbott GL. Asthma, then and now: are we treating it better? Ann Allergy 1979; 43:32–35.
44. Bullowa JGM, Kaplan DM. On the hypodermatic use of adrenalin chloride in the treatment of asthmatic attacks. Medical News 1903; 83:787–790
45. Camps PWL. A note on the inhalation treatment of asthma. Guy's Hosp Rep 1929; 79:496–498.
46. Chen KK, Schmidt CF. The action of ephedrine, the active principle of the Chinese drug, Ma Huang. J Pharmacol Exp Ther 1924; 24:339–357.
47. Rackemann FM. A clinical study of one hundred and fifty cases of bronchial asthma. Arch Intern Med 1918; 22:517–552.
48. Stedman TL. A Practical Medical Dictionary: of words used in medicine with their derivation and pronunciation, including dental, veterinary, chemical, botanical, electrical, life insurance and other special terms, anatomical tables of the titles in general use and those sanctioned by the Basle Anatomical Convention; pharmaceutical preparations, official in the U.S. and British pharmacopoeias and contained in the national formulary; chemical and therapeutic information as to the mineral springs of America and Europe, and comprehensive lists of synonyms. W. Wood & Co., New York, NY, 1920, p. 92.
49. Rackemann FM. Asthma in a Textbook of Medicine by American Authors (R. Cecil, ed), W.B. Saunders, Philadelphia, PA, 1927, pp. 481–489.
50. Rackemann FM. A clinical classification on asthma based upon a review of six hundred and forty eight cases. Am J Med Sci 1921; 162:802–811.
51. Schultze-Werninghaus G, Meier-Sydow J. The clinical and pharmacological history of theophylline: first report of the bronchospasmolytic action in man by S.R. Hirsch in Frankfurt (Main) 1922. Clin Allergy 1982; 12:211–215.
52. May CD. History of the introduction of theophylline into the treatment of asthma. Clin Allergy 1974; 4:211–217

53. Hermann G, Aynesworth MB, Martin J. Successful treatment of persistent extreme dyspnea "status asthmaticus." Use of theophylline ethylene diamine (aminophylline, U.S.P.) intravenously. J Lab Clin Med 1938; 23:135–148.
54. Solis–Cohen S. The use of adrenal substance in the treatment of acute asthma. JAMA. 1900; 34:1164–1166.
55. Bordley JE, Carey RA, Harvey AM, et al. Preliminary observations on the effect of adrenocortocotrophic hormone (ACTH) in allergic disease. Bull Johns Hopkins Hosp 1949; 85:396–398.
56. Rackemann FM. Allergy-histamine and ACTH: a review of the literature from August 1948 to September 1950. Arch Intern Med 1951; 87:598–621.
57. Carryer HM, Koelsche GA, Prickman LE, et al. The effect of cortisone on bronchial asthma and hay fever occurring in subjects sensitive to ragweed pollen. J Allergy 1950; 21:282–287.
58. Randolph TG Rollins JP. Effect of cortisone on bronchial asthma. J Allergy 1950; 21:288–295.
59. Segal MS, Herschfus JA. ACTH and cortisone in management of hypersensitivities with particular reference to bronchial asthma: review of clinical and laboratory studies. Ann Allergy 1950; 8:786–798.
60. Franklin W, Lowell FC, Schiller IW, et al. Clinical studies with cortisone by mouth, cortisone by injection, and ACTH in treatment of asthma. J Allergy 1952; 23:27–31.
61. Burrage WS, Irwin JW. The role of cortisone in the treatment of severe bronchial asthma. New Engl J Med 1953; 248:679–682.
62. Barach AL, Bickerman HA, Beck GJ. Clinical and physiological studies on the use of metacortandracin in respiratory disease. Dis Chest 1955; 27:515–527.
63. Sheldon JM, McLean JA, Mathews KP. Experiences with metacortandracin (Meticorten) in severe bronchial asthma. J Mich St Med Soc 1955; 54:1081–1083, 1093.
64. Pearson JEG. The treatment of asthma with corticotrophin. Br Med J 1955; 1:189–192.
65. Medical Research Council Subcommittee on Clinical Trials in Asthma. Controlled trial of the effects of cortisone acetate in status asthmaticus. Report to the Medical Research Council by the Subcommittee on Clinical Trials in Asthma. Lancet 1956; 2:803–806.
66. Grossman J. The evolution of inhaler technology. J Asthma 1994; 31:55–64.
67. Ahlquist RP. A study of adrenotropic receptors. Am J Physiol 1948; 153:586–600.
68. Lands AM, Arnold A, McAuliff JP, et al. Differentiation of receptor systems activated by sympathomimetic amines. Nature 1967; 214:597–598.
69. Brenner BE. Bronchial asthma in adults: Part I: Pathogenesis, clinical manifestations, diagnostic evaluation, and differential diagnosis. Am J Emerg Med 1983; 1:50–70.
70. Brenner BE. Bronchial asthma in adults: presentation to the emergency department. Part II Sympathomimetics, respiratory failure, recommendations for initial treatment, indications for admission, and summary. Am J Emerg Med 1983; 3:306–333.
71. Westerman DE, Benatar SR, Potgieter PD, et al. Identification of the high risk asthmatic patient: experience with 39 patients undergoing ventilation for status asthmaticus. Am J Med 1979; 66:565–572
72. Scoggin CH, Sahn SA, Petty TL. Status asthmaticus: a nine year experience. JAMA 1977; 238:1158–1162.
73. Chang G, Levison H. The effect of a nebulized bronchodilator administered with and without intermittent positive pressure breathing on ventilatory function in children with cystic fibrosis and asthma. Am Rev Respir Dis 1972; 106:867–872.
74. Karetzky MS. Asthma mortality: an analysis of one year's experience, review of the literature of the current modes of therapy and assessment . Medicine 1975; 54:471–484.
75. Brewer LA III. Respiration and respiratory treatment. Am J Surg 1979; 138:342–354.
76. Leigh JM. Variation in performance of oxygen therapy devices. Towards the rational employment of "The dephlogisticated air described by Priestly." Ann R Coll Surg Engl 1973; 52: 234–253.

77. Dobell AR. The origins of endotracheal intubation. Ann Thorac Surg 1994; 58:578–584.
78. Westhorpe R. O'Dwyer's tubes. Anaesth Intensive Care 1991; 19:157.
79. Hardy A. Tracheotomy versus intubation: surgical intervention in Europe and the United States, 1825–1930. Bull Hist Med 1992; 66:536–559.
80. Gilbertson AA. Before intensive therapy. J R Soc Med 1995; 88:459P–463P.
81. Wackers GL. Modern anaesthesiological principles for bulbar polio: manual IPPR in the 1952 polio-epidemic in Copenhagen. Acta Anaesthesiol Scand 1994; 38:420–431.
82. Lassen HCA. Management of life-threatening poliomyelitis, Copenhagen, 1952–1956, with a survey of autopsy findings in 115 cases. Livingstone, Edinburgh, Scotland, 1956, pp. ix–xi, 1–4, 147.
83. Somerson SJ, Sicilia MR. Historical perspectives on the development and use of mechanical ventilation. AANA J 1992; 60:83–94.
84. Ambiavagar M, Jones ES. Resuscitation of the moribund asthmatic. Use of intermittent positive pressure ventilation, bronchial lavage and intravenous infusions. Anaesthesia 1967; 22: 375–391.
85. Beam LR, Marcy JH, Mansmann HC Jr. Medically irreversible status asthmaticus in children: report of three cases treated with paralysis and controlled respiration. JAMA 1965; 194:120–124.
86. Iisalo EUM, Iisalo EI, Vapaavuori MJ. Prolonged artificial in severe status asthmaticus. Acta Med Scand 1969; 185:51–55.
87. Reisman RE, Friedman I, Arbesman CE. Severe status asthmaticus: prolonged treatment with assisted ventilation. J Allergy 1968; 37–48
88. Leonhardt KO. The resuscitation of the moribund asthmatic and emphysematous patient. N Engl J Med 1961; 264:785–790.
89. Cherniak RM. The recognition and management of respiratory insufficiency . Anesthesiology 1964; 25:209–216.
90. Alexander HL. A historical account of death from asthma. J Allergy 1963; 34:305–322.
91. Rackemann FM. Intrinsic asthma. J Allergy 1940; 11:147–162, 166–169.
92. Siegel S. History of asthma deaths from antiquity. J. Allergy Clin Immunol 1987; 80:458–462.
93. Speizer FE, Doll R. A century of asthma deaths in young people. Br Med J 1968; 3:245–246.
94. Haller JS. The beginning of urban ambulance service in the United States and England. J Emerg Med 1990; 8:743–755.
95. Marx JA. The history and future of emergency medicine. North Carolina Med J 1997; 58: 288–291.
96. Rupke JA, Wiegenstein JG, Fahrney PM, et al. Twenty-five Years on the Front Line. American College of Emergency Physicians, Dallas, TX, 1993.

2

Where Might We Go?
Trends in Emergency Asthma Research

Barry E. Brenner
The Brooklyn Hospital Center, member of New York–Presbyterian Hospitals, Weill Medical College of Cornell University, Brooklyn, New York

In 1994 a philanthropic group, the Josiah Macy, Jr., foundation, in collaboration with emergency physicians, medical practitioners in other specialists, and public health officials, reported on the state of emergency medicine. They noted that for emergency medicine to fulfill its goal as an academic specialty, research needed to be furthered. Some suggestions were specifically mentioned, i.e., collaborative, basic science, and health services related research (1). Research in emergency asthma offers all these opportunities.

The direction of acute asthma research has been recently discussed (2,3). This present discussion will endeavor not to duplicate the work or material that is also contained in this book. This chapter will hopefully stimulate interest in asthma research.

Basic science studies in emergency asthma have been hindered by difficulty in obtaining appropriate biologic materials. Serum and urinary markers are useful, but the most direct measures would come from the lung itself. In urine, leukotriene E4 has been a particularly useful marker for asthma severity (4). To obtain such material to study, many investigations on asthma have relied on bronchoalveolar lavage; however, this invasive process requires conscious sedation and is probably too risky to perform on acute asthmatics. Recently, spontaneous sputum production, as well as sputum induction with hypertonic saline, has been shown to be safe in patients with acute asthma (5,6). The role of several mediators of inflammation obtained from severe, acute asthmatics by sputum induction is under study. Markers that can be evaluated are eosinophilic cationic protein, albumin, fibrinogen, and interleukin 5 (7). Another approach to assess the level of bronchial inflammation measures the products of inflammation in the fluid that condenses after normal exhalation. Exhaled leukotrienes, hydrogen peroxide, and nitric oxide gas have been shown to be elevated in asthmatics and can serve as markers of inflammation (8–10). However, the equipment for this method of measuring exhaled products of inflammation presently is expensive.

Fundamental to emergency asthma is our method for diagnosing acute asthma in the emergency department (ED). The diagnosis is given to ED patients by the emergency physician, often without further follow-up studies. Some of these patients may have acute bronchitis and others vocal cord dysfunction or panic disorder (see Chapter 13 on clinical manifestations of acute asthma). Once the physician has given the patient the diagnosis, then the patient returns wheezing to the ED, states he has asthma, responds variably to inhaled β agonists and corticosteroids, and is diagnosed as an exacerbation of acute asthma. Is this physician–based clinical diagnosis accurate? Asthma is considered reversible airway disease and demonstrating improvement in expiratory flow rates is the cornerstone of the diagnosis in the ED. Does a 20% improvement in the expiratory flow rates help improve the accuracy of the diagnosis? Many patients with acute asthma, however, may not improve adequately with therapy. These patients are still considered to have acute asthma and are admitted to the hospital. On the other hand, patients with acute bronchitis may have reversible airway disease for up to the three months following an episode of viral bronchitis (see Chapter 13 on clinical manifestations). This entire subject of the ED diagnosis of acute asthma needs further clarification, such that an emergency physician can diagnose with confidence new onset asthma and an acute exacerbation of chronic asthma.

The identification of patients with acute asthma for national health statistics has depended on the billing records. The reliability of billing information on patients with acute asthma is poor (see Chapter 5, ''Epidemiology of Asthma''). At the Brooklyn Hospital Center, 34% of the admitted patients that were listed on billing records as having acute asthma, actually did not have acute asthma at all. To have meaningful national health statistics, a national database of emergency asthma should be developed. The database would avoid the limitations of relying on the billing records, since these acute asthmatics had physician-diagnosed acute asthma. The database would also be invaluable in planning national as well as local studies on acute asthma and measuring trends and the effects of national interventions, such as new therapies or educational programs.

Among the provocative factors for acute asthma, an association with menses may explain the increased frequency of adult female ED visits and admissions to the hospital. Likewise some patients seem particularly sensitive to the effects of indoor or outdoor air pollution. The ED can be used to identify these patients and in conjunction with pulmonologists or primary care physicians develop therapeutic strategies to treat and prevent these episodes. Identification of these patients from the ED is advantageous, since almost all patients with acute asthma that are admitted to the hospital, whether or not they have a primary care physician (PCP), are admitted after an ED visit. Therefore the ED can ''capture'' most of the information concerning patients that are admitted to the hospital with acute asthma.

New therapies will always require trials on acute asthmatics in the ED. The effect of a differential response according to gender, time of day, or route of administration has not been thoroughly investigated. From some preliminary work, certain asthma therapies may be more effective during the day than the night (see Chapter 11 on nocturnal asthma). In addition, different carriers for the administration of inhalants may be useful. For example β_2-agonists could be nebulized through Heliox (a 80/20 helium/oxygen mixture) instead of room air or oxygen, as is the current practice.

The evaluation of the acute asthmatic has been hindered by instrumentation that is highly effort dependent. Unless the test is obtained at the maximum vital capacity, the peak flow rate and FEV_1 are both effort dependent with the former test perhaps easier to perform in a highly tachypneic patient, since the peak flow requires less time to perform.

Both tests cause much coughing in the acute asthmatic. On the other hand, clinical appreciation of the severity of asthma is poor by both physicians and patients; peak flow and FEV_1 are the best objective tests available in the ED (see Chapter 14, "Pulmonary Function Testing"). New tests need to be developed to objectively assess the severity of the episode of acute asthma (see Chapter 16, "Pulse Oximetry and Other Noninvasive Monitors"). An assessment of the degree of inflammation of the bronchi can be achieved from the M/P ratio [the ratio of the expiratory flow between a forceful exhalation at a maximum inspiration (M) and one at partial inspiration (exhalation from the function residual capacity) (P)] (11). This ratio possibly could be used at the time of discharge of the asthmatic from the ED to evaluate the patient for their risk of relapse and need for glucocorticoids.

New therapies may affect the risk for relapse as well as the indications for admission. Admission criteria may be generated, but will frequently need to be changed as new therapies alter ED practices. Disposition and outcome questions will remain, independent of any changes in therapy. For example, asthmatics have increased bronchospasm during the night hours (see Chapter 11 on nocturnal asthma). Does an evening discharge from the ED increase the relapse rate as compared to a daytime discharge? Does the patient have a lower relapse rate if discharged with his medications in his hand (β-agonists, inhaled corticosteroids, oral corticosteroids) as opposed to receiving a prescription for them?

Probably the biggest change in admission/discharge criteria will come from utilizing observation units in acute asthma. At Cook County Hospital, these have reduced acute adult asthma admissions to the hospital from the ED by 60% after a 12-hr stay. Strikingly the relapse rate was 9% at two weeks in this study (see Chapter 33 on observation units). In contrast, a more nationally representative average relapse rate of 17% was noted in the Multicenter Asthma Research Collaboration series (12). Objective criteria need to be developed and validated for admission to an observation unit and subsequent discharge to home or admission to the hospital. The role of the observation unit needs to be clarified. In an ideal, efficient hospital environment, a prompt discharge of an acute asthmatic from the medicine wards should be achievable in the same time frame as the observation unit. Therefore, in a well-managed inpatient service, observations units for admitted patients with acute asthma would be unnecessary.

Assessment and treatment of the asthmatic patient needs further research in certain special situations such as prehospital care, where the diagnosis may be less certain and the therapeutic options more limited than in the ED. The pregnant asthmatic presents the special challenges of two patients: the mother and the fetus, as well as a diminished ability to monitor the fetus in the ED. In addition, the response of the uterus to different therapeutic agents varies with the trimester of pregnancy. Further studies need to be made on the treatment of the pregnant asthmatic. Most importantly the therapy of the refractory, severe asthmatic needs evaluation. These patients are not common and multicenter studies would be the most effective means to produce meaningful results. Particularly evaluations of ketamine and inhalational anesthetics, such as halothane, need thorough evaluation for their impact on avoiding endotracheal intubation or ameliorating the bronchospasm in the patient that is difficult to ventilate despite mechanical ventilation (13).

REFERENCES

1. Bowles LT, Sirica CM. The Josiah Macy Jr Foundation report: the role of emergency medicine in the future of American medical care. New York, Executive summary, April, 1994.

2. Nowak RM, Hurd SS, Skobeloff EM, et al. Asthma research: future directions for emergency medicine. Ann Emerg Med 1996; 244–249.
3. Geppert EF, Lester LA, Ober C. Prioritizing asthma research: the need to investigate childhood asthma. Am J Respir Crit Care Med 1995; 151:1294–1295.
4. Smith CM, Hawksworth RJ, Thien FCK, et al. Urinary leukotriene E4 in bronchial asthma. Eur Respir J 1992; 5:693–699.
5. Pizzichini E, Pizzichini MMM, Efthimiadis A, et al. Indices of airway inflammation in induced sputum: reproducibility and validity of cell and fluid-phase measurements. Am J Respir Crit Care Med 1996; 154:308–317.
6. Pizzichini MMM, Pizzichini E, Clelland L, et al. Sputum in severe exacerbations of asthma: kinetics of inflammatory indices after prednisone. Am J Respir Crit Care Med 1997; 155: 1501–1508.
7. in't Veen JCCM, de Gouw HWFM, Smits HH, et al. Repeatability of cellular and soluble markers of inflammation in induced sputum from patients with asthma. Eur Respir J 1996; 9:2441–2447.
8. Dohlman AW, Black HR, Royall JA. Expired breath hydrogen peroxide is a marker of acute airway inflammation in pediatric patients with asthma. Am Rev Respir Dis 1993; 148:955–960
9. Yates DH, Kharitonov SA, Robbins RA, et al. Effect of a nitric oxide synthetase inhibitor and a glucocorticoid on exhaled air nitric oxided. Am J Respir Crit Care Med 1995; 152:892–896.
10. Winsel K, Becher G, Beck E, et al. Leukotrienes in breathing condensate released during bronchial challenge test. Eur Respir J 1995; 8(suppl 19):s473.
11. Lim TK, Ang SM, Rossing TH, et al. The effect of deep inhalation on maximal expiratory flow during intensive treatments of spontaneous asthmatic episodes. Am Rev Respir Dis 1989; 140:340–343.
12. Camargo CA Jr, on behalf of the MARC Investigators. Management of acute asthma in US emergency departments: The Multicenter Asthma Research Collaboration [abstract]. Am J Respir Crit Care Med 1998; 157(3, Part 2):A623.
13. Saulnier FF, Durocher AV, Deturck RA, et al. Respiratory and hemodynamic effects of halothane in status asthmaticus. Intensive Care Med 1990; 16:104–107.

3

Asthma Production and Biochemistry

Phillip L. Rice Jr.
Kings County Hospital Center, Brooklyn, New York

I. INTRODUCTION

Advances in the treatment of asthma have, not surprisingly, paralleled advances in delineating the complex pathophysiology in asthma. Asthma was first viewed as a disease predominantly involving overactive smooth musculature, and treatment corresponded with this understanding. Our knowledge deepened to include a component of inflammation, but with the smooth muscle component continuing its dominance as the underlying problem. Later this view was reformulated to recognize the primacy of inflammation in the disease process, and the corresponding change in the primacy of steroids in the treatment of asthma followed. Additionally, even in the early literature on asthma, an allergic, as well as a genetic, component was known to contribute. The deepening of our base of knowledge of both genetics and more importantly immunology has led to important treatment modalities currently used in asthma treatment.

Currently accepted theory of asthma development considers it multifactoral in origin and progression and centers on the clinical triad of bronchial inflammation, hyperreactive smooth muscle activity, and reversible airflow obstruction. It includes immunological elements, neural components, genetic aspects, and, fundamentally, inflammatory components. The timing, as well as the qualitative and quantitative contribution of each to the process, is complex, but much is known. This chapter will present the biochemistry of this process.

The steps involved in biochemical production of asthma are complex and involve complex arrays of immune cell responses. Sensitization, stimulation, cellular cascade and migration, activation of intrapulmonary cellular matrix, tissue damages, and amelioration and return to a relative baseline characterize the different phases involved. Based on our understanding of the biochemical processes and the clinical manifestations, asthma is divided into two acute phases, an early phase and a late phase. The early phase is produced predominantly by the direct effect of preformed mediators residing within mast cells and platelets. In addition, the neural response is also part of this phase. The late phase is characterized by mechanisms that are a result of induction of gene expression.

The early phase consists of several components, which include smooth muscle contraction, edema of bronchial mucosa, and mucous secretion. Autonomic stimulation, as well as the release of the preformed leukotrienes, prostaglandins, thromboxane, platelet-aggregating factor, bradykinin, and histamine from IgE-ladened mast cells (as well as platelets) mainly bring about these events (1). However, these mediators have several functions that act in both the realms of the early phase and the late phase response (Table 1). For instance the mediator-induced leakiness of the endothelial vasculature produces the immediate edema, but also allows fibrinogen and fibronectin into the tissues, which forms scaffolding that facilitates leukocyte migration and subsequent retention in the extravascular tissues (2). In essence, most mediators serve to produce immediate effects while at the same time are involved in the late airway response involving the migration of inflammatory cells into the lung parenchyma.

Smooth muscle contraction is part of the picture of airway and airflow obstruction in asthma and a target of early intervention. Many of the mediators, especially the leukotrienes, are potent smooth muscle contractors, and upon degranulation of mast cells and platelets can produce severe contractions throughout the bronchial tree (3–7). Additionally, the autonomic nervous system clearly plays a role in smooth muscle tone and contraction, as well as the hyperresponsiveness to stimuli. There is evidence that mast cells may degranulate in response to neural transmitters such as acetylcholine (8). Hypertrophy of the bronchial smooth muscle and hyperresponsiveness characterize asthmatic anatomy and physiology; they are induced over time as part of chronic elements in the pathology of asthma, but are still factors in the degree of airway obstruction during an acute episode. For many decades focus was centered on smooth muscle contraction in asthma, and it continues to be a part of the treatment of all asthmatics. However, as the recognition of inflammation's role has grown, strategies to eliminate smooth muscle contraction as the main treatment have become secondary.

Another immediate factor that decreases airflow is the production of edema. Edema of the bronchial lumen and endothelium is induced by several of the aforementioned mediators, especially histamine and the leukotrienes. Endothelial cells loosen their attachments and change shape in response to these mediators, resulting in the movement of plasma and its proteins into or through the lamina propria. How edema produces immediate airflow

Table 1 Mediators Measured in Asthma

Early airway response	Late airway response
Leukotriene LTC_4, LTD_4	Leukotriene $LTC_4 + LTB_4$
Histamine	Histamine
Prostaglandin D_2	GM-CSF
Tryptase	Interleukin-5
Thromboxane	Prostaglandins $F_{2\alpha}$, D_2, E_2
	Kinins
	Eosinophil cationic
	Protein
	Major basic protein
	Eosinophil peroxidase

obstruction, in terms of the mechanics, is fairly straightforward, but the contribution of edema formation to the late phase should not be minimized, as it facilitates the subsequent cellular infiltration.

Mucous plugging, a feature of especially severe attacks, is also due to elements of both early and late airway responses. Some of the same mediators, especially the leukotrienes, are potent mucinogogues. They stimulate the goblet cells residing in the lumen of the bronchioles to secrete mucin, which form the plugs that decrease airflow and cause distal air trapping and atelectasis (8). Again, many of the degranulation elements of the mast cells induce late phase changes related to the production of mucous by stimulating the growth of goblet cells (9).

The early phase is marked by several elements that give rise to the clinical picture of early asthma. The effects of hyperresponsive smooth muscle contracting, edematous, mucous-filled bronchioles decrease airflow. Poiseuille's fourth-power law for flow relates flow to the radius of the lumen, but to the fourth power, and decreasing the lumen from mucous secretions and edema will clearly cause marked airflow problems: $V/t = \pi r^4(\Delta P)/8\eta L$, where L is the length of the tube and η is the coefficient of viscosity.

It is recognized, however, that even though the early phase elements produce such a marked airflow obstruction, the late airway response, characterized by inflammation, is the dominant factor in asthma. The results of mRNA transcription, new gene expression, mainly characterize this response with the resultant infiltration of leukocytes, predominantly eosinophils. This is signaled by cytokines (proteins by which immune cells communicate with and immumomodulate each other) released from several cell lines in response to antigens or other stimuli. The interleukins, also a cytokine, are critical in this step, as are several other cytokines such as tumor necrosis factor (TNF), granulocyte–monocyte colony stimulating factor (GM-CSF), and interferon (IFN)-γ (2).

After release, these cytokines induce genetic expression of adhesion molecules within the vascular lumen and cause eosinophils to be receptive to adhesion (10). Additionally, they promote eosinophil production and chemotaxis, and cause basement membrane remodeling and thickening (laying down of new collagen) (8). Clearly there is a time delay due to the necessity to transcribe genetic information. This is the reason that the inflammatory component predominates in the late phase.

Within one or two hours after the initial bronchial stimulus, TNF induces endothelial-leukocyte adhesion molecules in the capillary venules. Adhesion molecules enhance ability of endothelial cells to become ''sticky'' and capture passing leukocytes flowing through the venules. Venular endothelial cells regulate the infiltration of leukocytes into the inflammatory reaction site (2). Interleukin (IL)-4, a cytokine released by mast cells, stimulates the expression of vascular cell adhesion molecule-1 (VCAM-1), which selects for eosinophils, and to a lesser extent lymphocytes and monocytes. Both the intercellular adhesion molecule (ICAM-1) and VCAM-1 are induced in 4–6 hr. TNF in concert with IFN-g also causes the shape of the eosinophil to change from a round spherical shape to flatter one, i.e., a shape more conducive to navigating between cells. Likewise, TNF causes changes in the shape of the endothelial cells to allow passage of the inflammatory cells (2,11).

Again, events in both the early and late phases are working in concert to produce the inflammatory response. The early phase mediators along with mediators, such as nitric oxide and prostacyclin (PGI_2), produced by TNF-stimulated endothelial cells, increase blood flow and optimize delivery of eosinophils, lymphocytes, and monocytes to the lung. These cellular elements of inflammation in turn produce a wide range of effects on the local tissue environment through voluminous production of leukotrienes, prostaglandins, histamine, cytokines, and TNF. Eosinophils are the predominant cellular component in the inflammatory response in asthma and contain other proteins and enzymes that eliminate, along with the aforementioned mediators, cause tissue changes (12,13).

Eosinophilic infiltration of the lungs is followed by the destruction of the lung tissue and replacement by connective tissue and goblet cells. The basement membrane thickens consequently. Dead, destroyed tissue sloughs off into the airway, further contributing to the airflow obstruction. The faster-growing goblet cells become more numerous and the mucous production problem worsens. As the lining of the bronchioles thins and is replaced by connective tissue, the lungs become less compliant. In addition, with this loss, or thinning, of the lining, the nerve endings become more exposed with hyperirritability as a consequence.

Eosinophils continue to produce the mediators of inflammation long after the initiating insult has been removed. In particular, leukotriene production continues well into the late airway response time frame. Eosinophils are present in lung tissue during asthma, but while residing in the lung they continually produce mediators of inflammation that destroy tissue. This is a key point. In the early airway response there is a brief exposure to these mediators, but with eosinophilic infiltration, which characterizes the late airway response, the basis for a sustained exposure occurs. Sustained exposure to mediators is responsible for the chronic structural changes seen in asthmatics (14).

The focus of recent research has been on understanding how on a biochemical basis these mediators actually carry out their effects on the target organs, and in turn develop strategies to block their effects. There is evidence that in both the early and late airway responses a key element is leukotriene production. Blocking their effects may solve part of the puzzle. Clearly the ability to inhibit the transcription of genes that contribute to the late airway response is important in order to be able to decrease inflammation. Presently, glucocorticoid use is critical in the inhibition of the inflammation, but its long-term use is fraught with undesirable side effects. A more selective means to block this process has been heavily investigated and certain immunotherapies appear promising (15). In discussing the inflammation aspects of asthma, it is not to imply that reversing the smooth muscle contraction is not also key and a mainstay of current therapy of asthma, particularly with regard to the early airway response.

Blocking the mediators of inflammation has led to the focus on leukotrienes. Leukotrienes are the third group of lipid mediators produced, in addition to prostaglandins and platelet aggregating factor. Leukotrienes were discovered to be the main mediators of the slow-reacting substance of anaphylaxis in 1979 (16,17). The main leukotrienes are LTC_4, LTD_4, and LTE_4 in the cysteinyl group, and LTB_4 (Fig. 1) (18). There is now compelling evidence of the central and pivotal role of cysteinyl leukotrienes in the production of the clinical syndrome of asthma.

Various stimuli activate the phospholipases in the cell membrane to liberate arachidonic acid into the intracellular matrix. Leukotrienes are synthesized from arachidonic acid, which is a substrate for several enzymes (cyclooxygenase, 12-lipoxygenase, 5-lipoxygenase (5-LO), and 15-lipoxygenase enzymes) in many different tissues (Fig. 1) (19). Of the three lipoxygenases, the 5-lipoxygenase-enzyme pathway is crucial for the development of allergic inflammatory reaction in the lung. The 5-LO enzyme is an iron-containing enzyme consisting of 673 amino acids, which is dependent on Ca^{++}, adenosine triphosphate and several cofactors for maximal activity. 5-LO translocates from the cytosol to the nuclear cell membrane to initiate leukotriene biosynthesis (18,20).

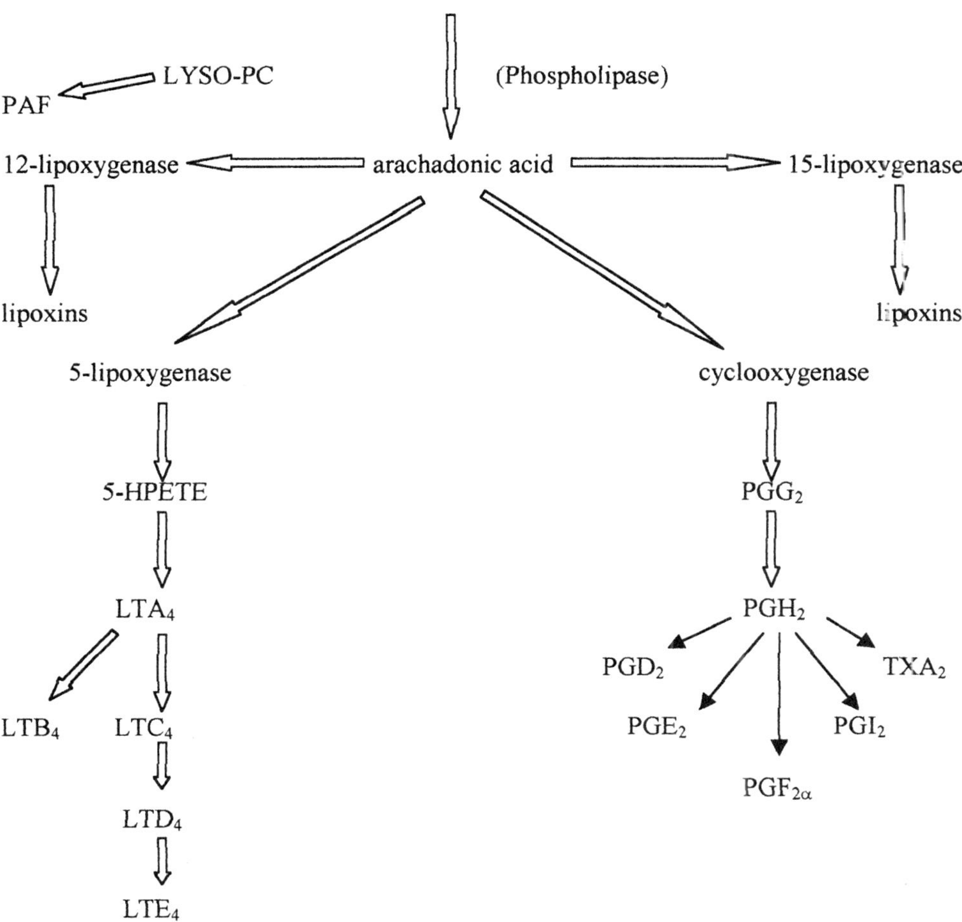

Figure 1 Phospholipid pathways producing leukotrienes, thromboxanes, and lipoxins.

Chemotaxis is an important step in the migration of inflammatory cells from the circulation to the site of inflammation. LTB_4 is produced mainly by neutrophils, and its predominant effect is one of neutrophil chemotaxis, although it has a lesser chemoattractant effect on eosinophils (21). It is transported out of the cell where it is metabolized further by endothelial cells and platelets. LTC_4 is further acted upon by α-glutamyltranspeptidase to form LTD_4 and LTE_4 (formed from LTD_4 by dipeptidase). LTD_4 represents the biologically most potent cysteinyl leukotriene (19,20).

The enzymes that take part in leukotriene synthesis are located in different cell lines. The 5-LO enzyme is limited to myeloid cells (neutrophils, eosinophils, basophils, monocytes, macrophages, and mast cells). LTC_4 synthase resides in mast cells and eosinophils, but also in endothelial cells and platelets. Being distributed among different cell types, various inflammatory cells can participate in the transcellular synthesis of leukotrienes. Cellular sources of cysteinyl leukotrienes are mast cells, macrophages and eosinophils. Eosinophils mainly produce LTC_4 (22).

The liver is the main organ for the metabolism of leukotrienes. Its metabolic byproducts are excreted in bile. Unmetabolized LTE_4 is excreted in the urine and can be measured. In the liver leukotrienes undergo beta-oxidation; these metabolic products are biologically less active or inactive than leukotrienes (23).

In the lung the cysteinyl leukotrienes are primarily responsible for the clinical picture of asthma (18). Their actions and properties are listed in Table 2, but importantly include vasoconstriction, bronchoconstriction, increase in vascular permeability (by contracting endothelial cells), and stimulation of mucus secretion. In fact, leukotrienes are the most potent bronchoconstrictors known. They are 1000 times more potent than histamines and 1000–5000 times more potent than histamine when inhaled. Intradermal application of LTC_4, LTD_4, and LTE_4 produces a flare-and-wheal reaction. Increased urinary measurements of LTE_4 have been noted following challenges to asthmatics with allergens, aspirin, and during acute asthmatic attacks. No increase was seen following exercise-induced asthma; however, leukotriene receptor antagonists blocked this response (19).

LTB_4 is also liberated in asthma but has only weak effects on smooth muscle. Most of the LTB_4 is derived from alveolar macrophages and neutrophils accumulated in asthmatic lung tissue, as well as from bronchial epithelial cells. Its promotion of expression of adhesion and transendothelial migration of leukocytes is a critical component of the late airway response. The amelioration of the symptoms of asthma correlates with a drop in the serum LTB_4 levels (24).

Table 2 Biological Effects of Leukotrienes

Cysteinyl leukotrienes	LTB_4
Vasoconstriction	Aggregation; chemokines
Increase of vascular permeability in postcapillary venules	Chemotaxis; release of lysosomal enzymes; stimulation of superoxide anion production
Bronchoconstriction	Adhesion and transendothelial migration of neutrophils
Stimulation of mucus secretion	Increase of vascular permeability (in the presence of PGE_2
Intestional contraction (ileum)	Enhancement of C3b receptor expression and complement-dependent cytotoxity
Plasma extravasation	Modulation of lymphocytic function
Reduction of myocardial contractility and coronary blood flow	Affector of the production and action of cytokines
Decrease of renal flow and GFR	Increase of cAMP and cGMP synthesis
Proliferation of glomerular endothelial cells	
Release of LH-releasing hormone	
Stimulation of prostacyclin synthesis (endothelium)	

II. STRATEGIES FOR TREATMENT

It is reasonable and prudent to assume that by either blocking leukotriene synthesis or blocking leukotriene receptors one could inhibit the production of symptoms related to asthma, and thus clinically ameliorate asthma.

A. Leukotriene Inhibitors

Production of leukotrienes can be inhibited by several mechanisms. Either the 5-LO or the 5-lipoxygenase activating protein (FLAP) can be inhibited, thereby blocking production of leukotrienes. Other strategies along that line involve blocking the LTC_4 synthase enzyme. The 5-LO inhibitor studies revealed that their effectiveness was good in muting the effects of cold air, dry air, and aspirin-induced asthma. It had little or no effect on muting the early airway response or the late airway response. However, while not effective in an acute attack, it was effective in chronic phases. It reduced β-agonist use, increased FEV_1, and decreased night asthma attacks. LTE_4 production was reduced by 39% (25).

The FLAP inhibitors were effective in blunting both the early airway response and late airway response, but had no effect on induced airway hyperresponsiveness. LTB_4 synthesis was almost completely blocked and LTE_4 urinary excretion was reduced 80%, and the number of acute attacks of asthma decreased (19).

The blocking of 5-LO has no effect on early airway response or late airway response for several probable reasons. Included is the possibility that since blockade is not 100%, a few molecules of leukotrienes are produced, and this small amount of leukotrienes is enough to produce the clinical picture of asthma. Also, any pathway inhibitor would not affect degranulation of preformed leukotrienes. Another theory is that since leukotrienes are not the only suspect in clinical asthma, and this disease is multifactoral, blocking only one aspect will not block the early or late airway response.

Currently the only 5-LO synthase inhibitor available for use in asthmatics is a product called zileuton (Zyflo®). It was approved in December 1996 at a dosing schedule of 600 mg four times per day (26). Other leukotriene biosynthesis inhibitors are currently in clinical trials (ZD-2138, MK-0591, and BAY-X-1005, FLAP inhibitors) (19,20). There have been no trials where the efficacy of both FLAP inhibitors and 5-LO inhibitors has been studied.

B. Receptor Antagonists

The second plan of attack is to block the receptors of the cysteinyl leukotrienes. This method would skirt around the problem of leukotriene production, i.e., any cysteinyl-leukotrienes produced will not have much effect because their receptors are saturated.

There are at least three cysteinyl-leukotriene receptors that are categorized by their receptance (cysteinyl-$leukotriene_1$ receptors) or resistance (cysteinyl-$leukotriene_2$ receptors) to blockade (there appears to be a subset of cysteinyl-$leukotriene_1$ receptors specific to LTE_4). All other cysteinyl-$leukotriene_1$ receptors are specific for LTC_4, LTD_4, and LTE_4 (19).

Studies have shown the receptor antagonists to have clinical benefit. In several studies, these antagonists inhibited exercise induced asthma by 50%. In allergen-induced asthma, the early and late airway responses were also inhibited, as was airway hyperresponsiveness. Aspirin doses used to induce asthma had to be increased over fivefold and airway conductance fell 59% less when exposed to platelet activating factor (19,27).

The first marketed leukotriene receptor antagonist was pranlukast, which was initially studied in Japan. Later trials were conducted in Europe and then North America. The only two approved drugs in the United States are zafirlukast (Accolate® 20 mg bid) and montelukast (Singulair® 10 mg bid). The other, pranlukast, is still in phase III trials (28,29).

Understanding the pathophysiology has led to the first new class of drugs with which to combat asthma in the last five years. It also gives us an understanding as to why earlier trials with antihistamines alone and prostaglandin inhibitors failed. As the medical community becomes more informed, these drugs have the potential to be included in the standard regimen of most asthmatics. The optimum regimen has yet to be determined. Whether it will include both inhibitors and receptor antagonists, or just one or the other awaits further clinical trials. Precisely because our understanding has taken a leap, antihistamines and prostaglandin inhibitors may very well merit study again, but clearly in conjunction with either the leukotriene inhibitors or receptor antagonists, or with both. The fine-tuning of each asthmatic becomes much more possible and an exciting era of treatment is unfolding.

REFERENCES

1. Flint KC, Leung K, Hudspith B, et al. Bronchoalveolar mast cells in extrinsic asthma: a mechanism for the initiation of antigen-specific bronchoconstriction. Br Med J 1985; 291:923–926.
2. Abbas A, Lichtman A, Pober J. Cellular and Molecular Immunology, Second Edition, WB Saunders Company, Philadelphia, PA, 1994, p. 240–291.
3. Dahlen S, Hedqvist P, Hammarstrom S, et al. Leukotrienes are potent constrictors of human bronchi. Nature 1980; 288:484–486.
4. Holroyde MC, Altounyan R, Cole M, et al. Bronchoconstriction produced in man by leukotrienes C and D. Lancet 1981; 2:17–18.
5. Cockcroft DW, Killian DN, Mellon JA, et al. Bronchial reactivity to inhaled histamine: a method and clinical survey. Clin Allergy 1977; 7:235–243.
6. Liu MC, Bleeker R, Lichtenstein LM, et al. Evidence for elevated histamine prostaglandin D2 and other bronchoconstricting prostaglandins in the airway of subjects with mild asthma. Am Rev Respir Dis 1990; 142:126–132.
7. Piper PJ. Leukotrienes: potent mediators of airway constriction. Int Arch Allergy Appl Immunol 1985; 76(suppl 1):43–48.
8. Lemanske RF, Busse WW. Asthma. JAMA 1997; 278:1855–1873.
9. Kirby JG, Hargreave FE, Gleich GJ, et al. Bronchoalveolar cell profiles of asthmatic and nonasthmatic subjects. Am Rev Respir Dis 1987; 136:379–383.
10. Albelda S, Buck C. Integrins and other cell adhesion molecules. FASEB J 1990; 4:2868–2880.
11. Wegner CD, Gundel RH, Reilly P, et al. Intercellular adhesion molecule-1 (ICAM-1) in the pathogenesis of asthma. Nature 1990; 247:456–459.
12. Corrigan C, Kay AB. Cells and eosinophils in the pathogenesis of asthma. Immunol Today 1992; 13:501–507.
13. Sanjar S, Aoki S, Kristersson A, Smith D, et al. Antigen challenge induces pulmonary airway eosinophil accumulation and airway hyperreactivity in sensitized guinea-pigs: the effect of anti-asthma drugs. Br J Pharmacol 1990; 99:679–686.

14. Roche WR, Beasley R, Williams JH, et al. Subepithelial fibrosis in the bronchi of asthmatics. Lancet 1989; 1:520–524.
15. Leff AR. Future directions in asthma therapy. Is a cure possible? Chest 1997; 111:61S–68S.
16. Murphy RC, Hammarstrom S, Samuelsson B. Leukotriene C: a slow-reacting substance from murine mastocytoma cells. Proc Natl Acad Sci USA 1979; 76:4275–4279.
17. Dahlen S, Hansson G, Hedqvist P, et. al. Allergen challenge of lung tissue from asthmatics elicits bronchial contraction that correlates with the release of leukotriene C4, D4, and E4. Proc Natl Acad Sci USA 1983; 80:1712–1716.
18. O'Byrne PM. Leukotrienes in the pathogenesis of asthma. Chest 1997; 111:27S–33S.
19. Chung KF. Leukotriene receptor antagonists and biosynthesis inhibitors: potential breakthrough in asthma therapy. Eur Respir J 1995; 8:1203–1213.
20. Ford-Hutchinson AW. Regulation of leukotriene biosynthesis. Cancer Metastasis Rev 1994; 13:257–267.
21. Konig W, Schonfeld W, Raulf M, et al. The neutrophil and leukotrienes: role in health and disease. Eicosanoids 1990; 3:1–22.
22. Mayatepek E, Hoffman G. Leukotrienes: biosynthesis, metabolism, and pathophysiologic significance. Pediatr Res 1995; 37:1–3.
23. Keppler D. Huber M. Weckbecker G. et al. Leukotriene C4 metabolism by hepatoma cells and liver. Adv Enzyme Regul 1987; 26:211–224.
24. Shindo K, Fukumura M, Miyakawa K. Leukotriene B4 levels in the arterial blood of asthmatic patients and the effects of prenisolone. Eur Respir J 1995; 8:605–610.
25. Israel E, Demarkarian R, Rosenberg M, et al. The effects of a 5-lipoxygenase inhibitor on asthma induced by cold air. N Engl J Med 1990; 323:1740–1744.
26. Bell RL, Young PR, Albert D, et al. The discovery and development of Zileuton: an orally active 5-lipoxygenase inhibitor. Int J Immunopharmacol 1992 14:505–510.
27. Snyder DW, Fleisch JH. Leukotriene receptor antagonists as potential therapeutic agents. Annu Rev Pharmacol Toxicol 1989; 29:123–124.
28. Barnes N, Jong B, Miyamoto T. Worldwide clinical experience with the first marketed leukotriene receptor antagonist. Chest 1997; 111:52S–60S.
29. Okudaira H. Challenge studies of a leukotriene receptor antagonist. Chest 1997; 111:46S–51S.

4

Asthma

Immunology and the Inflammatory Response

David M. Lang and Donald G. Raible
Allegheny University of the Health Sciences, Philadelphia, Pennsylvania

I. IMPORTANCE OF IMMUNOLOGY AND THE INFLAMMATORY RESPONSE IN ASTHMA

In the past, acute asthmatic relapse was viewed as a bronchospastic event. In recent years, the key role of immunology and the inflammatory response in promoting and perpetuating asthmatic exacerbation has been appreciated. Despite the realization that asthma is an inflammatory disorder, of which bronchospasm is a manifestation, many patients with asthma who merit treatment with anti-inflammatory agents unfortunately do not receive these drugs (1,2) and hence are undertreated.

The importance of inflammation in the pathophysiology of asthma, and the vital role of anti-inflammatory agents for asthma management, can be appreciated by considering what happens to asthmatic patients when asthma has been controlled with a regular inhaled steroid and these drugs are withdrawn. Gibson et al. (3) recruited 10 stable adults with moderate asthma receiving a regular inhaled steroid to gradually withdraw these medications at weekly intervals of 200 μg/day until asthmatic exacerbation occurred. At an average of 16 (range = 7–26) days after initiating an inhaled steroid taper in this graded fashion, each of these subjects experienced asthmatic exacerbation characterized by statistically and clinically significant changes in spirometric parameters, bronchial hyperresponsiveness, and circulating eosinophils; worsening asthma symptom scores; and diurnal variation in peak flow measurements. Five also developed sputum laden with eosinophils and metachromatic cells (mast cells and basophils). These changes reversed in nine with resumption of inhaled steroid use; one subject required oral prednisone.

In asthmatic children, withdrawal of regular inhaled steroids has also been associated with deterioration of asthma control marked by increased asthma symptoms, heightened bronchodilator reliance, and increased airway hyperresponsiveness (4). These data demonstrate that the therapeutic effects of anti-inflammatory agents can diminish quickly when treatment is withdrawn, and illustrate that asthmatic exacerbation which ensues is associated with evidence of immune system response and airway inflammation.

The important message from these studies is that anti-inflammatory medication is frequently required not only to reverse the inflammation of asthma, but also to maintain control of the inflammation and of asthma symptoms.

Recently released national (5) and international (6) guidelines for asthma management have encouraged more frequent use of pharmacotherapeutic agents that can exert an ''anti-inflammatory'' effect upon asthma. In the Guidelines for the Diagnosis and Management of Asthma, released by the National Heart, Lung, and Blood Institute in 1991, more frequent use of inhaled steroid was encouraged for severe as well as moderate asthmatics based on increasing evidence suggesting that ''airway inflammation is present in virtually *all* patients with asthma'' and demonstrating the utility of inhaled steroid for providing ''improved asthma care with minimal side effects'' (5). Recent data have shown that regular use of inhaled steroid prevents exacerbations of asthma (7), increases in bronchial hyperresponsiveness (8), accelerated loss of lung function (9), development of chronic airflow limitation (10), as well as fatal and near-fatal episodes of asthma (11). Moreover, regular use of inhaled steroid is cost-effective (12). The desirable effects of corticosteroids include inhibiting the cytokines involved with cell recruitment, activation, and proliferation; upregulation of β-adrenergic receptors; increasing synthesis of lipocortin-1; inhibiting mast cell degranulation, and eosinophil priming (13).

The goal of this chapter is to review the underlying immune mechanisms that lead to airway inflammation, which is a primary target of asthma treatment.

II. OVERVIEW OF IMMUNOLOGY

The immune system performs defense and surveillance functions, protecting the host organism from invasion by microorganisms and from neoplasia. Immune system elements are widely distributed in the body, and comprise a complex series of interrelating components. Major specific recognition systems are T cells and B cells; nonspecific systems include mononuclear phagocytes, polymorphonuclear leukocytes, and the complement system. Immune system ontogeny and differentiation have been reviewed extensively (14–16).

Key features of immune system function (14–18) include *specificity:* the capacity to distinguish foreign from self proteins; *memory:* the ability to respond to a specific stimulus upon re-exposure; *mobility:* the potential for influx and efflux into or out of areas based upon signaling, in this fashion local exposures can promote systemic response and/or sensitization; and *amplification:* based upon regulatory factors and capacity for cellular replication or traffic, optimal performance of the system is achieved through a net balance between influences that can promote or dampen amplitude of response.

B cells contribute to immune system function by producing immunoglobulin (16,19). Of the five classes of antibody, IgG (4 subclasses) is the most abundant and has important antibacterial properties; IgA (2 subclasses) is specialized for mucosal environments; IgM is the first immunoglobulin produced by activated B cells and is an efficient activator of complement; IgE is present in very small amounts, but has the potential to promote systemic response because of its high affinity binding to mast cells and basophils and capacity to trigger activation of these cells; and IgD is not well understood.

T cells exhibit a heterogeneous array of regulatory and effector functions within the immune system (14,16,18). T-cell subtypes include helper (CD4+ phenotype) and

Table 1 Mechanisms of Immune Reactions

Classification	Mechanism	Mediation	Clinical examples
Type I	Immediate hypersensitivity	IgE	Anaphylaxis, asthma, rhinitis
Type II	Cytotoxity	Autoantibody	Hemolytic anemia
Type III	Immune complex	Ag/Ab	Serum sickness
Type IV	Delayed hypersensitivity	Cellular	Allergic contact dermatitis

suppressor (CD8+ phenotype) cells. T cells play an important role in resistance to infection and also account for allergic contact dermatitis.

Phagocytic cells and the complement system are nonspecific elements that also participate in and can amplify host defense (14,16,20). Cellular participation in immune responses may be essential, as is the case with IgE-mediated reaction, which involves mast cell/basophil activation. The complement system consists of proteins that interact in a defined sequence to elaborate biologic activities that can promote host defense, and if not regulated appropriately will lead to host tissue injury. Activation of complement by antibody (IgG or IgM) proceeds by the classical pathway, in the absence of antibody by the alternate pathway. When activated, fragments of complement components are also generated. These fragments also can exert proinflammatory effects, including the minor fragments of C3 and C5 (C3a and C5a), which can trigger mast cell/basophil activation and are hence known as anaphylatoxins (20,21).

A variety of soluble mediators have been identified in recent years that are important for immune system performance (16,17,22). These nonspecific factors (discussed in more detail in Chapter 3) are produced by or act upon immune system elements, and are known as cytokines: lymphokines are factors produced by lymphocytes; interferons are a group of factors (α, β, γ) discovered in supernatants of virally infected cell cultures that interfered with superinfection of these cells; interleukins are mediators that act between leukocytes, are proinflammatory (IL-1, IL-6, IL-8), stimulate lymphocyte growth (IL-2, IL-9), induce immunoglobulin isotype switching (IL-4, IL-13), or provide negative feedback (IL-10).

Immunologic inflammatory response may occur in the airway (rhinitis, asthma), skin (urticaria, atopic dermatitis), gut (ulcerative colitis), joints (rheumatoid arthritis), eye (uveitis), or other sites. Improved understanding of immune mechanisms has great potential relevance for enhancing diagnosis and management of inflammatory disorders. Immune reactions can be approached from the standpoint of four basic mechanisms (14), which are shown in Table 1.

III. IMMEDIATE HYPERSENSITIVITY: IgE AND MAST CELLS

Type I (IgE-mediated) reactions are of greatest relevance for asthma care providers as the pathophysiology that results from IgE-mediated response accounts for clinical syndromes such as asthma, allergic rhinitis, atopic dermatitis, and anaphylactic reactions to foods, drugs, or insect stings (14,16,21,23). The term "immediate" is perhaps unfortunate, as it implies that reaction triggered by IgE-mediation is prompt but fleeting; however, clinical syndromes such as allergic rhinitis and asthma are characterized not only by episodic symptoms from allergen exposures, but also by chronic airway inflammation that waxes and wanes over time but is frequently persistent (24). The clinical features (and therapeutic responses) typically seen in asthma more closely reflect bronchial hyperreactivity, a correlate of ongoing airway inflammation, the pathophysiologic consequence of the late asthmatic response.

A factor was recognized in 1921 by Prausnitz and Kustner that accounted for allergic sensitization, but it was not until 1967 that IgE was identified by Ishizaka and Ishizaka (21). The most important biologic property of IgE is (high affinity) binding to receptors on mast cells and basophils to promote immediate hypersensitivity reactions. Recent evidence demonstrating the dependence of the late asthmatic reaction on presence of IgE (25) has furthered our appreciation of the pivotal role of IgE in the pathophysiology of asthma. Given this understanding, the genetic basis of IgE production and development of asthma has been the subject of ongoing investigation. The pattern of inheritance observed for asthma is consistent with a ''complex genetic disorder'' (26), which is similar to inheritance patterns observed for hypertension, atherosclerosis, diabetes mellitus, and arthritis. Clinical expression of the asthmatic phenotype may reflect a number of predisposing genes combined with exposures to relevant environmental influences (26,27); this suggests that expression of asthmatic potential can be modified by avoidance of exposures to allergens and tobacco smoke early in life (28).

Many studies have shown there is considerable overlap of serum IgE levels among atopic compared with nonatopic, as well as among asthmatic compared with nonasthmatic, individuals (23). Despite its importance for the pathophysiology of allergic and asthmatic response, the measurement of serum IgE, which lacks both specificity and sensitivity, has limited clinical utility. Indications for performing serum IgE quantitation include predicting IgE-mediated disorders among infants, evaluating (suspected) immunodeficient patients, screening for helminthic infestation, and managing patients with allergic bronchopulmonary aspergillosis.

Another essential component of the allergic response is the mast cell. The role of mast cells in airway inflammation has been extensively reviewed (29). Mast cells were first identified in tissues in the 1870s by Paul Ehrlich (30), and are well-suited based on their distribution, structure, biochemical contents, and other properties to serve a sentinel role in the allergic response. Mast cells possess on their surface 10,000–100,000 receptors for the Fc portion of IgE (31). Release of mediators from mast cells occurs when these cells are activated by cross-linking of two adjacent IgE molecules on the cell surface. In addition to IgE binding with antigen, a variety of other factors, including anaphylatoxins (see above), neuropeptides, and physical factors, can activate mast cells and lead to mediator release (21,23,29,31). The mediators released by mast cells can be categorized as those unique to mast cells (tryptase, heparin) and those that are shared with basophils (histamine) or other cells [leukotriene-C_4 (LTC_4)]. Mast cell mediators can also be subdivided into those that are preformed or secretory granule associated and those that are nonpreformed or newly synthesized following activation. Mast cell activation by allergen or other secretory triggers leads to release of the panoply of mediators shown in Figure 1, which have numerous and intertwined effects (discussed in detail in Chapter 3).

The immediate response to allergen results from rapid release of mediators, primarily from the mast cell (Fig. 2A). Preformed (histamine, adenosine, others) and rapidly synthesized mediators (prostaglandins, leukotrienes, platelet activating factor) induce vasodilatation, smooth muscle contraction, glandular secretion, and also exert other proin-

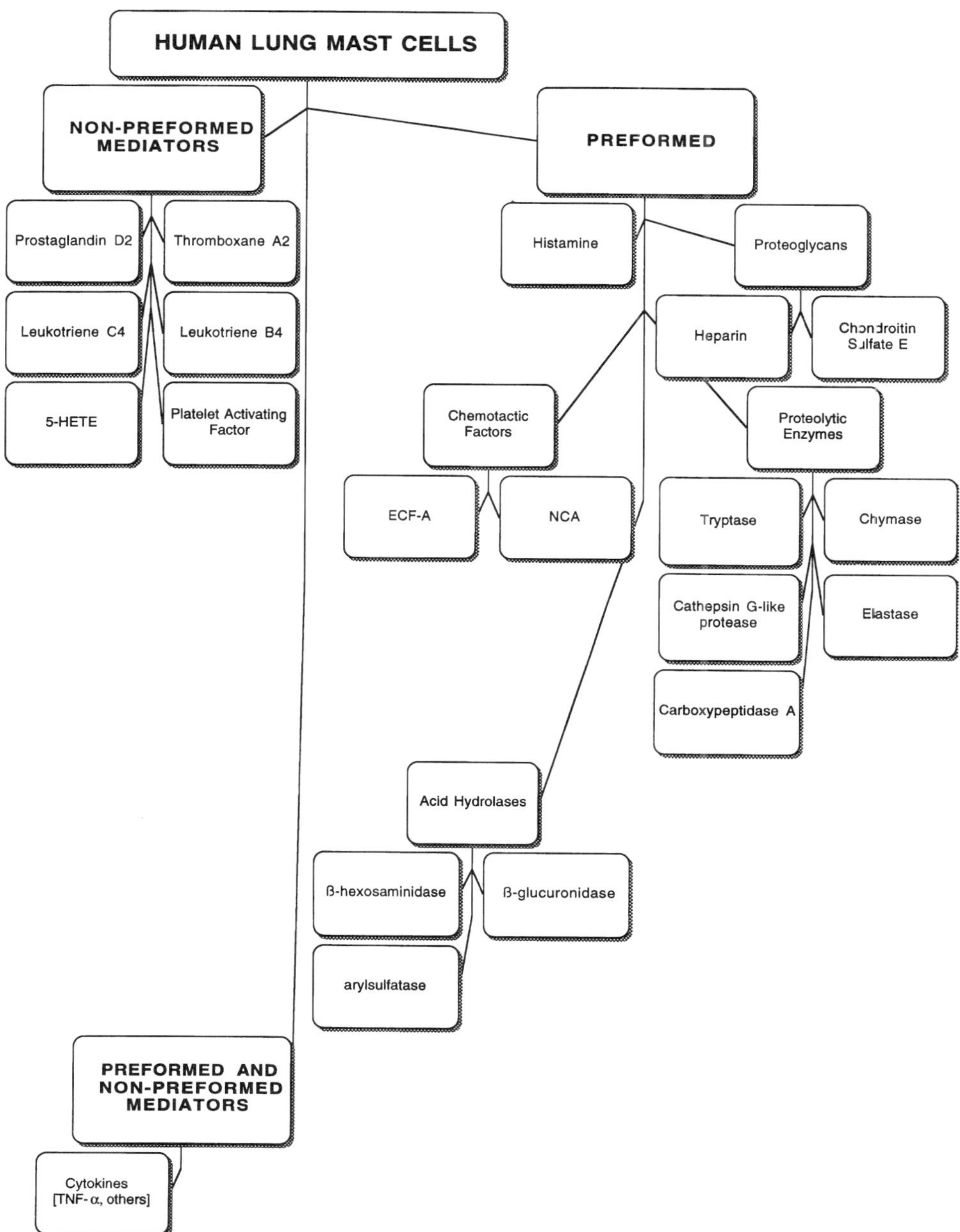

Figure 1 Mediators released from human lung mast cells. (From Ref. 29, with permission of Begell House, Inc.)

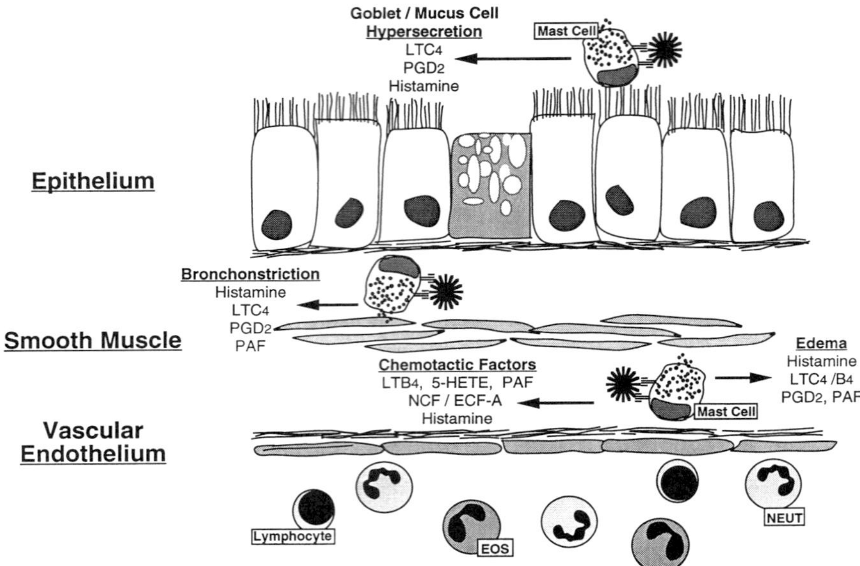

Figure 2 (A) Hypothetical representation of the immediate allergic response in the lung (see text). The lung mast cell is central to the initiation of the immediate response. Preformed and newly synthesized mast cell mediators produce the classic asthma response of bronchospasm, mucus production, and airway edema. (B) Hypothetical representation of the late allergic response in the lung (see text). Antigenic stimulation of mast cells and T cells results in the production of numerous cytokines that induce the expression of endothelial adhesion molecules. This process, combined with the chemotatic factors and chemokines, produces the influx of eosinophils and lymphocytes characteristic of asthma. These inflammatory cells release additional mediators that are bronchospastic, and lead to epithelial damage and bronchial hyperresponsiveness. (From Ref. 59.)

flammatory effects (14,16,17,24,29). Recent studies have expanded our understanding of the IgE-allergen reaction, and have established a view of such reactions as being far more complex than a one-shot stimulus–response event. Although mediators released during the immediate response are rapidly degraded, they also have proinflammatory effects. IgE-mediated reaction also entails a *late response* (24), consisting of cellular infiltration and in the case of asthma a state of bronchial hyperresponsiveness (Fig. 2B). Allergens can also interact with and activate T cells and monocytes, resulting in secretion of cytokines and other factors (16,17,29, 31). Mediators provide signals for recruitment of other inflammatory cells, which are then activated and in turn promote further inflammation. Recent findings indicate that circulating leukocytes respond to *adhesion molecules* (ICAM, selectins, and VCAM-1) expressed on vascular endothelium, which allow leukocyte adherence and migration to occur (32). Influx of eosinophils, neutrophils, and monocytes leads to an environment in which each population of cells contributes yet further to inflammation by release of more mediators and toxic substances.

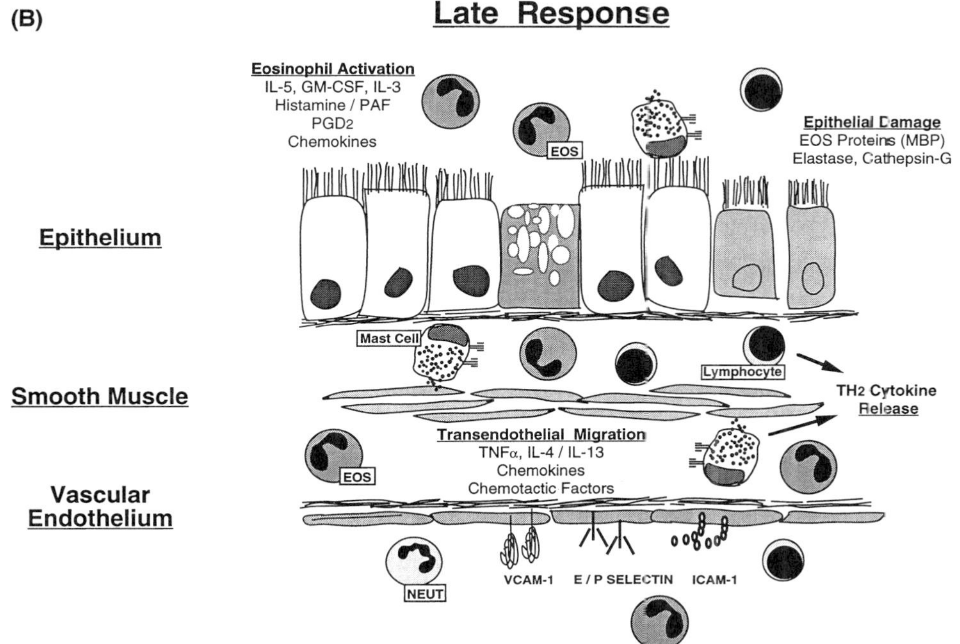

IV. EOSINOPHILS AND T CELLS

With the realization that airway inflammation underlies chronic asthma, intense investigation into its mechanisms has increased our understanding of this process. Much of this research effort has been directed at explaining the selective influx of eosinophils and lymphocytes seen in the lungs of asthmatics (33). The eosinophil was once thought to dampen the inflammatory response in allergic diseases, however it is now thought that eosinophil products directly contribute to pathogenesis (34,35).

Even though eosinophils are often thought of as circulating blood cells, it has been estimated that for every circulating eosinophil there are 100–300 eosinophils in the tissues. They have a tissue distribution similar to that of mast cells, being located below the epithelium in the lung, gut, and skin. Eosinophils develop into a fully differentiated granulocyte from precursor cells in the bone marrow. T-cell–derived hematopoetic growth factors such as interleukin-3 (IL-3) and granulocyte–macrophage colony stimulating factor (GM-CSF) contribute to the growth and differentiation of eosinophils (36). A key cytokine in this process appears to be interleukin-5 (IL-5), which supports the selective differentiation of progenitor cells to mature eosinophils, and also recruits eosinophils to the tissues. IL-5 has become an important target for pharmacologic intervention in eosinophil-associated diseases.

Eosinophils contain characteristic yellow-pink granules when stained with acidic aniline dyes (eosin or chromotrope-2R). The eosinophil specific (secondary) granules contain major basic protein (MBP), the predominant granule protein of eosinophils. MBP and the other unique eosinophil cationic granule proteins (eosinophil cationic protein, eosinophil derived neurotoxin) have been shown to have toxic effects on invading helminths and on normal lung cells (34,37). When airway epithelial cells are exposed to MBP, ciliary function is inhibited, and at higher MBP concentrations equivalent to those commonly found in sputum of asthmatics, epithelial damage occurs. MBP administration to primates results in airway hyperresponsiveness (38). An interesting finding is that MBP binds to inhibitory muscarinic M2 receptors on airway nerve endings (39). These M2 receptors function to decrease acetylcholine release from muscarinic nerves in the lung. By blocking the M2 receptors, MBP may enhance vagally mediated bronchoconstriction. Another eosinophil granule protein, eosinophil peroxidase (EPO) catalyses the conversion of H_2O_2 to the tissue toxic hypochlorous acid (HOCl). Eosinophil granules contain numerous other enzymes that may also contribute to airway damage in asthma.

How eosinophils (but not neutrophils) are selectively recruited to the lungs of asthmatics has been a mystery for many years. Understanding this process of eosinophil recruitment is essential since it has been shown that the late phase asthmatic response in humans occurs only in those patients who develop airway eosinophilia (40). Early research efforts focused on identification of factors that stimulated selective eosinophil chemotaxis. Eosinophil chemotactic factor of anaphylaxis (ECF-A) (41) and histamine proved to be very weak eosinophil chemotactic factors. Other mediators that can induce eosinophil chemotaxis includes newly synthesized lipid mediators (PAF, LTB_4), complement proteins (C3a, C5a), and numerous cytokines. These cytokines can act not only as chemotactic factors, but also as modulators of eosinophil recruitment through the vascular endothelium.

Significant advances have been made in our understanding of the mechanisms involved in recruitment of eosinophils through the vascular endothelium (42,43). Eosinophils express adhesion molecules common to many leukocytes, including LFA-1 (CD11a/CD18), MAC-1/CR3 (CD11b/CD18), and p150,95 (CD11c/CD18). These eosinophil surface receptors mediate adhesion through counter receptors on the endothelium, such as ICAM-1, E-selectin, and P-selectin. Eosinophils also express VLA-4 (CD49d/CD29), which binds to VCAM-1 on activated endothelium. Since neutrophils do not express VLA-4, this VLA-4/VCAM-1 pairing appears to be one mechanism mediating selective eosinophil recruitment into tissues. Evidence for this comes from animal models that have shown that antibodies to VLA-4 block antigen-induced airway eosinophilia, and also the associated antigen-induced bronchial hyperreactivity. Expression of adhesion molecules on endothelial cells occurs in response to cytokines such as IL-1 and TNF. It is interesting to note that VCAM-1 is expressed on vascular endothelium in response to the TH2 cytokines IL-4 and IL-13, which would lead to selective eosinophil recruitment.

A new class of cytokines, called chemokines, have taken center stage in many areas of immunology (44,45). Chemokines have potent chemotactic and stimulatory activity for inflammatory cells. The C-C class of chemokines have more activity toward eosinophils than the C-X-C chemokines, and include RANTES, MIP-1a, MCP-3, and LCF (IL-16). These chemokines are not eosinophil selective, but also attract basophils and lymphocytes. Eotaxin is a recently discovered chemokine that appears to selectively recruit only eosinophils (46,47), making it a promising target for pharmacological intervention in asthma. What remains unknown is how these various chemotactic agents and cytokines interact to produce eosinophil recruitment in vivo.

Once eosinophils are recruited to the lungs, they can be activated to release their granule proteins, and can also release other mediators that participate in the asthmatic response. Mast cells are an important source of IL-5 (48) and mast cell mediators activate eosinophils (49). Eosinophils are a rich source of leukotriene-C_4 (LTC_4), which is a potent bronchoconstrictor (50,51). Eosinophils also release PAF and synthesize their own cytokines. In addition, eosinophils produce superoxide and hydrogen peroxide, in larger quantities than neutrophils under in vitro conditions. All of these mediators are thought to contribute to the pathogenesis of the asthmatic response.

With the realization that eosinophils can potentially cause significant airway damage have come studies of pharmacological regulation of eosinophil recruitment and activation. It has been observed for years that the administration of glucocorticosteroids to patients with eosinophilia results in a rapid fall in circulating eosinophil numbers. The mechanisms underlying this decrease are thought to occur at several levels (52–54). Steroids inhibit mononuclear cell synthesis of IL-5 and other cytokines that are growth factors for eosinophil development. Glucocorticoids suppress production of cytokines responsible for increasing endothelial adhesion molecules such as VCAM-1, and recently it has been shown that glucocorticoids induce eosinophils to undergo apoptosis (55). Eosinophils express surface β_2-adrenergic receptors, that, when activated, result in an increase in cAMP levels (56). Agents that increase cAMP, such as theophylline, inhibit eosinophil degranulation.

The other inflammatory cell type implicated in the pathogenesis of chronic asthma is the T-lymphocyte. Studies of asthmatics using bronchoscopy and bronchoalveolar lavage (BAL) have shown that there are increased numbers of activated CD25+, CD4+ lymphocytes in asthmatics [reviewed in (57)]. These lymphocytes secrete cytokines characteristic of the TH2 subset of CD4+ T cells, such as IL-5 and IL-4. It has also been shown that corticosteroids decrease these CD4+ cells in asthmatics, suggesting this is one of the mechanisms of steroid action in asthma. Efforts are underway to determine why there is a preferential increase in these cells in asthmatics and how this process is initiated.

V. CONCLUSION

Allergen interaction with the immune system generates a complicated reaction cascade in the asthmatic patient that can promote and perpetuate chronic airway inflammation—the hallmark of asthma. Advances in our understanding of the intricate interrelationships between components of the immune system, of factors that allow communication to occur between cells, and identification of the soluble mediators that amplify inflammation provide greater opportunity to intervene with pharmacotherapeutic agents that can have "anti-inflammatory" effects. Agents that inhibit mediator release and mediator effects, or block expression of adhesion molecules may each have salutary effects upon asthma. Of the agents currently in use for these conditions, corticosteroids have been shown to have the most clinically significant impact on the late asthmatic reaction and on bronchial hyperreactivity. Based on the importance of immunology and the inflammatory response for asthmatic exacerbation, use of anti-inflammatory agents is appropriate and essential in management of asthma in the emergency department (58).

REFERENCES

1. Kemp JP, Approaches to asthma management. Realities and recommendations, Arch Intern Med 1993; 153:805–812.
2. Lang DM, Sherman MS, Polansky M, Guidelines and realities of asthma management—The Philadelphia story, Arch Intern Med 1997; 157:1193–1200.
3. Gibson PG, Wong BJ, Hepperle MJ, Kline PA, Girgis-Gabardo A, Guyatt G, Dolovich J,

Denburg JA, Ramsdale EH, Hargreave FE, A research method to induce and examine a mild exacerbation of asthma by withdrawal of inhaled corticosteroid, Clin Exp Allergy 1992; 22: 525–532.

4. Waalkens HJ, Van Essen-Zandvliet EE, Hughes MD, Gerritsen J, Duiverman EJ, Knol K, and Kerrebijn KF, Cessation of long-term treatment with inhaled corticosteroid (budesonide) in children with asthma results in deterioration. The Dutch CNSLD Study Group, Am Rev Respir Dis 1993; 148:1252–1257.
5. United States Department of Health and Human Services, Guidelines for the diagnosis and management of asthma, Washington, DC, 1991.
6. Global initiative for asthma. Global strategy for asthma management and prevention NHLBI/ WHO Workshop Report, Washington, DC, 1995.
7. Juniper EF, Kline PA, Vanzieleghem MA, Ramsdale EH, O'Byrne PM, Hargreave FE, Effect of long-term treatment with an inhaled corticosteroid (budesonide) on airway hyperresponsiveness and clinical asthma in nonsteroid-dependent asthmatics, Am Rev Respir Dis 1990; 142: 832–836.
8. Haahtela T, Jarvinen M, Kava T, et al., Comparison of a beta 2-agonist, terbutaline, with an inhaled corticosteroid, budesonide, in newly detected asthma, N Engl J Med 1991; 325:388–392.
9. Dompeling E, van Schayck CP, van Grunsven PM, van Herwaarden CL, Akkermans R, Molema J, Folgering H, van Weel C, Slowing the deterioration of asthma and chronic obstructive pulmonary disease observed during bronchodilator therapy by adding inhaled corticosteroids: A 4-year prospective study, Ann Intern Med 1993; 118:770–778.
10. Brown PJ, Greville HW and Finucane KE, Asthma and irreversible airflow obstruction, Thorax 1984; 39:131–136.
11. Ernst P, Spitzer WO, Suissa S, Cockcroft D, Habbick B, Horwitz RI, Boivin JF, McNutt M, Buist AS, Risk of fatal and near-fatal asthma in relation to inhaled corticosteroid use, JAMA 1992; 268:3462–3464.
12. Rutten-Van Molken MPMH, Van Doorslaer EKA, Jansen MCC, Van Essen-Zandvliet EE, Rutten FFH, Cost effectiveness of inhaled corticosteroid plus bronchodilator therapy versus bronchodilator monotherapy in children with asthma, Pharmacoeconomics 1993; 4:257–270.
13. Nimmigadda SR, Spahn JD, Leung DYM and Szefler SJ, Steroid-resistant asthma: evaluation and management, Ann Allergy Asthma Immunol 1996; 77:345–356.
14. Shearer WT and Huston DP, The immune system: An overview, In: Middleton EJ, Reed CE, Ellis EF, Adkinson NF, Yunginger JW, Busse WW, eds., Allergy, Principles and Practice, St. Louis: CV Mosby Co., 1993, p. 3.
15. Osmond DG, The ontogeny and organization of the lymphoid system, J Invest Derm 1985; 85:2s–9s.
16. Claman HN, The biology of the immune response, JAMA 1992; 268:2790–2796.
17. Arai KI, Lee F, Miyajima A, Miyatake S, Arai N, Yokota T, Cytokines: coordinators of immune and inflammatory responses, Ann Rev Biochem 1990; 59:783–836.
18. Reinherz EL, Schlossman SF, Current concepts in immunology: Regulation of the immune response–inducer and suppressor T-lymphocyte subsets in human beings, N Engl J Med 1980; 303:370–373.
19. Heiner DC, Significance of immunoglobulin G subclasses, Am J Med 1984; 76:1–6.
20. Fearon DT, Austen KF, Current concepts in immunology: the alternative pathway of complement–a system for host resistance to microbial infection, N Engl J Med 1980; 303:259–263.
21. Ishizaka T, Mechanisms of IgE-mediated hypersensitivity, In: Middleton EJ, Reed CA, Ellis EF, Adkinson NF, Yunginger JW, eds., Allergy: Principles and Practice, St. Louis: CV Mosby Co., 1988, p. 71.
22. Dinarello CA, Mier JW, Lymphokines, N Engl J Med 1987; 317:940–945.
23. Geha RS, Human IgE, J Allergy Clin Immunol 1984; 74:109–120.

24. Lemanske R Jr, Kaliner M, Late-phase IgE-mediated reactions, J Clin Immunol 1988; 8:1–13.
25. Kirby JG, Robertson DG, Hargreave FE, Dolovich J, Asthmatic responses to inhalation of anti-human IgE, Clin Allergy 1986; 16:191–194.
26. Sandford A, Weir T, Pare P, The genetics of asthma, Am J Respir Crit Care Med 1996; 153: 1749–1765.
27. Sporik R, Holgate ST, Platts-Mills TA, Cogswell JJ, Exposure to house-dust mite allergen (Der p I) and the development of asthma in childhood: A prospective study, N Engl J Med 1990; 323:502–507.
28. Arshad SH, Matthews S, Gant C, Hide DW, Effect of allergen avoidance on development of allergic disorders in infancy, Lancet 1992; 339:1493–1497.
29. Schulman ES, The role of mast cells in inflammatory responses in the lung, Crit Rev Immunol 1993; 13:35–70.
30. Erhlich P, Ueber die specifischen Granulationen des Blutes, Archiv fur Physiologie Physiologische Abtheilung des Archives fur Anatomie und Phsiologie 1879; 571–579.
31. Wasserman SI, Mast cell-mediated inflammation in asthma, Ann Allergy 1989; 636 (Pt 2): 546–550.
32. Springer TA, Adhesion receptors of the immune system, Nature 1990; 346:425–434.
33. Corrigan CJ, Kay AB, T cells and eosinophils in the pathogenesis of asthma, Immunology Today 1992; 13:501–507.
34. Gleich GJ, Adolphson, CR and Leiferman KM, The biology of the eosinophilic leukocyte, Ann Rev Med 1993; 44:85–101.
35. Leff AR, Hamann KJ, Wegner CD, Inflammation and cell-cell interactions in airway hyperresponsiveness, Am J Physiol 1991; 260:L189–L206.
36. Denburg JA, Woolley M, Leber B, Linden M, O'Byrne P, Basophil and eosinophil differentiation in allergic reactions, J Allergy Clin Immunol 1994; 946 (Pt 2):1135–1141.
37. Weller PF, The immunobiology of eosinophils, N Engl J Med 1991; 324:1110–1118.
38. Gundel RH, Letts LG, Gleich GJ, Human eosinophil major basic protein induces airway constriction and airway hyperresponsiveness in primates, J Clin Invest 1991; 87:1470—1473.
39. Jacoby DB, Gleich GJ, Fryer AD, Human eosinophil major basic protein is an endogenous allosteric antagonist at the inhibitory muscarinic M2 receptor, J Clin Invest 1993; 91:1314–1318.
40. De Monchy JG, Kauffman HF, Venge P, Koeter GH, Jansen HM, Sluiter HJ, De Vries K, Bronchoalveolar eosinophilia during allergen-induced late asthmatic reactions, Am Rev Respir Dis 1985; 131:373–376.
41. Wasserman SI, Goetzl EJ, Austen KF, Preformed eosinophil chemotactic factor of anaphylaxis (ECF-A), J Immunol 1974; 112:351–358.
42. Bochner BS, Schleimer RP, The role of adhesion molecules in human eosinophil and basophil recruitment, J Allergy Clin Immunol 1994; 943 (Pt 1):427–438.
43. Resnick MB, Weller PF, Mechanisms of eosinophil recruitment, Am J Respir Cell Molec Biol 1993; 8:349–355.
44. Taub DD, Oppenheim JJ, Chemokines, inflammation and the immune system, Therapeutic Immunology 1994; 1:229–246.
45. Lukacs NW, Strieter RM, Chensue SW, Kunkel SL, Activation and regulation of chemokines in allergic airway inflammation, J Leuk Biol 1996; 59:13–17.
46. Ponath PD, Qin S, Ringler DJ, Clark-Lewis I, Wang J, Kassam N, Smith H, Shi X, Gonzolo JA, Newman W, Gutierrez-Ramos JC, Mackay CR, Cloning of the human eosinophil chemoattractant, eotaxin: Expression, receptor binding and functional properties provide a mechanism for the selective recruitment of eosinophils, J Clin Invest 1996; 97:604–612.
47. Collins PD, Marleau S, Griffiths-Johnson DA, Jose PJ, Williams TJ, Cooperation between interleukin-5 and the chemokine eotaxin to induce eosinophil accumulation in vivo, J Exp Med 1995; 182:1169–1174.

48. Jaffe JS, Glaum MC, Raible DG, Post TJ, Dimitry E, Govindarao D, Wang Y, Schulman ES, Human lung mast cell IL-5 gene and protein expression: temporal analysis of upregulation following IgE-mediated activation, Am J Respir Cell Molec Biol 1995; 13:665–675.
49. Raible DG, Schulman ES, DiMuzio J, Cardillo R, Post TJ, Mast cell mediators prostaglandin-D_2 and histamine activate human eosinophils, J Immunol 1992; 148:3536–3542.
50. Henderson WR, Harley JB, Fauci AS, Arachidonic acid metabolism in normal and hypereosinophilic syndrome human eosinophils: generation of leukotrienes B4, C4, D4 and 15-lipoxygenase products, Immunology 1984; 51:679–686.
51. Weller PF, Lee CW, Foster DW, Corey EJ, Austen KF, Lewis RA, Generation and metabolism of 5-lipoxygenase pathway leukotrienes by human eosinophils: predominant production of leukotriene C4, Proc Natl Acad Sci USA 1983; 80:7626–7630.
52. Schleimer RP, Bochner BS, The effects of glucocorticoids on human eosinophils, J Allergy Clin Immunol 1994; 94:1202–1213.
53. Schleimer RP, An overview of glucocorticoid anti-inflammatory actions, Eur J Clin Pharm 1993; 45:S43–44
54. Schwiebert LA, Beck LA, Stellato C, Bickel CA, Bochner BS, Schleimer RP, Glucocorticosteroid inhibition of cytokine production: relevance to antiallergic actions, J Allergy Clin Immunol 1996; 971(Pt 2):143–152.
55. Stern M, Meagher L, Savill J, Haslett C, Apoptosis in human eosinophils Programmed cell death in the eosinophil leads to phagocytosis by macrophages and is modulated by IL-5, J Immunol 1992; 148:3543–3549.
56. Yukawa T, Ukena D, Kroegel C, Chanez P, Dent G, Chung KF, Barnes PJ, Beta 2-adrenergic receptors on eosinophils: Binding and functional studies, Am Rev Respir Dis 1990; 141:1446–1452.
57. Busse WW, Coffman RL, Gelfand EW, Kay AB, Rosenwasser LJ, Mechanisms of persistent airway inflammation in asthma: A role for T cells and T-cell products, Am J Respir Crit Care Med 1995; 152:388–393.
58. Cockroft DW, Management of acute severe asthma, Ann Allergy 1995; 75:83–89.
59. Schulman ES, Raible DG, Mast cells and eosinophils. In: Fishman AP, ed., Pulmonary Diseases and Disorders, New York: McGraw Hill, 1998.

5

Epidemiology of Asthma

Carlos A. Camargo Jr.
Massachusetts General Hospital and Harvard Medical School, Boston, Massachusetts

Lynne D. Richardson
Mount Sinai School of Medicine, New York, New York

I. INTRODUCTION

Asthma is a common disorder that accounts for 1.5 to 2 million emergency department (ED) visits in the United States each year (1,2). Over the past two decades, epidemiologists have made many important contributions to our understanding of this disorder. Most notably, they have documented a dramatic rise in asthma morbidity and mortality worldwide (3). The cause of this epidemic has become a focus of investigation. Likewise, epidemiologists are working to define genetic (4) and environmental (5) determinants or "risk factors" in the hope that timely interventions might prevent individuals from developing asthma. In this chapter, we highlight some of the major methodologic issues in asthma epidemiology, and summarize the influence of age, sex, race/ethnicity, and socioeconomic status on the distribution of asthma.

II. DEFINITION OF ASTHMA

Over the past 175 years, there has been remarkable consistency among medical writers on the major diagnostic criteria for asthma: episodic dyspnea generally associated with wheezing (6). Nonetheless, patients with asthma can exhibit tremendous heterogeneity in clinical features and severity of disease. Asthma can range from being an intermittent nuisance triggered by specific factors such as allergen exposure or exercise, to being a severe, progressive, and occasionally fatal disease without apparent external cause. Some patients may present with chronic cough as their sole manifestation of asthma (7). This clinical diversity has led to a growing appreciation that asthma, as currently defined, probably is not a specific disease, but rather a syndrome that derives from multiple precipitants leading to a common clinical presentation involving reversible airway obstruction. Thus, despite many formal attempts (8), a universally accepted definition of ''asthma'' is not available.

The most widely used definition was proposed by the American Thoracic Society (ATS) in 1987 (9). The ATS task group described a heterogeneous disorder characterized by: (1) airway obstruction (or airway narrowing) that is reversible (but not completely so in some patients) either spontaneously or with treatment; (2) airway inflammation; and (3) airway hyperresponsiveness to a variety of stimuli. All of these features need not be present to assign the diagnosis of asthma. Although the ATS criteria correctly characterize the pathophysiology of asthma, they are of remarkably little help in the acute setting since most of these features are not readily apparent to the clinician. Furthermore, in acute asthma, the absence of a clinically significant response to bronchodilator does not rule out asthma.

The National Asthma Education and Prevention Program (NAEPP) recently provided a more clinically useful approach to the diagnosis of asthma (10). The expert panel identified five ''key indicators'' for considering a diagnosis of asthma: (1) wheezing, especially in children; (2) history of cough (especially nocturnal), recurrent wheeze, recurrent dyspnea, or recurrent chest tightness; (3) reversible airflow limitation and diurnal variation as measured by using a peak flow meter; (4) symptoms occur or worsen in the presence of exercise, viral infection, animals with fur or feathers, house-dust mites, mold, smoke, pollen, changes in weather, strong emotional expression, airborne chemicals or dusts, or menses; and (5) symptoms occur or worsen at night, awakening the patient. These five key indicators are not diagnostic by themselves, but the presence of multiple indicators increases the probability of asthma. To establish a diagnosis of asthma, the expert panel requires formal spirometric testing (e.g., FEV_1 before and after the patient inhales a short-acting bronchodilator); the expert panel further advises that additional studies (e.g., bronchoprovocation with methacholine) should not be routine but may be useful when asthma is suspected and spirometry is normal or near normal. Thus, most outpatient clinicians (including emergency physicians) are unable to make an immediate and definite diagnosis of asthma by NAEPP criteria, but they may recognize a sufficient number of key indicators to make the diagnosis very likely.

Identification of *acute* asthma in an ED patient with a history of physician-diagnosed asthma usually is obvious to both the patient and emergency physician. Anecdotally, however, many ED ''asthma'' visits are made by patients without such a history. Once major competing diagnoses have been excluded, emergency physicians tend to label patients with dyspnea and wheezing as asthmatic, particularly when the patient is young and does not smoke. Thus, a ''soft'' ED diagnosis of asthma may later present to the ED as an exacerbation of ''known'' asthma; the magnitude (and importance) of this phenomenon is not known and merits study. Among middle-aged and elderly patients, the most important alternative diagnosis is exacerbation of chronic obstructive pulmonary disease (COPD). Emergency physicians should try to distinguish asthma from COPD since many acute interventions, such as systemic steroids and anticholinergic agents, appear to be more (or less) effective among asthmatics than patients with COPD (11,12). Clinical features that favor asthma rather than COPD include: younger age at onset of respiratory symptoms and at current ED presentation, nonsmoking status, and history of atopy. The optimal combination of factors and cut points is not known and is currently under investigation. Inevitably, however, the asthma vs. COPD dichotomy will fail in individuals who have lifelong, physician-diagnosed asthma but also smoke in quantities sufficient to develop COPD. Furthermore, some lifelong asthmatics have been shown to develop an irreversible component to their airway obstruction (13). For both scenarios, a combined diagnosis of ''asthma/COPD'' seems most appropriate.

The classification system used in the *International Classification of Diseases,* 9th revision (ICD-9), which took effect in 1979, sheds additional light on the term ''asthma'' (14). As shown in Table 1, asthma is distinct from tracheobronchitis, chronic bronchitis, emphysema, bronchiectasis, extrinsic allergic alveolitis, and chronic airway obstruction ''not elsewhere classified.'' Chronic obstructive asthma (with obstructive pulmonary disease) is considered a type of asthma (code 493.2). Unlike earlier classification systems, such as ICD-8, ''asthmatic bronchitis'' also is classified as asthma (code 493.9). The ICD-9 classification system keeps with tradition, however, by dividing uncomplicated asthma into either extrinsic or intrinsic types. According to this nosology (15), patients with extrinsic asthma tend to have childhood onset, atopy, and a family history of atopic disorders (including asthma), and they often have a predictable seasonal variation of their asthma. By contrast, intrinsic asthma usually begins in adulthood, is not associated with allergens, and exhibits little seasonal variation. Recent studies, however, have found that despite showing some distinct clinical features, most asthmatics have an atopic component (16) and bronchial biopsies reveal common immunopathologic mechanisms between ex-

Table 1 Overview of ICD-9 Classification of Asthma and Related Conditions

ICD-9		Disease
490		Bronchitis, not specified as acute or chronic (e.g., tracheobronchitis NOS): *excludes* allergic bronchitis NOS (493.9), asthmatic bronchitis NOS (493.9), bronchitis due to fumes and vapors (506.0)
491		Chronic bronchitis: *excludes* chronic obstructive asthma (493.2)
492		Emphysema
493		Asthma[a]
	493.0	Estrinsic asthma (e.g., allergic asthma with stated cause, atopic asthma, childhood asthma): *excludes* allergic asthma NOS (493.9), wood asthma (495.8)
	493.1	Intrinsic asthma (e.g., late-onset asthma)
	493.2	Chronic obstructive asthma (with obstructive pulmonary disease): *excludes* chronic asthmatic bronchitis (491.2), chronic obstructive bronchitis (491.2)
	493.9	Asthma, unspecified (e.g., allergic asthma NOS, allergic bronchitis, asthmatic bronchitis)
494		Bronchiectasis
495		Extrinsic allergic alveolitis (includes allergic alveolitis and pneumonitis due to inhaled organic dust particles of fungal, thermophilic actinomycete, or other origin)
496		Chronic airway obstruction, not elsewhere classified [e.g., chronic nonspecific lung disease, chronic obstructive lung disease, chronic obstructive pulmonary disease (COPD) NOS]

[a] A fifth-digit subclassification is used for category 493 to designate "without mention" (0) or presence (1) of status asthmaticus. "Without mention" does not always indicate absence of status asthmaticus since it may simply reflect the incompleteness of the clinical data used for coding.

Source: Modified from Ref. 14. ICD-9 denotes International Classification of Diseases, 9th revision; NOS, not otherwise specified.

trinsic and intrinsic asthmatics (17). These studies, and others like them, have cast doubts on the extrinsic vs. intrinsic classification. Furthermore, the distinction has not proven particularly useful to the clinical management of most asthmatic patients, especially adults. By contrast, the development of specific antagonists to the biochemical mediators of asthma (e.g., leukotrienes, cytokines) is refining current concepts about asthma and may lead to a more useful classification system based on clinical response to these specific interventions.

III. ASTHMA ASCERTAINMENT IN EPIDEMIOLOGICAL RESEARCH

Epidemiologists have used many approaches to ascertain ''asthma'' status: self-report questionnaires, clinical examination and physiologic measurements (e.g., spirometry, bronchoprovocation studies), and data from health information systems (e.g., vital statistics). Depending on the chosen definition of asthma, each approach may underestimate or overestimate the prevalence of the disorder. The advantages and disadvantages of each approach merit further consideration before proceeding to the literature review.

Most studies have relied on self-report questionnaires to identify individuals with ''asthma,'' and questions typically focus on respiratory symptoms or on prior physician-diagnosis of asthma. Interindividual, let alone intercultural, differences in symptom recall and interpretation complicate case identification. As a result, symptom questions (e.g., ''Have you ever wheezed?'') are generally less reliable than questions on prior asthma diagnosis. Two recent international studies have made great efforts to standardize questions and have made considerable progress in this regard (18,19). Further improvement in the reliability of symptom questions may be achieved by video questionnaire involving the audiovisual presentation of clinical asthma (20) but further research is warranted.

In addition to potential problems with reliability, self-reported ''asthma'' symptoms can be due to medical disorders besides asthma. Prior physician-diagnosis of asthma is preferred by most researchers because it relies on medical certification and because it is assumed that few people who do not have asthma will claim to have the condition. Diagnosis questions, however, make case identification highly dependent on the frequency of health care contacts and the diagnostic patterns of the individual providers. For example, physicians may tend to diagnose young, atopic, nonsmokers as having asthma while labeling older, nonatopic, smokers with identical symptoms as having COPD. Diagnosis questions are particularly misleading when health services are being evaluated since this approach will overestimate the proportion of asthmatics under treatment; mild cases are less likely to be counted in less vigilant health care settings. The latter phenomenon may result in mistaken associations with asthma prevalence for factors that actually are related to asthma severity.

More objective measures of airway function, such as clinical examination and physiological testing, are increasingly used in epidemiological studies. Auscultation for wheezing is the most useful physical sign of airway obstruction (21) but tends to miss mild intermittent cases; wheezing also is a fairly nonspecific finding that can be caused by a variety of cardiopulmonary and psychiatric conditions. Sole reliance on physiologic measurements suffers from similar problems. Moreover, different methods of assessing hyperresponsiveness give different results when applied to the same individuals (22) and standardization of challenge tests continues to be a problem. Lastly, common methods of bronchoprovocation (e.g., histamine challenge) give abnormal results in asymptomatic subjects that would not be conventionally regarded as having asthma (23). Clearly, there is no ''gold standard'' when it comes to asthma diagnosis in epidemiologic research.

Large health information systems (e.g., vital statistics, billing data) are another source of epidemiological data on asthma, particularly asthma mortality and lesser exacerbations that lead to health service utilization (i.e., clinic visits, ED visits, and hospitalizations). The particular strengths and weaknesses of using these pre-existing datasets are discussed in Section VI. In general, however, their greatest strengths are their large sample sizes and ready availability for statistical analysis; their greatest potential weakness is inaccurate or incomplete data (24). Although the diagnosis of asthma may be fairly obvious in younger patients, recognition of asthma in older patients is complicated by their much broader list of competing diagnoses, particularly COPD. Thus, older patients with so-called asthma may actually suffer from another condition, and older patients with true asthma may get diagnosed incorrectly as having another disorder. One recourse is to perform medical record review for all patients suspected of having asthma (25). An easier approach is to limit analyses to younger patients (e.g., age 5–34 years), but this precludes study of excluded groups. In both approaches, without the ability to question individual patients or to perform clinical examination or physiologic measurements, the investigator must somewhat blindly accept that previously collected data are correct.

In summary, the best approach to asthma ascertainment is, not surprisingly, quite similar to that recommended for clinical practice—that is, to question individual subjects about asthma symptoms or prior physician-diagnosis and then to perform physiologic measurements to ''confirm'' asthma status. Although this approach might miss some patients with mild intermittent asthma, it most effectively defines patients with clinically important asthma. Unfortunately, serial measurement of peak expiratory flow rate (PEFR) over 1–2 weeks (to demonstrate PEFR variability) requires a level of cooperation that may be difficult to achieve. Furthermore, formal spirometry and bronchoprovocation are not practical for most large-scale population studies. As a result, there currently are no studies that have used physiologic evidence to confirm asthma prevalence in a large, nationally representative U.S. population.

IV. INCIDENCE AND NATURAL HISTORY OF ASTHMA

Characterizing the epidemiology of asthma also requires an understanding of its *incidence* (i.e., the number of individuals who develop asthma in a defined population within a specified period of time) and its natural history. Unfortunately, there are few cohort studies that have examined these issues. The two best known studies come from Tecumseh, Michigan (26) and Tucson, Arizona (27). These relatively small prospective cohort studies enrolled individuals of all ages and followed them for approximately 4 years to determine asthma incidence. More recent estimates are available from the First National Health and Nutrition Survey (NHANES) Epidemiologic Follow-up Survey (28) and a 20-year retrospective cohort study from Rochester, Minnesota (29). Taken together, the cumulative incidence of asthma is approximately 0.2–0.4% annually, with approximately half of incident cases occurring before age 10. The generalizability of these results to nonwhites and inner city populations is uncertain.

Once an individual has developed asthma, the natural history of his/her disease is highly variable. In addition to having a broad spectrum of disease severity, asthma can be anything from a temporary affliction to a lifelong disorder. In general, however, childhood asthma is frequently self-limited and has a better prognosis than adult-onset asthma. Studies vary but somewhere between 30 and 70% of asthmatic children will be markedly improved or become symptom-free by early adulthood, whereas approximately 30% will have persistent, clinically significant asthma (30). Childhood asthmatics whose symptoms continue beyond the second decade show a low rate of remission (31). The severity of asthma in childhood correlates with the persistence of asthma into adulthood and with the severity of adult asthma (32,33).

Asthma in adulthood may be due to persistence (or re-emergence) of childhood asthma, but also may represent new-onset asthma; there are sparse data on the relative frequency of each type. Occupational asthma accounts for less than 15% of all newly diagnosed cases of adult asthma (34,35). As previously noted, the natural history of adult-onset asthma is characterized by a lower remission rate than childhood asthma. Nonetheless, a recent study found that approximately 40% of young adults with asthma were symptom-free after a 25-year follow-up (36); 11% of the cohort no longer was considered asthmatic at retesting. Furthermore, studies of patients with occupational asthma show that duration of symptoms before removal from exposure predicts long-term consequences irrespective of the causative agent; early removal from exposure increases the likelihood of asthma remission (34). For most adult asthmatics, however, asthma represents a lifelong disease. Compared to children with asthma, individuals with asthma starting after age 50 may have more severe disease, including less reversibility of bronchial obstruction (37). Adult asthma usually is not progressive but chronic asthma can cause irreversible airway obstruction in some patients (13); subbasement membrane fibrosis may underlie this subgroup's persistent abnormalities in pulmonary function (38).

V. ASTHMA PREVALENCE IN THE UNITED STATES

There are literally hundreds of reports in the literature on the distribution of asthma in various populations. The lack of a standard definition of asthma, and the variety of approaches to asthma ascertainment, make reliable estimates and comparisons between studies quite difficult. The most common summary measures provided by these epidemiologic studies is asthma *prevalence*, or the percentage of a defined population with asthma. More precise concepts, such as cumulative or lifetime prevalence (i.e., the total percentage of those who have ever had asthma) and point prevalence (i.e., the percentage with recently active asthma at a specific time) are not specified by many investigators and this ambiguity may explain some "inconsistencies" in the literature.

Despite these daunting methodologic challenges, one can make a gross estimate of asthma prevalence in the United States using data from several large epidemiologic surveys, including the National Health Interview Survey (NHIS) (39) and the NHANES (40,41). Studies of marginalized populations (e.g., inner city children) provide important supplementary data as they suggest that national surveys substantially underestimate asthma prevalence for these populations (42). Taken together, the overall lifetime prevalence in the United States is approximately 8–10%, while the overall point prevalence of asthma is approximately 4–8%. The latter estimate translates into approximately 10–20 million clinically active patients in the United States. Approximately 5 million of these

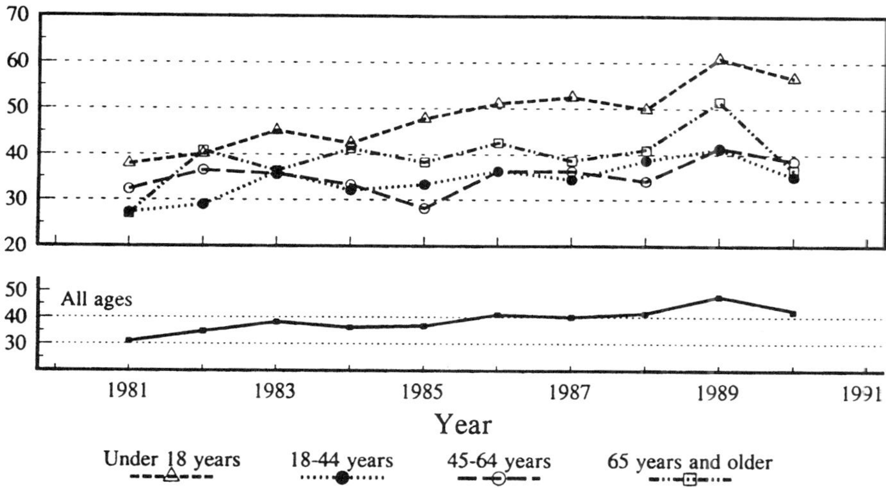

Figure 1 Prevalence rate (per 1000 persons) for self-reported asthma in past 12 months among persons of all ages—United States, 1981–1990. (From Ref. 3.)

individuals are less than 18 years old, making asthma the most common chronic disease of childhood (43) and the fourth leading cause of disability in children (44).

Over the last 20 years, the prevalence of asthma in the United States has increased dramatically. In 1970, a national survey by the Public Health Service estimated that 3% of the U.S. population had asthma (45); approximately 60% of these asthmatics had consulted a physician for asthma during the previous year and approximately 50% were using a medication or treatment for asthma. Figure 1 shows the steadily increasing *overall* prevalence of recent asthma from 1981 to 1990. More recent data from the NHIS show that the overall age-adjusted prevalence of asthma had risen to 4.9% by 1992 (46); this represents a more than 50% increase from 1980.

VI. ACUTE ASTHMA IN THE UNITED STATES

With the exception of asthma mortality, considerably less data are available about acute asthma—that is, asthma exacerbations that require modification of chronic asthma management. Although such exacerbations often can be managed by patients without contact with doctors or the hospital system (10), many (possibly most) asthma exacerbations in the United States continue to generate acute asthma "encounters" such as office visits, ED visits, and hospitalizations. Asthma deaths are an extreme but uncommon manifestation of acute asthma (47) and may not involve contact with the hospital system. To our knowledge, there is no large, nationally representative database that captures all of these acute asthma events and, therefore, their relative contribution and the overall magnitude of acute asthma are not known.

A large body of data are available concerning asthma mortality since vital statistics are collected routinely by many governments. For a variety of reasons, however, the accuracy of these data is suspect (24). The most important problem is the death certificate diagnosis. Coding is almost 100% accurate for asthma deaths among individuals under age 35, where the diagnosis is typically clear and the cause of death unambiguous, but accuracy declines with increasing age and is less than 70% by age 65 (48). Furthermore, a recent study found that death certificates identified only 42% of 339 asthma deaths as determined by an expert review panel (49). To increase the likelihood of drawing valid conclusions regarding asthma mortality, investigators often limit their analyses to younger age groups (e.g., age 5–34 years). Consequently, less is known about asthma mortality in older adults.

With these caveats in mind, asthma mortality in the United States appears to have increased steadily throughout the 1980s and early 1990s. The *overall* age-adjusted death rate from asthma rose from 13.4 deaths per million population (3154 deaths) in 1982 to 18.8 deaths per million population (5106 deaths) in 1991, an increase of 40% in only 10 years (46). For persons aged 5–34 years, the age group with more accurate data, asthma deaths increased by 42% over the same period (46). The most recent vital statistics, however, suggest that there has been a small but gradual *decline* in asthma mortality over the past few years (Fig. 2) (50). The cause of this surprising development is not clear, but we speculate that it might result from ongoing improvements in asthma management, such as the introduction of inhaled corticosteroid therapy and improvements in acute asthma care.

In 1985, asthma accounted for approximately 6.5 million visits to physicians' offices and an additional 1.5 million hospital-based outpatient visits, according to the National Ambulatory Medical Care Survey (NAMCS) (51). The majority of these visits (75% and 71%, respectively) involved adults, and most of the office visits (65%) were to physicians in primary care specialties (i.e., general practice/family medicine, pediatrics, and internal medicine). Only two years later, the National Medical Expenditure Survey (NMES), which relied largely on self-reported data from patients, estimated more than 13 million office

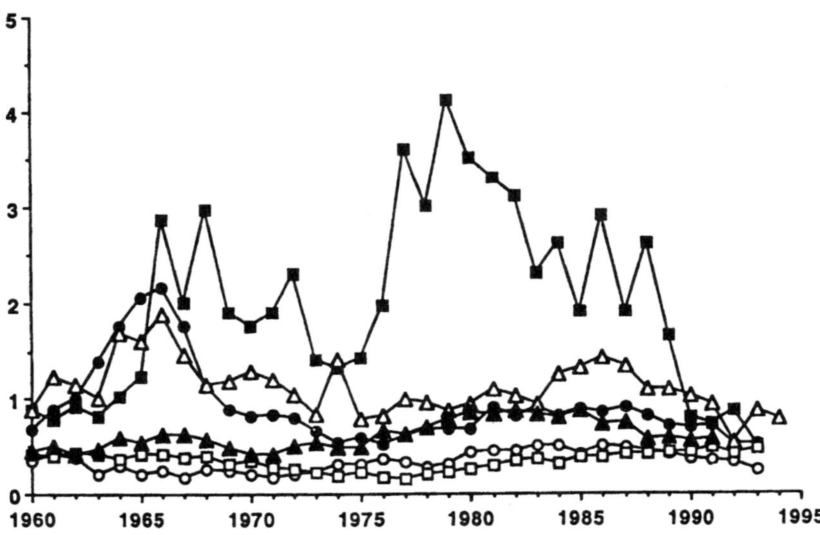

Figure 2 International patterns of annual asthma mortality (deaths per 100,000 persons) among persons age 5–34 years, by country and year—1960–1994. ■—■, New Zealand; ●—●, England and Wales; △—△, Australia; ▲—▲, West Germany; ○—○, Canada; □—□, United States. (From Ref. 50.)

visits and more than 1.5 million hospital-based outpatient visits related to asthma (52). These differences do not reflect changes in asthma burden but rather large differences in study design. Indeed, from 1975 to 1990, the annual rate of office visits for asthma increased by only 5% from 2.71 to 2.85 visits per 100 population (3). Moreover, all of these figures reflect a combination of ''urgent'' visits for acute asthma and ''routine'' visits for chronic stable asthma (e.g., medication refill, patient education). Unfortunately, billing data do not permit accurate separation of ''urgent'' from ''routine'' asthma visits due to incomplete ICD-9 coding (see Table 1).

ED asthma visits are more clearly related to acute asthma but their generalizability is unclear; ED patients differ considerably from the general population and it is not clear what percentage of all asthma exacerbations involve the ED. Nonetheless, one study estimated that there were more than 1.8 million ED asthma visits in the United States in 1985, and that 52% of ED visits involved adults (1). The NMES estimated approximately 1.2 million ED visits in 1987 (52). More recent data from the National Hospital Ambulatory Medical Care Survey (NHAMCS) suggested that asthma was the primary diagnosis for almost 1.5 million ED visits in 1992 . Although ED visits accounted for only 1.6% of all ED visits nationwide in NHAMCS, dramatic sociodemographic differences between ED catchment areas may explain why up to 10% of some inner city ED's visits are related to asthma (53). Preliminary data from the Multicenter Asthma Research Collaboration (54) suggest that, on an annual basis, between 10 and 30% of ED asthma visits are repeat visits. Frequent ED use is associated with greater asthma severity and with poor asthma self-management skills (55). There are no readily available data concerning trends in ED asthma, and only sparse data on the test characteristics of using ED billing data for case identification. A recent study found that the primary billing diagnosis identified only 68% of ED asthma visits at one teaching hospital and introduced significant selection bias (56). If confirmed by other investigators, it would appear that billing data may significantly underestimate the number of asthma visits in some EDs.

Approximately 10–30% of ED asthma visits in this country result in hospital admission (54), which is about half the admission rate reported from the United Kingdom (57). Regardless, combined data from the 1983 to 1987 National Hospital Discharge Surveys (NHDS), as well as 1987 NMES data (52), suggest that acute asthma accounts for approximately 460,000 hospital admissions annually in the United States. The majority of these hospitalizations (65%) involved adults (1). On an annual basis, approximately 18% of all asthma admissions among children and young adults are readmissions (58); comparable adult data are not available. Hospital admissions for asthma as the primary diagnosis more than tripled from 1970 to 1983 (59), but were essentially constant between 1982 and 1992 (46); the latter finding contrasts with concomitant increases in asthma prevalence and mortality. The stable asthma hospitalization rates also contrast, however, with dramatic declines in hospitalization rates for other conditions during this period (60). The stable (or falling) asthma hospitalization rate between 1982 and 1992 may reflect fundamental changes in the ED management of asthma and not a decline in severe asthma exacerbations (61).

As previously noted, several factors limit the usefulness of health care utilization data (24) and we suggest cautious interpretation and generalization of the preceding results. Discrepancies of literally millions of asthma visits between one source and another are reason enough for caution. We also expect major changes in acute asthma statistics in upcoming years as a result of dramatic and ongoing changes in health care delivery. For example, increasing market penetration by health management organizations (HMOs) may lead to significant decreases in ED asthma visits (and concomitant increases in "urgent" office visits) if ED visits are denied reimbursement by the patient's HMO. Also, the introduction of ED-based observation units may have a dramatic impact on asthma hospitalization rates. Such scenarios highlight the need for asthma surveillance programs that collect comprehensive and internally consistent data concerning health care utilization (62).

VII. GEOGRAPHIC VARIATION IN ASTHMA

Geographic variation in the prevalence or severity of asthma may provide important clues regarding the etiology of asthma, and assist health planners charged with controlling the current asthma epidemic. For example, asthma has been noted to be a largely urban phenomenon (63). More than 20% of U.S. asthma deaths in 1985 occurred in New York City and Chicago (Cook County), yet these places accounted for only 7% of the population at risk; these cities had such a disproportionate number of asthma deaths that they were, to some extent, driving the national increase in the 1980s (64). Small area analysis of New York City itself revealed that the highest rates of asthma hospitalization and asthma mortality are concentrated in the city's poorest neighborhoods (65) (Fig. 3). Similar findings have been reported from Philadelphia, where increases in asthma mortality from 1969 to 1991 were most pronounced in areas with poor socioeconomic status (SES) and high in minority populations (66). These and other small-area analyses have led to repeated calls for the design and implementation of public health policies aimed to reduce the disproportionate asthma burden borne by inner city inhabitants (63).

Migrant studies offer another perspective on the asthma problem. Populations that move from a rural to urban setting appear to adopt the increased asthma burden of the urban environment. For example, exercise-induced asthma in the offspring of migrants to Cape Town was 20 times greater than in the migrants' rural community of origin (67). Likewise, asthma symptoms in the offspring of Tokelauans who had migrated to New Zealand were twice as common as reported by Tokelauans who remained in Tokelau (68). These studies provide persuasive evidence that environmental factors play an important role in the etiology of asthma.

At a more global level, many studies have compared the asthma experience of the United States with that of the rest of the world. Previously discussed methodologic issues present an even greater challenge when looking across countries than when looking at U.S. data alone. Nonetheless, the prevalence of asthma in different populations has been shown to vary from less than 1% to greater than 30% (Table 2) (69); these differences cannot be entirely explained by differences in methodology. Asthma tends to be more common in developed nations and, consequently, common attributes of developed nations (e.g., urbanization, westernization, and increased affluence) are correlated with increased asthma prevalence (70). Some groups have speculated that the key factor may be the "cleanness" of living—that is, the increased time indoors and lack of exposure to childhood infections and resultant increase in expression of the asthma phenotype (71). Although this hypothesis appears quite attractive, a multifactorial environmental explanation seems most likely with the predominant reason varying by location.

As in the United States, asthma prevalence is increasing in many countries, including Australia, England, Finland, France, New Zealand, and the United Kingdom (69). Asthma hospitalizations for children age 0–14 reflect this increase with three–10-fold increases

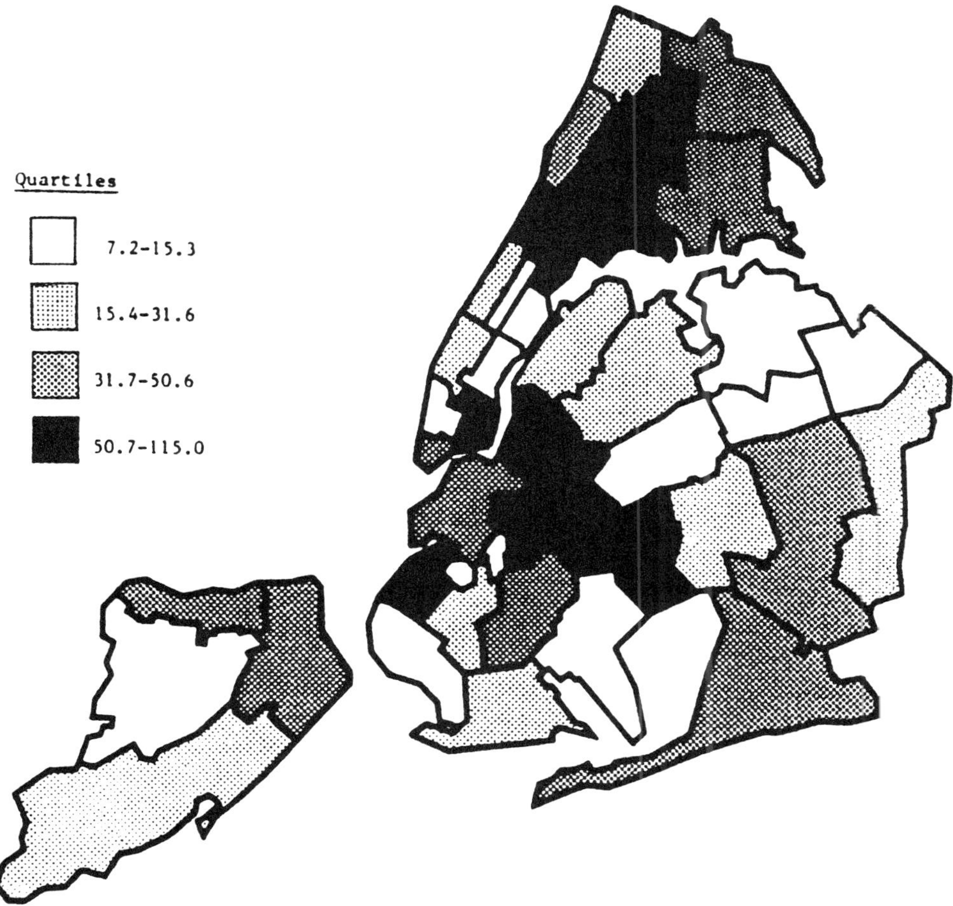

Figure 3 Average annual asthma hospitalization rate (per 10,000 persons) among persons age 0–34 years, by neighborhood—New York City, 1982–1986. (From Ref. 65; © 1992, American Public Health Association.)

noted between the 1960s and 1980s in several countries around the world (72). Additional evidence for a worldwide asthma epidemic may be found in vital statistics data, which show that the increase in asthma mortality also has been observed in countries such as Australia, Canada, England, Germany, Japan, Singapore, Sweden, and Switzerland (50). Interestingly, the most recent mortality figures show a small decline in asthma mortality in several of these countries (see Fig. 2), including England and Wales (73).

VIII. INFLUENCE OF AGE AND SEX

As previously noted, asthma can begin at any age, including infancy. Numerous epidemiological studies suggest that the most rapid rise in asthma incidence and prevalence has occurred in children (3). Population-based data from Rochester, Minnesota (29) show that

Table 2 Prevalence of Asthma in Selected Population Studies from Around the World

Country	Year	Age (years)	Recent asthma (%)	Lifetime asthma (%)
Australia				
general	1991	8 to 11	10	31
aborigines	1991	7 to 12	0	0
China	1988	11 to 17	2	2
Denmark	1987	7 to 16	5	—
England	1980	NA	8	—
France				
Paris	1982	21	—	5
Tahiti	1984	13	—	14
Germany	1990	9 to 11	4	8
Indonesia	1981	7 to 15	1	2
Kenya	1991	9 to 12	3	11
New Zealand	1989	12	8	17
	1989	12 to 18	—	34
Papua New Guinea	1985	6 to 20	0	0
United States (multiple studies)	1990s	all ages	4–8	8–10
Wales	1989	NA	5	12

Source: Modified from Figures 2-1 and 2-2 in the Global Initiative for Asthma (Ref. 69).

the 55% increase in annual age- and sex-adjusted incidence of asthma from 1964 to 1983 occurred only in children age 1–14; incidence rates for infants (age < 1) and for adults remained constant. NHANES data concerning children age 6–11, revealed an almost 60% increase in lifetime asthma prevalence for 1971–1974 (4.8%) and 1976–1980 (7.6%) (59). The trend continued during the 1980s: NHIS data show that asthma prevalence increased by more than 50% from 3.5% in 1982 to 5.3% in 1992 among persons age 5–34 (46). U.S. asthma hospitalization rates among children age 0–14 reflect this increased asthma burden as they have increased three-fold from the 1960s to 1980s in this age group alone (72). More recently, from 1980 to 1993, asthma hospitalization rates have continued to climb among children age 0–4 (Fig. 4). There are sparse epidemiologic data on trends in asthma prevalence among persons over age 65 because of legitimate concerns about disease misclassification in this age group.

A consistent observation across numerous epidemiological studies is an interaction between age and gender in terms of asthma burden. Asthma prevalence is higher among boys than girls before adolescence, but there is a slight female predominance thereafter (26,27,29). This gender difference is much larger for acute asthma. For example, Skobeloff and colleagues (74) examined all asthma admissions in southeastern Pennsylvania and found that males were admitted nearly twice as often as age-identical females in the 0–10 year age group, just as often at age 11–20, but then only 30-40% as often after age 20 (Fig. 5); hospital length of stay was greater for females than males after 30 years of age. Overall hospital admissions for asthma have been consistently higher for females than for males (46). Likewise, there is a female predominance among adults age 18–54 who present to the ED with acute asthma (54). Some population-based studies have found

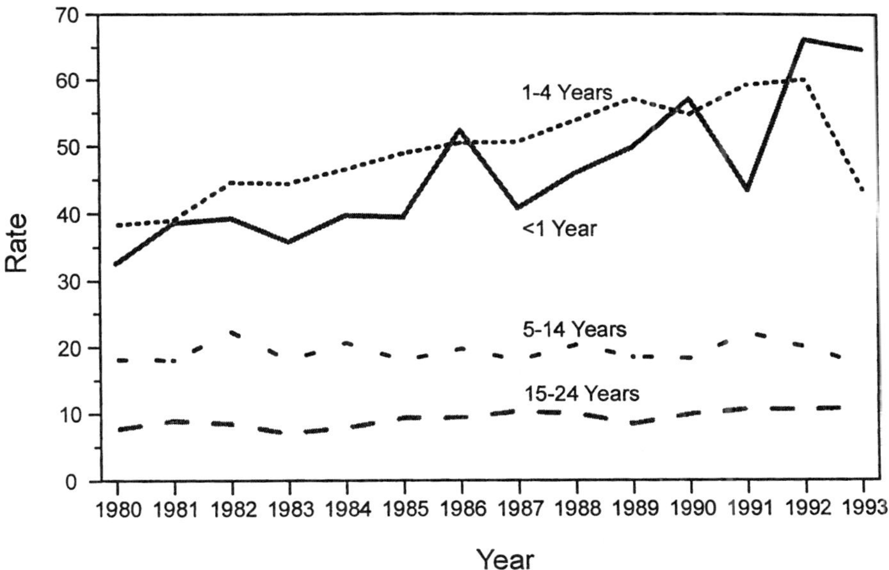

Figure 4 Annual asthma hospitalization rate (per 10,000 persons) among persons age 0–24 years, by age group and year—United States, 1980–1993. (From Ref. 43.)

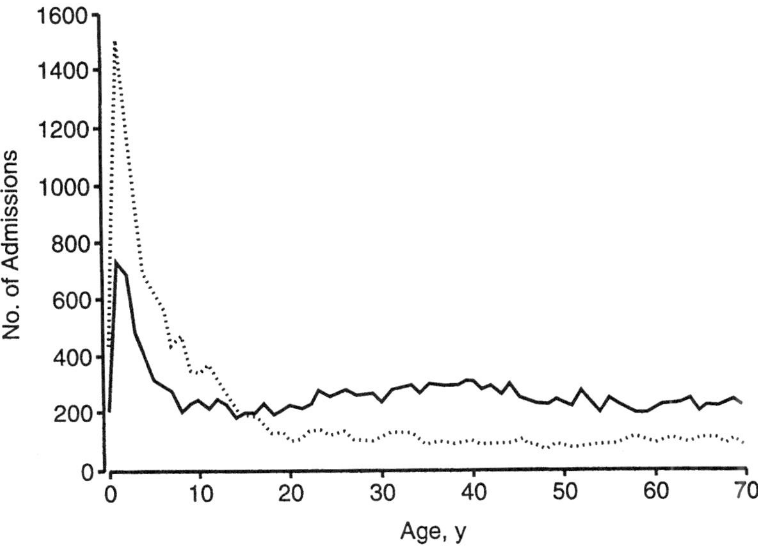

Figure 5 Number of asthma admissions by age for males (dotted line) and females (solid line)—southeastern Pennsylvania, 1986–1989. (From Ref. 74; © 1992, American Medical Association.)

a slight male predominance among elderly asthmatics (27,29) but this finding awaits confirmation.

Over the past few decades, the asthma burden has increased more among women than men. For example, asthma prevalence increased by 80% between 1982 and 1992 for females (from 2.9% to 5.4%) but increased only 29% for males (from 4.0% to 5.1%) (46). Likewise, asthma mortality during 1982–1991 increased 59% for females (from 15 to 25 deaths per million population) versus 34% for males (from 12 to 16 deaths per million population) (46). Taken together, there is ample evidence that, despite roughly comparable asthma prevalence rates, women are more severely affected by asthma than are men, and this gender difference is increasing over time.

IX. INFLUENCE OF RACE, ETHNICITY, AND SOCIOECONOMIC STATUS

Race and ethnicity are complex and imprecise concepts in epidemiological research (75,76). Typically, members of a specific ethnic group share some combination of geographic origins, language, social structures, cultural norms, religious traditions, literature, music, dietary preferences, and employment patterns. Although ethnic groups may share a range of physical characteristics due to their shared ancestry, the term is typically used to highlight these sociocultural characteristics instead of the biological ones. By contrast, race is biologically determined, and denotes people who share common physical characteristics, usually skin color. A common phenotype is often taken to imply a common genotype, an assumption that provides a biological basis for disease resistance or susceptibility. The basic assumption of this research, however, has been invalidated by genetic studies demonstrating that intraracial biological variation far exceeds interracial differences (77). Moreover, the genes that are associated with physical characteristics are not necessarily associated with those that determine disease susceptibility. Thus, classifying populations by ethnic (rather than racial) backgrounds is preferable since it acknowledges probable differences in culture and lifestyle as well as in genetic composition.

Nonetheless, most U.S. epidemiological studies to date have focused on differences between three racial groups: blacks, Hispanics, and whites. These studies reveal a consistently higher asthma burden among blacks compared to the other racial groups. For example, NHANES data show that the prevalence of asthma in blacks is more than twice the prevalence among whites; this asthma excess was found in both males and females (78). Blacks also have consistently higher asthma hospitalization rates than whites (46), as well as a greater proportion of asthma readmissions each year (58). Lastly, asthma mortality has been consistently highest among blacks compared to other racial groups, and this difference appears to be growing (46,43) (Fig. 6). Little research has focused on role of ethnic differences within the African-American community.

Likewise, sparse data are available concerning Hispanics (i.e., all people who trace their origins to a Spanish-speaking country or culture). The asthma prevalence rates of this large group are often considered intermediate between blacks (high) and whites (low), but this widespread view does not take into account important ethnic differences within the Hispanic community. Indeed, the most recent data from NHANES-III (1988–1991) showed that asthma prevalence was lower among Mexican Americans (5%) than among blacks (7%) or whites (8%) (41). Another study found that Puerto Rican children had

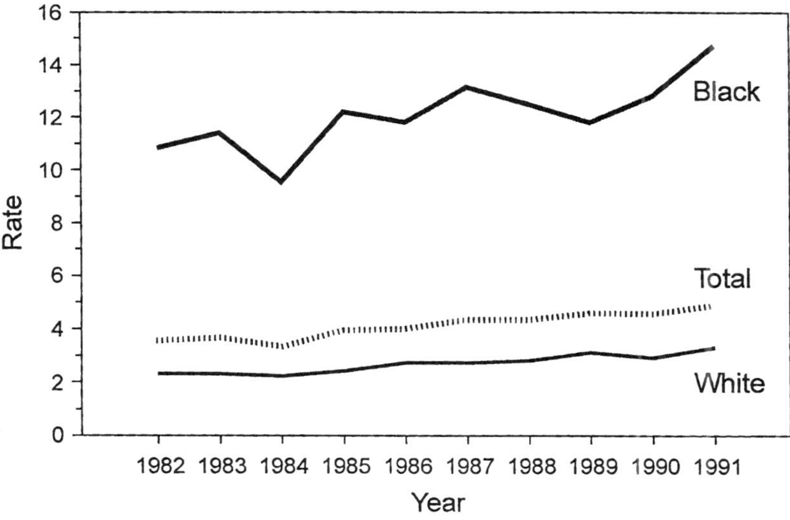

Figure 6 Age-adjusted annual mortality rate (per 1 million persons) for asthma as the underlying cause of death among persons age 5–34 years, by race and year—United States, 1982–1991. (From Ref. 46.)

a much higher prevalence of active asthma (11%) than blacks (6%), Cubans (5%), whites (3%), and Mexican Americans (3%) (79). Clearly, categorization of individuals as ''Hispanic'' alone does not capture the genetic and environmental characteristics that confer increased risk for asthma.

The most plausible explanation for the observed racial differences is that being black or Hispanic does not increase risk per se but instead serves as a marker for another factor, such as socioeconomic status (SES), that is thought to influence health. In other words, nonwhite Americans may bear a disproportionate amount of the asthma burden compared to white Americans, because, on average, blacks and Hispanics tend to have lower SES (e.g., lower family incomes, fewer years of formal education, suboptimal housing conditions) and some aspect of SES may increase the likelihood of having or dying from asthma. The convergence of all of these factors probably underlies the phenomenon of ''inner city'' asthma (63). Like ethnicity and race, however, SES is a difficult and imprecise concept (80). Furthermore, the relation of SES to asthma prevalence is complex: within the United States, individuals with low SES are more likely to have diagnosed asthma, but within other countries the opposite may be true (81). Ecologic studies support the latter association—that is, asthma is more prevalent in affluent countries than in nonaffluent countries (69).

Returning to asthma epidemiology in the United States, several statistical analyses of the relationship between race and asthma, controlling for SES, suggest that race is not a simple proxy for SES (78,82); furthermore, the persistent, albeit small, prevalence difference does not explain the much larger disparity in hospital admissions and asthma mortality. Nonetheless, given the strong association between SES and health, and our remarkably crude methods of measuring SES, it remains possible (indeed likely) that the persistent association between race and asthma is due, in large part, to ''residual confounding'' by SES or related factors (e.g., low birthweight, unfavorable housing conditions, psychosocial stressors, limited access to primary care). Racism (i.e., discrimination or prejudice based on race) may exacerbate some of these risk factor differences (e.g., by worsening already limited access to high-quality primary care). The relative contributions of these SES-related factors need to be studied in ethnic groups with increased asthma burden. Factors which are responsible for a significant portion of the excess morbidity and mortality could then be targeted for intervention (63).

X. POTENTIAL EXPLANATIONS FOR INCREASING ASTHMA MORBIDITY AND MORTALITY

Since the early 1980s, there have been many attempts to explain the worldwide increase in asthma morbidity and mortality. The most fundamental question, of course, is whether the overall trend is real or simply an artifact of the way we diagnose asthma or record health statistics. Weiss et al. (3) have carefully reviewed the subject, and their observations on the most likely explanations are summarized below.

A. Changes in Diagnostic Recognition

Changes in asthma prevalence could be due to a change in diagnostic recognition of asthma by either the general population or by health care providers. Since much asthma is undiagnosed (83), particularly in milder cases and in children, increasing asthma awareness could have led to an increased number of asthma diagnoses without a true increase in disease prevalence. Most repeated cross-sectional surveys are consistent with this hypothesis (84). One would expect, however, that changes in asthma hospitalization and mortality would be less affected by such a phenomenon. Moreover, recent prevalence studies with more rigorous case ascertainment do not support this explanation. For example, an analysis of asthma prevalence among Finnish military conscripts undergoing clinical examination between 1926–1989 suggests that if the apparent increase in asthma was due entirely to changes in diagnostic recognition that some 95% of cases must have gone undiagnosed in the years before 1966 (85); this seems inconceivable and suggests that much of the observed increase in asthma prevalence was real.

B. Diagnostic Transfer

Another explanation invokes changes in the way diseases are classified where specific diseases (e.g., bronchitis) are now being classified as ''asthma.'' Changes in ICD coding provide a clearcut example of such a phenomenon; indeed, the 1979 coding change involving ''asthmatic bronchitis'' (see Section II) resulted in a dramatic 1-year increase in asthma events (59). It is difficult, however, to attribute the continued rise in asthma burden throughout the 1980s to the ICD-9 revision.

More subtle examples of diagnostic transfer offer a more plausible explanation. For example, more gradual changes in ''diagnostic fashion'' might dictate that a diagnosis of asthma be substituted for bronchitis, in which case the substitution would lead to an inflated estimate of asthma prevalence. Analysis of annual hospitalization rates for both asthma and bronchitis show, however, that asthma hospitalizations steadily increased during a time period when bronchitis figures remained essentially constant (3).

C. Changes in Asthma Risk Factors

The most attractive hypothesis for the observed increase in asthma burden relates to possible widespread changes in asthma risk factors, such as increased rates of prematurity (and premature infant survival), decreased rates of breastfeeding, unfavorable changes in the outdoor environment (e.g., air pollution), unfavorable changes in the indoor environment (e.g., smoking, indoor allergens, irritant gases), changes in socioeconomic status, and changes in the medical care environment (e.g., access to medical care, pharmacotherapy). We agree with Weiss and colleagues (3) that premature births, indoor air quality, and medical care issues are the most likely explanations from the preceding list. Widespread changes in asthma risk factors continue to be a focus of intense research activity, with recent interest directed toward the roles of high-dose β-agonist therapy (86), cockroach allergen (87), and childhood infections (88).

Thus, although some portion of the observed increase in morbidity and mortality is undoubtedly artifactual, it appears that asthma morbidity and mortality truly are rising. Simultaneous changes in multiple asthma risk factors appear to be the most likely explanation; these factors include probable causes of asthma (e.g., indoor allergens) and features of the health care delivery system (e.g., access to primary care).

XI. IMPLICATIONS FOR PATIENT CARE, RESEARCH, AND HEALTH POLICY

The lack of a standard definition of asthma, apparent overall increase in asthma morbidity and mortality, and differential asthma burden in specific sociodemographic groups all have important implications for clinical care, research, and health policy.

At a patient level, our inability to refine the definition of asthma, particularly *acute* asthma, has led us to provide relatively unfocused pharmacotherapy for a remarkably diverse group of patients. Indeed, one might marvel at how well current therapies work for what is, undoubtedly, a heterogeneous condition. More sophisticated definitions (e.g., based on genetic factors, biochemical mediators, natural history, and character of exacerbation) would allow us to divide patients into more distinct asthma subtypes that might respond better to specific types of interventions. Identification of the factors that have led to the current asthma epidemic and, more specifically, to the increased burden in specific sociodemographic groups, also may have direct implications for clinical care (e.g., asthma prevention in high-risk individuals). Clearly, more research is needed in this arena.

At a societal level, the current definition of asthma is sufficiently detailed to provide us with gross estimates of the asthma burden but little more. The problem is of sufficient magnitude that it merits increased attention from the health policy planners. In monetary terms alone, the cost of illness related to asthma was estimated to be $6.2 billion in 1990, or nearly 1% of all U.S. health care costs (1). A more recent analysis, which did not include a mortality component, estimated a total cost of $5.8 billion in 1994 (52). These are crude estimates but, taken together, approximately 50% of the economic impact was associated with emergency department visits, hospitalization, and death (i.e., expenditures related to acute rather than chronic asthma). Better asthma surveillance data are needed to assist effective health policy planning, including the provision of adequate access to health care. Current epidemiologic data suggest that specific groups (i.e., children, women, blacks, Hispanics, and inner city inhabitants) bear a disproportionate percentage of the

U.S. asthma burden, and that public health efforts might be best focused on these high-risk populations. Research is needed on the most effective educational and interventional strategies for each group.

XII. SUMMARY

Despite numerous methodologic challenges, such as the lack of a standard definition of asthma, there is persuasive evidence that asthma prevalence is rising worldwide. The frequency of *acute* asthma (including fatal asthma) paralleled this increase until recent years when preliminary data suggest a leveling off or even gradual decline. The distribution of asthma varies dramatically by age, sex, race, and socioeconomic status. Although every sociodemographic group is affected, certain groups (i.e., children, women, blacks, Hispanics, and inner city inhabitants) appear to bear a disproportionate percentage of the asthma burden in the United States. It is difficult, and probably incorrect, to ascribe the current asthma epidemic to any single underlying factor. Taken together, these epidemiologic observations have important implications for patient care, research, and health policy concerning asthma.

ACKNOWLEDGMENTS

Dr. Camargo is supported by grant HL-03533 from the National Institutes of Health, Bethesda, MD.

REFERENCES

1. Weiss KB, Gergen PJ, Hodgson TA. An economic evaluation of asthma in the United States. N Engl J Med 1992; 326:862–866.
2. McCaig LF. National Hospital Ambulatory Medical Care Survey: 1992 emergency department summary. Advance data from vital and health statistics; no. 245. Hyattsville, MD: National Center for Health Statistics, 1994.
3. Weiss KB, Gergen PJ, Wagener DK. Breathing better or wheezing worse? The changing epidemiology of asthma morbidity and mortality. Annu Rev Publ Health 1993; 14:491–513.
4. Sandford A, Weir T, Paré P. The genetics of asthma. Am J Respir Crit Care Med 1996; 153: 1749–1765.
5. Newman-Taylor A. Environmental determinants of asthma. Lancet 1995; 345:296–299.
6. Guidotti TL. Consistency of diagnostic criteria for asthma from Laënnec (1819) to the National Asthma Education Program (1991). J Asthma 1994; 31:329–338.
7. Corrao WM, Braman SS, Irwin RS. Chronic cough as the sole presenting manifestation of bronchial asthma. N Engl J Med 1979; 300(12):633–637.
8. Scadding JG, Moser KM. Definition of asthma. In: Weiss E, Stein M, eds. Bronchial Asthma: Mechanisms and Therapeutics. 3rd ed. Boston: Little, Brown, 1993:3–14.
9. American Thoracic Society. Standards for the diagnosis and care of patients with chronic obstructive pulmonary disease (COPD) and asthma. Am Rev Respir Dis 1987; 136:225–243.
10. National Asthma Education and Prevention Program. Expert Panel Report II: Guidelines for the Diagnosis and Management of Asthma. Bethesda, MD: National Institutes of Health, 1997.

11. Chapman KR. Therapeutic approaches to chronic obstructive pulmonary disease: An emerging consensus. Am J Med 1996; 100(suppl 1A):5s–10s.
12. Keatings VM, Jatakanon A, Worsdell YM, Barnes PJ. Effects of inhaled and oral glucocorticoids on inflammatory indices in asthma and COPD. Am J Respir Crit Care Med 1997; 155: 542–548.
13. Braman SS, Kaemmerlen JT, Davis SM. Asthma in the elderly: A comparison between patients with recently acquired and long-standing disease. Am Rev Respir Dis 1991; 143:336–340.
14. Anonymous. International Classification of Diseases, 9th Revision, Clinical Modification. Washington, DC: U.S. Government Printing Office; publication no. 91-1260, 1991.
15. Rackeman FM. A working classification of asthma. Am J Med 1947; 3:601–606.
16. Burrows B, Martinez FD, Halonen M, Barbee RA, Cline MG. Association of asthma with serum IgE levels and skin-test reactivity to allergens. N Engl J Med 1989; 320(5):271–277.
17. Humbert M, Durham SR, Ying S, et al. IL-4 and IL-5 mRNA and protein in bronchial biopsies from patients with atopic and nonatopic asthma: Evidence against "intrinsic" asthma being a distinct immunopathologic entity. Am J Respir Crit Care Med 1996; 154:1497–1504.
18. European Community Respiratory Health Survey. Variations in the prevalence of respiratory symptoms, self-reported asthma attacks, and use of asthma medications in the European Community Respiratory Health Survey (ECRHS). Eur Respir J 1996; 9:687–695.
19. Pearce N, Weiland S, Keil U, et al. Self-reported prevalence of asthma symptoms in children in Australia, England, Germany, and New Zealand: An international comparison using the ISAAC protocol. Eur Respir J 1993; 6:1455–1461.
20. Shaw R, Woodman K, Ayson M, et al. Measuring the prevalence of bronchial hyperresponsiveness in children. Int J Epidemiol 1995; 24:597–602.
21. Holleman DRJ, Simel DL. Does the clinical examination predict airflow limitation? JAMA 1995; 273:313–319.
22. Higgins BT, Britton JR, Chinn S, Cooper S, Burney PGJ, Tattersfield AE. Comparison of bronchial reactivity and peak expiratory flow variability measurements for epidemiologic studies. Am Rev Respir Dis 1992: 145:588–593.
23. Burney PGJ, Britton JR, Chinn S, et al. Descriptive epidemiology of bronchial reactivity in an adult population: Results from a community study. Thorax 1987; 42:38–44.
24. Vollmer WM, Osborne ML, Buist AS. Uses and limitations of mortality and health care utilization statistics in asthma research. Am J Respir Crit Care Med 1994; 149(2 pt 2):S79–87; discussion S88–90.
25. Beard CM, Yunginger JW, Reed CE, O'Connell EJ, Silverstein MD. Interobserver variability in medical record review: an epidemiological study of asthma. J Clin Epidemiol 1992; 45: 1013–1020.
26. Broder I, Higgins MW, Matthews KP, Keller JB. Epidemiology of asthma and allergic rhinitis in a total community, Tecumseh, Michigan: IV. Natural history. J Allergy Clin Immunol 1974; 54:100–110.
27. Dodge RR, Burrows B. The prevalence and incidence of asthma and asthma-like symptoms in a general population sample. Am Rev Respir Dis 1980; 122:567–575.
28. McWhorter WP, Polis MA, Kaslow RA. Occurence, predictors, and consequences of adult asthma in NHANES1 and Follow-up Survey. Am Rev Respir Dis 1989; 139:721–724.
29. Yunginger JW, Reed CE, O'Connell EJ, Melton JL, III, O'Fallon WM, Silverstein MD. A community-based study of the epidemiology of asthma: Incidence rates, 1964–1983. Am Rev Respir Dis 1992; 146:888–894.
30. Weiss ST, Speizer FE. Epidemiology and natural history. In: Weiss, Stein M, eds. Bronchial Asthma: Mechanisms and Therapeutics. Boston: Little, Brown, 1993:15–25.
31. Bronnimann S, Burrows B. A prospective study of the natural history of asthma. Chest 1986; 90:480–484.
32. Blair H. Natural history of childhood asthma. Arch Dis Child 1977; 52:613–619.

33. Martin AJ, McLennan LA, Landau LI, Et al. The natural history of asthma to adult life. Br Med J 1980; 1:1397–1400.
34. Chan-Yeung M, Malo J-L. Occupational asthma. N Engl J Med 1995; 333:107–112.
35. Meredith S, Nordman H. Occupational asthma: Measures of frequency from four countries. Thorax 1996; 51:435–440.
36. Panhuysen CIM, Vonk JM, Koëter GH, et al. Adult patients may outgrow their asthma: A 25-year follow-up study. Am J Respir Crit Care Med 1997; 155:1267–1272.
37. Vergnenegre A, Antonini MT, Bonnaud F, Melloni B, Mignonat G, Bousquet J. Comparison between late onset and childhood asthma. Allergol Immunopathol (Madr) 1992; 20:190–196.
38. Roche WR. Fibroblasts and asthma. Clin Exp Allergy 1991; 21:545–548.
39. Adams PF, Marano MA. Current estimates from the National Health Interview Survey, 1994. Vital Health Stat 1995; 10:94.
40. Gergen PJ, Mullally DI, Evans R. National survey of prevalence of asthma among children in the United States, 1976–1980. Pediatrics 1988; 81:1–7.
41. Bang KM, Kim JH. Prevalence of asthma in the U.S. Population, 1988–1991 [abstract]. Am J Epidimiol 1996; 143(suppl):S17.
42. Crain EF, Weiss KB, Bijur PE, Hersh M, Westbrook L, Stein RE. An estimate of the prevalence of asthma and wheezing among inner-city children. Pediatrics 1994; 94:356–362.
43. Centers for Disease Control. Asthma mortality and hospitalization among children and young adults—United States, 1980–1993. MMWR 1996; 45:350–353.
44. Centers for Disease Control. Disabilities among children aged 5–17 years—United States, 1991–1992. MMWR 1995; 44:609–613.
45. Anonymous. Prevalence of Selected Chronic Respiratory Conditions—United States, 1970. U.S. Department of Health, Education, and Welfare; Series 10, No. 84. Washington, DC: U.S. Government Printing Office, 1973.
46. Centers for Disease Control. Asthma—United States, 1982–1992. MMWR 1995; 43:952–955.
47. Silverstein MD, Reed CE, O'Connell EJ, Melton LJ, III, O'Fallon WM, Yunginger JW. Long-term survival of a cohort of community residents with asthma. N Engl J Med 1994; 331:1537–1541.
48. Sears MR, Rea HH, de Boer G, et al. Accuracy of certification of deaths due to asthma: A national study. Am J Epidemiol 1986; 124:1004–1011.
49. Hunt LW, Silverstein MD, Reed CE, et al. Accuracy of the death certificate in a population-based study of asthmatic patients. JAMA 1993; 269:1947–1952.
50. Beasley R, Pearce N, Crane J. International trends in asthma mortality. In: Chadwick DJ, Cardew G, eds. The Rising Trends in Asthma (Ciba Foundation Symposium 206). Chichester, England: John Wiley & Sons, 1997:140–156.
51. Nelson C, McLemore T. The National Ambulatory Medical Care Survey: United States, 1975–81 and 1985 trends. Vital and health statistics. Series 13, No. 93. Washington, DC: U.S. Government Printing Office, 1988.
52. Smith DH, Malone DC, Lawson KA, Okamoto LJ, Battista C, Saunders WB. A national estimate of the economic costs of asthma. Am J Respir Crit Care Med 1997; 156:787–793.
53. Richardson LD, Ford JG. Use of the emergency department by patients with asthma in an indigent urban African-American community. Poster presented at the Tenth Annual Meeting of the Association for Health Services Research. Washington, DC: June 1993.
54. Camargo CA, Jr. First Multicenter Asthma Research Collaboration (MARC-1) [abstract]. Acad Emerg Med 1997; 4:470.
55. Richardson LD, McLean DE, Ford JG, Findley SE, Misra DP, Zhang W. Factors associated with frequent ED use for asthma in an urban black population [abstract]. Acad Emerg Med 1996; 3:434–435.
56. Camargo CA Jr, Emond SD, Lee EY. Case identification by administrative claims data vs. ED logbooks: experience with the acute asthma [abstract]. Acad Emerg Med 1996; 3:458.

57. Partridge MR, Latouche D, Trako E, Thurston JG. A national census of those attending UK accident and emergency departments with asthma. The UK National Asthma Task Force J Accid Emerg Med 1997; 14:16–20.
58. Centers for Disease Control. Asthma hospitalizations and readmissions among children and young adults—Wisconsin, 1991–1995. MMWR 1997; 46:726–729.
59. Evans R, Mullally DI, Wilson RW, et al. National trends in the morbidity and mortality of asthma in the US—Prevalence, hospitalization and death from asthma over two decades: 1965–1984. Chest 1987; 91(suppl):65S–74S.
60. National Center for Health Statistics. Health, United States, 1990. Hyattsville, MD: Public Health Service, 1991.
61. Vollmer WM, Osborne ML, Buist AS. Temporal trends in hospital-based episodes of asthma care in a health maintenance organization. Am Rev Respir Dis 1993; 147:347–353.
62. Centers for Disease Control. Asthma surveillance programs in public health departments—United States. MMWR 1996; 45:802–804.
63. Weiss KB, Gergon PJ, Crain EF. Inner city asthma: The epidemiology of an emerging US public health concern. Chest 1992; 101(suppl 6):362S–367S.
64. Weiss KB, Wagener DK. Changing patterns of asthma mortality: Identifying target populations at high risk. JAMA 1990; 264:1683–1687.
65. Carr W, Zeital L, Weissw K. Variations in asthma hospitalizations and deaths in New York City. Am J Public Health 1992; 82(1):59–65.
66. Lang DM, Polansky M. Patterns of asthma mortality in Philadelphia from 1969 to 1991. N Engl J Med 1994; 331:1542–1546.
67. van Niererk CH, Weinberg EG, Shore SC, Heese HD, van Schalkwyk DJ. Prevalence of asthma: A community study of urban and rural Xhosa children. Clin Allergy 1979; 9:319–324.
68. Waite DA, Eyles EF, Tonkin Sl, O'Donnell TV. Asthma prevalence in Tokelauan children in two environments. Clin Allergy 1980; 10:71–75.
69. Anonymous. Global Initiative for Asthma: Global Strategy for Asthma Management and Prevention, NHLBI/WHO Workshop Report. Bethesda, MD: National Institutes of Health; publication no. 95-3659, 1995.
70. Cookson JB. Prevalence rates of asthma in developing countries and their comparisons with those in Europe and North America. Chest 1987; 91(6 suppl):97S–103S.
71. Woolcock AJ, Peat JK. Evidence for the increase in asthma worldwide. In: Chadwick DJ, Cardew G, eds. The Rising Trends in Asthma (Ciba Foundation Symposium 206). Chichester, England: John Wiley & Sons, 1997:122–139.
72. Mitchell EA. International trends in hospital admission rates for asthma. Arch Dis Child 1985; 60:376–378.
73. Campbell MJ, Cogman GR, Holgate ST, Johnston SL. Age specific trends in asthma mortality in England and Wales, 1983–95: Results of an observational study. BMJ 1997; 314:1439–1441.
74. Skobeloff EM, Spivey WH, St. Clair SS, Schoffstall JM. The influence of age and sex on asthma admissions. JAMA 1992; 268(24):3437–3440.
75. Senior PA, Bhopal R. Ethnicity as a variable in epidemiological research. BMJ 1994; 309: 327–330.
76. Williams DR. Race and health: Basic questions, emerging directions. Ann Epidemiol 1997; 7:322–333.
77. Jones JS. How different are human races? Nature 1981; 293:188–190.
78. Schwartz J, Gold D, Dockery DW, Weiss ST, Speizer FE. Predictors of asthma and persistent wheeze in a national sample of children in the United States: Association with social class, perinatal events, and race. Am Rev Respir Dis 1990; 142:555–562.
79. Carter-Pokras OD, Gergen PJ. Reported asthma among Puerto Rican, Mexican-American, and Cuban children, 1982 through 1984. Am J Public Health 1993; 83:580–582.

80. Blane D. Social determinants of health—socioeconomic status, social class, and ethnicity. Am J Public Health 1995; 85:903–905.
81. Gergen P. Social class and asthma—Distinguishing the disease and the diagnosis. Am J Public Health 1996; 86:1361–1362.
82. Cunningham J, Dockery DW, Speizer FE. Race, asthma, and persistent wheeze in Philadelphia schoolchildren. Am J Public Health 1996; 86:1406–1409.
83. Speight AN, Lee DA, Hey EN. Underdiagnosis and undertreatment of asthma in childhood. Br Med J 1983; 286:1253–1256.
84. Magnus P, Jaakkola JJK. Secular trend in the occurance of asthma among children and young adults: Critical appraisal of repeated cross sectional surveys. BMJ 1997; 314:1795–1799.
85. Haahtela T, Lindholm H, Björkstén F, Koskenvuo K, Laitinen LA. Prevalence of asthma in Finnish young men. Br Med J 1990; 301:266–268.
86. Ernst P, Habbick B, Suissa S, et al. Is the association between inhaled beta-agonist use and life-threatening asthma because of confounding by severity? Am Rev Respir Dis 1993; 148: 75–79.
87. Rosenstreich DL, Eggleston P, Kattan M, et al. The role of cockroach allergy and exposure to cockroach allergen in causing morbidity among inner-city children with asthma. N Engl J Med 1997; 336:1356–1363.
88. Cookson WO, Moffatt MR. Asthma: An epidemic in the absence of infection? Science 1997; 275:41–42.

6

Allergic Asthma

Michael A. Kaliner
Washington Hospital Center, Washington, D.C.

I. INTRODUCTION

It is estimated that 9–12 million Americans currently have asthma and that the incidence has increased by about 60% in the past decade (1), not only in the United States but worldwide (2). Asthma was estimated to cost approximately $6.2 billion in 1990 (3), to be the number one cause for hospitalizations in pediatric hospitals nationwide, to be the sixth most common cause for all hospitalizations, and to cause nearly 5000 deaths per year (an increase of nearly 80% in the past decade).

Asthma was derived from the Greek meaning for panting, or breathlessness, and thus might be considered a description of the primary symptom of this disease. Asthma can be defined clinically as recurrent airflow obstruction causing intermittent wheezing, breathlessness, and sometimes cough with sputum production. The National Asthma Education Panel, developed in conjunction with the National Heart, Lung, and Blood Institute, defined asthma in 1991 (4) as having three components:

1. Airflow obstruction that is reversible either spontaneously or in response to therapy
2. Airway inflammation
3. Increased airway responsiveness to a variety of stimuli

About 90% of asthmatics between the ages of 2 and 16 years are allergic, 70% of asthmatics less than 30 years are allergic, and about 50% of asthmatics older than 30 years of age are concomitantly allergic (5). Thus, coincidental allergies are far and away the most common underlying condition contributing towards developing asthma.

One should suspect allergy as a contributing factor when (1) there is a family history of allergic diseases; (2) the clinical presentation includes seasonal exacerbations or exacerbations related to exposures to recognized allergens; (3) there is concomitant allergic rhinitis, other allergic disease, or a family history of allergic disease; (4) a slight-to-moderate eosinophilia is present (300 to 1000/mm^3) or eosinophilia in the sputum is observed; or (5) the patient is less than 40 years old, although many mature asthmatics are concomitantly allergic. Skin testing confirms IgE directed against the incriminated allergen but does not establish a cause-and-effect relationship. The inhalation of allergens by bronchial provocation testing will be positive in subjects who have positive prick-type skin test results but many of these patients do not exhibit clinical asthma during the relevant pollen seasons. Thus, the presence of a positive skin test (or in vitro test for IgE antibodies) must always be confirmed with a good history (6). Levels of total IgE may be somewhat useful but are not diagnostic; about 60% of allergic asthmatic subjects have elevated IgE levels while the IgE in the remaining 40% is normal. Because limiting exposure to allergens by avoidance techniques and treating patients with specific allergy immunotherapy are both extremely helpful in treating allergic asthmatic subjects, a careful search for possible allergies is indicated in nearly all asthmatics.

Current recommendations are that all asthmatics who wheeze more than 2 days per week should be evaluated by an allergist, or other physician skilled in identifying allergic disease, in order to institute prophylactic allergen avoidance measures (7,8). Thus, any asthmatic with persistent symptoms, who uses medications on a regular basis, or who has nocturnal wheezing should be evaluated for possible allergies. It was once thought that allergic asthma was associated with a relatively milder form of disease but this contention has not been borne out. Allergic asthma is as severe as any other cause of asthma, and allergen exposures can complicate or contribute to asthma of all severities (9). Onset of asthma between the ages of 2 years and puberty generally has a good prognosis, while asthma appearing before age 2 may be of a more severe nature (10). While childhood asthma may spontaneously remit during teenage years, we now recognize that many of these patients become asthmatic again in adulthood. Moreover, the philosophy of ignoring asthma in a child is a serious error in judgment for many reasons, including the availability of excellent medications, the impairment of body image that an asthmatic child may develop and lasts throughout life, the long-range effects of restricted physical activity on mental and physical health, and the loss of school and recreation time due to a treatable problem. Current recommendations include conditioning of the asthmatic to better prepare him for strenuous exercise, choosing swimming or biking in place of running, and using prophylactic medications to prevent exercise-related airflow obstruction (4,8).

II. THE ALLERGIC REACTION

The essential components of allergic reactions include: allergens, IgE antibodies directed at antigenic determinants on the allergen, and activated mast cells that generate and release mediators and cytokines. In order to initiate allergic responses, exposure to an appropriate antigen and a genetically determined capacity to respond with IgE production are required. Antigen presentation requires access of antigens to the mucous membrane, uptake by antigen presenting cells, antigen processing, and stimulation of local antibody production. IgE production occurs in the same local environment as antigen presentation, probably in the draining lymph nodes. IgE production is regulated by locally produced helper factors, thought to include interleukin (IL)-4 and IL-10 produced by local helper T lymphocytes (TH-2 cells). The IgE that is produced sensitizes mast cells in the same environment by binding to high affinity receptors for IgE on the cell surface. Although no one is certain of the precise time involved, the production of sufficient IgE to render a subject allergic is thought to take several years or more. However, children less than 1 year old with unquestionable allergic diseases are not uncommon.

Once sensitized, mast cells may degranulate upon subsequent allergen exposure. The bridging of IgE receptors by aggregation of IgE molecules bound to multivalent allergens initiates a biochemical reaction that leads to the secretion of a range of chemical mediators from mast cells (11). These mediators then stimulate the surrounding tissues to elicit the allergic response, the nature of which is determined by the local environment. Thus, mast cell degranulation and mediator production may cause rhinitis, conjunctivitis, sinusitis, cough, asthma, abdominal cramping, diarrhea, urticaria, eczema, headaches, hypotension, laryngeal edema, and other syndromes depending upon the local environment (12).

In humans, the mast cell is found in the loose connective tissues of all organs, most notably around blood vessels, nerves, and lymphatics (13). In the lung, mast cells are found beneath the basement membranes of airways, near blood vessels in the submucosa, adjacent to submucous glands, scattered throughout the muscle bundles, in the intra-alveolar septa, and in the bronchial lumen (11). Mast cells appear in increased numbers in the epithelium after allergen exposure and are predominant in biopsies obtained during the allergy season. In the airways, there are about 20,000 mast cells/mm^3 (12), and the mast cell represents 1–2% of alveolar cells.

Mast cells may be divided into two types. In the skin, the predominant mast cell (known as the MC_{tc} type) contains tryptase, chymase, and cathepsin G; the granules have a pattern described as lattice-like or crystalline; and the cells degranulate in response to neuropeptides such as substance P or morphine. By contrast, lung mast cells (known as the MC_t type) contain tryptase but not other proteases, have a granule pattern described as scroll-like, and do not respond to substance P or morphine with degranulation (14). Of interest is the recent observation that nasal mucosal mast cells are predominantly of the MC_{tc} type, while the epithelial mast cells are of the MC_t type (15). Thus, it is not possible to predict the exact phenotype of the resident mast cells based solely upon their location in the mucosa or epithelium.

There are four sources of mediators generated during the process of mast cell degranulation: preformed soluble molecules stored within the granules, newly formed molecules generated de novo during the degranulation process, newly synthesized proteins transcribed over a period of hours after the initiation of degranulation, and macromolecular materials that derive from the granule matrix that may cause actions lasting for a prolonged period after degranulation (Table 1). The consequences of mediator release occur within minutes (immediate hypersensitivity) or may require hours to develop (late-phase allergic reactions). Research has revealed an expanding list of mediators whose actions may contribute to the pathological changes seen in asthma (Table 2). In addition to the granule-derived mediators, the process of degranulation leads to transcription, synthesis, and secretion of additional inflammatory materials, including a number of potent cytokines, over several hours that likely contribute to the late-phase allergic response. Thus, mast cells synthesize and release IL-3, IL-4, IL-5, and IL-6 in addition to tumor necrosis factor (TNF) and other inflammatory cytokines (16). Mast cells store IL-4 and secrete it as one of the granule mediators, as well (17). As IL-4 helps regulate IgE production, mast cell activation and release of IL-4 might actually upregulate IgE production (18).

Table 1 Mast Cell–Derived Mediators

Preformed mediators that are rapidly released under physiological conditions
Histamine
Eosinophil and neutrophil chemotactic factors
Kininogenase
TNF-α
Endothelin-1
Arylsulfatase A
Exoglycosidases
Mediators formed during the degranulation process
Superoxide and other reactive oxygen species
Leukotrienes C_4, D_4, E_4
Prostaglandins, HETEs, HHT
Prostaglandin-generating factor of anaphylaxis
Adenosine
Bradykinin
Platelet-activating factor
Mediators closely associated with the granule matrix
Heparin, chondroitin sulfate E
Tryptase
Chymase
Cathepsin G
Carboxypeptidase
Peroxidase
Arylsulfatase B
Inflammatory factors
Superoxide dismutase
Cytokines transcribed after activation
Interleukins-1, 2, 3, 4, 5, 6
Granulocyte–macrophage colony-stimulating factor
Macrophage inflammatory proteins 1 and 1β
Monocyte chemotactic and activating factor
TNF-α
TCA-3
Endothelin-1

Source: Modified from Refs. 12 and 16.

III. ALLERGENS

Inhalant allergens are most frequently involved in allergic respiratory diseases such as allergic rhinitis and asthma. These antigens, which directly impact on the respiratory mucosa, are usually derived from natural organic sources such as house dust, pollens, mold spores, and insect and animal emanations. Chemicals and irritants from the work place have been increasingly recognized as a cause of rhinitis, asthma, or both. These chemicals can act as allergens or irritants, or could influence the mucosal environment in such a manner as to predispose the individual towards developing an allergic response. It appears that most particulate materials from which aeroallergens are derived are between 2 and

Table 2 Pathological Changes in Asthma and the Putative Mediators Responsible

Pathological changes	Mast cell mediators responsible
Bronchial smooth-muscle contraction	Histamine
	Leukotrienes C_4, D_4, E_4
	Prostaglandins and thromboxane A_2
	Bradykinin
	Platelet-activating factor
Mucosal edema	Histamine
	Leukotrienes C_4, D_4, E_4
	Prostaglandin E_2
	Bradykinin
	Platelet-activating factor
	Chymase
	Reactive oxygen species
Mucosal inflammation	Inflammatory factors
	Cytokines
	Eosinophil and neutrophil chemotatic factors
	Leukotriene B_4
	Platelet-activating factor
	IL-1, IL-6, TNF
Mucus secretion	Histamine
	Prostaglandins
	HETEs
	Leukotrienes C_4, D_4, E_4
	Chymase
Desquamation	Reactive oxygen species
	Proteolytic enzymes
	Inflammatory factors and cytokines

Source: Modified from Ref. 5.

60 μm in diameter, and their allergenic constituents usually are water soluble proteins with a molecular weight between 10,000 and 40,000 daltons (19,20).

Inhalant allergic diseases may be episodic, seasonal (such as hay fever), or perennial. The most important seasonal allergens are pollens, such as ragweed. Most tree pollens are released during the early spring, and in most parts of the country the height of the grass pollen season is late spring to midsummer. Although some species of weed pollen are airborne in spring and early summer, the greatest difficulty from weeds is in late summer and early fall. In the eastern and midwestern United States, ragweed is by far the worst offender. Despite popular belief, the heavy, sticky pollens of brightly colored flowers seldom cause allergy symptoms, as these pollen are spread by insects and not by wind currents. Inhalant allergens are most often responsible for rhinitis, conjunctivitis or asthma, although occasionally urticaria, eczema or systemic anaphylaxis may occur.

Exposure to nonseasonal allergens, mainly through inhalation but in some instances by ingestion, accounts for year-round allergies. Among the inhalants, dust mites, mold allergens, cockroaches, and animal emanations are responsible for most perennial allergic rhinitis and asthma (21). House dust itself is a mixture of lint, mites, mite derived feces, danders, insect parts, fibers, and other particulate materials. Overwhelming evidence indicates that certain mites, *Dermatophagoides farinae* and *D. pteronyssinus*, are the principal sources of antigen in house dust. The mites themselves are small, but can be noted by the naked eye as a speck if placed on a dark cloth. These arachnids encase their fecal materials in a coating rich in intestinal enzymes, and it is a protease within this coating that is the primary allergen. Mite fecal balls are large and heavy compared to other allergens, and thus only float in the air briefly after disturbance. Mites living in bedding, mattresses and carpets feed on human skin dander, and require a warm, relatively humid environment to proliferate (65–70° and >50% relative humidity). They survive best in carpets, bedding and upholstery. Disturbance of the carpet, perhaps by vacuuming, leads to a brief (approximately 30 min) episode of airborne mite feces, leading to inhalation and possible initiation of allergic reactions (19,20).

Cat allergens derive both from salivary and skin sources, are much smaller and lighter than dust allergens, are found constantly in the air in households with cats, and are a potent source of allergen. Dog allergens are also found in saliva, skin dander, and urine, but not hair. Thus, short-haired or long-haired breeds may be equally allergenic. Cockroaches are another major allergen in urban environments, which should be suspected in any perennially allergic patient living in or around a city. Cockroaches are an especially important allergen in inner city, relatively poor populations (23). Commercial spraying and eradication are the only measures that have been shown to reduce cockroach related disease, although immunotherapy is also useful.

Among the inhalant antigens, fungi occupy a unique position because they are found in both outdoor and indoor environments (20). *Alternaria* and *Cladosporium* are the major outdoor mold allergens. The smut and rust fungi, both members of the class Basidiomycetes, can also cause allergic problems, especially near granaries. *Penicillium* and *Aspergillus* are the most prevalent molds found in basements, bedding, and damp interior areas. *Rhizopus nigricans* (''black bread mold''), *Saccharomyces cerevisiae* (''bakers' yeast''), *Chaetomium, Curvularia, Helminthosporium, Spondylocladium, Stemphylium, Rhodotorula,* and the slime molds *Fusarium*, *Phoma*, *Pullularia*, and *Trichoderma* also are frequent allergens in certain locations. Although pollen allergens typically become windborne during dry weather and are removed from the air during rain, high mold-spore counts are found in clouds and mist, and many upper respiratory tract allergy symptoms during periods of high humidity are probably attributable to favorable conditions for mold growth. When indoor mold exposures are important, installing a dehumidifier in a damp area may be helpful. In general, use of a bleach works as well as any other product to remove fungi and mold from the walls in damp areas such as bathrooms and basements.

IV. SKIN TESTING AND IgE

Despite the development of in vitro methods of detecting IgE antibodies, skin testing (prick or intradermal) with appropriate allergens is the least time-consuming, most sensitive, most useful, and also the most inexpensive method employed to confirm the presence of allergen-specific IgE (22,24). Skin testing can be performed on infants as young as 1–4 months of age, although age dictates both the choice of allergens used and the clinical conditions for which they can be used. Under the age of 1, food antigens are the likely offenders, causing eczema or asthma. Inhalant allergens are more likely to be involved after 2–4 years of exposure, although sensitization to indoor allergens can occur much more quickly. In exceptional cases, such as in patients with extensive eczema or marked dermatographism that negates use of skin tests, in vitro assays for serum IgE antibodies by radioallergosorbent, fluorescent-allergosorbent, multiple-thread allergosorbent, or enzyme-linked immunosorbent test techniques might be substituted for direct testing. With either in vitro testing or skin tests, however, it is essential that the relevance of the results be correlated to the patient's current clinical problems and their detailed history.

Since total IgE levels are elevated in only about two-thirds of allergic asthmatics, and increased total IgE levels also occur in nonallergic conditions, an elevated level does not make a diagnosis of allergy, and a normal level does not rule it out. Thus, the clinical value of determining total serum IgE levels is limited.

Prick skin tests correspond very closely to seasonal- or exposure-related symptoms, responses to provocations, and eventual response to treatment (22). Intradermal skin tests are less exact in their relationship to both symptoms and provocations. Thus, patients with histories suggestive of allergic disease and positive prick tests may receive instructions for allergen avoidance and consideration for immunotherapy. We usually do not prescribe immunotherapy to patients who only are positive by intradermal testing. Patients with seasonal asthma, or whose asthma appears to be related to specific exposures, should be referred to an allergy specialist for a careful history, skin testing, and detailed instruction on allergen avoidance. Immunotherapy is usually reserved for those patients who cannot avoid allergens, and in whom pharmacotherapy is not completely effective.

V. ALLERGIC ASTHMA AND THE EMERGENCY DEPARTMENT

The emergency physician should treat the airflow obstruction of asthma irrespective of underlying precipitating factor(s). However, upon discharge, it is helpful to direct the patient appropriately. Thus, patients with seasonal disease, allergen-precipitated symptoms, those with pale boggy nasal mucous membranes, allergic changes to their conjunctiva, allergic shiners, positive family histories of allergies, high eosinophil counts, and other signs and symptoms of allergy should be told that allergy might play an important part in their disease and that an allergy evaluation is appropriate. Once evaluated, specific information on avoiding allergens confirmed by both history and skin testing should be provided to the patient. Patients whose disease is severe enough to warrant an emergency department (ED) visit should be discharged on corticosteroids, both oral and inhaled. There is no need to start antiallergy medications such as cromolyn or nedocromil in the ED, but providing corticosteroids may prevent the need for return visits to the ED. Consideration for the use of depot corticosteroids by injection should include an assessment of the reliability of the patient, their past history of ED usage, and whether the physician considers the patient reliable in regards to follow up visits.

In compliant patients properly managed by a knowledgeable primary care physician or by an asthma or allergy expert, nearly all asthma can be managed satisfactorily, with very limited needs for ED visits. Proper outpatient management includes patient education; the use of anti-inflammatory agents, particularly inhaled corticosteroids as primary agents; identification of allergens and careful education of the patient in allergen avoidance techniques; the use of peak flow monitors in order to identify exacerbations early enough to treat without the need for the ED; and establishing a rapport with the patient that will encourage the patient to seek medical care before an exacerbation become emergent. In most contemporary studies, done both by asthma experts and by managed care companies, following these principles reduces the need for emergency visits by 50–75% within one year (7,25). The emergency physician is responsible to make certain that the asthma patient is directed to expert care and that he is provided appropriate medications to carry him over until such follow-up can be arranged.

REFERENCES

1. Nelson C, McLemore T. The National Ambulatory Care Survey, United States, 1975–81 and 1985 Trends. Vital and Health Statistics, Series 13, No. 93. HHS pub. no. (PHS)88-1754. Washington DC: US GPO, Oct. 88.
2. Sears MR: Epidemiological trends in bronchial asthma, In: Kaliner MA, Persson C, Barnes P, eds., Asthma: Its Pathology and Treatment, New York: Marcel Dekker, 1990; 1–49.
3. Weiss KB, Gergen PJ, Hodgson TA. An economic evaluation of asthma in the United States, N Engl J Med 1992; 326:862–866.
4. Sheffer AL, Bailey WC, Bleeker ER, et al. Guidelines for the diagnosis and management of asthma. U.S. Department of Health and Human Services, National Institutes of Health, Publication No. 91-3042, Bethesda, MD, Aug. 1991.
5. Kaliner MA, Lemanske R: Rhinitis and asthma, *JAMA,* 268;2807-2829 (1992).
6. Spector SL. Antigen inhalation challenges, In Spector SL, ed., Provocative Testing in Clinical Practice, New York: Marcel Dekker, 1995, 325–368.
7. Kaliner MA. Allergy care in the next millennium: Guidelines for the specialty. J Allergy Clin Immunol 1997; 99:729–734.
8. Murphy S, Bleecker ER, Boushey H, et al. Guidelines for the diagnosis and management of asthma, expert panel report 2, U.S. Dept of Health and Human Services, National Institutes of Health, NIH Publication 97-4051, April 1997.
9. Platts-Mills TAE, Pollart S, Chapman MD, Luczynska CM. Role of allergens in airway hyperresponsiveness: Relevance of Immunotherapy and allergy avoidance, In: Kaliner MA, Persson C, Barnes P, eds., Asthma: Its pathology and treatment, New York: Marcel Dekker, 1990, 595–632.
10. Evans R. Epidemiology and natural history of asthma, allergic rhinitis, and atopic dermatitis, In: Middleton E, Reed CE, Ellis EF, Adkinson NF Jr, Yunginger JW, Busse WW, eds., Allergy: Principles and practice, 4th Ed., St. Louis: CV Mosby Co, 1993, 1109–1136.
11. White MV, Kaliner, MA. Mast cells and asthma, In: Kaliner MA, Persson C, Barnes P, eds., Asthma: Its Pathology and treatment, New York: Marcel Dekker, 1990, 409–440.
12. Scott T, Kaliner MA. Mast cells in asthma, In: Kaliner MA, Metcalfe DD, eds., The mast cell in health and disease, New York: Marcel Dekker, 1992, 575–608.
13. Dvorak AM. Human mast cells: Ultrastructural observations of in situ, ex vivo, and in vitro sites, sources, and systems, In: Kaliner MA, Metcalfe DD, eds., The mast cell in health and disease, New York: Marcel Dekker, 1992, 1–90.
14. Schwartz, LB. Heterogeneity of human mast cells, In: Kaliner MA, Metcalfe DD, eds., The mast cell in health and disease, New York: Marcel Dekker, 1992, 219–236.
15. Igarashi Y, Goldrich MS, Kaliner MA, Irani AMM, Schwartz LB, and White MV. Quantification of inflammatory cells in the nasal mucosa of allergic rhinitis and normals subjects. J Allergy Clin Immunol 1995; 95:716–725.
16. Costa JJ, Metcalfe DD. Mast cell cytokines, In: Kaliner MA, Metcalfe DD, eds., The mast cell in health and disease New York: Marcel Dekker, 1992, 443–466.

17. Bradding P, Feather IH, Howarth PH, Mueller R, Roberts J, Britten K, Bews JPA, Hunt TC, Okayama Y, Heusser CH, Bullock GR, Church MK, Holgate ST. Interleukin 4 is localized to and released by human mast cells. J Exp Med 1992; 176:1381–1386.
18. Gauchat JF, Henchoz S, Mazzei G, Aubry JP, Brunner T, Blasey H, Life P, Talabot D, Flores-Romo L, Thompson J, Kishi K, Butterfield J, Dahinden C, Bonnefoy JY. Induction of human IgE synthesis in B cells by mast cells and basophils. Nature 1993; 365;340–343.
19. Marsh DG, Norman PS. Antigens that cause atopic disease, In: Samter M, ed., Immunological diseases, 4th Ed., Boston: Little Brown & Co, Inc, 1988, 981–1008.
20. Solomon WR, Platts-Mills TAE. Aerobiology of inhalant allergens, In: Middleton E, Reed CE, Ellis EF, Adkinson NF Jr, Yunginger JW, Busse WW, eds., Allergy: Principles and practice, 4th Ed., St Louis: CV Mosby Co, 1993, 469–528.
21. Platts-Mills TAE, Heymann PW, Longbottom JL, et al. Airborn allergens associated with asthma: Particle sizes carrying dust mite and rat allergens measured with a cascade impactor, J Allergy Clin Immunol 1986; 77:850–857.
22. Nelson HS, Oppenheimer J, Buchmeier A, Kordash TR, Freshwater LL. An assessment of the role of intradermal skin testing in the diagnosis of clinically relevant allergy to timothy grass. J Allergy Clin Immunol 1996; 97:1193–1201.
23. Rosensteich DL, Eggleston P, Kattan M et al. The role of cockroach allergy and exposure to cockroach allergen in causing morbidity among inner-city children with asthma, N Engl J Med 1997; 336:1356–1363.
24. Nelson HS, Clinical application of immediate skin testing, In: Spector SL, ed., Provocation testing in clinical practice, New York: Marcel Dekker, 1995, 703–728.
25. Westley CR, Spiecher B, Starr L, et al. Cost effectiveness of an allergy consultation in the management of asthma, Allergy Asthma Proc 1997; 18:15–18.

7

Rhinitis, Sinusitis, and Acute Asthma

Susan M. Brugman
University of Colorado Health Sciences Center, Denver, Colorado

Although acute asthma is often the presenting complaint to the emergency department (ED), upper airway inflammation such as rhinitis and sinusitis may be the engine driving the more obvious lower airway disease. Given the contiguity between the upper and lower respiratory tracts, it should not be surprising that these two anatomic structures might influence each other. There is much debate as to whether upper airway conditions actually "cause" asthma or, conversely, whether the coexistent inflammation is merely an extension of the airways dysfunction that characterizes asthma. It is known that attacks of asthma are frequently precipitated by viral upper respiratory tract infections (URIs) and that chronic rhinosinusitis is associated with poor asthma control. Thus, inflammatory processes of the nose and sinuses should be investigated, particularly when asthma is recalcitrant or incompletely responsive to the usual therapies in the ED.

I. VIRAL UPPER RESPIRATORY TRACT INFECTIONS

The propensity of viral respiratory tract infections to trigger asthma episodes is well recognized and the subject of a chapter in itself. Approximately 30% of children will have a wheezing illness sometime in the first five years of life, with respiratory syncytial virus (RSV) the most common cause (1). Of the children previously infected with RSV, 30–50% will wheeze with subsequent viral URIs (2). In known young asthmatic children, viral URIs were discovered as the etiology of 42% of the acute wheezing episodes over a 2-year period (3). RSV, parainfluenza virus, coronavirus, and adenovirus were the causative agents. Of interest, no bacterial infections could be identified to cause asthmatic episodes. In two other similarly designed studies of childhood asthmatics, 29% (4) to 69% (5) of the asthma exacerbations were found to be associated with either rhinovirus, RSV, or influenza.

In adults, viral infections appear to precipitate asthma exacerbations only about 11% of the time (6,7). However, viral-induced episodes are more often severe and prolonged in adults when compared to noninfectious episodes of acute asthma (7,8). Interestingly, viruses, particularly adenovirus, have been recently implicated in chronic obstructive pulmonary disease (COPD) as well (9). Future studies may expand this hypothesis, giving more credence to the etiologic role of viruses in both acute and chronic airflow obstruction.

Viruses likely precipitate asthma by the following mechanisms: (1) enhancement of airways hyperresponsiveness; (2) damage to bronchial epithelium with sensitization of rapidly adapting sensory vagal fibers; (3) stimulation of vagus-mediated bronchoconstriction; (4) down regulation of β_2-adrenergic responsiveness; (5) propagation of virus-specific IgE antibodies; and (6) increased bronchospastic and inflammatory mediator release from pulmonary mast cells and basophils (10). Since effective antiviral therapies for airway diseases are sparse, the best treatment for viral-induced asthma in the ED setting is vigorous antiasthma medications.

II. *MYCOPLASMA/CHLAMYDIA* INFECTIONS

Other nonbacterial causes of acute asthma deterioration have been recognized and may be causative in the patient presenting emergently. *Mycoplasma pneumoniae* is a motile, filamentous, free-living organism without a cell wall that constitutes 20% of the nonviral or "walking" pneumonias in children and adults (11). In two studies of acute asthma, *M. pneumoniae* infection accounted for 20–25% of the wheezing episodes in adults compared with an isolation rate of 5.7% in normals (12,13). *M. pneumoniae* lower respiratory tract disease typically presents as an indolent prodrome of fever, malaise and headache followed in 3–5 days by cough and pharyngitis. Upper respiratory complaints are not common and pneumonia occurs in 10% of patients. Extrapulmonary manifestations are unusual but may be severe and involve gastrointestinal, hematologic, musculoskeletal, dermatologic, cardiac and neurologic organ systems.

Chlamydia pneumoniae (previously called Strain TWAR), an obligate intracellular parasite, has also been implicated in acute asthma. Nearly half of 19 wheezing adults and children studied prospectively were documented to have *C. pneumoniae* infection (14). Of these patients, four had their first attack of asthma and four had exacerbations of underlying asthma precipitated by *C. pneumoniae*. In another study of 74 adult outpatients with acute attacks of asthma, 9% were found to have *C. pneumoniae* infection by seroconversion (14a). Symptoms with this organism mimic those seen with *M. pneumoniae* infection although extrapulmonary involvement is not a feature.

If either of these organisms is highly suspected in the acutely wheezing patient, then antibiotic treatment with erythromycin, tetracycline (in older children and adults), or the newer macrolide antibiotics should be added to appropriate antiasthma therapy.

III. SINUSITIS

A. Prevalence

Sinusitis is a common disorder, affecting 14.7% of the U. S. population overall (15) and complicating 0.5–5% of upper respiratory infections in children (16). Since the average child experiences six to eight colds per year and since many children are in group daycare, which is more apt to result in protracted respiratory symptoms, the frequent occurrence of sinusitis in normal children is understandable (17). Furthermore, in pediatric patients presenting to allergy clinics with chronic respiratory complaints, 63% had documented sinusitis by computed tomographic (CT) imaging, evenly divided between allergic and nonallergic individuals (18). The financial burden of sinusitis is substantial, estimated at $2 billion dollars in over-the-counter drugs and $150 million in prescription medications (18a). The unmeasured cost in terms of diminished quality of life, pain, malaise, altered social functioning, and lost productivity at work has been documented as well (19,19a).

B. The Sinusitis/Asthma Link

The association between asthma and sinusitis has long been recognized although the precise nature of this relationship remains contentious. There are several lines of evidence linking these two entities (Table 1). Very early observations documented the common coprevalence of sinusitis and asthma. Approximately 26% of asthmatic adults and up to 70% of asthmatic children were found to have sinusitis (20,21). More recent investigators have concurred with these observations, finding a 50% incidence of abnormal sinus radiographs in a pediatric allergy clinic population (22) and in severe, inpatient asthmatic children (23). Radiographic and symptomatic sinusitis among adult patients presenting with acute asthma exacerbations has been reported to occur in 50–87% (24,25).

The demonstration of a nasobronchial reflex by early physiologists spurred interest in the connection between nasal and pulmonary pathology. Nasal stimulation of animals with a number of irritants (26,27) or with electricity (28) resulted in demonstrable increases in lower airways resistance. Likewise in humans, sensory excitement of the nose has been found to increase lower airways resistance and worsen asthma symptoms (29–31). That this reflex arc is vagally mediated is suggested by its obliteration with vagal sectioning (28,32) and with anticholinergics (31,32). The extension of these observations to allergic nasal inflammation and asthma in humans has been debated. Several investigators failed to observe any change in lung function in allergic asthmatics in whom histamine or ragweed particles were applied to the nose (33–35). However, a significant drop in FEV_1 following intranasal histamine could be demonstrated in half the patients with active rhinitis, indicating that perhaps a certain baseline nasal inflammation is necessary to "prime" this reflex (36). Furthermore, it appears that while lung function may remain unchanged after nasal allergen challenge, lower airways responsiveness increases measurably in allergic asthmatics (37,38). This increase has been shown to be blocked by intrana-

Table 1 Evidence to Suggest a Link Between Rhinosinusitis and Asthma

1. Coprevalence of asthma and sinusitis and/or rhinitis
2. Abnormal sinus radiographs in asthma patients
3. Demonstration of a nasobronchial reflex
4. Demonstration of postnasal drip in association with lower airways hyperresponsiveness
5. Improvement in airways hyperresponsiveness following nasal treatment
6. Improvement in asthma following medical and/or surgical treatment of sinusitis

sal steroids given during natural allergen exposure (39,40). In a study comparing the effectiveness of various intranasal anti-inflammatory agents on allergic rhinitis symptoms in 120 adults, Welsh remarked that "surprisingly, we also found that these intranasal treatments considerably reduced the symptoms of seasonal asthma" (42). A subsequent randomized, placebo-controlled, crossover study corroborated this observation in 23 children, finding a decrease in asthma scores as well as rhinitis scores among subjects treated with intranasal steroids (42a). Other investigators report that asthma symptoms also improve with this nasal anti-inflammatory treatment, further lending credence to the theory that a nasobronchial reflex is likely contributory to allergic asthma (40–42).

Perhaps the most convincing evidence for disease association is documented improvement in asthma when concurrent sinusitis is treated. Indeed, several studies have demonstrated this phenomenon. Medical treatment of chronic sinusitis (including three 6-week courses of antibiotics, intranasal steroids and oral decongestants) in 48 asthmatic children resulted in an impressive amelioration of asthma symptoms, medication requirements, and pulmonary functions abnormalities. In 80% of these patients, cough, wheezing, and rhinorrhea disappeared and 79% were able to discontinue all daily antiasthma therapy and oral corticosteroids (22). Several other studies, mostly uncontrolled, corroborated these findings in both children (43) and adults (44). Cummings et al. performed a double-blind, placebo-controlled trial of medical sinusitis treatment in 42 children with severe asthma. This study documented improvement in asthma and a trend toward a lowered airways responsiveness after three weeks of oral antibiotics, oral and intranasal decongestants, and intranasal steroids when compared to identical placebos (45).

Surgery appears to be of benefit in intractable asthma where sinusitis is circumstantially related. Slavin reported an improvement in asthma symptoms in 65% of adults who underwent aggressive surgical treatment of sinusitis (46). This effect was sustained for up to 5 years in 60% of the original patients, most of whom also reported significant relief of nasal symptoms (47). With the advent of less invasive surgical approaches, specifically, functional endoscopic sinus surgery (FESS), the outcome for even less severely affected asthmatics appears even better. In an uncontrolled retrospective analysis of 52 children, ages 7 months to 17 years, 46% had coexisting asthma (48). From 12 to 38 months following FESS, 96% had fewer or no episodes of asthma, 58% were asymptomatic, and there was a 79% decrease in ED visits per year. There was no information, however, about the severity of asthma, the use of medications or the degree of pulmonary function impairment in these children. In a similar retrospective study, 20 of 32 asthmatic adults who had undergone FESS for chronic sinusitis responded to a mailed questionnaire (49). Comparing the year before surgery to the year after, patients reported a decrease in the frequency of their asthma symptoms (95%), a diminished severity of asthma (80%), a decrease in routine asthma medications (54%), less need for intermittent or daily steroids (54%), and a substantial reduction in hospitalizations (75%) and ED visits (81%). Prospective studies are needed to corroborate these results, which support the notion that sinusitis is causally linked to asthma.

C. Definition

Another more recent report classifies sinusitis as follows (19a): Sinusitis has been aptly described as the "cold that doesn't go away" (50). In truth, even acute, uncomplicated colds in normal adults have been associated with abnormalities in the sinuses by highly sensitive computed tomographic imaging in nearly 90% of the cases (51). Sinusitis is part and parcel of allergic rhinitis as well (52). The diagnosis of sinusitis can thus be problematic since there is so much symptom overlap with these entities. However, the time course of persistent or worsening symptoms appears to be the best indicator of significant sinus disease. However, there remains controversy regarding the chronologic classification of sinusitis. A recent consensus panel has proposed the following definitions of sinusitis based upon symptom endurance: (1) *acute*: between 7 and 14 days; (2) *subacute*: 2–12 weeks; and (3) *chronic*: greater than 3 months (53). This same panel proposed symptom criteria upon which to base a clinical diagnosis of sinusitis (Table 2). It should be noted that no one symptom is an accurate marker for this disease. Acute sinusitis of a severe nature is likely to be present if high fever (>39°C), lethargy, and/or periorbital edema accompany typical cold symptoms, in which case prompt treatment is reasonable (54).

1. *Acute*: symptoms present for less than eight weeks in adults and less than twelve weeks in children.

Table 2 Symptoms of Sinusitis

Signs and Symptoms
Major criteria
Purulent nasal discharge
Purulent pharyngeal drainage
Cough
Minor criteria
Periorbital edema[a]
Headache[b]
Facial pain[b]
Tooth pain[b]
Earache
Sore throat
Foul breath
Increased wheeze
Fever
Diagnostic Tests
Major criteria
Waters' radiograph with opacification, air fluid level, or thickened mucosa filling ≥ 50% of antrum
Coronal CT scan with thickening of mucosa or opacification of sinus
Minor criteria
Nasal cytologic study (smear) with neutrophils and bacteremia
Ultrasound studies
Probable Sinusitis
Signs and symptoms: 2 major criteria or 1 major and ≥ 2 minor criteria
Diagnostic tests: 1 major = confirmatory. 1 minor = supportive

[a] More common in children.
[b] More common in adults.
Source: From Ref. 53, with permission.

2. *Subacute*: indeterminate period of mild to moderate symptomatology.
3. *Chronic*: symptoms beyond 8–12 weeks and documented with sinus imaging after four weeks of medical treatment.

It is apparent that precise time courses of symptoms for making the diagnosis of sinusitis are still not agreed upon.

Most children with sinusitis present with chronic or recurrent cough, purulent rhinorrhea, or recurrent acute otitis media. Headache, facial pain, toothache, and facial fullness are not the common complaints they are in adults (53). A history of halitosis can be elicited from the parents although it is not usually volunteered as a problem. Painless periorbital swelling is also reported by parents. There are several conditions predisposing to sinusitis that should be considered and remedied when possible (Table 3).

D. Pathophysiology

The sinuses are air-filled cavities that develop as evaginations of the nasal mucous membranes and are part of the continuos mucosal-lined surface of the upper respiratory tract. Numerous functions have been ascribed to the sinuses including: (1) lessening the density

Table 3 Predisposing Factors for Sinusitis

- Systemic disorders
  - Ciliary dysmotility syndromes (including Kartagener's Syndrome)
  - Cystic fibrosis
  - Down's syndrome
  - Immunodeficiency (including AIDS)
  - Aspirin sensitivity
  - Wegener's granulomatosis
  - Young's syndrome (bronchiectasis and obstructive azoospermia)
  - Pregnancy
- Local Disorders
  - Recurrent viral respiratory tract infections
  - Dental infections
  - Swimming
  - Diving (barotrauma)
  - Facial trauma
  - Nasal obstruction
    - foreign body
    - septal deviation
    - polyps
    - tumors
    - adenoid hypertrophy
      - nasogastric or nasotracheal intubation
      - anatomic intranasal variants (e.g., concha bullosa, Haller cells, variant uncinate process)
  - Allergic or nonallergic rhinitis
  - Rhinitis medicamentosa
  - Cocaine abuse
  - Environmental tobacco smoke exposure

and weight of the skull; (2) improving voice resonance; (3) equalizing pressure differences in the nasal cavity; (4) aiding olfaction; (5) regulating the temperature and humidity of the ambient air; and (6) providing an air buffer to concussive effects of trauma (55). The sinuses are lined by a membrane consisting of pseudostratified, ciliated, columnar epithelium covered with a 10–15 micron thick mucus blanket. This mucus blanket absorbs gases and traps microbes and particulate matter as it is constantly propelled toward the sinus ostia (in an antigravitational manner in the maxillary sinuses) by ciliary beating at a rate of 6 mm/min. The mucus enters the nasal cavity, where it can either drain and be swallowed or blown out.

That the sinuses function in such a highly efficient manner is largely dependent upon the patency of the sinus ostia. Of particular importance is the structure known as the ostiomeatal complex. This structure is the confluence of the anterior ethmoid sinuses, the ostia of the frontal and maxillary sinuses, and the middle meatus (Figure 1). The obstruction of this complex by mucosal edema, mucus, or structural anomalies is now believed to be the original event in the cascade that leads to all sinus inflammation. Mucus stagnation and hypoxemia within the sinuses then predisposes to overgrowth of resident nasal bacteria. Ciliated cells are damaged, thus disabling the ''mucociliary escalator'' from its function of secretion clearance. Other factors such as immunoglobulin A, antimicrobial proteins, and surface enzymes also play a part in sinus homeostasis (56).

Sinusitis is an inflammation of the sinus membranes. Mucosal swelling is an early manifestation, followed by mucus hypersecretion and fluid accumulation in the obstructed sinus. This is apparent on the Water's view x-ray as air-fluid levels or complete opacification of the maxillary sinuses. When this inflammatory process becomes chronic, the lining

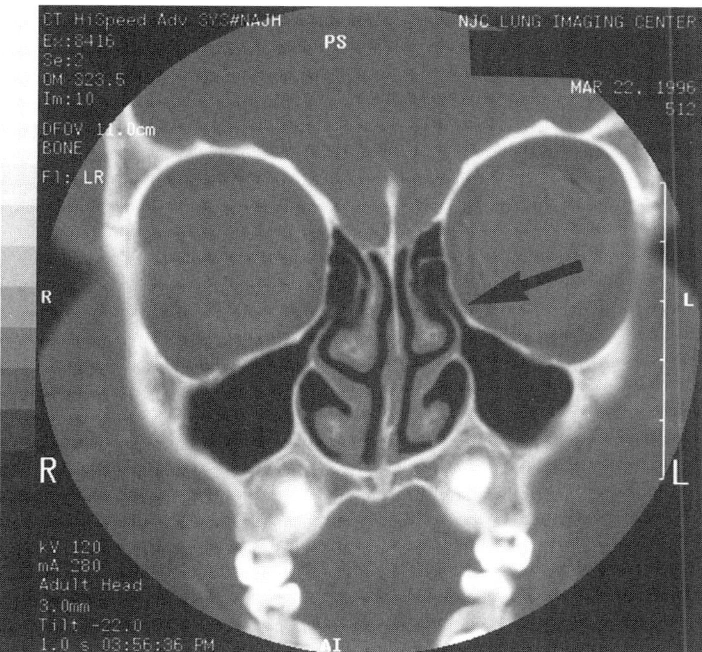

Figure 1 The ostiomeatal complex. (See text for details.)

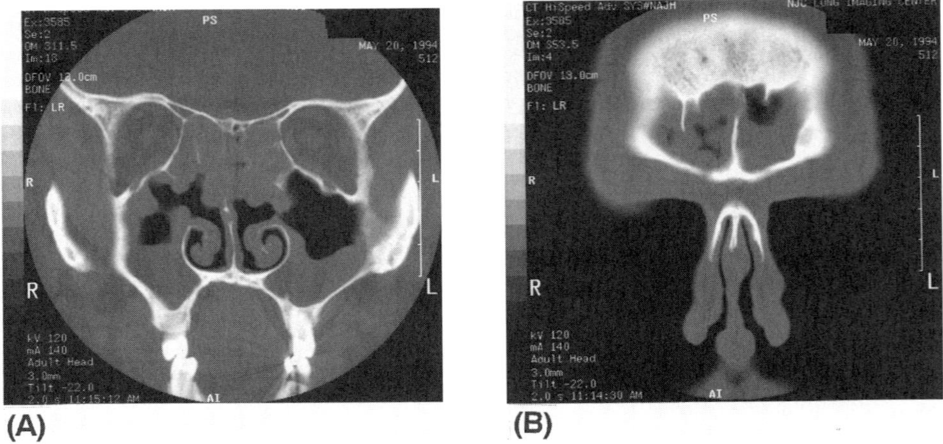

Figure 2 X-rays showing sinusitis. (See text for details.)

mucosa thickens, becomes ''heaped up'' in appearance, and may proliferate into polyps (Fig. 2). Polyps complicate rhinosinusitis in about 7% of asthmatics and are seen frequently in aspirin sensitive individuals (discussed below) (57). Other complications of chronic sinusitis include mucus retention cysts (inflammatory obstruction of seromucinous glands within the sinus mucosa) and mucoceles (dilated, mucus-engorged sinus whose ostium is completely blocked). Thickened bone adjacent to the sinuses or frank osteomyelitis are occasionally seen in chronic sinusitis but are usually indicative of fungal pathology (58).

Bacterial pathogens have been recovered in high density ($>10^{-4}$ cfu/ml) from maxillary puncture in up to 70% of children and 25–59% of adults with acute maxillary sinusitis (59,60). Although not similarly quantitated, bacteria have also been identified in 93% of children with chronic, surgically treated sinusitis (61). The failure to recover bacteria in some cases may, as Gwaltney speculates, be due to involvement of sinuses other than the maxillary antra, prolonged viral infection, or infection with unusual organisms (62). On the contrary, eosinophilic infiltration of sinus mucosa has been seen more often in allergic rhinitis and asthma than in uncomplicated chronic sinusitis, raising the possibility of noninfectious eosinophil toxicity to the tissue as a primary pathogenic factor (62a). The sinuses are sterile under usual circumstances even though the major bacterial pathogens causing sinusitis (Table 4) can be normal ''residents'' of the nose or posterior nasopharynx (62). It has been speculated that viral colds predispose to sinusitis through inflammatory obstruction of the ostiomeatal complex and by damage to the lining epithelium, the sum of which compromises normal sinus drainage and promotes bacterial overgrowth.

E. Diagnosis

Although sinusitis is primarily a clinical diagnosis, other tools can be helpful in establishing the presence and extent of disease. These include: nasal cytology, radiographic imaging, transillumination, ultrasonography, and bacterial sampling of the sinuses.

Table 4 Pathogens in Sinusitis (Generally in Order of Frequency)

	Adult[a]	Childhood[b]
Acute	*S. pneumoniae*	*S. pneumoniae*
	H. influenzae	*M. catarrhalis*
	Anaerobes	*H. influenzae*
	Streptococcal sp.	
	M. catarrhalis	
	S. aureus	
Chronic	Aerobes	Aerobes (38%)
	H. influenzae	Alpha-hemolytic strep
	Coagulase negative *S. aureus*	Group A β-hemolytic strep
	Corynebacerium sp.	Group F β-hemolytic strep
	Alpha hemolytic strep	*S. aureus*
	S. aureus	*S. epidermidis*
	Other	*E. coli*
		H. influenzae
		H. parainfluenzae
	Anerobes	Anaerobes (100%)
	Bacteroides	
	Veillonella	
	Peptostreptococcus sp.	
	Hemolytic strep	

Sources: [a] From Refs. 60, 102, 103; [b] from Ref. 104.

1. *Nasal Cytology*

The cellular milieu within the nose can be sampled by having the patient blow his or her nose into cellophane wrap, then smearing the mucus on a glass slide and staining it. Normal nasal mucus is comprised of ciliated and nonciliated columnar epithelial cells, goblet cells, and basal cells. Neutrophils are sparse and there are usually no basophils or eosinophils present (63). Large numbers of neutrophils and intracellular bacteria are frequently present in nasal smears of sinusitis patients. A 79% correlation between radiographic sinusitis and a positive nasal cytology (defined as a nasal smear showing greater than 6 neutrophils per high-power field) has been reported (64). In a population of 300 allergic rhinitis patients, sinusitis was found radiographically more often when the nasal smear showed more than 5 neutrophils or 5 eosinophils per high-power field (65). That nasal eosinophilia closely reflects active allergic rhinitis has been seen in both children and adults (66,67). The clinical context is most important to the interpretation of the nasal smear since neutrophils are present in uncomplicated colds as well. Furthermore, there is no study that correlates nasal cytology to bacterial aspirates of the sinuses so this procedure has yet to be validated against the "gold standard."

2. *Radiographic Imaging*

Three plain x-ray views of the sinuses have been the traditional standard for diagnosing sinusitis. Lateral, occipitomeatal (Water's), and anteroposterior (Caldwell) views are obtained to visualize the sphenoid, maxillary, and ethmoid and frontal sinuses respectively. The presence of an air-fluid level, complete opacification of the sinuses, and mucosal thickening of greater than 4 mm correlates with bacterial recovery from the sinuses nearly 75% of the time (16,68). Plain sinus films are readily available, relatively inexpensive, and do not require much patient cooperation or sedation.

Despite long experience with plain radiography, there are numerous disadvantages: (1) inadequate specificity in infants less than one year of age in whom crying, sinus asymmetry and underdevelopment, or redundancy of sinus mucosa may manifest as sinus opacification (69); (2) frequent false positives and false negatives in both children and adults (70,71); and (3) superimposition of sinus structures preventing adequate visualization of the posterior ethmoids, the ostiomeatal complex and the sphenoid sinus. A recent task force report from the American College of Radiology suggests that the usefulness of plain sinus radiography in acute sinusitis of all ages is marginal and should be discouraged (72).

CT imaging demonstrates fine sinus detail and is the technique of choice in evaluating sinusitis. Multiple, thin section images (approximately 5 mm thickness at 3–5 mm intervals) in the coronal plane are typical (Fig. 3). Axial plane images may be easier to obtain in children although they are not as useful in evaluating the ostiomeatal complex. A screening sinus CT involves fewer cuts at greater intervals and has the advantage of less cost (often similar to that of plain radiography), less radiation dose, and shorter study time. The screening study is not particularly helpful in children because it does not obviate the need for sedation and because it frequently misses the ostiomeatal complex and thus gives suboptimal information.

Accepting sinus CT as the gold standard is complicated by the frequent overestimation of clinical sinusitis. Incidental maxillary and/or ethmoid abnormalities have been

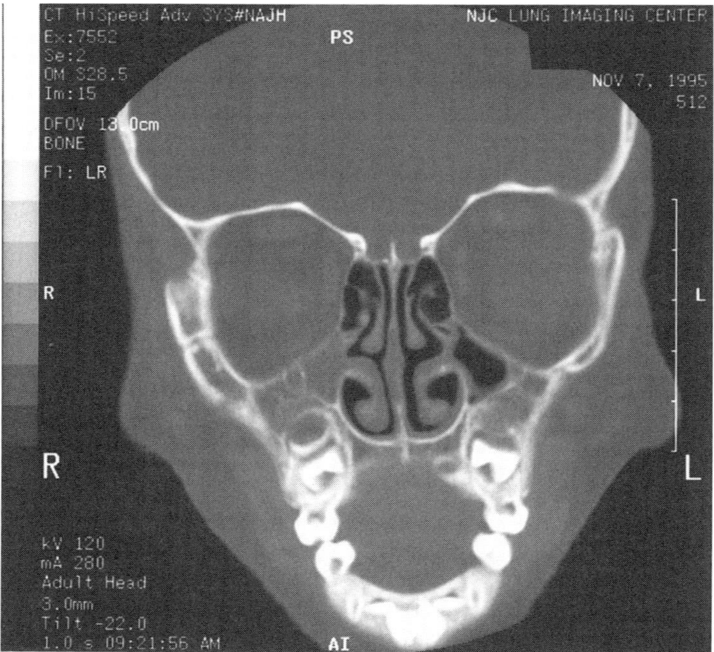

Figure 3 Computed tomographic (CT) imaging showing sinusitis. (See text for details.)

reported in 14–55% of children less than 13 years of age undergoing CT scanning of the head for nonrespiratory reasons (73). The common cold is known to cause CT-evident sinus inflammation that is self-limited in both adults and in infants younger than one year of age (51,69). The clinical context is essential in the proper ordering and interpreting of sinus CTs. They are rarely necessary in the management of acute sinusitis (72).

Magnetic resonance imaging (MRI) uses radiofrequency waves in a magnetic field to produce sinus images. MRI gives superior soft-tissue imaging and is the technique of choice if tumor or extensive infection of the paranasal sinuses is suspected. The expense, long examination time, need to sedate pediatric patients, and poor resolution of bony structures, especially the ostiomeatal complex, limits the usefulness of MRI in sinus disease.

For the emergency physician, sinus imaging of any sort is rarely indicated, except when acute complications of sinusitis are a concern (see Table 5). Patients who fail medical management of their acute or chronic sinusitis in the ED should probably be referred to an otolaryngologist for further diagnostic evaluation.

3. *Transillumination*

This technique consists of examining the patient in a darkened room and shining a light (usually from an otoscope) against the inferior orbital ridge. Transmission of light through the hard palate is assessed at the open mouth of the patient (74). A failure of transillumination is interpreted to mean fluid or mucosal swelling of the respective maxillary sinus. Unfortunately, this technique is not sensitive enough nor used often enough to be of any value to most practitioners, including those in the ED.

4. *Ultrasound Evaluation*

A-mode ultrasonography of the sinuses has the advantages of being radiation-free, rapid, and not requiring sedation in pediatric patients. This technique was reported on in Scandinavia in the 1980s and was found to correlate well with the presence of maxillary fluid on puncture (75,76). However, as reviewed by Druce, there are other reports that are conflicting as to its usefulness (77). Ultrasonography appears to be highly specific (93%) but not very sensitive (29–61%) (78,79). It is not useful for evaluating frontal disease and, indeed, ultrasound cannot provide the detailed view of intranasal and sinus structure that is needed in the evaluation of chronic sinusitis. At present, the only reasonable clinical

Table 5 Indications for High Resolution CT Imaging of the Sinuses in Children and Adults

1. Persistent symptoms after two 3-week courses of antibiotics and adjunctive treatments
2. Evidence of complications of sinusitis
   - orbital celluitis
   - intracranial abscess
   - osteomyelitis
   - toxic shock syndrome
3. Preoperative assessment of anatomy
4. Difficult-to-treat asthma with persistent rhinosinal symptoms
5. Unilateral symptoms or suspicion of a tumor

application for ultrasound is in diagnosing sinusitis in pregnant women in whom avoidance of ionizing radiation is prudent. The need for this in the ED would be quite unusual.

5. Sinus Puncture

This technique is truly the gold standard for diagnosing infectious sinusitis. A trocar is passed transnasally into the maxillary sinus and fluid is either directly aspirated or else sterile saline in injected and aspirated. Aerobic and anaerobic cultures and Gram's stain of the fluid is undertaken. A finding of one bacterial organism per high-power field on a Gram's stain correlates with growth of bacteria $>10^4$ colony-forming units per milliliter (74). Sinus puncture is usually reserved for the patient with evidence of complications, severe facial pain, associated immunosuppression, or disease unresponsive to repeated treatment. This technique usually requires sedation in the pediatric patient and should only be done by a skilled operator.

F. Childhood Sinusitis

There is a common misconception that young children cannot have sinusitis because they do not have sinuses. Although there is wide variability among children, most have aerated maxillary and ethmoid sinuses at birth with later development of the sphenoid and frontal sinuses (see Table 6) (Fig. 3) (80). There appears to be a predilection among younger children for chronic sinusitis. Among 58 children with chronic sinusitis by CT imaging, 48% were 2–6 years of age and 34% were 6–10 years of age (81). In fact, young age was the single most significant risk factor for sinusitis in children presenting with chronic respiratory symptoms (81).

Purulent nasal discharge has often been referred to as ''bacterial'' or ''purulent'' rhinitis or ''adenoiditis.'' The publication in 1981 of Dr. Wald's first treatise on bacterial sinusitis in children allowed this diagnosis to be legitimately entertained in place of the less precise ones mentioned above (82). Sinusitis has become the fifth most common diagnosis for which antibiotic therapy is prescribed among adults (83), a trend that is no doubt similar for children as well.There is debate, however, as to whether sinusitis is being overdiagnosed and overtreated in children (84). Diagnosis by symptom constellation is difficult, given the overlap with viral upper respiratory tract infections. The symptom duration parameters are inexact in that some uncomplicated URIs may last three weeks or more (17). As discussed previously, radiographic diagnosis is expensive, sometimes technically complicated (i.e., requiring sedation) and too sensitive to be the gold standard (see Section III. E. 2). Treatment of suspected sinusitis with antibiotics raises issues of

Table 6 Development of the Paranasal Sinuses

Sinus	Present	Developed
Ethmoid	Birth	3 yr
Maxillary	Birth	3 yr
Sphenoid	3 yr	12 yr
Frontal[a]	8 yr	12 yr

[a] Absent in approximately 10% of the population.
Source: Ref. 80.

expense, uncertainty as to duration of therapy, only modest improvement in cure rate, and the risk of generating more or different strains of resistant bacterial pathogens. On the other hand, one could argue that complications from sinusitis, while infrequent, can be severe and costly. With a huge proportion of children in out-of-home daycare, treatment of bacterial sinusitis will likely hasten their return to daycare and their parents' return to the workplace. For the asthmatic child, there is the important potential for ameliorating asthma symptoms, restoring normal sleep patterns, decreasing medical utilization, and enhancing quality of life by effectively treating the sinusitis.

G. Medical Treatment

Once the diagnosis of sinusitis is made in the acute asthmatic, treatment for both disorders should be instituted promptly. Follow-up is advisable in 2–3 days if there is no improvement in either asthma or sinusitis symptoms; otherwise it should be arranged for two weeks hence.

1. Antibiotics

Antibiotics are the cornerstone of medical management of sinusitis in both adults and children. Studies in adults using sinus puncture and culture before and after antibiotic therapy have shown successful eradication of bacteria along with symptomatic improvement (74). Similar documentation in pediatric patients is lacking although numerous studies have shown resolution of clinical symptoms of sinusitis with antibiotic treatment (74). The choice of antibiotic follows from the bacteriology of acute and chronic sinusitis (Table 6). Since there is a 45% spontaneous cure rate for acute sinusitis in all age groups, the first rule of therapy should be safety (85,86). Thus, amoxacillin is the preferred first-line antibiotic for adults and children (Table 7). In spite of a high rate of beta-lactamase producing *Hemophilis influenzae* in most communities, the clinical cure rate for amoxacillin is 93–100% in adults and 67–100% in children (74). Whether the emergence of penicillin-resistant pneumococci will alter this success rate for amoxacillin remains to be seen.

The first choice antibiotic for patients hypersensitive to penicillin is trimethoprim-sulfamethoxasole or erythromycin-sulfasoxazole. In the setting of severe, acute sinusitis (high fever, periorbital swelling, and systemic toxicity), a broader spectrum, beta-lactamase resistant drug such as amoxacillin/clavulanate or a second- or third-generation cephalosporin (cefuroxime or cefprozil) should be initially instituted. Likewise, a lack of clini-

Table 7 Antibiotics for the Treatment of Sinusitis

Drug	Pediatric dosage	Adult dosage
1. Amoxacillin	40 mg/kg/d in 3DD	1500 mg/d in 3DD
2. Amoxacillin/clavulanate	40/10 mg/kg/d in 3DD	750/1500 mg/d in 3DD
3. Trimethoprim-sulfamethoxazole	8/40 mg/kg/d in 2DD	320/1600 mg/d in 2DD
4. Cefaclor	40 mg/kg/d in 3DD	2000 mg/d in 4DD
5. Cefuroxime axetil	250 mg/d in 2DD (<2 yr) 500 mg/d in 2DD (2–12 yr)	500–1000 mg/d in 2DD
6. Cefprozil	30 mg/kg/d in 2DD	500 mg/d in 1 dose
7. Erythromycin/sulfasoxazole	50/150 mg/kg/d in 4DD	—

DD = divided doses.

cal response within three days in any patient should also prompt a return visit to the ED and a change in antibiotics.

The first-line agents for chronic sinusitis are the same as for acute sinusitis with the proviso that a second, three-week course of a broader spectrum antibiotic should follow if there is a suboptimal response to the initial treatment.

The newer macrolide antibiotics (azithromycin, clarithromycin) have excellent antimicrobial coverage for usual sinusitis organisms. Only clarithromycin has approved for acute sinusitis.

The optimal duration of therapy has not been systematically studied. For acute sinusitis, significant improvement is usually seen within four days and a 10–14 day course of treatment is recommended (74). However, at least one study found comparable efficacy from a three-day vs. a 10-day course of trimethoprim-sulfamethoxasole in acute sinusitis (87). It has been argued that entry criteria for this study were vague and that many individuals with common colds were included, thus casting doubt on the conclusions (87a). For chronic sinusitis, there are no studies determining the ideal duration of therapy. It is generally agreed that 21 days of antimicrobials is indicated (88). Multiple short (7–10 days) courses of different and increasingly expensive broad-spectrum antibiotics have no advantage over more prolonged therapy with a first-line antimicrobial.

2. Saline Nasal Lavage and Steam Inhalation

Salutary effects of steam inhalation and nasal irrigation have been touted as folk remedies for sinusitis although the scientific proof is not robust (88,89). Steam generated in a hot shower or inhaled from a pan of boiling water with a towel draped around the head are two methods of inhalation. The addition of astringents or aromatics (pine oil, menthol, oil of eucalyptus) may enhance the sensation of nasal patency. Saline nasal lavage can be accomplished by one of several methods (Table 8). Both of these techniques allow for removal of adherent, dried mucus, and blood; moisturization of the nasal mucosa; and cleansing of the mucus membrane prior to instilling intranasal decongestants or topical steroids. The soothing and symptomatic relief provided by these methods may be enough to recommend them in spite of little data proving their efficacy.

Table 8 Techniques for Saline Nasal Lavage

1. Mix a solution of one-fourth to one-half teaspoon of noniodized table salt and a pinch of baking soda with 8 ounces of tepid tap water. This solution should be prepared fresh with every treatment.
2. Fill a 2-ounce bulb syringe (available at most pharmacies) with saline and, while leaning over a sink or bathtub, squeeze the contents into one side of the nose under pressure. Saline will drip down the back of the throat and from both sides of the nose. Alternate in opposite nares until saline is gone. Blow nose afterwards to evacuate all the liquid (nose may drip for up to 10 min after lavage).
3. Bottled saline nose spray may be used as an alternative. Spray each nostril alternately several times while sniffing the saline, then blow nose.
4. The "snuffing" technique consists of pouring the saline solution into the hand and snuffing it up one nostril at a time.
5. A Water Pik® device fitted with a nasal adapter (Hydro Med Inc., Los Angeles, CA) is especially helpful in paients who have had sinus surgery. Saline is washed ito each nostril at the lowest Water Pik® pressure.

3. Decongestants and Antihistamines

Decongestants are vasoconstrictors that are the mainstay of over-the-counter cold and sinus remedies. Oral formulations have been shown to enlarge sinus ostia in chronic sinusitis by as much as 50% (90). One study of the effectiveness of phenylpropanolamine in acute sinusitis found a poorer outcome in patients in whom this drug was added to the regimen (91). Controlled studies are unavailable to corroborate or refute this finding. Decongestants are remarkably well tolerated for extended periods of time in adults but hypertension may be a significant concern. In children, hyperactivity and insomnia are frequent adverse effects. Topical decongestants are very effective in relieving nasal mucosal swelling but must be limited to 3–5 days to avoid serious rebound rhinitis. These agents are indicated for acute colds, as prophylaxis for barometric pressure changes during air travel, and as short-term adjuncts to intranasal steroids.

Oral decongestants are often combined with antihistamines for a dual effect. Histamine-mediated symptoms include sneezing, watery rhinorrhea, and nasal itching in addition to nasal obstruction. Antihistamines are only beneficial in the setting of allergy-associated sinus inflammation and should be reserved for those specific patients. Newer, nonsedating, selective H1-antihistamines are preferable because they are less likely to result in dried, inspissated secretions. The caution that antihistamines may dry lower airway secretions and thus should not be used in asthma has not been substantiated (92).

4. Intranasal Steroids

Applying topical steroids to the nasal mucosa has the theoretic advantage of subduing inflammation at the critical ostiomeatal complex. These agents (beclomethasone, triamcinolone, budesonide, flunisolide, dexamethasone) have gained wide usage in allergic rhinitis and in patients with nasal polyposis (93). There are recent data to support their use as adjunctive treatment of sinusitis (94). Typically, intranasal steroids are added after nasal decongestion has been achieved with topical vasoconstrictors for 3–5 days. There is no prohibition to the long-term use of intranasal steroids and they may be prophylactic in patients prone to recurrent or chronic sinusitis. The risk of septal perforation is minimal, especially when patients are instructed to deliver the spray to each nostril with the opposite hand, thereby directing the drug away from the septum. Intranasal steroids can be used safely in young children although they are labeled for use only over the age of 5 years.

5. Oral Corticosteroids

Oral prednisone or methylprednisolone provides potent anti-inflammatory therapy for the patient failing other therapy or for the patient with severe, obstructive polyposis. Treatment should be limited to 1–2 weeks.

6. Prevention

Allergically mediated sinusitis should be investigated with history and prick skin testing to determine what allergens can be eliminated or avoided in the environment. Viral-induced sinusitis may be decreased by close attention to viral vectors (children, especially in daycare settings; hands and surfaces in home, school, and work environments) and by timely influenza vaccination.

H. Surgical Treatment

Referral of an ED patient for surgical treatment of sinusitis would be an unusual occurrence. The primary acute indication for sinus surgery is an infectious complication, particularly orbital cellulitis, intracranial abscess, osteomyelitis, or toxic shock syndrome. Other surgical indications are not emergent and include: (1) chronic sinusitis that has failed prolonged medical therapy; (2) coexistent, severe, steroid-dependent asthma, especially if improvement in asthma is demonstrable when the sinus disease is controlled; (3) severe polyposis unresponsive to oral or topical steroids; and (4) obstructive anatomic variants within the nose that are surgically remediable. The understanding of the critical role of the ostiomeatal complex in sinus pathophysiology has revolutionized sinus surgery. Thus, radical procedures (e.g., Caldwell–Luc) that stripped sinus mucosa and created artificial maxillary ostia have given way to endoscopic techniques that preserve the mucous membrane and open existing ostia to improve natural drainage (95). The role of sinus surgery in improving underlying asthma has been addressed above.

I. Associated Upper Respiratory Tract Conditions

1. Aspirin Sensitivity and Nasal Polyps

Sinusitis is so integral a part of typical "triad asthma" (asthma, nasal polyposis, and aspirin intolerance) that it has been suggested this syndrome be called "tetrad asthma" (57). Nasal polyposis is rare in childhood and its presence in anyone under age 20 should prompt an evaluation for cystic fibrosis where the incidence is 6.7–27% (96). Tetrad asthma predominantly affects adults over age 40 years and is often associated with severe, usually nonallergic, and steroid-dependent asthma. Other characteristics of these patients include a normal serum IgE level, peripheral and nasal eosinophilia, and acute bronchospasm, rhinorrhea, and sometimes anaphylaxis with the ingestion of aspirin, indomethacin, ibuprofen, and other nonsteroidal antiinflammatory medications. A predilection to sinusitis is thought to result from both the obstruction of the ostiomeatal complex by the nasal polyps as well as by the toxic effects of eosinophilic mediators that retard ciliary clearance within the nose and sinuses (57).

In addition to standard sinusitis treatment, oral corticosteroids in decreasing doses over 7–10 days should be considered and may be repeated. Intranasal steroids are a mainstay over the long term and intrapolyp injection of systemic steroids may be helpful in selected cases (97). Polypectomy is effective in the short term but is rarely a permanent cure. Of 143 patients undergoing polypectomy, 40% had three or more procedures to treat recurrent disease (98). Another form of therapy is aspirin desensitization that may benefit both the sinusitis and asthma. The 1–3 day, medically supervised protocol involves ingesting increasing doses of oral aspirin until a reaction occurs or until the patient tolerates the maximum dose of 650 mg. The patient must continue to take aspirin daily to maintain the desensitization or risk recurrent aspirin intolerance (99).

2. Vocal Cord Dysfunction

Among other upper airway abnormalities is vocal cord dysfunction (VCD), a functional disorder of the larynx that is frequently mistaken for asthma (100). Patients present to the ED with acute, often severe, respiratory distress along with inspiratory and/or expiratory wheezing. They complain of choking, suffocating, "not getting enough air in," hoarseness, and throat or chest tightness (100a,101). VCD results from a paradoxical closure of the vocal cords, primarily on inspiration, with consequent obstruction of the upper airway. VCD is frequently seen in conjunction with asthma, although the rapid onset of attacks, the inspiratory stridor, and the normal pulse oximetry in the face of apparent severe distress helps to differentiate these two entities. Upper airway inflammation is thought to predispose certain individuals to attacks of VCD, presumably because of the laryngeal irritation brought on by postnasal drip of secretions and possibly by the breathing of cold, dry air due to nasal obstruction. The importance of recognizing VCD cannot be overemphasized. Asthma medications are usually ineffective and the mistaken diagnosis of an organic upper airway obstruction has resulted in inappropriate intubation and even cricothyrotomy to treat this functional disorder (100,100a). Treatment of VCD in the ED starts with a calm, reassuring manner and breathing exercises coached by a speech therapist if this is available. Inhalation of a helium-oxygen gas mixture (70–80% helium, 20–30% oxygen) by face mask at 6–10 LPM may abort the upper airway obstruction by decreasing the resistance in an area of turbulent airflow (100,101a). Because heliox also overcomes lower airways obstruction in a like manner, a response to this therapy alone will not differentiate asthma from VCD. The inhalation of nebulized lidocaine (2 cc of 2% liquid lidocaine) has been used anecdotally to anesthetize laryngeal afferents but this therapy has never been studied. It is paramount that underlying conditions that may result in an irritable upper airway (e.g., rhinitis, sinusitis, gastroesophageal reflux) as well as psychosocial stress and anxiety be recognized and treated appropriately as well.

J. Conclusion

Upper airway processes are frequently comorbid with asthma and may contribute to the severity of disease in patients who present to the ED. Viruses constitute a common provocation for attacks of asthma and, of themselves, require only symptomatic treatment. *Mycoplasma pneumoniae* and *Chlamydia pneumonie* are less well studied but potential causes of acute asthma exacerbations and should be considered and treated. Bacterial sinusitis, either acute or chronic, is linked to poorly controlled asthma. A high index of suspicion can guide appropriate historical questioning that can lead to a clinical diagnosis and treatment. Follow-up is important to determine resolution of both the acute asthma and upper airway symptoms.

REFERENCES

1. Henderson FW, Clyde WA Jr, Collier AM, Denny FW, Senior RJ, Sheaffer CI, Conley WG III, Christian RM. The etiology and epidemiologic spectrum of bronchiolitis in pediatric practice. J Pediatr 1979; 95:183–190.
2. Zweiman B, Schoenwetter WF, Papano JE, et al. Patterns of allergic respiratory disease in children with a past history of bronchiolitis. J Allergy 1971; 48:283–289.
3. McIntosh K, Ellis EF, Hoffman LS, Lybass TG, Eller JJ, Fulginiti VA. The association of viral and bacterial respiratory infections with exacerbations of wheezing in young asthmatic children. J Pediatr 1973; 82:578–590.
4. Minor TE, Dick ED, DeMeo AN, Ouellette JJ, Chen M, Reed CE. Viruses as precipitants of asthmatic attacks in children. JAMA 1974; 227:292–298.
5. Carlsen KH, Orstavik I, Leegaard J, Hoeg H. Respiratory virus infections and aeroallergens in acute bronchial asthma. Arch Dis Child 1984; 59:310–315.
6. Hudgel DW, Langston L, Selner JC, McIntosh K. Viral and bacterial infections in adults with chronic asthma. Am Rev Respir Dis 1979; 120:393–397.
7. Beasley R, Coleman ED, Hermon Y, Holst PE, O'Donnell TV, Tobias M. Viral respiratory tract infection and exacerbation of asthma in adult patients. thorax 1988; 43:679–683.
8. Kava T. Acute respiratory infection, influenza vaccination and airway reactivity in asthma. Eur J Respir Dis 150; 1987; 150(suppl):7–38.

9. Hogg JC. Latent viral infections in airway epithelium. Chest 1992; 101(suppl):80–82S.
10. Busse WW. The precipitation of asthma by upper respiratory infections. Chest 1985; 87(suppl):44–48S.
11. Azimi PH, Chase PA, Petru AM. Mycoplasmas: their role in pediatric disease. Curr Prob Pediatr 1984; 14:1–46.
12. Seggev JS, Lis I, Siman-Tov R, Gutman R, Abu-Samara H, Schey G, Naot Y. *Mycoplasma pneumoniae* is a frequent cause of exacerbation of bronchial asthma in adults. Ann Allergy 1986; 57:263–265.
13. Gil JC, Cedillo RL, Mayagoitia BG, Paz MD. Isolation of *Mycoplasma pneumoniae* from asthmatic patients. Ann Allergy 1993; 70:23–25.
14. Hahn DL, Dodge RW, Bolubjatnikov R. Association of *Chlamydia pneumoniae* (Strain TWAR) infection with wheezing, asthmatic bronchitis, and adult-onset asthma. JAMA 1991; 266:225–230.
14a. Allegra L, Blasi F, Centanni S, Cosentini R, Denti F, Raccanelli R, Tarsia P, Valenti V. Acute exacerbations of asthma in adults: role of Chlamydia pneumoniae infection. Eur Respir J 1994; 7:2165–2168.
15. Benson V. Marano MA, National Center for Health Statistics. Current estimates for the National Health Interview Survey—1993. Vital and health statistics. 10(190). Washington, DC: Government Printing Office, 1995.
16. Wald ER. Sinusitis. Pediatrics in Review 1993; 14:345–351.
17. Wald ER, Guevra N, Byers C. Upper respiratory tract infections in young children: duration of and frequency of complications. Pediatrics 1991; 87:129–133.
18. Nguyen KL, Corbett ML, Garcia DP, Eberly SM, Massey EN, Le HT, Shearer LT, Karibo JM, Pence HL. Chronic sinusitis among pediatric patients with chronic respiratory complaints. J Allergy Clin Immunol 1993; 92:824–830.
18a. Williams JW Jr. Sinusitis-beginning a new age of enlightenment? West J Med 1995; 163: 80–82.
19. Gliklich R, Metson R. Asthma and sinusitis as comorbidities on SF-36 testing. Otolaryngol Head Neck Surg 1995; 113:104–109.
19a. Kaliner MA, Osguthorpe JK, Fireman P, Anon J, Georgitis J, Davis ML, Naclerio R, Kennedy D. Sinusitis: bench to bedside. Current findings, future directions. J Allergy Clin Immunol 1997; 99:S829–848.
20. Gottlieb MJ. Relation of intranasal disease in the production of bronchial asthma. JAMA 1925; 85:257–267.
21. Chobot R. Asthma in children. Am J Dis Child 1933; 45:25–31.
22. Rachelefsky G, Goldberg M, Katz RM, Boris G, Gyepes MT, Shapiro MJ, Mickey MR, Finegold SM, Siegel SC. Sinus disease in children with respiratory allergy. J Allergy Clin Immunol 1978; 61:310–314.
23. Adinoff AD, Wood RW, Buschman D, et al. Chronic sinusitis in childhood asthma: correlations of symptoms, x-rays, culture and response to treatment. Pediatr Res 1983; 17:264.
24. Schwartz HJ, Thompson JS, Sher TH, Ross RJ. Occult sinus abnormalities in the asthmatic patient. Arch Intern Med 1987; 147:2194–2196.
25. Rossi OVJ, Pirila T, Laitinen J, Huhti E. Sinus aspirates and radiographic abnormalities in severe attacks of asthma. Int Arch Allergy Immunol 1994; 103:209–213.
26. Kratchmer Z. Cited in Kiyoshi A. Physiologic relationships between nasal breathing and pulmonary function. Laryngoscope 1966; 76:30.
27. Whicker JH, Kern EB. The nasalpulmonary reflex in the awake animal. Ann Otolaryngol 1973; 82:355–358.
28. Dixon WE, Brodie TG. The bronchial muscles, their innervation and the action of drugs upon them. J Physiol (Lond)1903; 29:93–97.
29. Kaufman J, Wright GW. The effect of nasal and nasopharyngeal irritation on airways resistance in man. Am Rev Respir Dis 1969; 100:626–630.

30. Sluder G. Asthma as a nasal reflex. JAMA 1919; 73:589–591.
31. Nolte D, Berger D. On vagal bronchoconstriction in asthmatic patients by nasal irritation. Eur J Respir Dis 1983; 64(suppl 128):110–114.
32. Kaufman J, Chen JC, Wright GW. The effect of trigeminal resection on reflex bronchoconstriction after nasal and nasopharyngeal irritation in man. Am Rev Respir Dis 1970; 101: 768–769.
33. Hoehne JH, Reed CE. Where is the allergic reaction in ragweed asthma? J Allergy Clin Immunol 1971; 48:36–39.
34. Rosenberger GL, Rosenthal RR, Norman PS. Inhalation challenge with ragweed pollen in ragweed sensitive asthmatics. J Allergy Clin Immunol 1983; 71:302–310.
35. Schumacher MJ, Cota KA, Taussig LM. Pulmonary response to nasal challenge testing of atopic subjects with stable asthma. J Allergy Clin Immunol 1986; 78:30–35.
36. Yan K, Salome C. The response of the airways to nasal stimulation in asthmatics with rhinitis. Eur J Rispir Dis 1983; 64(suppl 128):105–108.
37. Corren J, Adinoff A, Irvin C. Changes in bronchial responsiveness following nasal provocation with allergen. J Allergy Clin Immunol 1992; 89:611–618.
38. Plotkowski LM, Dessanges TF, Larand F, Hahaert B, Lockhart A. Nasal pollen challenge causes bronchial hyperresponsiveness to methacholine in patients with allergic rhinitis. Am Rev Respir Dis 1990; 141:A652.
39. Corren J, Adinoff AP, Buchmeier AD, Irvin CG. Nasal beclomethasone prevents the seasonal increase in bronchial responsiveness in patients with allergic rhinitis and asthma. J Allergy Clin Immunol 1992; 90:250–256.
40. Watson WTA, Becker AB, Simons FER. Treatment of allergic rhinitis with intranasal corticosteroids in patients with mild asthma: effect on lower airway responsiveness. J Allergy Clin Immunol 1993; 91:97–101.
41. Henriksen JM, Wenzel A. Effect of an intranasally administered corticosteroid (budesonide) on nasal obstruction, mouth breathing, and asthma. Am Rev Respir Dis 1984; 130:1014–1018.
42. Welsh PW, Stricker WE, Chu CP, et al. Efficacy of beclomethasone nasal solution, flunisolide and cromolyn in relieving symptoms of ragweed allergy. Mayo Clin Proc 1987; 62:125–134.
42a. Wade T, Watson A, Becker AB, Simons FE. Treatment of allergic rhinitis with intranasal corticosteroids in patients with mild asthma: effect on lower airway responsiveness. J Allergy Clin Immunol 1993; 91:97–101.
43. Friedman R, Ackerman M, Wald E, Cassellrant M, Friday G, Fireman P. Asthma and bacterial sinusitis in children. J Allergy Clin Immunol 1984; 74:185–189.
44. Slavin RG, Cannon RE, Friedman WH, Palitang E, Sundaram M. Sinusitis and bronchial asthma. J Allergy Clin Immunol 1980; 66:250–257.
45. Cummings NP, Wood RN, Lere JL, Adinoff AP. Effect of treatment of rhinitis/sinusitis on asthma: results of a double-blind study. Pediatr Res 1983; 17:373–378.
46. Slavin RG. Relationship of nasal disease and sinusitis to bronchial asthma. Ann Allergy 1982; 49:76–80.
47. Mings R, Friedman WH, Linford P, Slavin RG. Five-year follow-up of the effects of bilateral intranasal sphenoethmoidectomy in patients with sinusitis and asthma. Am J Rhinol 1988; 71:123–132.
48. Parsons DS, Phillips SE. Functional endoscopic surgery in children: a retrospective analysis of results. Laryngoscope 1993; 103:899–903.
49. Nishioka GJ, Cook PR, Davis WE, McKinsey JP. Functional endoscopic sinus surgery in patients with chronic sinusitis and asthma. Otolaryngol Head Neck Surg 1994; 110:494–500.
50. Druce HM. The diagnosis of sinusitis in adults: history, physical examination, nasal cytology, echo and rhinoscopy. J Allergy Clin Immunol 1992; 90:436–441.

51. Gwaltney JM, Phillips CD, Miller RD, Riker DK. Computed tomographic study of the common cold. N Engl J Med 1994; 330:25–30.
52. Shapiro GG. Role of allergy in sinusitis. Pediatr Infect Dis 1985; 4:55–58.
53. Shapiro GG, Rachelefsky GS. Introduction and definition of sinusitis. J Allergy Clin Immunol 1992; 90:417–418.
54. Fireman P. diagnosis of sinusitis in children: emphasis on the history and physical examination. J Allergy Clin Immunol 1992; 90:433–436.
55. Wagenmann M, Naclerio RM. Anatomic and physiologic considerations in sinusitis. J Allergy Clin Immunol 1992; 90:419–423.
56. Kaliner MA. Human nasal host defense and sinusitis. J Allergy Clin Immunol 1992; 90:424–430.
57. Settipane GA, Settipane RA. Tetrad of nasal polyps, aspirin sensitivity, asthma, and rhinosinusitis. In: Druce HM, ed., *Sinusitis: pathophysiology and treatment*. New York: Marcel Dekker, Inc., 1994, 227–246.
58. Benson ML, Oliverio PJ, Zinreich SJ. Imaging techniques: conventional radiography, computed tomography, magnetic resonance and ultrasonography of the paranasal sinuses. In: Gershwin ME, Incaudo GA, eds., *Diseases of the sinuses. A comprehensive textbook of diagnosis and treatment*, NJ: Humana Press, Totowa, 1996, 63–83.
59. Wald ER, Reilly JS, Casselbrant M, et al. Treatment of acute maxillary sinusitis in childhood: a comparative study of amoxicillin and cefaclor. J Pediatr 1984; 104:297–302.
60. Gwaltney JM, Scheld WM, Sande MA, Sydnor A. The microbial etiology and antimicrobial therapy of adults with acute community-acquired sinusitis: a fifteen-year experience at the University of Virginia and review of other selected studies. J Allergy Clin Immunol 1992; 90:457–462.
61. Brook I. Bacteriologic features of chronic sinusitis in children. JAMA 1981; 246:967–969.
62. Gwaltney JM. Microbiology of sinusitis. In: Druce HM, Ed. *Sinusitis: pathophysiology and treatment*. NY: Marcel Dekker, Inc., 1994, 41–56.
62a. Baroody FM, Hughes CA, McDowell P, Hruban R, Zinreich SJ, Naclerio RM. Eosinophilia in chronic childhood sinusitis. Arch Otolaryngol Head Neck Surg 1995; 121:1396–1402.
63. Howarth PH, Holgate ST. Basic aspects of allergic reactions. In: Naspitz CK, Tinkelman DG, Eds. *Childhood rhinitis and sinusitis: pathophysiology and treatment*. NY: Marcel Dekker, Inc., 1990, 1–35.
64. Wilson NW, Jalowayski AA, Hamberger RN. A comparison of nasal cytology with sinus x-rays for the diagnosis of sinusitis. Am J Rhinol 1988; 2:55–59.
65. Gill FF, Neiburger JB. The role of nasal cytology in the diagnosis of chronic sinusitis. Am J Rhinol 1989; 13–15.
66. Miller RE, Paradise JL, Friday GA, Fireman P, Voith D. the nasal smear for eosinophils. Its value in children with seasonal allergic rhinitis. Am J Dis Child 1982; 136:1009–1011.
67. Pipkorn U, Karlsson G, Ennerback L. The cellular response of the human allergic mucosa to natural allergen exposure. J Allergy Clin Immunol 1988; 82:1046–1054.
68. Arruda LK, Mimica IM, Sole D, Weckx LLM, Schoettler J, Heiner DC, Naspitz CK. Abnormal maxillary sinus radiographs in children: do they represent bacterial infection? Pediatrics 1990; 85:553–558.
69. Glasier CM, Mallory GB, Steele RW. Significance of opacification of the maxillary and ethmoid sinuses in infants. J Pediatr 1989; 114:45–50.
70. McAlister WH, Lusk R, Muntz HR. Comparison of plain radiographs and coronal CT scans in infants and children with recurrent sinusitis. Am J Roentgenol 1989; 153:1259–1264.
71. Fascenelli FW. Maxillary sinus abnormalities; radiographic evidence in an asymptomatic population. Arch Otolaryng 1969; 90:98–101.
72. American College of Radiology Task Force report on appropriateness criteria for imaging and treatment decisions. Reston, VA, 1995, 6.1–6.14.

73. Diament MJ, Senac MO Jr, Gilsanz V, et al. Prevalence of incidental paranasal sinuses opacification in pediatric patients: a CT study. J Comp Assist Tomog 1987; 11:426.
74. Wald ER. Sinusitis in children N Engl J Med 1981; 326:319–323.
75. Revonta M. Ultrasound in the diagnosis of maxillary and frontal sinusitis. Acta Otolaryngol 1980; 370 (suppl):1–54.
76. Jannert M, Andreasson L, Holmer N-G, et al. Ultrasonic examination of the paranasal sinuses. Acta Otolaryngol 1982; 389(suppl):1–51.
77. Druce HM. Diagnosis of sinusitis in adults: history, physical examination, nasal cytology, echo, and rhinoscope. J Allergy Clin Immunol 1992; 90:436–441.
78. Shapiro GG, Furukawa CT, Pierson WE, et al. Blinded comparison of maxillary sinus radiography and ultrasound for diagnosis of sinusitis. J Allergy Clin Immunol 1986; 77: 59–64.
79. Rohr AS, Spector SL, Siegel SC, et al. Correlation between A-mode ultrasound and radiography in the diagnosis of maxillary sinusitis. J Allergy Clin Immunol 1986; 78:58–61.
80. Dunham ME. New light on sinusitis. Contemporary Pediatr 1994; 11:102–117.
81. Nguyen KL, Corbett ML, Garcia DP, Eberly SM, Massey EN, Le HT, Shearer LT, Karibo JM, Pence HL. Chronic sinusitis among pediatric patients with chronic respiratory complaints. J Allergy Clin Immunol 1993; 92:824–830.
82. Wald ER, Milmoe GJ, Bowen A, et al. Acute maxillary sinusitis in children. N Engl J Med 1981; 304:749–754.
83. McCaig LF, Hughes JM. Trends in antimicrobial drug prescribing among office-based physicians in the United States. JAMA 1995; 273:214–219.
84. Abbasi S, Cunningham AS. Are we overtreating sinusitis? Contemporary Pediatr 1996; 13: 49–62.
85. Wald ER, Chiponis D, Ledesma-Medina J. Comparative effectiveness of amoxicillin and amoxicillin-clavulanate in acute paranasal sinus infections in children: a double-blind, placebo-controlled trial. Pediatrics 1986; 77:795–800.
86. Sykes DA, Wilson R, Chan KL, Mackay IS, Cole PJ. Relative importance of antibiotic and improved clearance in topical treatment of chronic mucopurulent rhinosinusitis. A controlled study. Lancet 1986; 2:359–360.
87. Williams JW, Holleman DR, Samsa GP, Simel DL. Randomized controlled trial of 3 vs 10 days of trimethoprim/sulfamethoxazole for acute maxillary sinusitis. JAMA 1995; 273: 1015–1021.
87a. Wald ER. Dr. Wald on sinusitis (letter). Contemporary Pediatr 1997; 14:30.
88. Druce HM. Medical management of sinusitis in the adult. In: Druce HM. *Sinusitis: pathophysiology and treatment.* NY: Marcel Dekker, Inc., 1994; 73–85.
89. Van Bever HPS, Bosmans J, Stevens WJ. Nebulization treatment with saline compared to bromhexine in treating chronic sinusitis in asthmatic children. Allergy 1987; 42:33–36.
90. Melen I, Friberg B, Andreasson L, et al. Effects of phenylpropanolamine on ostial and nasal patency in patients treated for chronic maxillary sinusitis. Acta Otolaryngol 1986; 101:494–500.
91. Axelsson A, Jensen C, Melin O, et al. Treatment of acute maxillary sinusitis. V. Amoxicillin, azidocillin, phenylpropanolamine, and pivampicillin. Acta Otolaryngol 1981; 91:313–318.
92. Sly RM, Kemp JP. The use of antihistamines in patients with asthma. J Allergy Clin Immunol 1988; 82:481–482.
93. Mygind N. Topical steroid treatment of allergic rhinitis and allied conditions. Clin Otolaryngol 1982; 7:343–347.
94. Meltzer EO, Orgel A, Backhaus JW, et al. Intranasal flunisolide spray as an adjunct to oral antibiotic therapy for sinusitis. J Allergy Clin Immunol 1993; 92:812–823.
95. Lusk RP. Endoscopic approach to sinus disease. J Allergy Clin Immunol 1992; 90:496–505.
96. Stern RC, Boat TF, Wood RE, et al. Treatment and prognosis of nasal polyps in cystic fibrosis. Am J Dis Child 1982; 136:1067–1070.

97. McCleve D, Gatos L, Goldstein J, Silvers S. Corticosteroid injections of the nasal turbinates: past experience and precautions. ORL J Otorhinolaryngol Rel Spec 1978; 86:851–857.
98. Settipane GA, ed. Nasal polyps. In: *Rhinitis,* 2nd ed., Providence: Oceanside Publications, 1991; 178.
99. Stevenson DD. Oral challenge: aspirin, NSAID, tartrazine and sulfites. N Engl Reg Allergy Proc 1984; 5:111.
100. Christopher KL, W.R., Eckert RC, Blager FB, Raney RA, Souhrada JF. Vocal cord dysfunction presenting as asthma. N Engl J Med. 1983; 308:1566–70.
100a. Newman KB, Mason UG, Schmaling KB. Clinical features of vocal cord dysfunction. Am J Respir Crit Care Med 1995; 152:1382–1386.
101. Skinner DW, Bradley PJ. Psychogenic stridor. J Laryngol Otol 1989; 103:383–385.
101a. Ramirez J, Leon I, Rivera LM. Episodic laryngeal dyskinesia. Clinical and psychiatric characterization. Chest. 1986; 90:716–721.
102. Evans KL. Diagnosis and management of sinusitis. Br Med J 1994; 309:1415–1422.
103. Newman LJ, Platts-Mills TA, Phillips CD, Hazen KC, Gross CW. Chronic sinusitis. Relationship of computed tomographic findings to allergy, asthma, and eosinophilia. JAMA 1994; 271:363–367.
104. Wald ER. Microbiology of acute and chronic sinusitis in children. J Allergy Clin Immunol 1992; 90:452–460.

8

Respiratory Infections
The Major Cause

Jill M. Baren
University of Pennsylvania School of Medicine, Philadelphia, Pennsylvania

I. INTRODUCTION

It has long been recognized that respiratory infections are closely associated with exacerbations of asthma (1). Patients that present to the ED with acute exacerbations of asthma often give a history of antecedent cold symptoms, which has lead many investigators to try to determine a causal link between acute respiratory infections and the development of acute symptoms of asthma (2,3,4). The etiology of acute respiratory infections may be either viral or bacterial, and range from a simple "cold" to a consolidated lower airway pneumonic process. Viral respiratory infections have been shown to be far more important in provoking exacerbations of asthma than bacterial infections. In the pediatric population, viral infections are the most important trigger for acute asthma, and although studies have shown conflicting results, this is likely to be true for adults as well (5). This chapter will review the historical and epidemiological data that have established viral infections as a leading precipitant of acute asthma attacks and will discuss mechanisms and theories for viral provocation of attacks.

II. HISTORICAL FACTORS

Initially, observations by investigators in the 1950s showed that certain illnesses like mumps, chicken pox, or measles caused an exacerbation of "bronchial allergic diseases" (6,7). It was also noted that the resolution of these illnesses corresponded to the resolution of the symptoms of allergic disease, both of which were facilitated by the use of antibacterial medications. This perpetuated the concept that the exacerbation of asthma was due to a bacterial allergy (6). In all likelihood, these investigators were describing viral respiratory infections possibly complicated by bacterial superinfection. Later, careful prospective studies of adults (8) and children (9–11) with chronic asthma showed that the incidence of bacterial infection during wheezing exacerbations was not increased over the incidence of bacterial infections during asymptomatic periods. Although potential bacterial pathogens, such as *Hemophilus influenzae* and *S. pneumoniae* were cultured frequently from the respiratory tracts, there was no correlation with wheezing episodes. The authors concluded that the respiratory tract in some asthmatic patients may be colonized with pathogenic bacteria, but this did not produce an increased frequency of asthma exacerbations (8). These results give little justification for the use of routine antibacterial treatment in acute asthma as is noted in general practice today.

The first reports implicating viral infections, specifically influenza, as triggers of asthma attacks appeared in the 1950s (12,13). This was coincident with the discovery of the respiratory syncytial virus (RSV) in the oral cavity of infants with bronchiolitis and bronchopneumonia (14). Throughout the 1960s and 1970s a series of investigations began to delineate which viruses were responsible for exacerbations of wheezing or asthma when the role of bacteria in triggering exacerbations became less important (15–27).

III. VIRAL INFECTIONS AND ASTHMA

A. Epidemiology

1. Overview

There is a great deal of evidence that links respiratory virus infections with acute exacerbations of asthma but, to fully understand this relationship, several questions must be answered: Which viral etiologic agents are responsible for acute respiratory infections? Which etiologic agents produce a greater frequency of obstructive symptoms (i.e., wheezing)? What is the viral identification rate during acute asthma exacerbations or acute wheezing illnesses? Do asthmatic patients have a higher frequency of respiratory virus infections than non asthmatics? How does respiratory virus infection cause an acute exacerbation of asthma symptoms?

This topic has been studied most intensively in the pediatric population. Epidemiological studies of children have attempted to answer many of these questions and can be broadly divided into two categories. The first category includes studies of children with acute respiratory infections that define the spectrum of viral etiologies for acute respiratory infections and document the presence of symptoms of airway obstruction along with infection. The second category includes studies that look at viral identification rates in patients already diagnosed with recurrent wheezing or chronic asthma.

2. Etiology of Acute Respiratory Infections in Children and the Occurrence of Wheezing

General epidemiological studies of children with acute lower respiratory infection are important, because subjects are not selected based on the presence or absence of atopic disease or known asthma. They describe the influence of age, sex, and etiologic agent on the occurrence of wheezing in all children with respiratory infections. Host factors such as age and its relationship to airway size are important because they may influence the frequency and severity of airway obstruction in children (15). If acute viral illnesses in young children are antecedent events of chronic asthma, which many authors have suggested (28), it is still unclear which children will go on to develop recurrent wheezing episodes (29,30).

To answer the first several questions it is useful to review some early studies. A large population based study of 3000 clinically defined lower respiratory illnesses in a pediatric practice, viral pathogens were isolated in 28% of cases (25). Seventy-five percent of the isolates were either RSV, parainfluenza virus (PIV), or Mycoplasma pneumoniae (MP). All isolates were associated with a range of clinical illnesses, but RSV was associated with bronchiolitis and pneumonia more often than other agents (25). Subsequent studies confirmed these results with varying percentages (18–34%) and added rhinovirus (RV), adenovirus (AV), influenza (IFV), and coxsackie virus (CSV) to the list of etiologic agents (18,23,24). In addition, RV infection was highly associated with episodes of wheezing as well as RSV infection (18,23).

In a large 11-year prospective study of the causes and patterns of occurrence of wheezing in children seeking care for acute respiratory infection showed that wheezing was present in 1851 of the 6165 episodes of acute respiratory disease, most of them single episodes by individual children (15). The incidence of wheezing associated infection was highest in the first year of life, with the highest proportion of cases between 2 and 10 months (15). Male children experienced wheezing associated infections 1.25 times as frequently as female children across all age groups but this eventually equalized after age 9 years (15). Viral pathogens were isolated during wheezing episodes 21% of the time, and the etiologic agents did not vary markedly amongst age groups (15). RSV, PIV, AV, RV, and MP accounted for 87% of the pathogens isolated (15). RSV was again the most important agent isolated from infants and preschool children with wheezing, and MP the most common agent isolated from school aged children. The seasonal occurrence of wheezing was related to the seasonal occurrence of infections with the various causative agents (15).

3. *Viral Identification During Episodes of Acute Asthma in Children*

There are numerous prospective studies of asthmatic children that have enabled us to learn about the viral identification rate during asymptomatic and symptomatic periods. Despite technical difficulties with viral isolation and inconsistencies in the selection of patients and controls, most studies show a viral identification rate ranging from 14% to 63% during acute episodes of wheezing compared with 1% to 23% during nonwheezing periods or in nonwheezing controls with symptoms of acute respiratory infection (10,11,19,21,22,26,31–34). When a decrease in baseline forced expiratory volume in 1 sec (FEV_1) or peak expiratory flow rate (PEF) were used in addition to clinical exam findings of wheezing to define an acute episode of asthma, the viral identification rates in several studies were even higher at 80–89% (35,36).

The profile of viral isolates from acute asthmatic subjects is very similar to that found in studies of children with acute respiratory infections. The most common isolates in most studies were RSV and RV in varying proportions, with IFV and PIV also noted (11,19,21,22,31–36). The range of viruses uncovered shows that acute asthma is not associated with a specific virus or a small range of viruses, but with many of the recognized respiratory viral pathogens (33). Overall, the low isolation rates of viruses in asthmatics during asymptomatic periods supports the role of viruses as triggers of acute asthma.

4. Temporal Relationship Between Acute Viral Infection and Onset of Wheezing in Children

Viruses have not only been simply identified in relation to acute exacerbations of asthma in children but have been shown to have a distinct temporal relationship to the onset of wheezing symptoms. Seasonal variations in wheezing among asthmatic children have been shown to correspond to identifiable peaks of various viruses (1,10), particularly with RSV infection (15). Once an acute respiratory infection has subsided, viral identification rates tend to decrease making it less likely that virus identification during acute wheezing episodes is occurring by chance (1,11). Other studies have shown that virus identification during wheezing coincides with the need for additional asthma medication, higher ratings of asthma symptoms, and decreases in baseline pulmonary function performance (10,22,36). One group of investigators described a characteristic pattern of wheezing associated with an acute respiratory infection amongst their subjects. Wheezing began at a mean of 43 hours after respiratory symptoms began and lasted for a mean of 3.8 days in those patients who were ultimately proven to have viral infections (31). This pattern of wheezing is clearly different from that seen with the more abrupt onset of wheezing that occurs with allergen challenge and again supports the role of viruses in the provocation of asthma attacks (1).

5. The Role of Viral Precipitants in Acute Asthma Compared to Other Precipitants

Very few studies have examined the relative importance of viruses as triggers of asthma when compared to other precipitants. There was no correlation found in a prospective study of 80 children—40 asthmatic and 40 nonasthmatic—between hospital admissions for asthma and meteorological changes, changes in pollen counts, or known allergen exposure (37). However, a strong correlation existed between admission and viral infection (37). Similarly, there was no significant correlation between asthma attacks in patients with known allergies and known exposure to the offending agents in a study of 169 children over a two year-period. However, the single most important precipitating factor for acute asthma in this study was respiratory virus infection (34). An investigation of yearly admissions for asthma over an 11-year period showed a repeated yearly pattern with a large autumn peak and a small spring peak. The large autumn peak was preceded by a late summer trough. The peaks and troughs in admissions coincided with the timing of school holidays. The authors postulated that holidays disrupt the spread of viral infections throughout the community and synchronized subsequent attacks (32). All of these studies support the hypothesis that viral infections play a major role in exacerbations of asthma in children.

6. Correlation Between Acute Viral Infection and Severity of Wheezing in Children

In addition to documenting the association of viruses to acute asthma exacerbations, some studies have examined the relationship of viruses to the severity of the exacerbation. Although they classified acute asthma episodes retrospectively, Horn et al. found that virus isolation rates were higher in episodes that were classified as severe (63%) compared to episodes that were classifies as mild (17%) or moderate (54%) (11). In episodes that required corticosteroid treatment, the viral identification rate was 64% (11). In a more recent study, Johnston et al. found a very high viral detection rate in all patients with wheezing (77%) but the highest detection rate occurred in patients who reported a combination of more severe symptoms including wheezing, cough, and upper respiratory symptoms, and a decrease in baseline PEF (35).

7. *Viruses as Triggers of Acute Asthma in Adults*

While the preceding evidence clearly establishes the role of viruses as precipitants of acute asthma attacks in children, the exact same conclusions cannot be drawn based on literature regarding adult asthma patients. First, there is a paucity of data compared to the pediatric population, and second, studies have shown conflicting results. Several studies support the role of viruses in the development of wheezing exacerbations. For example, 19 adult asthma patients were examined for organisms during acute wheezing episodes and on a routine monthly basis when asthma was under control. In this study only 8 viral infections were identified during 243 routine visits (3.3%) and 8 during 84 wheezing exacerbations (11%), a statistically significant greater incidence (8). In a study of similar design, 31 adult asthma patients were followed prospectively. There were 178 exacerbations of asthma over 6 months and 28 were classified as severe. Viruses were identified on 30 occasions, 18 associated with wheezing exacerbations and 10 of those during severe wheezing exacerbations (38). The authors of both studies conclude that viruses are clearly associated with asthma exacerbations despite the low identification rates and stress the importance of the association of viral infections and severe exacerbations (38). However, they acknowledge the contrast with the data in children and suggest that other factors may account for most episodes of asthma in adults (8,38).

Three additional studies provide data that viruses do not play a major role in triggering attacks of acute asthma in adults. A study comparing 19 asthmatics and their spouses at monthly intervals during one year showed that the asthmatic patients reported a larger number of symptoms describing a cold than nonasthmatics but had significantly fewer of these episodes confirmed as viral infections (16). In addition, less than 10% of the asthma exacerbations experienced were associated with respiratory infections (16). Viruses were isolated in only 4 of 27 exacerbation sputum specimens provided by 51 asthmatic patients over 18 months. The study concluded that the great majority of exacerbations of asthma in those patients were not due to respiratory infections (16). Only one study to date has looked exclusively at adult asthmatic patients presenting to an emergency department for an acute exacerbation to determine the role of viral infections (39). Not a single viral culture or rapid antigen detection for IFV, PIV, RSV, AV, or RV was positive. Despite the fact that 56% of the 33 patients studied complained of acute respiratory infection symptoms, viral pathogens could not be identified (39). These results strongly suggest that viral infection may not be as prevalent a precipitant of asthma in adults requiring emergency department treatment for acute asthma, although additional studies of a larger sample size should be done for confirmation.

Although specific viruses predominate in one study versus another, the spectrum of viruses isolated from studies on adult asthmatics are similar to those found in children (8,16,17,20,38,40). RV is a frequent pathogen of the ''common cold'' and seems to be the predominant virus in many studies of adult asthmatics. When RV infection was experimentally induced in 19 asthmatic adults, only a minority of patients had a wheezing exacerbation while 17 of 19 developed typical coryza symptoms (40). Additional studies are needed to truly delineate the role of viral precipitants in the adult population.

8. Do Asthmatics Get More Respiratory Infections Than Their Nonasthmatic Counterparts?

It is unclear if asthmatics have a greater susceptibility to respiratory infections or if they simply manifest infection more overtly (1). Based on the evidence presented for children, it is obvious that they get more viral infections than adults; however, asthma may be a risk factor for more symptomatic infections. For adults with asthma, there is still far too little data to draw any conclusions regarding increased susceptibility to viral infections.

9. Summary

Viruses are often associated with acute wheezing episodes, especially in children, and are far more commonly found in relation to acute exacerbations of wheezing than bacteria. Viruses are also unlikely to be isolated in asthmatics during asymptomatic periods. The major types of viruses isolated in children during wheezing are RV, RSV, and PIV but this profile may vary with age. Adults are less likely to have high viral identification rates during acute wheezing episodes although current data is sparse.

B. Mechanism of Virus-Induced Asthma Exacerbations

1. Overview

Epidemiological evidence presented above confirms an association between exacerbations of asthma and viral infections. The exact mechanisms by which viruses induce or contribute to an acute exacerbation of asthma are currently unknown, but a large body of evidence has accumulated to support a growing number of theories (41). Theories proposed thus far fall into two categories: (1) those in which a virus infection involves both the upper and lower respiratory tracts, and leads to direct pathophysiologic changes observed in the airways, and (2) those in which a virus infection is confined only to the upper respiratory tract but, by indirect means, results in changes in the lower respiratory tract (41). It is likely that there is no single mechanism that can account for all viral induced asthma exacerbations and that the effects of viruses are likely to be multifactorial and interrelated (42). The most well studied and supported mechanisms are discussed in more detail below.

2. Mechanisms with Direct Effects on the Lower Respiratory Tract

Epithelial Damage/Increased Cholinergic Sensitivity

Certain viruses can cause severe abnormalities in the lower airways. Influenza A induces diffuse inflammation coupled with submucosal edema and cellular infiltrates (43). Damaged epithelium might result in increased exposure of rapid adapting sensory parasympathetic fibers that cause bronchoconstriction by a vagal reflex mediated pathway. Direct support for this theory comes from a study where healthy volunteers with uncomplicated upper respiratory infections showed increased airway resistance to histamine inhalation when compared to healthy controls (44). This increased airway resistance was prevented by the prior administration of aerosolized atropine (44). Damage to epithelial cells might also result in greater penetration of allergen and increased allergic inflammation (41). Repeated viral infections might cause cumulative epithelial damage leading to irreversible changes in airway structure and function (45).

Release of Inflammatory Mediators

Release of tissue damaging substances from macrophages, neutrophils, eosinophils, and mast cells may be another mechanism by which viruses induce airway inflammation. Substances found to be experimentally released in response to respiratory viruses include histamine, interferon, bradykinin, complement, lipoxins, and superoxide (42,46–52).

Activation of Immune Responses

Humoral and cellular immune responses have been shown to play a role in an augmented response to viral infections in asthmatic patients. Asthmatic subjects have higher baseline IgA and IgG and a greater response to influenza infection than normal subjects (53). Viral-induced release of cytokines may enhance IgE response and recruitment of eosinophils to the bronchial mucosa (54–56). Another study noted increased lymphocyte activation in subjects who wheezed compared to subjects who did not wheeze 6 months after an acute RSV infection (42,57).

Decreased β-Receptor Function

Viruses may exacerbate an already impaired adrenergic function found in asthmatic patients creating an imbalance between parasympathetic and adrenergic responses. This observation has been primarily confirmed in vitro and as yet has little clinical relevance (41).

Synthesis of Viral-Specific IgE

As previously stated, patients with detectable RSV-IgE after acute infection had a higher incidence of wheezing than those with undetectable levels of RSV-IgE (58). Specific IgE produced in response to acute PIV infection was detected earlier and in greater magnitude in patients with wheezing and croup compared with patients who had upper respiratory symptoms alone, suggesting an immunologic mechanism for more severe infection (59). If viral infections can trigger enhanced production of IgE, then certain atopic individuals may be at considerable risk for an exaggerated and even life-threatening response to a routine cold (41).

3. *Selected Mechanisms with Indirect Effects on the Lower Airways*

Nasal Blockage and Mouth Breathing

During an acute upper respiratory infection, patients tend to breathe through the mouth because of temporary nasal blockage. Inspired air that does not go through the nasal passages is delivered to the lower airways at a lower temperature and humidity and without being filtered. The combination of these factors may contribute to increased penetration of allergens and increased bronchospasm in sensitized individuals (41).

Release of Proinflammatory Mediators into the Circulation

During an acute viral infection, cytokines may be released into the general circulation causing the nonspecific symptoms of fever, fatigue, and malaise. In addition, inflammatory cells such as leukocytes are released resulting in an ''upregulation'' of inflammatory responses in general, which may cause a sensitized individual with asthma to have an exacerbation of their disease (41). Hard evidence is lacking to support either of these last two theories.

4. *Summary*

Acute respiratory infections of the upper airways frequently trigger a response in the lower airways that can lead to increased morbidity in patients with pre-existing airway disease (41). Viruses likely induce a sequence of events that ultimately result in airway obstruction in asthmatics but only in a mild cold in nonasthmatic individuals. The inflammatory changes brought on by viruses may be both additive and synergistic with inflammatory processes inherent in individuals with asthma (41).

C. Recent Advances with Human Rhinovirus (RV) Infection

Many respiratory viruses are exceedingly difficult to isolate because of technical problems in obtaining, preserving, growing, and identifying them in the laboratory. Overall, this contributes to a very low false-positive rate for identification of respiratory viruses in general in clinical studies (1). However, there is also likely to be a significant false negative identification rate for the more fastidious viruses, such as RV. RV, as previously noted, is one of the top two or three etiologic agents responsible for respiratory infections both in asthmatic and nonasthmatic individuals (1). In a study of children with recurrent wheezing, rhinoviruses were actually found to account for half of the episodes of respiratory illness, which was six times more frequent than the next most common virus (60).

Conventional methods for the isolation of rhinovirus have primarily involved culturing nasopharyngeal secretions on human epithelial cells. For maximal isolation, secretions need to be obtained within 1–2 days of the onset of symptoms and even then, underdiagnosis is likely (61). Serological tests have also been tried but have not been useful because of the large number of distinct RV serotypes (62). Recent advances in molecular biology have lead to a greater understanding of the genomic and protein structure of RVs, and recent advances in the techniques for RV identification have lead to more rapid and accurate diagnosis. Both have enabled the development of potential treatment strategies aimed at either prophylaxis or attenuation of infection. Specifically, the polymerase chain reaction (PCR) technique has been employed to provide a sensitive and specific method for the diagnosis of RV infection and appears to be superior to viral culture techniques (63–66).

IV. TREAMENT AND PREVENTION OF VIRAL-INDUCED WHEEZING

A. Treatment

Other than symptomatic and supportive therapy, no treatment modality has been routinely applied to individuals with viral respiratory infections that trigger acute asthma. A number of specific treatments have been attempted in clinical studies; most are not found to be universally effective and many are associated with undesirable side effects. In addition, the application of specific therapies may be limited by the ability to diagnose the virus in a timely manner (within 1–2 days of symptom onset), so that the therapy has a reasonable chance of being successful.

Specific therapies that have been studied include the following: First, intranasal interferon (not yet approved for use in the United States) has effectively prevented RV colds if given shortly before or after exposure and is well tolerated for short courses (67). If used more long term, bleeding and excess nasal discharge have been noted (68). Second, drugs that interfere with different essential steps in the viral replication process have been tested in humans but unfortunately drug resistant strains have emerged (62). Other drugs that inhibit attachment of RV to cells have been tested in vivo and show promising results for anti-RV activity (69). Third, monoclonal antibodies directed against RV receptor sites have been preliminarily studied in humans, showing reduction in clinical illness and infection without undesired effects, however, more intensive study is needed (70). Fourth, compounds that antagonize the effects of inflammatory mediators have also undergone clinical trials with mixed results. Nedocromil sodium, salicylic acid, and acetaminophen have all been examined for these properties and for their usefulness in ameliorating the clinical effects of RV infection (61). And fifth, corticosteroids are well known for their broad spectrum of anti-inflammatory effects. Although the use of nasal and oral steroids during viral respiratory infections has been shown to reduce nasal obstruction, mucus production, and the concentration of inflammatory mediators in nasal secretions, the apparently minimal benefits of such use must be weighed against cost and possible adverse effects of long term or recurrent steroid administration (1,41,71).

In individuals with viral-induced asthma exacerbations, current treatment is therefore aimed at reducing the symptoms of wheezing and dyspnea using the standard regimen of bronchodilators and anti-inflammatory medications.

B. Prevention

The issue of prevention of viral induced wheezing can be examined in two ways: primary prevention of respiratory illness through the development of antiviral vaccines and secondary prevention of severe viral induced wheezing attacks by early identification of infection and use of early directed therapy. Antiviral vaccine development, in the case of RVs, for example, has been difficult because of the known antigenic diversity of the many serotypes of the RV (72). Much more work is needed before an effective vaccine is designed and tested. If available, a vaccine might be administered to patients with increased morbidity associated with viral-induced asthma exacerbations.

A number of specific therapeutic strategies for the amelioration of viral-induced wheezing were described in the preceding section; none, however, have been applied routinely. Corticosteroids are the most frequently used of all the therapies mentioned. A few studies examined how inhaled corticosteroids, when applied at the first sign of an upper respiratory tract illness, might successfully reduce the symptoms of asthma in children. Compared to placebo, both studies showed a decrease in symptoms scores and an increased parental preference for the inhaled steroid (61,73). Such studies are logistically difficult as they require early reporting of symptoms, accurate diagnostic techniques, and high subject compliance to demonstrate efficacy of the treatment. Additional studies are needed in both adults and children to define the role of corticosteroid prophylaxis against viral-induced wheezing.

V. RESPIRATORY ILLNESS IN INFANCY AND THE DEVELOPMENT OF ASTHMA

Asthma is a complex clinical problem. Individuals with asthma have a heterogeneous presentation and course and a multiplicity of risk factors for the development of disease (28). To further complicate this issue, many infants and children experience wheezing illnesses that closely resemble asthma but may not ultimately lead to the presence of chronic airway hyperresponsiveness (28). Although, the focus of this chapter has been to examine the relationship between acute viral illness and acute asthma exacerbations, it is worthwhile to explore how respiratory infection in infancy and childhood might contribute to the subsequent development of wheezing or asthma.

Prospective studies of infants and children with wheezing episodes due to respiratory infections have shown that, in some cases, early infection leads to diminished lung function and recurrent episodes of wheezing later in life (2); in other cases, there is no relationship to subsequent wheezing (28). In addition, some of these studies were able to show that other factors, such as family history of atopy, passive cigarette smoke exposure, and bottle feeding, all increased the risk of developing asthma independent of prior wheezing associated respiratory illness (28,74,75). In an effort to predict which children might be at risk for recurrent wheezing after acute infection, many indices have been studied, such as the magnitude of IgE responses at the time of infection or the need for hospitalization for treatment of bronchiolitis. However, more studies need to be done to determine the children who will subsequently have chronic asthma (28,76).

A recent study evaluated the effectiveness of inhaled anti-inflammatory therapy on subsequent wheezing episodes and admissions for bronchiolar obstruction in 100 consecutively hospitalized infants with bronchiolitis who were followed for 8 weeks (77). There was a 16% and 19% decrease in physician diagnosed wheezing episodes in the groups treated with budesonide and cromolyn sodium, respectively, compared to controls, and a significant reduction in admissions in the budesonide group and among children with atopy in both treatment groups (77). More studies similar to this one need to be carried out to ascertain the true value of preventative anti-inflammatory therapy.

In the last decade there have been enormous strides in the understanding of asthma pathophysiology and treatment; it is likely that parallel gains will be made in the understanding of how asthma begins, who is at risk, and how individuals at risk will be identified. Viral respiratory infections will continue to be recognized as a major precipitant of acute exacerbations of asthma and efforts to reduce the severity and frequency of these infections will hopefully lead to decreased asthma morbidity and improved quality of life for affected individuals.

REFERENCES

1. Pattemore PK, Johnston SL and Bardin PG, Viruses as precipitants of asthma Symptoms. I. Epidemiology, Clin. Exp. Allergy 1992; 22:325–336.
2. Hill M, Szefler SJ, et al, Asthma Pathogenesis and the Implications for Therapy in Children, Ped Clin of North Am 1992; 39(6):1205–1224.
3. Sterk PJ, Virus–induced airway hyperresponsiveness in man, Eur. Respir. J. 1993; 6:894–902.
4. Gregg I, Provocation of airflow limitation by viral infection: implication for treatment, Eur. J. Respir. Dis. 1983; 64(suppl 128):369–379.
5. Abramson MJ, Marks GB, and Pattemore PK, Are non–allergenic environmental factors important in asthma? Med. J. Aust. 1995; 163:542–545.
6. Stevens FA, Acute asthmatic episodes in children caused by upper respiratory bacteria during colds, with and without bacterial sensitization, J Allergy 1952; 24:221–226.
7. Feingold BF, Infection in bronchial allergic disease: bronchial asthma, allergic bronchitis, asthmatic bronchitis, Ped Clin North Am 1959; 6:709–724.
8. Hudgel DW, Langston L, Jr., Selner JC, et al., Viral and bacterial infections in adults with chronic asthma, Am. Rev. Respir. Dis. 1979; 120:393–397.
9. Disney ME, Matthews R, and Williams D, The role of infection in the morbidity of asthmatic children admitted to hospital, Clin. Allergy 1971; 1:399–406.
10. McIntosh K, Ellis EF, Hoffman LS, et al, The association of viral and bacterial respiratory

infections with exacerbations of wheezing in young asthmatic children, J. Pediatr. 1973; 82(4): 578–590.

11. Horn MEC, Reed SE, Taylor P, Role of viruses and bacteria in acute wheezy bronchitis in childhood: a study of sputum, Arch. Dis. Child. 1979; 54:587–592.
12. Podosin RL, Felton WL, The clinical picture of Far-East influenza occurring at the 4th National Boy Scout Jamboree, NEJM 1958; 258:778–782.
13. Rebhan AW. An outbreak of Asian influenza in a girls' camp, Can Med Assoc J 1957; 77: 797–799.
14. Chanock R, Fineberg L, Recovery from infants with respiratory illness if a virus related to chimpanzee coryza agent. II. Epidemiologic aspects of infection in infants and young children, Am J Hyg 1957; 66:291–300.
15. Henderson FW, Clyde WA, Jr., Collier AM, et al, The etiologic and epidemiologic spectrum of bronchiolitis in pediatric practice, J Pediatr 1979; 95(2):183–190.
16. Tarlo S, Broder I, and Spence L, A prospective study of respiratory infection in adult asthmatics and their normal spouses. Clin Allergy 1979; 9:293–301.
17. Clarke CW, Relationship of bacterial and viral infections to exacerbations of asthma, Thorax 1979; 34:344–347.
18. Horn MEC, Brain EA, Inglis JM, et al., Respiratory viral infection and wheezy bronchitis in childhood, Thorax 1979; 34:23–28.
19. Mitchell I, Inglis JM, and Simpson H, Viral infection as a precipitant of wheeze in children. Combined home and hospital study, Arch Dis Child 1978; 53:106–111.
20. Minor TE, Dick EC, and Baker JW, et al, Rhinovirus and Influenza Type A Infections as Precipitants of Asthma, Am Rev Respir Dis 1976; 113:149–153.
21. Mitchell I, Inglis H, and Simpson H, Viral infection in wheezy bronchitis and asthma in children, Arch Dis Child 1976; 51:707–711.
22. Minor TE, Dick EC, DeMeo AN, et al., Viruses as Precipitants of Asthmatic Attacks in Children, JAMA 1974; 227(3):292–298.
23. Richardson JB, Hogg JC, Bouchard T, et al., Electron Microscopic Localization of Antigen in Experimental Bronchoconstriction in Guinea Pigs, Chest 1973; 63(4) (Suppl.):44S–48S.
24. Maletzky AJ, Cooney MK, Luce R, et al., Epidemiology of viral and mycoplasma agents associated with childhood lower respiratory illness in a civilian population, J Pediatr 1971; 78(3):407–414.
25. Glezen P, Loda FA, Clyde WA, Jr., et al., Epidemiologic patterns of acute lower respiratory disease of children in a pediatric group practice, J Pediatr 1971; 78(3):397–406.
26. Berkovich S, Millian SJ, and Snyder RD, The association of viral and mycoplasma infections with recurrence of wheezing in the asthmatic child, An Allergy 1970; 28(2):43–49.
27. Freeman GL, Wheezing Associated With Respiratory Tract Infections In Children. The Role of Specific Infectious Agents in Allergic Respiratory Manifestations, Clin Pediatr 1966; 5(10): 586–592.
28. Morgan WJ and Martinez FD, Risk Factors For Developing Wheezing and Asthma in Childhood, Pediatr Clin North Am 1992; 39(6):1185–1203.
29. Kellner G, Popow-Kraupp T, Kundi M, et al., Clinical manifestations of respiratory tract infections due to respiratory syncytial virus and rhinoviruses in hospitalized children, Acta Paediatr Scand 1989; 78:390–394.
30. Carlsen KH and Orstavik I, Bronchopulmonary obstruction in children with respiratory virus infections, Eur J Respir Dis 1984; 65:92–98.
31. Mertsola J, Ziegler T, Ruuskanen O, et al., Recurrent wheezy bronchitis and viral respiratory infections, Arch Dis Child 1991; 66:124–129.
32. Storr J and Lenney W, School holidays and admissions with asthma, Arch Dis Child 1989; 64:103–107.
33. Jennings LC, Barns G, Dawson KP, et al., In Practice. The association of viruses with acute asthma, NZ Med J 1987; 100:488–490.

34. Carlson KH, Orstavik I, Leegaard J, et al., Respiratory virus infections and aerollergens in acute bronchial asthma, Arch Dis Child 1984; 59:310–315.
35. Johnston SL, Pattemore PK, Sanderson G, et al., Community study of role of viral infections in exacerbations of asthma in 9–11 year old children, Br Med J 1995; 310:1225–1228.
36. Roldaan AC and Masural N, Viral respiratory infections in asthmatic children staying in a mountain resort, Eur J Respir Dis 1982; 63:140–150.
37. Potter PC, Weinberg E, and Shore SCL, Acute severe asthma. A prospective study of the precipitating factors in 40 children, S Afr Med J 1984; 66(15):397–402.
38. Beasley, ED Coleman, Hermon Y, et al., Viral respiratory tract infection and exacerbations of asthma in adult patients, Thorax 1988; 43:679–683.
39. Sokhandan M, McFadden ER, Huang YT, et al., The Contribution of Respiratory Viruses to Severe Exacerbations of Asthma in Adults, Chest 1995; 107:1570–1575.
40. Halperin A, Eggleston PA, Beasley P, et al., Exacerbations of Asthma in Adults during Experimental Rhinovirus Infection, Am Rev Respir Dis 1985; 132:976–980.
41. Bardin PG, Johnston SL, and Pattemore PK, Viruses as precipitants of asthma symptoms II. Physiology and mechanisms, Clin Exp Allergy 1992; 22:809–822.
42. Busse WW, Lemanske RF, and Dick EC, The Relationship of Viral Respiratory Infections and Asthma, Chest 1992; 101(6)(Suppl.):385S–388S.
43. Hers JF, Disturbances of ciliated epithelium due to influenza virus, Am Rev Respir Dis 1966; 93:162–171.
44. Empey DW, Laitinen LA, Jacobs L, et al., Mechanisms of bronchial hyperreactivity in normal subjects after upper respiratory tract infection, Am Rev Respir Dis 1976; 113:131–139.
45. Jakab GJ, Sequential virus infections, bacterial superinfections, and fibrogenesis, Am Rev Respir Dis 1990; 142:374–379.
46. Busse WW, Swenson CA, Bordon EC, et al., Effect of influenza A virus on leukocyte histamine release, J Allergy Clin Immunol 1983; 71:382–388.
47. Ida S, Hooks JJ, Siraganian RP, et al., Enhancement of IgE mediated histamine release from human basophils by viruses: role of interferon, J Exp Med 1977; 145:892–906.
48. Chonmaitree T, Lett-Brown MA, Tsong Y, et al., Role of interferon in leukocyte histamine release caused by common respiratory viruses, J Inf Dis 1988; 157:127–132.
49. Kimira I, Tanizaki Y, Saito K, et al., Appearance of basophils in the sputum of patients with bronchial asthma, Clin Allergy 1975; 1:95–98.
50. Naclerio RM, Proud D, Lichtenstein LM, et al, Kinins are generated during experimental rhinoviral colds, J Inf Dis 1987; 157:133–142.
51. Kaul TN, Welliver RC, Ogra PL, Appearance of complement components and immunoglobulins on nasopharyngeal epithelial cells following naturally acquired infection with respiratory syncytial virus, J Med Virol 1982; 9:149–158.
52. Volovitz B, Welliver RC, De Castro G, et al., The release of leukotrienes in the respiratory tract during infection with respiratory syncytial virus: role in obstructive airway disease, Pediatr Res 1988; 24(4):504–507.
53. Alvarado CA, Canesco C, Wentz–Murtha P, et al., Serum and secretory antibody response of normal and asthmatic subjects to influenza vaccine, J Allergy Clin Immunol 1991; 87(abstr): 287.
54. Pene J, Rousset F, Briere F, et al., IgE production by normal lymphocytes is induced by interleukin 4 and suppressed by interferons and prostaglandin E2, Proc Natl Acad Sci 1988; 85:6880–6884.
55. Vritis R, Schrader L, Dick EC, et al., Development of low density eosinophils following in vitro incubation with respiratory viruses, J Allergy Clin Immunol 1990; 85(abstr):165.
56. Garofalo R, Kimpen JL, Welliver RC, et al., Role of respiratory syncytial virus-induced eosinophil degranulation in bronchiolitis, J Allergy Clin Immunol 1991; 87(abstr):24.
57. Welliver RC, Kaul A, and Ogra PL, Cell-mediated immune response to respiratory syncytial

virus infection: Relationship to the development of reactive airway disease, J Pediatr 1979; 94(3):370–375.
58. Welliver RC, Wong DT, Sun M, et al., The development of respiratory syncytial virus-specific IgE and the release of histamine in nasopharyngeal secretions after infection, N Engl J Med 1981; 305(15):841–846.
59. Welliver RC, Wong DT, Middleton E, et al., Role of parainfluenza virus-specific IgE in pathogenesis of croup and wheezing subsequent to infection, J Pediatr 1982; 101(6):889–896.
60. Johnston S, Pattemore PK, Smith S, et al., Viral infections in exacerbations in school children with cough or wheeze: a longitudinal study, Am Rev Respir Dis 1992; 145:A546.
61. Johnston SL, Bardin PG, and Pattemore PK, Viruses as precipitants of asthma symptoms III. Rhinoviruses: molecular biology and prospects for future intervention, Clin Exp Allergy 1993; 23:237–246.
62. Dearden C, Al-Nakib W, Andries K, et al., Drug resistant rhinoviruses from the nose of experimentally treated volunteers, Arch Virol 1989; 109:71–81.
63. Hyypia T, Auvinen P, Maaronen P, Polymerase chain reaction for human picornaviruses, J Gen Virol 1989; 70:3261–3268.
64. Gama RE, Horsnell PR, Hughes PJ, et al., Amplification of rhinovirus specific nucleic acids from clinical samples using the polymerase chain reaction, J Med Virol 1989; 28:73–77.
65. Olive DM, Al-Mufti S, Al-Mulla W, et al., Detection and differentiation of picornaviruses in clinical samples following genomic amplification, J Gen Virol 1990; 71: 2141–2147.
66. Johnston S, Sanderson G, Pattemore PK, et al., Use of polymerase chain reaction for diagnosis of picornavirus infection in subjects with and without respiratory symptoms, J Clin Microbiol 1993; 31:11–117.
67. Sperber SJ, Hayden FG, Chemotherapy of rhinovirus colds, Antimicro Agents Chemother 1988; 32:409–419.
68. Hayden FG, Mills SE, Johns ME, Human tolerance and histopathologic effects of long term administration of interferon-alpha 2, J Inf Dis 1983; 148:914–921.
69. Andries K, DeWindt B, Snoeks J, et al., In Vitro activity of Pirodavir (R77975), a substituted phenoxy-pyridazinamine with broad spectrum antipicornaviral activity, Antimicrob Agents Chemother 1992; 36:100–107.
70. Hayden FG, Gwaltney JM, Colonno RJ, Modification of experimental rhinovirus colds by receptor blockade, Antiviral Res 1988; 9:233–247.
71. Webb MS, Henry RL, Milner AD, Oral corticosteroids for wheezing attacks under 18 months, Arch Dis Child 1986; 61:15–19 (1986).
72. Russell SM, Trowbridge M, Appleyard G, et al., Mapping of neutralization epitopes on human rhinovirus type 2 with monoclonal antibodies, Vaccines 1989; 89:431–436.
73. Connet G and Lenney W, Prevention of viral induced asthma attacks using inhaled budesonide, Arch Dis Child 1993; 68:85–87.
74. Welliver RC, Wong DT, and Sun M, et al., Parainfluenza virus bronchiolitis. epidemiology and pathogenesis, Am J Dis Child 1986; 140:34–40.
75. Frick OL, German DF, and Mills J, Development of allergy in children. I. Association with virus infections, J Allergy Clin Immunol 1979; 63(4):228–241.
76. Welliver RC, Sun M, and Rinaldo D, et al., Predictive value of respiratory syncytial virus-specific IgE responses for recurrent wheezing following bronchiolitis, J Pediatr 1986; 109(5): 776–780.
77. Reijonen T, Korppi M, Kuikka L, et al., Anti-inflammatory therapy reduces wheezing after bronchiolitis, Arch Pediatr Adolesc 1996; 150:512–517.

9

The Relationship Between Acute Asthma and Air Pollution

George D. Thurston
New York University School of Medicine, New York, New York

Mark J. Leber
The Brooklyn Hospital Center, member of New York–Presbyterian Hospitals, Weill Medical College of Cornell University, Brooklyn, New York

I. INTRODUCTION

Why is it so important to further our understanding of the connections between air pollution and asthma? Asthma incidence is growing in the general population. Increasing numbers of annual emergency department visits, hospital admissions, and deaths related to asthma are being recorded annually (1). One of the etiologies that may be contributing to the asthma incidence rate is air pollution, which has been shown to aggravate asthma and increase the likelihood of an exacerbation among those who have asthma. Research studying the association between air pollution and asthma is needed to determine the specific populations most affected and the pathophysiology and biological markers that determine patients' sensitivities to air pollution. Once these aspects are better understood, preventative public health and medical care measures may be more effectively instituted. These measures might include the following:

- Coordinated efforts through public policy to reduce ambient concentrations of key air pollutants
- Intensive educational efforts geared to specific locales and populations
- More effective warnings to especially susceptible individuals to avoid their exposures to air pollution
- The development of better medications and medication protocols that will reduce the effects of air pollution on the asthma patient's respiratory and immune systems

This chapter discusses the available evidence regarding the epidemiological associations between asthma and air pollution, the culpable components of air pollution, the especially susceptible populations, and the pathophysiology and mechanisms underlying individual susceptibilities to air pollution's adverse effects.

II. WHAT IS THE EVIDENCE OF A RELATIONSHIP BETWEEN AIR POLLUTION AND HEALTH?

A. Background

Major past pollution episodes have dramatically increased morbidity and mortality in affected communities. For example, the incidence of both daily hospital admissions and mortality increased precipitously during a 4-day pollution-laden London Fog Episode in December 1952, with some 4000 premature deaths being associated with this one air pollution episode (2). During a 1948 pollution episode in the industrialized valley town of Donora, PA, 19 people died, 50 were hospitalized, and thousands became ill in a community of 14,000 (3,4). These episodes were each associated with a stagnant air mass, caused by a dispersion-inhibiting weather pattern that persists over a region for multiple days, causing local air pollution to build up to high levels.

Patients with underlying cardiopulmonary disease were among those most severely affected during the Donora incident (3). Most of the hospitalized people suffered from asthma, and 80% of those in the community who had asthma became symptomatic. In addition, in Donora asthma was found to play a role in 5 of the 12 deaths for which a cause was confirmed. Thus, an epidemiological association exists between extreme air pollution and adverse health effects, especially among those with pre-existing respiratory diseases such as asthma, but the question has been raised as to whether these kinds of air pollution effects occur at present-day ambient air pollution levels.

B. Present-Day Studies of Air Pollution and Adverse Health Effects

At present, assessment of the effects of air pollution on asthmatics have focused largely on particulate matter (PM) and ozone (O_3) air pollution. Particulate matter is composed of two major components: primary particles, or ''soot,'' emitted directly into the atmosphere by pollution sources such as industry, electric power plants, diesel buses, and automobiles; and ''secondary particles'' formed in the atmosphere from pollutant gases, such as sulfur dioxide (SO_2) and nitrogen oxides (NO_x), emitted by many combustion sources, including coal-burning electric power plants. Ozone is a highly irritant gas that is formed in our atmosphere in the presence of sunlight from other ''precursor'' air pollutants, including nitrogen oxides and hydrocarbons. These precursor pollutants, which cause the formation of O_3, are emitted by pollution sources including automobiles, electric power plants, and industry.

Epidemiological studies that follow a population over time, called time-series studies, have provided valuable information relating variations in present-day pollution to changes in human health. For example, the epidemiological evidence indicating an association between present-day PM and the increased incidence of mortality and morbidity has been documented in the literature by numerous investigators studying populations in various locales. In 1997, Schwartz compared various studies that reported relative risks (RR) resulting from an increase of 100 $\mu g/m^3$ in ambient PM_{10} (inhalable particles less than 10 μm in diameter), that is, the ratio of the number of problems reported on days when subject populations were exposed to elevated pollution versus the number reported on clean days (5). Examining multiple studies conducted around the globe (e.g., across 17 studies of mortality), Schwartz found consistency for all respiratory hospital admissions (average RR = 1.13), chronic obstructive pulmonary disease (COPD) hospital admissions (average RR = 1.19), pneumonia hospital admissions (average RR = 1.13) and mortality (average RR = 1.09). The fact that these epidemiological pollution-health effect associations have been so consistently shown, both across outcomes and from place to place, supports the conclusion that ambient particulate matter air pollution and adverse human health effects are causally related.

While specific causal mechanisms (i.e., the ''smoking guns'') of the PM-health effects associations are not yet known at this time, there are biologically plausible mechanisms that could account for the associations. For example, PM exposure stresses the lung (e.g., by inducing inflammation and/or edema), and places an extra burden on the heart, which could induce fatal complications for cardiac patients. Recent animal experiments by Godleski and coworkers at Harvard University confirm that exposures to elevated concentrations of ambient PM can result in cardiac related death in animals (6,7). In addition, controlled exposure studies of animals have demonstrated significant adverse pulmonary effects from combustion-related fine particles ($PM_{2.5}$, or those particles less than 2.5 μm in diameter). These include diminished respiratory defense mechanisms and the opening of the lung to illness from other causes. In addition, repeated exposures to acidic fine particulate matter, a portion of the fine $PM_{2.5}$ that the newly promulgated ambient PM standards of the Environmental Protection Agency (EPA) will focus on in future control strategies (8), has been shown to affect lung clearance in a manner similar to the effects of tobacco smoke, suggesting that these fine particles may have analogous long-term exposure implications to the development of COPD (9).

Epidemiological evidence has also accumulated over recent years indicating a role by O_3 in daily human morbidity and mortality, including for asthma. In a summary of the published literature, Schwartz showed that O_3 has consistently been found to acutely increase hospital admissions: average RR = 1.06 for all respiratory admissions; average RR = 1.10 for COPD admissions; and average RR = 1.07 for COPD admissions, given a 50 parts per billion (ppb) rise in daily maximum O_3 concentration (5). Such O_3 pollution increases are common in the summer months, when O_3 concentrations rise above 100 ppb in many U.S. cities on polluted days.

The Schwartz (5) review did not address the potential effects of O_3 on mortality, perhaps because fewer studies of this were available in the published literature, but evidence is mounting that O_3 can also cause premature deaths. For example, Verhoeff et al. (10) used Poisson regression to analyze associations between daily mortality and air pollution concentrations in Amsterdam, The Netherlands, during 1986–1992, and found a daily mortality RR = 1.10 per 100 ppb 1-hr daily maximum O_3, even after controlling for weather and copollutants. Anderson et al. (11) investigated whether outdoor air pollution levels in London, England, influenced daily mortality during 1987–1992, finding a daily mortality RR = 1.10 per 100 ppb 8-hr O_3 (RR = 1.08 per 100 ppb 1-hr O_3), even after controlling for weather and copollutants. Samet et al. (12) considered total daily mortality and environmental data for Philadelphia during 1973–1980, finding that, when pairs of pollutants were considered simultaneously, only the O_3 effect consistently remained unchanged and statistically significant, with a total mortality RR of 1.02 for a 20 ppb increase in 24-hr daily average O_3. An evaluation of specific causes of death indicated the largest O_3 RR for respiratory deaths, consistent with biological plausibility. More recently, Thurston (13) found that daily mortality also rises after high O_3 days in the U.S. cities of New York City, Atlanta, Detroit, Chicago, St. Louis, Minneapolis, San Francisco, Los Angeles, and Houston, even after accounting for other factors such as season and weather. These studies indicate that the overall population's risk of death, albeit low on any one day, rises by about 6–10% following days having a 1-hr maximum of O_3 that is 100 ppb above the average (i.e., after high summertime pollution days).

Time-series studies have shown that present-day pollution can also exacerbate asthma. For example, Thurston and colleagues have documented associations between ambient summertime haze air pollutants, such as O_3, and increased daily numbers of asthma and respiratory admissions to the hospital (14). In that work, hourly O_3 data were recorded by the New York State Department of Environmental Conservation, while daily particle samples were collected by New York University at three urban sites in New York Sate over three years (1988–1990). The ambient air particle samples were analyzed for acidity and for sulfate levels. Hospital admission records were obtained from the N.Y. State Department of Health's Statewide Planning and Research Cooperative System (SPARCS). Results indicated that there was a direct relationship between summertime respiratory admissions in New York City and both O_3 and sulfate levels (14). In this study, summer haze pollution was associated with both total respiratory and asthma admissions. Even after controlling for temperature, the association remained significant ($p \leq 0.05$). Summer haze pollution accounted for 6–24% of adult asthma admissions in Buffalo and New York City. Asthma admission relative risks ranged from RR = 1.19–1.43 on the highest atmospheric pollution days, relative to an average day, indicating that asthma admission rates were raised by on the order of 20–40% by high pollution days.

On the other hand, in a study done in England by Devereux, comparing an industrialized section of England (high pollution) with a rural section (low pollution), no real differences in the incidence of asthma was found between the two studied populations (15). These and several other negative findings regarding air pollution and asthma have cast some doubt over the role of pollution in asthma. However, asthma is caused by multifactorial agents, and there may be interactions required between air pollution and allergens that may not have been present at the time of this negative study. Such apparent epidemiological inconsistencies may be therefore be explained by the fact that air pollution can act to enhance the reactivity of asthmatics to other environmental factors, such as allergens, which are not always present in the environment at the same time as air pollution. Indeed, Koren and Bromberg (16) noted that inflammatory changes in the respiratory tract induced by air pollution augment the responses of allergic asthmatics to nasal and inhalation challenge by antigens, and that this may explain the findings of air pollution–asthma associations by epidemiological field studies.

Excess hospital admissions and premature deaths are only the tip of the iceberg of air pollution's effects that can be eliminated by cleaning the air. In order to give some insight into the much larger numbers of other effects lurking beneath the surface of the O_3 hospital admissions effects noted in Table VI-2(revised) of the Ozone OAQPS Staff Paper (17), working estimates have been made of the other documented adverse impacts of O_3 exposure that will also be reduced in New York City, when the EPA's recently promulgated new O_3 standard are achieved (18).

The results of the analyses are presented in Figure 1 (19). Note that the figure could not be drawn to scale, because if it were the New York City (NYC) asthma admissions triangle would not even be visible, since it accounts for only approximately 0.01% of the total number of 0_3 related impacts noted for NYC. However, despite the fact that it visually overstates the relative size of the NYC hospital asthma admissions, and the fact that still other O_3 effects cannot be considered in these calculations due to a lack of data, this figure clearly shows that New York City asthma admissions counts represent only a small frac-

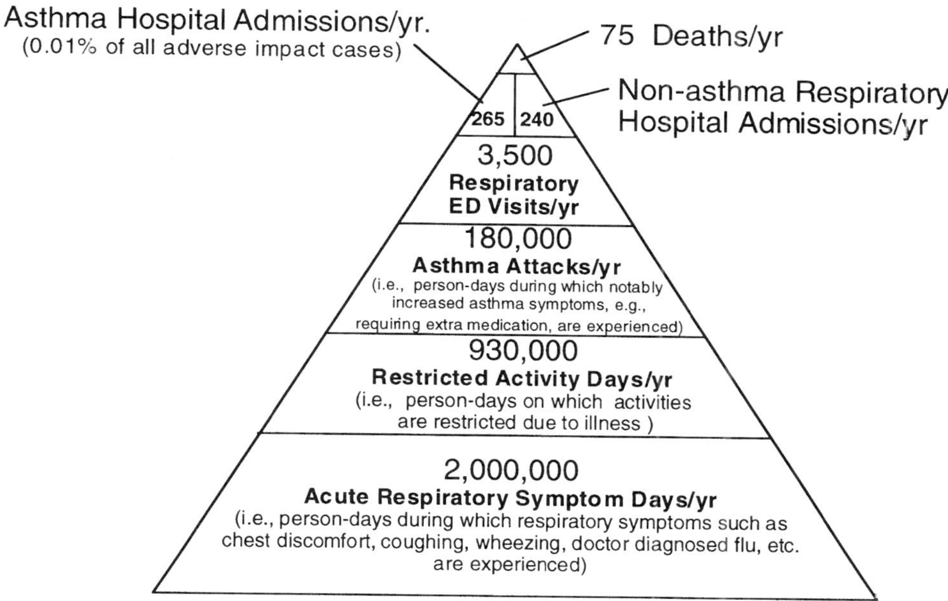

Figure 1 Pyramid of New York City annual adverse ozone impacts avoided by the implementation of the proposed new standard (vs. "as is"). (Figure section sizes not drawn to scale.)

tion (far less than 1%) of the adverse effects of air pollution which will be avoided after implementation of the new U.S. EPA O_3 standard.

This analysis, developed for testimony before Congress (19), used as its starting point the 265 New York City asthma admissions estimated to be avoided as a result of the implementation of the EPA's standard (i.e., 385 − 120 = 265 admissions), as estimated by the U.S. EPA (18). First, as noted above, there are also nonasthma respiratory admissions effects. Based upon the average O_3 impacts derived from the published O_3-admissions regression results for New York City and Buffalo, this indicated that the nonasthma respiratory admissions avoided (for causes such as pneumonia and bronchitis) will be about 90% of the size of the asthma admissions, or 240/yr (14). Then, based on a report that New York City hospital records indicate that 12.6% of pediatric asthma emergency department (ED) visits result in an asthma hospital admission (20), it was estimated that the ED visits associated with the 505 O_3-related respiratory admissions would amount to approximately 3500 O_3-induced ED visits (i.e., 505 × 1/.126). Furthermore, based on the O_3 adverse health effect coefficients reported in the published literature, effects for other outcomes were also derived (21). In this way, estimated annual effects to be avoided in New York City each year were also obtained for:

- Premature mortality
- Asthma attacks
- Restricted activity days (i.e., the total number of person-days during which some normal activities were curtailed)

- Acute respiratory symptom days (i.e., the total number of person-days during which additional respiratory symptoms would be experienced)

Some may quarrel with the specific coefficients chosen here to model the other effects, but the overall point remains that these other effects collectively represent large multiples of the hospital admissions benefits previously noted for New York City. Note that the numbers in this figure have been corrected to avoid double counting of adverse health "events." For example, the number of unscheduled hospital admissions has been subtracted from the total number of ED visits, since patients would likely have first passed through the ED before being admitted.

Finally, although there are about 7 million persons in New York City, there are a total of some 122 million persons throughout the United States, who now live in areas exceeding the EPA's new O_3 standard and will therefore also benefit from that new standard (18). Thus, the hospital admissions and mortality effects resulting from air pollution are best viewed as an indicator of a much broader spectrum of avoidable adverse health effects experienced by the public.

Prospective epidemiological studies of panels of individuals confirm the epidemiological asthma–air pollution association. For example, in a recent study of individuals with asthma, Thurston and colleagues (22) followed the effects of air pollution on children at a summer "asthma" camp in Connecticut over time, rather than focusing on aggregated citywide counts of asthma events. This study of a group of moderate to severely asthmatic children over three summers (1990–1992) showed that these children experience diminished lung function, increased asthma symptoms, and increased use of unscheduled asthma medications as O_3 pollution levels rose. As shown in Figure 2, the risk of a child having an asthma attack was found to be approximately 40% higher on the highest O_3 days than on an average study day, with these adverse effects extending to below the old 120 ppb O_3 air quality standard.

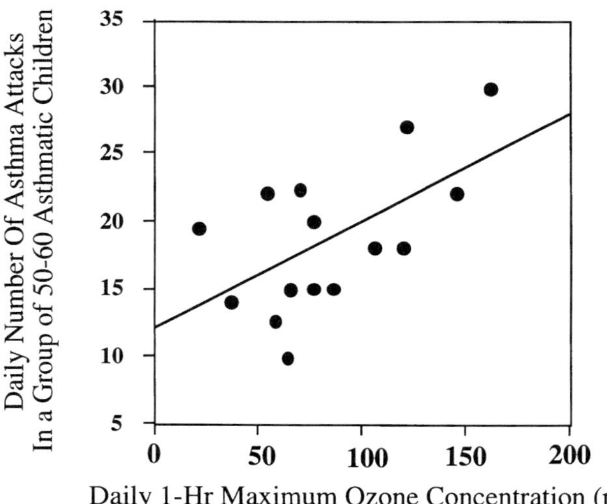

Figure 2 Daily asthma attacks in children increase as ozone levels rise. (From Ref. 23.)

III. WHAT ARE THE RESPONSIBLE AIR POLLUTION AGENTS?

As discussed above, numerous studies of metropolitan areas have shown associations between acute increase in the incidence of asthma exacerbations and levels of air pollution. In particular, strong epidemiological associations have been noted between the level of outdoor particulate matter smaller than 10 μm in diameter (PM_{10}), and O_3 air pollution and the incidence of respiratory morbidity and mortality. The pollutants affecting asthmatics can be thought of as falling into two classes: summertime haze air pollutants formed in the atmosphere (i.e., secondary pollutants) and predominantly wintertime pollutants emitted directly into the atmosphere (i.e., primary pollutants).

A. Summer Haze Pollutants: O_3 and $SO_4^=$

Probably the largest hospital admissions database analyzed to date came from the series of studies by Bates and Sizto (23–26) in which O_3 and particulate sulfates ($SO_4^=$) in southern Ontario, Canada, were most strongly associated with increased asthma admissions above expected rates for summertime. A re-analysis of this database by Lipfert and Hammerstrom indicated that 20% of summertime respiratory admissions were associated with outdoor air pollution (27). Burnett and colleagues, also examining the southern Ontario area, found significant asthma hospital admissions associations in all four seasons for $SO_4^=$, and for O_3 in the summer months only (28). Cody et al. and Weisel et al. also showed significant associations between summertime O_3 concentrations and ED visits for asthma in New Jersey (29,30). Thurston and colleagues reported associations between asthma hospital admissions and elevated summertime haze air pollution, especially for O_3 and particulate aerosol acidity in Toronto, Ontario, during the summers of 1986–1988. Stronger associations with admissions were found for fine and acidic particulate matter than for coarse particles. Consistent with biological plausibility, no such air pollution associations were found for control disease categories (e.g., digestive disease admissions) (31). Similar results were found by Thurston et al. for Buffalo, NY, and New York City during the summers of 1988 and 1989 (14). Thus, acute increases in summertime haze air pollutants, including O_3 and acidic $SO_4^=$, have been found to increase the incidence of both daily asthma hospital visits and admissions in metropolitan areas.

B. Predominantly Winter Pollutants: Black Smoke and SO_2

In a study of adult asthmatics in France over a six-month period, Diakite and colleagues found that asthma symptoms in mild and moderate asthmatics increased with increasing concentrations of PM (measured as black smoke) and SO_2 (32). Forsberg et al. (33) followed a panel of 31 asthmatic patients residing in the town of Piteá in northern Sweden. Severe symptoms of shortness of breath, wheeze, cough, and phlegm were recorded in an asthma diary together with suspected causes. Daily variations in the concentrations of PM had significant effects on the risk of developing severe symptoms of shortness of breath (33).

In a panel study by Ostro and colleagues, conducted during the winter in Denver, Colorado, 207 adult asthmatics recorded respiratory symptoms, frequency of medication use, and related information in daily diaries (34). Airborne particulate acidity (H^+) was found to be significantly associated with several indicators of asthma status, including moderate or severe cough and shortness of breath. Cough was also associated with increases in fine particles ($PM_{2.5}$), and shortness of breath was associated with increases in $SO_4^=$. Incorporating the participants' time spent outside and exercise intensity into the daily measure of exposure strengthened the association between these pollutants and asthmatic symptoms.

Pope et al. found, in a 1991 diary study of a group of persons with asthma (8–72 years of age) living in an industrialized valley in Utah, that the probability of the use of asthma medication on the day with the highest concentration of thoracic PM (PM_{10}) was six times that of the lowest pollution day (35). Roemer et al. found consistent positive associations between PM_{10} and SO_2 air pollution and both wheeze symptoms and bronchodilator use by schoolchildren with chronic respiratory symptoms (36).

Thus, PM, O_3, and $SO_4^=$ are the pollutants that appear to most exacerbate asthma, and these effects can occur throughout the year.

IV. ARE THERE PLAUSIBLE BIOLOGICAL MECHANISMS FOR THESE AIR POLLUTION–ASTHMA ASSOCIATIONS?

Although the mechanism(s) by which air pollution causes the aforementioned adverse health effects are not fully understood, biologically plausible hypotheses exist that are supported by a large body of data from controlled exposure studies. For example, clinical studies have demonstrated decreases in lung function, increased frequencies of respiratory symptoms, heightened airway hyperresponsiveness, and cellular and biochemical evidence of lung inflammation in exercising adults exposed to O_3 concentrations at exposures as low as 80 ppb for 6.6 hr [e.g., Follinsbee et al. (37) and Devlin et al. (38)].

Most hypothesized mechanisms for the induction of an asthma attack by air pollution involve an enhancement of an asthmatic's reactivity to environmental antigens, rather than a direct triggering by air pollution. Gordon and Fine recently summarized the possible physiological mechanisms by which air pollution may enhance the likelihood of an asthma attack, including increased lung permeability; altered pollutant clearance; lymphocyte effects; and influences on antigen-presenting cells (39). Increased lung lining permeability can occur when air pollution exposure causes epithelial cell damage in the lung. This may increase the penetration of inhaled antigenic particles to immune system cells located beneath the airway epithelial lining and to the lymphatic system serving the lung. Alteration of lung clearance by air pollution exposure can result in increased retention of inhaled antigens, thereby increasing the probability of an antigen-antibody interaction. Air pollution–induced changes in the numbers of T lymphocytes in the lung may alter the immune system balance, enhancing asthmatic responses to antigens. Air pollution exposure may also stimulate antigen-presenting (or accessory) cells, which are involved in the initiation of most immune responses. Thus, air pollution affects several aspects of the asthma response to environmental antigens, such as pollens, and may thereby precipitate asthma attacks when they would not otherwise occur, or worsen the severity of attacks initiated by other causes.

Air pollution may also act to counteract the intended effects of preventative anti-inflammatory asthma medications, such as corticosteroids, reducing their effectiveness. Airway inflammation in the lung is among the adverse effects that have been demonstrated by controlled human studies of O_3 at typical ambient levels (40). Airway inflammation is especially a problem for children and adults with asthma, as it makes them more susceptible to having asthma attacks. For example, controlled human studies have indicated that prior exposure to O_3 enhances the reactivity of asthmatics to aeroallergens, such as pollens, which can trigger asthma attacks (41). Thus, O_3 exposures may exert their greatest effects on asthma by increasing inflammation in the lung, which heightens the responsiveness of asthmatics' lungs to all other environmental agents that may cause an exacerbation.

Combustion-related fine particles ($PM_{2.5}$) have also been shown by recent controlled exposure studies to have significant adverse effects on the lung, including diminished respiratory defense mechanisms, opening the lung to illness from other causes. For example, repeated exposures to acidic fine particulate matter has been shown to affect particle clearance from the lung in a fashion similar to tobacco smoke, suggesting that these fine particles may have analogous long-term exposure effects on the development of COPD (9).

In other work, Li and colleagues (42) conducted bronchioalveolar lavages on rats exposed to PM_{10}. They reported increasing free radical activity that caused lung inflammation and epithelial injury. These free radicals, they theorized, may be responsible for airway disease in asthmatic patients (42). Scannell and colleagues (43) performed bronchioalveolar lavages on human subjects in order to compare asthmatic and nonasthmatic responses to exposure to O_3. They found both increased neutrophil and total protein in asthmatic patients, as compared to nonasthmatics, when exposed to O_3 (43). These two studies indicate that enhanced inflammation resulted when asthmatics were exposed to O_3 or PM_{10}.

Thus, based on recent clinical studies, there is mounting evidence that air pollutants are involved in worsening and exacerbating acute asthma, and there are biologically plausible physiological mechanisms for these effects.

V. WHAT ASTHMA SUBPOPULATIONS ARE MOST AFFECTED BY AIR POLLUTION?

A. Background

It is well established that both asthma mortality and asthma hospital admissions increased during the 1980s [e.g., Buist and Vollmer (44) and Taylor and Newacheck (45)], and that the highest rates are associated with inner city residence [Carr et al. (46) and Weiss and Wagener (47)], and being of Latino or African-American origin [Carter-Pokras and Gergen (48); Coultas et al. (43), and Weiss and Wagener (47)]. In the words of Weiss and Wagener: ''whatever the reason for the increases, both asthma mortality and hospitalization continue to affect non-whites, urban areas, and the poor disproportionately.'' For example, the hospitalization rate for asthma is higher in New York City than anyplace else in the United States (46).

Pollution-asthma admissions associations were found by Thurston and colleagues to be weaker in the less urbanized Albany population area and in the NYC suburbs than in the inner city (14). This study employed total citywide daily counts, and did not specifically monitor the inner city minority population, which was a limitation in this regard. However, the work did suggest that cities with large minority populations (e.g., New York City) had the strongest associations between pollution and respiratory admissions.

Factors that might cause residents of low-income underprivileged urban neighborhoods to be more affected by air pollution may include:

1. Enhanced individual susceptibility of minority populations to pollution effects (i.e., more compromised health status, due either to greater genetic predetermination or severity of underlying disease)
2. Exposures to atmospheric pollution that may be greater than those of the general population, due to the greater concentration of some types of pollution in the center of cities, combined with a lower prevalence of protective air conditioning
3. Potentially enhanced exposures to a variety of residential risk cofactors such as cockroaches, dust mites, and indoor pollution sources (e.g., gas stoves used for space heating purposes)
4. A greater likelihood of poverty and resulting reduced access to routine health care

The roles of these various factors in defining who in these urban populations are most likely to react strongly enough to air pollution resulting in a visit to an ED are not yet understood.

Children are among those most likely to be adversely affected by pollution, based on both their behavioral patterns and physiology (50). With regard to air pollution, youngsters spend significantly more time outdoors, especially in the summertime, when O_3 air pollution levels are the highest. In addition, children spend approximately three times as much time engaged in sports and vigorous activities as do adults. This extra activity results in breathing in more air, and therefore more pollution being breathed into the lungs. Also, during exercise, children and adults breathe with both their nose and mouth rather than just their noses. When the nose is bypassed during the breathing process, the filtering effects of the nose are lost, thereby allowing more air pollution to reach the lung. Moreover, because of their larger surface-to-volume ratio, children's metabolic rates are higher, and their air consumption is greater per pound of body weight. Thus, while the average adult oxygen consumption is 3.5 ml/kg body weight/min., a 6-month-old child averages 7 ml/kg body weight/min., or double that of an adult (51). Children's developing lungs may also be especially susceptible targets. For example, it has been found that the growth rate of lung function in children exposed to environmental tobacco smoke (ETS) is significantly lower than that of children with no exposure (52). Thus, children can be more impacted by air pollution than adults because of their greater pollutant exposure, absorption, and target organ susceptibility.

Available evidence suggests that the aforementioned epidemiological associations between air pollution and asthma may be driven by a subpopulation of people with asthma who are ''pollution responders,'' rather than by all asthmatics having been affected equally. This phenomena has been demonstrated most clearly for O_3, which has been shown to elicit responses, in terms of respiratory symptoms and lung function decrements, in some persons but not in others. For example, in groups of healthy volunteers who underwent multiple O_3 exposures (2-hr duration, with exercise) at various time intervals ranging from 3 weeks to 14 months, individual physiological responses were reproducible at concentrations from 180 to 400 ppb O_3 (53). This indicated that high or low reactivity to O_3 is a persistent biological characteristic of individuals. Silverman (54) exposed 17 adults with asthma to 250 ppb O_3 for 2 hr while they were quietly resting. Paired t-tests showed no demonstrable overall changes in lung function, but effects were significant in 6 of the 17 asthmatics, again indicating that there was a more susceptible sector of the asthma population (54).

In an effort to further understand individual differences in susceptibility to O_3, Linn and colleagues exposed 59 adult volunteers from the L.A. area to 180 ppb O_3 for 2 hr with intermittent exercise in the spring of 1986 (55). Not all subjects had asthma, but preference was given to selecting subjects who had asthma or who were atopic. Responsiveness was determined on the basis of lung function change and respiratory symptoms. Eight of the 12 responders were either atopic or asthmatic. Of the original 59 subjects, 12 persons who were unusually responsive to O_3 and 13 subjects who were unusually nonresponsive were retested in the fall and in the spring of the following year. By fall, it was found that the responders lost much of their responsiveness, confirming the adaptation process known to occur with repeated exposures to O_3. However, by the following spring, the responders and nonresponders were again distinctly different in their responsiveness to O_3, indicating that O_3 responsiveness as measured by lung function and respiratory symptoms is a persistent individual characteristic.

Sulfur dioxide (SO_2), a known bronchoconstrictor at elevated concentrations, has also shown individual-to-individual variability in the air pollutant concentration required to elicit a response. Linn and colleagues, for example, found that a 15-min exposure to 600 ppb SO_2 elicited a significant (15%) reduction in $FEV_{1.0}$ in most, but not all, mild to severe asthmatics in their study, but a reduction was even elicited well below this level in some of these subjects (56). Airway responsiveness of reactive subjects were highly reproducible over time intervals ranging from 1 to 7 weeks. It is interesting to note that variations in individual responsiveness to SO_2 could not be predicted by asthma status. A 1995 World Health Organization (WHO) report concluded that, ''a wide range of sensitivity has been demonstrated, both among normal subjects and among those with asthma, who form the most sensitive group'' (57). Thus, it has been demonstrated for O_3 and SO_2, and it is also thought to be true for other air pollutants, that certain asthmatics are more sensitive than others with asthma to the effects of air pollution.

B. Atopy and Air Pollution Effects

Based on available evidence, it is widely held today that air pollution effects in asthmatics are largely due to air pollution enhancement of allergic reactions (i.e., in atopics). This belief is based largely on the work of Molfino and colleagues (58), who reported that atopic asthmatics showed increased sensitivity to inhaled allergens after exposure to O_3. However, Chen and colleagues (59) exposed 14 atopic asthmatics to doubling doses of dust mite allergen (*Dermatophygoides Farinae*) after exposure to either air or 200 ppb O_3, finding there was a nonsignificant trend ($p = 0.42$) in the group toward increased sensitivity to allergen after O_3 exposure, but that individual responsiveness changes varied widely among the group. The authors speculated that ''a group of asthmatic individuals who are more O_3-sensitive may be at even greater risk for an increase in allergen sensitivity due to ozone'' (59).

VI. HAS AIR POLLUTION CONTRIBUTED TO THE RISE IN ASTHMA PREVALENCE OVER THE LAST TWO DECADES?

As discussed previously, asthma incidence has risen in the United States over the past decade. This rise is not fully understood, which has led to speculation as to whether environmental factors, including air pollution, might be involved in this trend. However, a report by Lang and Polansky reported that, ''the rates of death from asthma have increased in Philadelphia, whereas concentrations of major air pollutants have declined'' (60). Some have mistakenly concluded that these and similar overall trends elsewhere mean that air pollution cannot be related to asthma. However, this conclusion would ignore the fact that much of this increase in the incidence of asthma hospital admissions and deaths is accounted for by a rise in asthma prevalence during the 1980s. For example, the prevalence of asthma among persons 5–24 years of age was approximately 30/1000 in 1982, but rose to approximately 55/1000 by 1992 (61). This nearly doubling in the absolute numbers of persons who have asthma would clearly swamp the beneficial effects of the relatively modest reductions that have been achieved in air pollution in the United States during the past decade (e.g., U.S. O_3 levels dropped only 8% between 1982 and 1991) (62). Such a relatively small decline in air pollution and, in turn, in the number of exacerbations caused by ozone in a year, could not possibly offset a doubling of the overall numbers of people with this disease.

Thus, although it seems clear that air pollution cannot be behind the widely reported increased induction of new asthma cases (i.e., the nearly doubling of the number of people with asthma), Lang and Polanski's (60) Philadelphia results are not at all inconsistent with air pollution as a causal agent in exacerbating the asthma of persons who already have the disease. Moreover, as the number of persons with asthma rises, the pool of persons ''available'' to be adversely affected by air pollution grows each year, implying that the negative impacts of air pollution also grows each year, despite the modest improvements we have made in air pollution levels in recent years. Indeed, the extent of the present O_3-asthma threat was made clear in a recent report finding that 27 million, or 54%, of all U.S. children 13 years of age or less were exposed, on four or more occasions during 1991–1993, to O_3 levels above the newly promulgated EPA legal limit of 80 ppb 8-hr average O_3 (63).

VII. THE THEORETICAL PATHOPHYSIOLOGY OF INDIVIDUAL ASTHMATIC SENSITIVITY TO AIR POLLUTION

Although air pollution has been shown by epidemiological studies and controlled chamber experiments to exacerbate asthma, there is no skin-prick or blood test that can test whether a person is especially affected by air pollution. Indeed, since air pollution heightens the likelihood of atopic subjects reacting to an allergen (i.e., relative to when air pollution is not present), it can appear that another cause (e.g., pollen) acted alone in precipitating an asthma exacerbation, even though elevated pollution may have contributed to the triggering of that exacerbation. However, indirect measures of the immune system response, such as cytokines, or mixtures of cytokines) may help identify when air pollution has been a contributing factor.

Cytokines include chemicals that modulate and modify a patient's inflammatory response and are thought to influence the individual variation in response to asthmatic stimuli. They provide the extracellular signal to stimulate the production and differentiation of different types of immunocompetent cells. There are basically two different extracellular signals that can be generated, and each signal is associated with different characteristic cytokines. The tissue histocompatibility 2 (TH2) signal is the atopic signal and is responsible for urticaria, allergic rhinitis, asthma, and anaphylaxis. The cytokines that support the TH2 signal are interleukin-4 (IL-4) and its congeners IL-5, IL-6, IL-9, IL-10, and IL-13. The TH1 signal is the cytotoxic signal, and it is responsible for the fever, chills, anorexia, and myalgias that are seen in many immune situations. The cytokines associated with the TH1 response include interferon-γ (IFN-γ), IL-2, and tumor necrosis factor-β (TNF-β) (64). The balance between these two cell phenotypes has been thought to play an important role in human immune response, especially in asthma (65).

Important among the candidate cytokines representing the TH1 and TH2 phenotypes of cells in studies examining asthmatics are IL-4 and IFN-γ, respectively. In recent work with human subjects, the ratio of these two cytokines (IL-4/IFN-γ) has been found to be a significant predictor of asthma status (66). This is likely to be because the balance between IL-4 and IFN-γ is important to the regulation of human IgE synthesis in vivo (67). While the ratio of IL-4/IFN-γ appears to be useful in discriminating between atopics and nonatopics, the absolute levels of IFN-γ may also help discriminate those most at risk of hyperreactivity. Kimura et al. showed that IFN-γ plays an important role in the pathogenesis of nonatopic severe asthmatics, finding that IFN-γ production in nonatopic severe asthmatics was significantly higher than in both healthy subjects and atopic mild to moderate asthmatics (68). Furthermore, Tsnoda et al. found that subjects with higher IFN-γ levels in their serum displayed greater hyperresponsiveness, as indicated by a 20% fall in FEV_1 (PD20) after exposure to methacholine (69). Methacholine is a cholinergic agent that causes bronchoconstriction in sensitive asthmatics, and if a patient has a 20% fall in FEV_1 after exposure to methacholine, that is considered a positive test. Tollerud et al. found that the rate of decline in the FEV_1 of asthmatics over time was significantly associated with their IFN-γ serum levels (70).

Among asthmatics, and especially in adults (for whom atopy plays a lesser role than in children), those subjects with characteristically elevated IFN-γ may well prove to be those asthmatics manifesting the greatest autonomous responses to nonallergic asthma stimuli like air pollution. Thus, attempts to quantitatively discriminate among the various types of asthmatics on an individual level should consider incorporating various potential biomarkers of asthma status, especially IL-4 and IFN-γ, as they may well provide a key to identifying asthmatics who are most at risk to air pollution effects.

VIII. FUTURE PROSPECTS

The recognition of the role of air pollution in predisposing asthmatics to exacerbations, along with an identification of especially at-risk populations and the subsequent prevention of pollution-induced morbidity in patients with asthma, could then yield health care cost-containment benefits (71). In particular, it is possible that:

1. Improved recognition of the temporal relationships between exposures to pollutants and exacerbations of asthma might provide improved physician diagnosis, more refined patient education (to avoid or reduce exposures and/or to better manage the effects of unavoidable exposures), and, ultimately, reductions in the individual health impacts and collective societal costs associated with pollution-induced responses. Indeed, recent evidence suggests that certain adverse asthma symptoms from air pollution are reduced by asthma medications (72). The ED is well positioned to play a leading role in the identification of at-risk individu-

als, the documentation of the pollutants associated with increased ED visits and hospital admissions, and in-patient education management.

2. Better identification of those most at risk to the adverse risks of air pollution could help focus patient recruitment strategies for future controlled human exposure studies aimed at better understanding the underlying mechanisms behind air pollution effects on the most relevant populations.
3. Studies of exposure-response in the particularly susceptible populations may lead to the establishment of better targeted, more effective, and more efficient means for intervening, via both public policy and improved health care, to better control air pollution exposures and their adverse effects among persons with asthma.

IX. CONCLUSIONS

Available epidemiological and clinical research indicates that air pollution exposures can have significant adverse effects on patients with asthma, causing them to be more likely to display symptoms, experience an exacerbation, need medical attention at an ED, and even to be admitted to a hospital for asthma. However, air pollution's contribution to a specific asthma exacerbation is unlikely to be noted by the attending physician because of asthma's multifactorial nature, and because there are no diagnostic skin-prick tests or radioallergosorbent tests (RASTs) for sensitivity to air pollutants. Indeed, it now appears that air pollution exposures can predispose asthmatics to be more likely to react to ambient aeroallergens than they would without air pollution, and, when they have an asthma exacerbation, pre-exposure to air pollution may make that exacerbation more severe. For example, ozone pollution induces inflammation in the lung, which can potentially reduce the efficacy of preventative anti-inflammatory drugs, such as corticosteroids, increasing the chances of an asthma attack after a pollution exposure. In effect, air pollution exposures can apparently lower a patient's ''threshold'' for having an exacerbation by other causes (e.g., pollens), irrespective of that patient's individual triggers (although all asthmatics may not be affected equally). Thus, patients with asthma are generally more likely to experience an exacerbation during, or immediately after, high outdoor air pollution days.

Of those adversely impacted by air pollution, children and inner city populations have been identified as among the most affected. The reasons for greater effects in the inner city are not yet clear, but may be related to the higher prevalence of underprivileged populations in the urban core. The reasons for enhanced effects among children are better understood. Children tend to have greater pollution exposures than adults, per pound of body mass, as a result of their greater amount of exercise, greater amount of time spent outdoors, and their higher metabolic rates, all of which tend to increase their doses of air pollution relative to adults in the same populations. In addition, lung development in children may be adversely affected by pollution. These enhanced impacts of air pollution on such sensitive subgroups as children and the disadvantaged make all the more compelling the need to better understand, diagnose, and address air pollution–induced asthma problems.

REFERENCES

1. Morbidity and Mortality Weekly Report. Asthma-United States, 1982–1992. Vol. 43, 952–955, Jan. 6, 1995.

2. Ministry of Health of Great Britain. Reports on Public Health & Medical Subjects: Mortality and Morbidity during the London Fog of 1952. London, England: Her Majesty's Stationery Office, 1954.
3. Wardlaw AJ. The role of air pollution in asthma. Clin Exper Allergy 1993; 23:81–96.
4. Committee of the Environmental and Occupational Health Assembly of the American Thoracic Society. Health effects of outdoor pollution. Am J Respir Critical Care Med 1996; 153(1): 3–50.
5. Schwartz J. Health effects of air pollution from traffic: Ozone and particulate matter. In: Fletcher T, McMichael AJ, eds. Health at the Crossroads: Transport Policy and Urban Health, New York: John Wiley and Sons, 1997, 61–82.
6. Godleski JJ, Sioutas C, Katler M, Catalano P, Koutrakis P. Death from inhalation of concentrated ambient air particles in animal models of pulmonary disease. Proceedings of the Second Colloquium on Particulate Air Pollution and Human Health, Park City, Utah, May 1–3, 1996.
7. Godleski JJ, Sioutas C, Verrier RL, Killingsworth CR, Lovett E, Murthy GG, Hatch V, Wolfson JM, Ferguson T, Koutrakis P. Inhalation exposure of canines to concentrated ambient air particles (abstr). Am J Respir Crit Care Med 1997; 155(4):A246.
8. US Federal Register. National Ambient Air Quality Standards for Particulate Matter. 40 CFR Part 50. Vol. 62, No. 138:38651–38701, July 18, 1997.
9. Lippmann M, Gearhart JM, Schlesinger RB. Basis for a particle size-selective TLV for sulfuric acid aerosols. Appl Ind Hyg 1987; 2:188–199.
10. Verhoeff AP, Hoek G, Schwartz J, Wijnen JH. Air pollution and daily mortality in Amsterdam. Epidemiology 1996; 7:225–230.
11. Anderson HR, Ponce de Leon A, Bland JM, Bower JS, Strachen DP. Air pollution and daily mortality in London: 1987–92. Br Med J 1996; 312:665–669.
12. Samet JM, Zeger SL, Kelsall JE, Xu J, Kalkstein LS. Air pollution, weather, and mortality in Philadelphia 1973–1988. Analyses of the Effects of Weather and Multiple Air Pollutants. The Phase IB Report of the Particle Epidemiology Evaluation Project. Cambridge, MA: Health Effects Institute, March 1997.
13. Thurston GD. Ozone air pollution and human mortality. Paper 97-MP9.04, For presentation at the Air and Waste Management Association's 90th Annual Meeting and Exhibition, Toronto, Ontario, Canada, June 8–13, 1997.
14. Thurston, GD, Ito K, Kinney PL, Lippmann M. A multi-year study of air pollution and respiratory hospital admissions in three New York State metropolitan areas: Results for 1988 asthma and 1989 summers. J Expos Anal Environ Epidemiol 1992; 2:429–450.
15. Devereux G, Ayatollahi T, Ward R, Bromly C, Bourke SJ, Stenton SC, and Hendrick DJ. Asthma, airways responsiveness and air pollution in two contrasting districts of Northern England. Thorax 1996; 51(2):169–174.
16. Koren HS, Bromberg PA. Respiratory responses of asthmatics to ozone. Int Arch Allergy Immunol 1995; 107:236–238.
17. US EPA. Review of National Ambient Air Quality Standards for Ozone. Assessment of Scientific and Technical Information. OAQPS Staff Paper. Research Triangle Park, NC: Office of Air Quality Planning and Standards, EPA-452/R-96-007, 1996.
18. US Federal Register. National Ambient Air Quality Standards for Ozone. 40 CFR Part 50, Vol. 62, No. 138:38856–38896, July 18, 1997.
19. Thurston, GD. Testimony before the U.S. House of Representatives. Joint Hearings before the Subcommittee on Health and the Environment and the Subcommittee on Oversight and Investigations of the Committee on Commerce: Review of EPA's Proposed Ozone and Particulate Matter NAAQS Revisions-Part 2. Serial No. 105–24, p. 148, Washington, DC: USGPO, 1997.
20. Barton, DJ, Teets-Grimm K, Kattan M. Emergency room visit patterns of inner city children for asthma (abstr). Am Rev Respir Dis 1993; 147:A577.

21. Empire State Electric Energy Research Corporation (ESEERCO). The New York State Environmental Externalities Cost Study. Dobbs Ferry, NY: Oceana Publications, Inc., December 1995.
22. Thurston GD, Lippmann M, Scott MB, Fine JM. Summertime haze air pollution and children with asthma. Am J Respir Crit Care Med 1997; 155:654–660.
23. Bates DV, Sizto R. Relationship between air pollutant levels and hospital admission in Southern Ontario. Can J Public Health 1983; 74:117–122.
24. Bates DV, Sizto R. A study of hospital admissions and air pollutant levels in southern Ontario. In: Lee SD, Schneider T, Grant LD, Verkerk, PJ, eds. Aerosols Research, Risk Assessment Management and Control Environmental Strategies, Chelsea, Michigan: Lewis Publishers, 1986, 767–780.
25. Bates DV, Sizto R. Air pollution and hospital admissions in Southern Ontario: The acid summer haze effect. Environ Res 1987; 43:317–331.
26. Bates DV, Sizto R. The Ontario air pollution study: Identification of the causative agent. Arch Environ Health 1989; 79:69–72.
27. Lipfert FW, Hammerstrom T. Temporal patterns in air pollution and hospital admissions. Environ Res 1992; 59:374–399.
28. Burnett RT, Dales RE, Raizenne E, Krewski D, Summers PW, Roberts GR, Raad-Young M, Dann T, Brooke T. Effects of low ambient levels of ozone and sulfates on the frequency of respiratory hospital admissions to hospitals. Environ Res 1993; 65:172–194.
29. Cody RP, Weisel CP, Birnbaum G, Lioy PJ. The effect of ozone associated with summertime major photochemical smog on the frequency of visits to hospital emergency departments. Environ Res 1992; 58:184–194.
30. Weisel CP, Cody RP, Lioy PJ. Relationship between summertime ambient ozone levels and emergency department visits for asthma in central New Jersey. Environ Health Perspect 1995; 103(suppl 2):97–102.
31. Thurston GD, Ito K, Hayes CG, Bates DV, Lippmann M. Respiratory hospital admissions and summertime haze air pollution in Toronto, Ontario: Considerations of the role of acid aerosols. Environ Res 1994; 65:271–290.
32. Diakite B, Aubier M, Korobaeff M, Quenel P, LeMoullec Y, Neukirch F. Relationships of air pollution levels to asthma symptoms and peak flow variability recorded daily during six months. Preliminary results (abstr). Am J Respir Crit Care Med 1994; 149(4):A662.
33. Forsberg B, Stjernberg N, Wall, S. People Can Detect Poor Quality well below guideline concentrations: a prevalence study of annoyance reactions and air pollution from traffic. Occup Environ Med 1997; 54(1):44–48.
34. Ostro BD, Lipsett MJ, Wiener MB, Selner, JC. Asthmatic response to airborne acid aerosols. Am J Public Health 1991; 81:694–702.
35. Pope CA III. Respiratory hospital admissions associated with PM10 pollution in Utah, Salt Lake, and Cache Valleys. Arch Environ Health 1991; 46:90–97.
36. Roemer W, Hoek G, Brunekreef B. Effect of ambient winter air pollution on respiratory health of children with chronic respiratory symptoms. Am Rev Respir Dis 1993; 147:118–124.
37. Follinsbee LJ, McDonnell WF, Horstman DH. Pulmonary function and symptom responses after 6.6 hour exposure to 0.12 ppm ozone with moderate exercise. JAPCA 1988; 38:28–35.
38. Devlin RB, McDonnell WF, Mann R, Becker S, House DE, Schreinemachers D, Koren HS. Exposure of humans to ambient levels of ozone for 6.6 hours causes cellular and biochemical changes in the lung. Am J Respir Cell Mol Biol 1991; 4:72–81.
39. Gordon T, Fine J. The contribution of ambient air pollution to allergic asthma. Toxicol Environ Notes 1997; 4:20–24.
40. Balmes JR. The role of ozone exposure in the epidemiology of asthma. Environ Health Perspect 1993; 101(suppl 4):219–224.
41. Molfino NA, Wright SC, Katz I, Tarlo S, Silverman F, McClean PA, Szalai JP, Raizenne M,

Slutsky AS, Zamel N. Effect of low concentrations of ozone on allergen responses in asthmatic subjects. Lancet 1991; 338:199–203.
42. Li XY, Gilmour PS, Donaldson K. Free radical activity and proinflamatory effects of particulate air pollution (PM10) in vivo and vitro. Thorax 1996; 51(12):1216–1222.
43. Scannell C, Chen L, Aris RM, Tager I, Christian D, Ferrando R, Welch B, Kelly T, Balmes JR. Greater ozone- induced inflammatory responses in subjects with asthma. Am J Respir Crit Care Med 1996; 154:24–29.
44. Buist AS, Vollmer VM. Reflections on the rise in asthma morbidity and mortality. J Am Med Assoc 1990; 264:1719–1720.
45. Taylor WR, Newacheck PW. Impact of childhood asthma on health. Pediatrics 1992; 90:657–662.
46. Carr W, Zeitel L, Weiss K. Variations in asthma hospitalizations and deaths in New York City. Am J Public Health 1992; 82:59–65.
47. Weiss KB, Wagener DK. Changing patterns of asthma mortality. Identifying target populations at high risk. J Am Med Assoc 1990; 264:1683–1687.
48. Carter-Pokras OD, Gergen PJ. Reported asthma among Puerto Rican, Mexican-American, and Cuban children, 1982 through 1984. Am J Public Health 1993; 83:580–582.
49. Coultas DB, Gong H Jr, Grad R, Handler A, McCurdy AS, Player R, Rhoades ER, Samet JM, Thomas A, Westley M. Respiratory diseases in minorities of the United States. Am J Respir Crit Care Med 1993; 149:S93–S131.
50. Bearer CF. How are children different from adults? Environ Health Perspect 1995; 103(suppl 6):7–12.
51. Tager IB, Weiss ST, Munoz A, Rosner B, Speizer FE. Longitudinal study of the effects of maternal smoking on pulmonary function in children. N Engl J Med. 1983; 309:699–703.
52. World Health Organization (WHO). Environmental Health Criteria 59: Principles for Evaluating Health Risks from Chemicals during Infancy and Early Childhood: The Need for a Special Approach. Geneva, Switzerland, 1986.
53. McDonnell WF, Horstman DH, Abdul-Salaam S, House DE. Reproducibility of individual responses to ozone exposure. Am Rev Respir Dis 1985; 131:36–40.
54. Silverman F. Asthma and respiratory irritants (ozone) Environ Health Perspect 1979; 29:131–136.
55. Linn WS, Avol EL, Shamoo DA, Peng RC, Valencia LM, Little DE, Hackney JD. Repeated laboratory ozone exposures of volunteer Los Angeles residents: An apparent seasonal variation in response. Toxicol Ind Health 1988; 4:505–520.
56. Linn WS, Linn WS, Avol EL, Peng RC, Shamoo DA, Hackney JD. Replicated dose-response study of sulfur dioxide effects in normal, atopic, and asthmatic volunteers. Am Rev Respir Dis 1987; 126:1127–1134.
57. World Health Organization (WHO). Update and revision of the air quality guidelines for Europe, EUR/ICP/EHAZ 94 05/PB01. Regional Office for Europe, Copenhagen, Denmark, 1995, p. 11.
58. Molfino NA, Wright SC, Katz I, Tarlo S, Silverman F, McClean PA, Szalai JP, Raizenne M, Slutsky AS, Zamel N. Effect of low concentrations of ozone on inhaled allergen responses in asthmatic subjects. Lancet 1991; 338:199–203.
59. Chen L L, Scannell C, Tager I, Peden DB, Christian DL, Ferrando RE, Welch BS, Kelly TJ, Balmes JR. The effect of ozone on the inflammatory response to inhaled attergen in allergic asthmatic subjects. Submitted for publication.
60. Lang, D.M, Polansky, M. Patterns of asthma mortality in Philadelphia from 1969 to 1991. N Engl J Med 1994; 331:1542–1546.
61. Morbidity and Mortality Weekly Report. Asthma-United States, 1982–1992. Vol. 43, 952–955, Jan. 6, 1995.

62. US EPA. National Air Quality and Emissions Trend Report. Publ. No. 450-R-92-001, Research Triangle Park, NC: OAQPS, October 1992.
63. Morbidity and Mortality Weekly Report. Children at Risk From Ozone Air Pollution-United States, 1991–1993. Vol. 44, 309–312, April 28, 1995.
64. Toews GB. Regulation of pulmonary immune responses. In: Inflammatory Mechanisms in the Lung and Airways: Cells, Cytokines, and Mediators. American Thoracic Society (ATS) Postgraduate Course 7 Text, New Orleans, LA: ATS, 1996.
65. National Institutes of Health (NIH). Global Strategy for Asthma Management and Prevention. NHLBI/WHO Workshop, Publ. No. 95-3659, Bethesda, MD, p. 42, 1993.
66. Hoekstra MO, De Reus D, Hoekstra Y, Rutgers B, Gerritsen J, Kauffman, HF. Interleukin-4 (IL-4), interferon-γ (IFN-γ) and IL-5 in serum and supernants of cultured PBMC's of children with moderate asthma compared with healthy controls (abstr). Am J Respir Crit Care Med 1996; 153:A215.
67. Pene J. Seasonal variations of interleukin-4 and interferon-gamma release by peripheral blood mononuclear cells from atopic subjects stimulated by polyclonal activators. J Allergy Clin Immunol 1995; 96:932–940
68. Kimura G, Ogurusu K. Soda R, Tada S. Takahashik. Kimuta I. Studies on IFN-gamma production by peripheral blood mononuclear cell cultured with Candida antigen in asthmatics. Arerugi-Japan J Allergology 1992; 41(12):1717–1721.
69. Tsnoda M, Kuniak MP, Weiss ST, Satoh T, Guevarra L, Tollerud DJ. Serum interferon-γ (IFN-γ) and airway responsiveness (abstr). Am J Respir Crit Care Med 1995; 151:A565.
70. Tollerud DJ, Sparrow DW, Guevarra L, O'Connor GT, Weiss ST. Serum cytokines and longitudinal change in pulmonary function among asthmatics (abstr). Am J Respir Crit Care Med 1995; 151:A566.
71. Weiss KB, Gergen PJ, Hodgson TA. An economic evaluation of asthma in the United States. New Engl J Med 1992; 326:862–866.
72. Peters A, Dockery DW, Heinrich J, Wichmann HE. Medication use modifies the health effects of particulate sulfate air pollution in children with asthma. Environ Health Perspect 1997; 105: 430–435.

10

Premenstrual Asthma

Emil M. Skobeloff
MCP-Hahnemann Medical College, Crozer-Chester Medical Center, Philadelphia, Pennsylvania

I. INTRODUCTION

This chapter presents an area of research that has only recently gained acceptance as an important focus of attention in the chronic and emergent management of asthma. For many years, asthma had been assumed to be a disease seen in near equal frequency among adult males and females. However, new understandings suggest that gender may play a significant role in the pathophysiology of adult asthma.

In 1931, Frank first introduced the concept of premenstrual asthma as one of several symptoms of "premenstrual tension" (1). Since then, several case reports and small, mostly retrospective studies have suggested "circamenstrual" worsening of asthma symptoms in adult females (2–6). However, nearly all of the clinical studies were retrospective and based on patient-recorded recollections of subjective data without any objective finding of increased asthma severity. Other investigations have postulated that there may be an increase in hospitalizations, greater morbidity, and more frequent intubations, intensive care unit admissions, and deaths (7) in females with perimenstrual asthma. Despite these various observations, the case for perimenstrual exacerbation is the substance of ongoing debate and research.

Current belief is that 30–40% of asthmatic women experience premenstrual worsening of their asthma symptoms. Rees et al. evaluated 81 adult female asthma patients who were of reproductive potential and found that 33% demonstrated a "clear tendency for attacks during the week to ten days prior to the onset of menses with a peak incidence during the two to three days before menses" (6).

Eliasson reported the results of an analysis of 632 subjects admitted in one year to an urban teaching hospital. He found a 1.9:1 male predominance in asthma admissions for patients under the age of 10 and a 2.6:1 female predominance in asthma admissions in subjects between the age of 22 and 40. He also noted a 1.2:1 female predominance between age 40 and 55. After age 55, female predominance increased to 2.2:1. He concluded that pre- and postpubertal differences in rate of admission and length of stay might be a result of hormonal differences between sexes before and after puberty (8).

Gibbs, et al (9) reported the results of their survey of 91 asthmatic adult females in 1984. When asked, ''Does your asthma ever seem worse before your menstrual period?'' 40% answered in the affirmative. Evaluating his objective data, Gibbs noted, ''falls in peak expiratory flow rate were modest and of a degree that would not be expected to result in increased breathlessness.'' These authors concluded that it was a heightened awareness of symptoms and not a significant decrease in peak expiratory flow rates that might be the core issue (9). However, Hanley demonstrated statistically significant premenstrual reductions in peak expiratory flow rates in asthmatic women who said they had regular asthma exacerbations during their premenstrual interval when compared to asthmatics who had noted no such premenstrual asthma worsening (10).

On the other hand, Juniper and colleagues examined the influence of menstrual cycle timing on changes in airway response to methacholine in 17 stable asthmatics 1 week before and 1 week after the onset of menses. His group found no objective deterioration in forced expiratory volume in 1 sec (FEV_1), increased response to methacholine, or increased medication use during this interval. However, there was a significant increase in the reported severity of subjective asthma symptoms during the days just prior to and during menses (11). Weinmann et al reported no increased pathologic changes in FVC, FEV_1, or airways response to histamine during the same interval (12).

To attempt to clarify these conflicting findings, Skobeloff et al. reported the results of a retrospective study of 33,576 admissions for acute exacerbations of asthma describing demographic data from 67 hospitals in 5 counties of southeastern Pennsylvania over four years (1986–1989). This study found that adult females are more severely affected by asthma than age-identical males. In fact, this study demonstrated that both pre- and postmenopausal adult females are admitted to hospitals more than age-identical males by nearly 3:1 with an average length of stay that was nearly 1 day longer for females (13).

A prospective study (14) involving 182 adult female asthmatics, age 13 to menopause, demonstrated that there is a fourfold increase in emergency department (ED) presentations by adult females for asthma during the 7 perimenstrual days of the menstrual cycle, when serum estradiol levels fall sharply after a 7-day sustained peak. While that study demonstrated a fourfold increase in asthma presentations to the ED during the perimenstrual interval, no difference in objective measurement of disease severity was noted among the four menstrual-interval groups that were evaluated (14). That 50% of the women asthmatics were seen during a single 7-day window of the estrous cycle, without any significant difference in disease severity when compared with the asthmatic women seen during the other three 7-day intervals, suggests that far less provocation may be necessary to create clinically significant asthma exacerbations during the perimenstrual interval. It may be reasonable to conclude that there is a heightened perimenstrual pathological potential in asthmatic women that may underlie a majority of the asthma presentations seen in the ED by the group who account for 75% of adult asthma hospital admissions and the associated health care costs that result.

Brenner et al. (15) examined the records of 190 consecutive adult females presenting to an inner city ED for acute exacerbations of asthma. They found a significantly greater number of overall ED visits, a higher incidence of ED asthma presentations, and a twofold greater frequency of asthma-related hospitalizations in the preceding two years for adult female asthmatic patients presenting during and after the menstrual interval associated with rapid decline of serum estradiol levels (perimenstrual and preovulatory) (15).

Huovinen and colleagues (16) have also reported the results of a 16-year cohort study which was performed to assess the overall survival of adult patients with asthma who were also twins whose siblings did not have asthma. Mortality for all causes was increased among the asthmatic siblings and significantly higher in females asthmatics compared to males (16).

In summary, research demonstrates that far more than 30–40% of women asthmatics have the potential to decompensate their asthma during the perimenstrual window with a significantly increased risk of death. As such, this may be a health problem whose magnitude has been significantly underestimated and largely ignored for decades.

II. HORMONAL VARIATION OF ESTROGEN DURING THE MENSTRUAL CYCLE

During the monthly estrous cycle, estrogen and progesterone rise and fall with a brief peak in serum estrogen levels during ovulation (days 14 and 15), and a sustained week-long elevation between days 19 and 25. Thereafter, serum estrogen levels fall sharply to baseline, reaching a nadir just before the onset of menses and remaining at low levels until ovulation. In men, there is no such day to day, or week to week, variation in testosterone levels. Rather, testosterone peaks during a boy's adolescent years and then serum levels fall very gradually through adulthood into old age. It is possible that this difference between men's and women's serum hormone variations may play a significant role in making women more susceptible to severe exacerbations of asthma, requiring ED presentations, hospital admissions, and an increased risk of death.

To facilitate an evaluation of the clinical and scientific effects of estrogen variation, Skobeloff et al. (14) divided the cycle into four 7-day intervals based on dynamic fluctuations in serum levels of estradiol by 7-day groups during an idealized, normal menstrual cycle. The intervals were: preovulatory (days 5–11), periovulatory (days 12–18), postovulatory (days 19–25), and perimenstrual (days 26–4) (5). By plotting time of the menstrual cycle, without actually measuring serum estradiol levels, a novel concept was proposed, not only in the consideration of asthma in adult women, but possibly in the evaluation of women's disease in general. They postulated that it is not the *static* state of serum estradiol levels that may dictate airway responsiveness. Instead, they proposed that it may be the *dynamic* fluctuation of estrogen after a sustained elevation, which may impact adversely on airway mediators (14).

Cydulka and colleagues have confirmed this hypothesis. They prospectively studied an observational cohort of 69 women presenting to a university-affiliated county hospital ED for asthma. Their investigation found that *absolute* serum estradiol levels had no correlation with severity of bronchospasm, response to bronchodilator therapy, or likelihood of hospital admission for asthma (17).

The rise and fall of serum estradiol has other important features as well. The first 14 days of the monthly estrous cycle, classically known as the follicular phase is fairly well conserved among adult women. The duration of the luteal phase may be longer or shorter than 14 days. However, once the postovulatory serum estrogen plateau ends, a precipitous interval of estrogen withdrawal begins. It is this phenomenon of estrogen withdrawal that appears to be a crux of the pathology that has been heretofore observed in connection with the asthmatic process. By applying a four-interval concept of the menstrual cycle, rather than the traditional two-interval menstrual cycle, the evaluation of the effects of estrogen withdrawal are easier to conceptualize.

III. THE EFFECT OF ESTROGEN ON IMMUNE MEDIATORS AND RECEPTOR SPECIES

Bronchial hyperresponsiveness observed after estradiol withdrawal may be mediated by an agent or agents whose synthesis is affected by estradiol but released from sites outside of the genitalia. Several potential sources for such mediators are the adrenals, bronchial epithelium, and the immune system. These tissues produce cortisol, corticosterone, progesterone, various interleukins, tumor necrosis factor (TNF), granulocyte monocyte–colony stimulating factor (GM-CSF), prostaglandins, leukotrienes, and other soluble regulators and mediators of inflammation.

Estradiol has been shown to enhance the production of prostaglandins. In female rat lungs, prostaglandin production has been shown to be at a maximum when estradiol levels are at maximum (18). In the lung, prostaglandin levels increase with hypoxia causing pulmonary hyperemia and increased bronchoconstriction (19). It would be expected that estradiol withdrawal after prolonged elevation may attenuate these effects. However, the timing of such changes, if they occur, is unclear.

Estradiol increases β-adrenergic receptor sites in rabbit lung tissue. Progesterone, a steroid secreted by the adrenals and ovaries, decreases β-adrenergic receptor effects (20) but relaxes smooth muscle and stimulates respiratory drive and the response of central chemoreceptors to hypercarbia (21). Progesterone is known to cause upregulation of lymphocyte β-adrenergic receptors in healthy, normal female subjects when serum estrogen levels are maintained at normal levels (22). Tan et al. (23) have shown that in adult female asthmatics progesterone causes a paradoxical *down*regulation of β-adrenergic receptors on lymphocytes. This downregulation of receptors is also accompanied by a trend towards a lower cyclic adenosine monophosphate responsiveness to isoproterenol. These authors propose that ''this paradoxical effect of progesterone in female asthmatics suggests an abnormal regulation of β-adrenoreceptors, and might be a possible mechanism for 'premenstrual' asthma when progesterone levels are high during this period of the cycle'' (23).

Corticosterone is a steroid secreted by the adrenal gland that inhibits the secretion of progesterone (24). Inhibition of progesterone secretion is negated by the presence of estradiol (25). Estrogen withdrawal through ovariectomy increases the concentration of corticosterone in plasma (26).

Other sections of this text will discuss the effects of endogenous and exogenous corticosteroids on asthma, its response, and therapy. However, we will briefly examine the effect of estrogen and its absence on cortisol, a steroid manufactured by the adrenals. It has been shown that cortisol (1) primes β-adrenergic receptors, making them more responsive to β-adrenergic agonists; (2) stimulates the conversion of norepinephrine to epinephrine in the adrenal medulla; (3) stimulates the production of lipomodulin, which blocks phospholipase activity, interfering with arachidonic acid metabolism and the production of bronchospastic agents such as the leukotrienes and some prostaglandins; and (4) has primary anti-inflammatory effects. These anti-inflammatory effects include inhibition of lymphocyte, granulocyte, and monocyte populations, decreasing the level of TNF in serum; interference with chemotaxis and phagocytosis; stabilization of lysosomal membranes; inhibition of nonlysosomal proteolytic enzyme release; and a vasoconstrictive inhibition of the effects of histamine and kinins (27). The absence of estradiol does not appear to effect the serum level of endogenous cortisol (28). However, estradiol treatment of gonadectomized males and female rats causes increased ACTH production and a blunting of the deleterious effects of ether-induced stress (29).

The late-phase asthmatic reaction is accompanied by the influx of inflammatory cells (lymphocytes and alveolar macrophages) and into both the proximal and distal airways along with bronchial hyperresponsiveness. It has been demonstrated that interleukin-1 (IL-1) and TNF cause the release of gonadotropin releasing hormone (GnRH) from the pituitary and IL-6 from macrophages, T-lymphocytes, endothelial and epithelial cells, and fibroblasts. Interleukin-6 also induces cell growth and differentiation of T-lymphocyte stem cells into cytotoxic T-lymphocytes (30,31). Production of IL-1, IL-6, and TNF by alveolar macrophages has been shown to be elevated when collected 18–20 hr after allergen challenge (32). Increases in serum estradiol suppresses IL-6 production in vitro (33). Conversely, low serum estradiol causes maximal proliferation of IL-1 and TNF (32,34).

In animals, estradiol has been shown to increase acetylcholine concentration (35), cholinesterase activity (36), mucus secretion (37), prostaglandin production (38), and α-, β_1-, and β_2-adrenergic receptor densities in the lung (39,40). Progesterone decreases β-adrenergic receptor density to baseline when given to animals previously treated with estradiol (41). The effect of estrogen withdrawal on these manifestations in normal or asthmatic animals has never been demonstrated.

IV. THE EFFECT OF ESTROGEN WITHDRAWAL ON WHITE BLOOD CELL POPULATIONS AND INFLAMMATORY MEDIATORS OF THE LATE-PHASE ASTHMATIC RESPONSE

The late-phase reaction of the asthmatic response is largely mediated by leukotrienes. Asthmatic airways have been shown to have a disproportionate hyperresponsiveness to LTE_4 (42) as compared to normal airways. Estradiol has been shown to inhibit eosinophil mobilization and degranulation while stimulating the release of substances that suppress the reactivity of leukotrienes and enhancing suppressor T-lymphocyte function (43). Recent animal studies have demonstrated that estrogen withdrawal increases the proportion of circulating neutrophils and decreases the percent of circulating lymphocytes in blood. Estrogen withdrawal increases the neutrophil : lymphocyte ratio in blood and increases the percent of circulating monocytes in blood (44).

V. THE EFFECT OF ESTROGEN WITHDRAWAL ON MUSCARINIC-CHOLINERGIC–INDUCED BRONCHOCONSTRICTION

An initial study by Skobeloff and colleagues (46) showed that bronchial rings from intact male rabbits treated over 7 days with 70 mcg/Kg per day of 17-β-estradiol demonstrated a greater contractile response to increasing doses of the cholinergic, contractile agonist bethanechol when compared to male controls. Comparisons were then made of the contractile and relaxation response of bronchial smooth muscle obtained from male rabbit controls, untreated castrated male rabbits, castrated males treated daily for 14 days with 30 mcg/kg of estradiol, and castrated male rabbits injected for 7 days with 17-β-estradiol with a 1-, 3-, 7-, or 10-day recovery period. That investigation demonstrated statistically significant changes in bronchial smooth muscle contraction and relaxation responses, which were observed at 1, 3, and 7 days after cessation of a 7-day continuous interval of estradiol injection, when compared to male and female controls, castrated males, and castrated males injected with estradiol daily for two weeks (45). It is hypothesized that the observed variations were mediated through reflex increases in serum and bronchiolar levels of mediators derived from inflammatory cells of the immune system due to decreasing levels of serum estradiol in the 10 days after a sustained elevation as well as estradiol-withdrawal mediated changes in postsynaptic receptor densities and intracellular second messenger system modulations. Subsequent studies in an asthmatic rabbit model demonstrated that estrogen-withdrawal caused a similar increase in bronchoconstriction in the asthmatic rabbit model that was maximal after 3 days of the cessation of estrogen dosing (46).

Increased intracellular calcium induces bronchoconstriction by activating calmodulin. Potassium chloride (KCl) causes increased intracellular influx of exogenous calcium into bronchial smooth muscle cells. Estrogen withdrawal causes a significant increase in contractile response to equal doses of KCl in the asthmatic model when compared to the (1) uncastrated asthmatic rabbits, (2) castrated asthmatic rabbit, and (3) untreated normal male controls. Estrogen withdrawal has been shown to cause significant increases in the response of bronchial smooth muscle to calcium chloride, but not histamine (47).

To summarize, in the absence of endogenous sex steroids, estrogen withdrawal increases bronchoconstriction in both normal and asthmatic animals in response to cholinergic stimulation and calcium. These changes are maximal at 3 days after estrogen withdrawal. This in vitro interval coincides nearly identically with the peak of adult female asthma presentations to the emergency department during the perimenstrual interval (44–50).

VI. EFFECT OF ESTROGEN WITHDRAWAL ON THE DENSITY AND KINETICS OF MUSCARINIC-CHOLINERGIC RECEPTORS

In the smaller caliber, distal airways, estrogen withdrawal causes a greater increase in total contractile muscarinic-cholinergic receptors than that observed in the early generations of bronchi. This increased bronchoconstrictive potential creates a milieu in which mucous plugging can cause significant atelectasis, air trapping, and loss of surface area for gas exchange. The impact of these changes has yet to be explored. Skobeloff et al. have shown that, in the asthmatic state, contractile receptors in bronchi are increased compared to normal controls. The airway then compensates by decreasing the kinetics of the receptor. In the estrogen withdrawal, asthmatic state, contractile receptors are increased more than either the normal or asthmatic controls, and the kinetics at these contractile receptors is restored to their original, higher level of responsiveness to cholinergic stimulation. The end result is a significant heightening of bronchoconstriction due to an increase in both the number and efficiency of muscarinic-cholinergic receptors and a heightened state of muscarinic-cholinergic responsiveness (48,49).

VII. EFFECT OF ESTROGEN WITHDRAWAL ON BRONCHODILATOR RESPONSE

Early investigations by Skobeloff and colleagues showed that in normal, gonadectomized, sex-steroid–free rabbits, estrogen withdrawal caused significant increases in the response of bronchial smooth muscle to isoproterenol when compared to normal controls (50). However, when asthmatic rabbits were exposed to estrogen withdrawal, no increase in β-adrenergic responsiveness was observed. This would suggest a down regulation of β-adrenergic receptor density and/or kinetics in response to estrogen withdrawal and a resulting diminished ability of the airways to respond to β-agonist therapy during the perimenstrual interval (51). Brenner et al. (15) noted a one-third less response to *initial* β-agonist intervention during emergency department treatment, observed during the periovulatory interval of the menstrual cycle, when estrogen levels were elevated. However, those authors noted a higher, *overall* bronchodilation response to subsequent treatment in the ED during that high estradiol interval (15).

Ipratropium bromide is an anticholinergic bronchodilator similar to atropine. Ipratropium differs from atropine in that it has a quaternary ammonium ion, which prevents significant systemic absorption, thus preventing systemic, anticholinergic side effects. Estrogen withdrawal decreases the response to ipratropium bromide10-fold (52).

Magnesium sulfate is an effective bronchodilator in patients who are refractory to nebulized β-agonist therapy. Silverman and colleagues have demonstrated that magnesium sulfate is most effective in asthmatics whose FEV_1 is less than 28% of predicted (53). In vitro studies have shown that estrogen withdrawal increases the bronchodilator response to magnesium chloride (54).

VIII. PRIOR INVESTIGATIONS INTO PREVENTIVE THERAPEUTIC INTERVENTIONS

Investigations into possible therapies for perimenstrual or premenstrual asthma have involved limited numbers of asthmatic females and have met with varying degrees of success. Benyon et al. (55) described data about three such patients who consistently had perimenstrual worsening of their asthma as manifested by a significant decrease in observed peak expiratory flow rates. Despite the addition of inhaled corticosteroids and aggressive conventional therapy, none of his reported subjects noted significant clinical improvement. In those patients, Benyon described the successful treatment of their asthma with intramuscular injections of Depo-Provera. However, their numbers were limited (55). Chandler and colleagues (56) described the results of a recent small crossover study in which 14 adult asthmatic female asthmatic patients were told to record subjective and objective measures of asthma severity, including ED visits and hospitalizations. At the time of enrollment into the study, only five of the 14 subjects reported premenstrual worsening of their asthma. However, all 14 had a 20% decrease in peak expiratory flow rate (PEFR) and/or increased symptoms premenstrually during the study. Chandler also reported that asthma symptoms and PEFR appeared to be best during intervals of high estrogen and worst during low estrogen intervals. After a one-month run-in phase, all 14 were given estradiol therapy from day 23 to day 7 of two successive menstrual cycles. Thirteen of the 14 patients in this small study noted statistically significant improvement in dyspnea scores and asthma symptoms. A trend towards increases in responsiveness to terbutaline, beta-2 receptor density and function, and catecholamine concentrations were observed. Although these results are promising, estrogen therapy in women with child-bearing potential is fraught with the danger of increased likelihood of endometrial and breast cancers (56). To date, no large studies have examined interventions specifically targeted towards adult female asthmatics.

Tan et al. (57) compared airway reactivity to adenosine monophosphate (AMP) challenge in female asthmatics with natural menstrual cycles and those who were taking an oral, combined contraceptive pill. These authors evaluated lung function during the follicular and luteal phases of subjects in both groups by measuring (1) response to AMP and (2) AM and PM PEFR. The untreated asthmatics demonstrated a fourfold increase in airway reactivity during the luteal phase. The treated group demonstrated no significant change in airway responsiveness. The untreated group demonstrated significant diurnal variation in AM/PM PEFRs at follicular phase and luteal phase visits. The treated group demonstrated no significant diurnal variation in AM/PM PEFRs at either visit (57).

Other therapies hold promise for the future but are as yet unproven. In vitro studies would suggest that magnesium sulfate may be a more effective fail-safe therapy in the perimenstrual phase. The observed effect of estrogen withdrawal on leukotrienes C_4, D_4, and E_4 also suggests that zileuton (Zyflo®), a leukotriene inhibitor, and zafirlukast (Accolate®), a leukotriene receptor blocker, may also prove effective during the perimenstrual phase. To date, however, no clinical trials have demonstrated any conclusive effect.

IX. THE IMPORTANCE OF ASTHMA EDUCATION

We have described significantly increased pathological potential for perimenstrual worsening of asthma in adult female asthmatics. However, clinicians should not ignore the overall lack of knowledge that women asthmatics and their health care providers may have about proper day-to-day asthma management. It is imperative that adult women, their physicians, and other health care providers be educated about the current state of the art in asthma prevention and care, with an emphasis on the knowledge that a significant increased risk of morbidity and mortality exists for these patients during the 7 perimenstrual days. Hopefully, a greater awareness of the increased pathological potential during the perimenstrual interval will spur both patients and their caregivers to manage asthma more aggressively to diminish risk behaviors and remove known asthma triggers to the greatest realistic extent possible. Beyond these universal guidelines, which are clearly relevant for all asthmatics, the issue of therapy is wide open.

X. CONCLUSION

This chapter has presented an area of ongoing research, which has only recently gained acceptance as an important focus of attention in the chronic and emergent management of asthma. New understandings suggest that gender may play a significant role in the pathophysiology of adult asthma in women through changes mediated by the immune system and its soluble products and changes in receptor densities and efficiencies. These variations lead to increased pathological response to provocation and a decreased response to most therapeutic intervention. Prior research into therapeutic and preventive treatments has been limited, though promising. Substantial effort into a widened understanding of the effect of sex steroids on the pathological basis of asthma and its appropriate treatment is essential due to the significantly heightened pathological potential in asthmatic women. This potential may be at the root of the majority of asthma presentations seen in the ED by that segment of the population, who account for 75% of adult asthma hospital admissions and the associated health care costs that result. Because women represent 75% of the adult admissions and 65% of the ED visits, this segment of the American asthmatic population appears to be a very important focus for asthma prevention, therapy, and education.

Perimenstrual worsening of asthma may not be limited to a subset of women who experience asthma exacerbations solely during one week of their cycle. Rather, it is possible that *every* asthmatic woman has the potential to decompensate her asthma during the perimenstrual window. Because nearly 50% of ED visits for asthma occur during a single, 7-day menstrual interval by a heterogeneous population of adult female asthmatics, it is compelling evidence that this is a health problem that should command much greater attention for future asthma research.

REFERENCES

1. Frank RT, The hormonal causes of premenstrual tension. Arch Neurol Psychiatr 1931; 26: 1053
2. Dodge RR, Burrows B. The Prevalence and incidence of asthma and asthma-like symptoms in a general population sample, Am Rev Respir Dis 1980; 122:567–575.
3. Green R, Dalton K. The premenstrual syndrome. Br Med J 1953; 1:1007.
4. Dalton K. The premenstrual syndrome and progesterone therapy. Chicago: Year Book Medical Publishers, Inc., 1984, 45–100.
5. Eliasson O, Scherzer HH. Morbidity in asthma in relation to the menstrual cycle. J Allergy Clin Immunol 1988; 77:87–94.
6. Rees L. An etiological study of premenstrual asthma. J Psychosom Res 1963; 7:191–197.
7. Hanley SP. Asthma variations with menstruation. Br J Dis Chest 1981; 75:306.
8. Eliasson O. The male-female ratio of hospital admissions for asthma, Am Rev Respir Dis 1985; 131(4):A110.
9. Gibbs CJ, Coutts H, Lock R, et al. Premenstrual exacerbation of asthma, Thorax 1984; 39: 833–836.
10. Hanley SP. Asthma variations with menstruation, Br J Dis Chest 1981; 306–308.
11. Juniper EF, Kline PA, Roberts RS, et al. Airway responsiveness to methacholine during the natural menstrual cycle, Am Rev Respir Dis 1987; 135:1039–1042.
12. Weinmann GG, Zacur H, Fish JE. Absence of changes in airway responsiveness during the menstrual cycle, J Allergy Clin Immunol 1987; 79:634–638.
13. Skobeloff EM, Spivey WH, StClair SS, Schoffstall J. The influence of age and sex on asthma admissions, JAMA 1992; 268:3437–3440.
14. Skobeloff EM, Spivey WH, Silverman R, Eskin BA, Harchelroad F, Alessi TA. The effect of the menstrual cycle on asthma presentations in the emergency department, Arch Intern Med 1996; 156:1837–1840.
15. Brenner BE, Yates JD, Rogove V. The effect of the menstrual cycle on emergency department visits and response to therapy in patients with acute asthma, Acad Emerg Med 1997; 4:481.

16. Huovinen E, Kapiro J, Vesterinen E, Koskenvuo M. Mortality of adults with asthma, Thorax 1997; 52:49–54.
17. Cydulka RK, Emerman CL. Serum estradiol levels in women with acute exacerbations of asthma, Acad Emerg Med 1997; 4:481.
18. Bakhle YS, Zakrzewski JT. Effects of the oestrus cycle on the metabolism of arachidonic acid in rat isolated lung, J Physiol Lond. 1982; 326:411–423.
19. Gordon JB, Wetzel RC, McGeady ML et al. Effects of indomethacin on estradiol-induced attenuation of hypoxic vasoconstriction in lamb lungs, J Appl Physiol 1986; 61:2116–2121.
20. Moawad AH, River LP, and Kilpatrick SJ. The effect of estrogen and progesterone on β-adrenergic receptor activity in rabbit lung tissue, Am J Obstet Gynecol 1982; 144:608–613.
21. Weinberger SE, Weiss ST, Cohen WR, et al. Pregnancy and the lung, Am Rev Respir Dis, 1980; 121:559–581.
22. Tan KS, McFarlane LC, Coutie WJ, et al. Effects of exogenous female sex-steroid hormones on lymphocyte beta$_2$-adrenoreceptors in normal females, Br J Clin Pharmaacol 1996; 41:414–416.
23. Tan KS, McFarlane LC, Lipworth BJ. Beta$_2$ adrenoreceptor regulation and AMP reactivity during the menstrual cycle in female asthmatics, Thorax 1995; 50(suppl):A60.
24. Sugino N, Tamura H, Nakamura Y. Different mechanisms for the inhibition of progesterone secretion by ACTH and corticosterone in pregnant rats, J Endocrinology 1991; 129:405–410.
25. Grassman M, Crews D. Ovarian and adrenal function in the parthenogenetic whiptail lizard *cnemidophorus uniparens* in the field and laboratory, Gen Comp Endocrinol 1989; 76:444–450.
26. Scanlon R. Asthma: a panoramic view and a hypothesis, Ann Allergy 1984; 53:203–212.
27. Waage A, Bakke O. Glucocorticoids suppress the production of tumor necrosis factor by lipopolysaccharide-stimulated human monocytes, Immunology 1988; 63:299–302.
28. Dowsett M, MacNeill F, Mehta A, et al. Endocrine, pharmacokinetic and chemical studies of the aromatase inhibitor 3-ethyl-3-(4-pyridyl)piperidine-2,6-dione ('Pyridoglutethimide') in postmenopausal breast cancer patients, Br J Cancer 1991; 64:887–894.
29. Leoniewska B, Myokowiak B, Nowak M. Sex differences in adrenocortical structure and function: The effect of ether stress on ACTH and corticosterone in intact, gonadectomized, and testosterone- or estradiol-replaced rats, Res Exp Med (Berlin) 1990; 190:95–103.
30. Yamaguchi M, Yoshimoto Y, Komura H, et al. Interleukin-1β tumor necrosis factor-α stimulate the release of gonadotropin-releasing hormone and interleukin-6 by primary cultured rat hypothalamic cells, Acta Endocrinol (Copenh) 1990; 123:476–480.
31. Snyers L, Dewit L, Content J. Glucocorticoid up-regulation of high affinity interleukin-6 receptors on human epithelial cells, Proc Natl Acad Sci USA, 1990; 87:2838–2842.
32. Mamata D, Sanford TR, Wood GW. Interleukin-1, interleukin-6 and tumor necrosis factor-are produced in the mouse uterus during the estrous cycle and are induced by estrogen and progesterone, Developmental Biol, 1992; 151:297–305.
33. Jilka RL, Hangoc G, Girasole G, et al. Increased osteoclast development after estrogen loss: Mediation by interleukin-6, Science 1992; 257:88–91.
34. Polan ML, Danieli A, Kuo A. Gonadal steroids modulate human monocyte interleukin-1 activity, Fertil Steril 1988; 49:964–968.
35. Abdul-Karim RW, Marshall LD, Nesbitt RE. Influence of estradiol-17$_B$ on the acetylcholine content of the lung in the rabbit neonate, Am J Obstet Gynecol 1970; 107:641–644.
36. Abdul-Karim RW, Drucker M, Jacobs RD. The influence of estradiol-17$_B$ on cholinesterase activity in the lung, Am J Obstet Gynecol 1970; 108:1098–1101.
37. Vidic B, Kapur SP, Jenkins DP. Estrogen and tracheal secretion: The effect of estrogen on the epithelial secretory cells of the rat trachea, Cytobiologie 1970; 10–21.
38. Eliasson O, Scherzer HH, DeGraff AC. Morbidity in relation to the menstrual cycle, J Allergy Clin Immunol 1986; 77:87–94.
39. Johansson U, Waldeck B. Beta$_1$-adrenoceptors mediating relaxation of the guinea-pig trachea:

Experiments with prenalterol, a $Beta_1$-selective adrenoceptor agonist, J Pharm Pharmacol 1981; 33:353–356.
40. Konno A, Terada N, Okamoto Y. Effects of female hormones on the muscarinic and $alpha_1$-adrenergic receptors of the nasal mucosa, Otorhinolaryngology J 1986; 48:45–51.
41. Moawad AH, River LP, Kilpatrick SJ. The effect of estrogen and progesterone on beta-adrenergic receptor activity in rabbit lung tissue: Am J Obstet Gynecol 1982; 144:608–613.
42. Arm JP, O'Hickey S, Hawksworth RJ, et al. Asthmatic airways have a disproportionate hyperresponsiveness to LTE_4 as compared to normal airways, but, not LTC_4, LTD_4, methacholine and histamine, Am Rev Respir Dis, 1990; 142:1112–1118.
43. Tchernitchin AN, Carter W, Soto J, et al. Effect of eosinophil-degranulating estrogens on spleen eosinophils and white pulp/red pulp ratio, Agents Actions, 1990; 31:249–256.
44. Skobeloff EM, Jacobson M, Mu A, Eskin BA. Estrogen withdrawal alters the neutrophil: lymphocyte ratio in rabbits, Acad Emerg Med 1994; 1:2
45. Skobeloff EM, Spivey WH, McNamara RM, Levin RM. The influence of estrogen administration on the contractile and relaxation response of rabbit bronchial smooth muscle, Ann Emerg Med 1992; 21(abstr):647.
46. Skobeloff, EM, Mu A, Satz WA. Estrogen withdrawal alters bronchial smooth muscle response in a rabbit asthmatic model, Ann Emerg Med 1995; 25:128.
47. Skobeloff EM, Satz WA, Eskin BA, Mu A. Estrogen-withdrawal modulates the response of bronchial smooth muscle to calcium but not histamine, Acad Emerg Med 1996; 3:459.
48. Skobeloff EM, Mu A, Luthin G, Eskin BA, Roberts J. Estrogen withdrawal alters the Density of Cholinergic-muscarinic receptor subtypes in asthmatic rabbit trachea, bronchi and whole lung, Acad Emerg Med, 1997; 4:514.
49. Skobeloff EM, Mu A, Luthin G, Eskin BA, Roberts J. Estrogen withdrawal alters the kinetics of muscarinic-cholinergic receptor subtypes in asthmatic rabbit trachea, bronchi and whole lung, Acad Emerg Med, 1997; 4:480.
50. Skobeloff EM, Spivey WH, Connolly C. Estradiol withdrawal alters bronchial smooth muscle response, Ann Emerg Med, 1993; 22:943.
51. Satz WA, Skobeloff EM, Mu A. Estrogen withdrawal alters the bronchodilation response in the rabbit asthmatic, Acad Emerg Med 1995; 2:361.
52. Satz WA, Skobeloff EM, Mu A. Estrogen withdrawal diminishes the effectiveness of ipratropium in the asthmatic rabbit, Acad Emerg Med 2:393.
53. Bloch H, Silverman R, Mancherje N, Grant S, Jagminus L, Scharf SM. Intravenous magnesium sulfate as an adjunct therapy in the treatment of acute asthma, Chest 1995; 107:1576–1581.
54. Satz WA, Skobeloff EM, Mu A. An in-vitro analysis of magnesium as a bronchodilator in normal, asthmatic and estrogen-withdrawal asthmatic rabbits, Acad Emerg Med 1995; 2(5): 393.
55. Benyon HL, Garbett ND, Barnes PJ, Severe premenstrual Exacerbations of Asthma: Intervention with Intramuscular Progesterone, Lancet 1988; 2:370–334.
56. Chandler MH, Schuldheisz S, Phillips BA, Muse KN. Premenstrual asthma: The effect of estrogen on symptoms, pulmonary function and beta 2-receptors, Pharmacotherapy 1997; 17: 224–234.
57. Tan KS, McFarlane LC, Lipworth BJ. Modulation of airway reactivity and peak flow variability in asthmatics receiving the oral contraceptive pill, Am J Respir Crit Care Med 1997; 155: 1273–1277.

11

Nocturnal Asthma

Monica Kraft and Richard J. Martin
National Jewish Medical and Research Center and University of Colorado Health Sciences Center, Denver, Colorado

I. INTRODUCTION

Nocturnal symptoms from bronchial asthma were acknowledged as far back as 1698 by Floyer (1) and in 1882 by Salter (2). Insightful and interesting statements were made by both physicians. Dr. Floyer said, "I have observed the fit always to happen after sleep in the night where nerves are filled with windy spirits and the heat of the bed has rarefied the spirits and humors!" Dr. Salter felt that, "this fact is that sleep favours asthma—that spasm of the bronchial tubes is more prone to occur during the insensibility and lethargy of sleep than during the waking hours."

Drs. Floyer and Salter are not alone in their observations. Nocturnal worsening of asthma has become a recognized and important aspect of asthma, and must be considered in the management of the disease process. It is certainly prevalent, as Turner-Warwick found in her survey of 7729 outpatient asthmatics in the United Kingdom (3). Ninety-four percent responded that they awoke at least one night a month with symptoms of asthma. Seventy-four percent awakened at least one night a week, 64% at least three times per week, and 39% every night. The occurrence of these symptoms is also reflected in mortality statistics. For all age groups, 83 of 168 (53%) asthma mortality cases over a 1-yr period occurred at night (4). For the population of 168 patients, 79% had premortem complaints of asthma affecting their sleep, and this occurred every night in 61 patients (42%). Cochrane and Clark found that 68% of all asthmatic deaths occurred between midnight and 8 AM, and Hetzel et al. found that 8 of 10 ventilatory arrests occurred between midnight and 6 AM (5,6). Bagg and Hughes also found morning decreases in peak expiratory flow rates in 30 of 40 stable asthmatics (7). In a wash-out phase of a pharmacological study, 1525 of 1631 dyspneic episodes in 3129 asthmatic patients occurred between 10 PM and 7 AM (Fig. 1) (8). Storms and colleagues noted a 67% incidence of nocturnal asthma in their allergy practice as determined by a questionnaire sent to 2019 patients

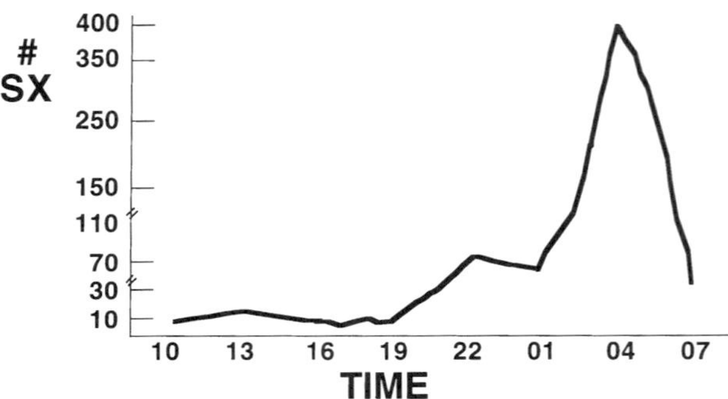

Figure 1 There is a marked frequency of nocturnal symptoms (SX) in 3129 mainly asthmatic patients. (Adapted from Ref. 8.)

with 560 responders (9). This observation is of unique importance to the emergency physician because it is he or she who often takes care of these patients when they present during the nighttime and early morning hours. However, Karras and colleagues found no difference in time of presentation to the emergency department (ED) for treatment of asthma (10). In addition, they found no difference in the time of symptom onset. As the authors point out, patients were required to remember when their symptoms began, and one-third of patients could not recall this information. Despite these conclusions, 28% of asthmatics presented from midnight to 8 AM, suggesting that emergency physicians are taking care of these patients. Further study is needed in the ED population before this conclusion can be drawn.

The important topic called chronobiology underlies understanding of the pathophysiology of nocturnal asthma. Chronobiology is the understanding of biological processes that have time-related rhythms, and human bioprocesses and functions that manifest predictable and recurring variability in time at every level of organization. These rhythms may occur yearly, monthly, or on a 24-hr cycle. Many organ functions exhibit chronobiological variation, such as heart rate (11), blood pressure, and gastrointestinal motility (12). Consequently, disease processes can also exhibit their signs and symptoms in circadian fashion: allergic rhinitis (13), angina, myocardial infarction, stroke (14), acid-peptic disease (15), and arthritis (16). These concepts assist the emergency physician in understanding why patients with asthma often present during the nighttime and early morning hours. The following discussion will focus upon the concept of circadian rhythms and pathophysiological mechanisms involved in nocturnal asthma. Also discussed are factors contributing to the presentation of nocturnal asthma, which can be recognized and potentially treated by the emergency physician.

II. CIRCADIAN RHYTHMS RELATED TO ASTHMA

A. Lung Function

In asthma, the 24-hr cycle is extremely important. For the asthmatic patient, a circadian pattern in lung function occurs, with peak lung function occurring at approximately 4 PM

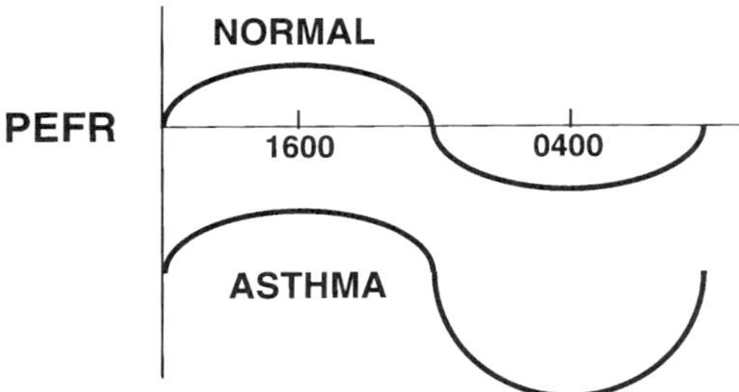

Figure 2 Both normal subjects and asthmatic patients have circadian alterations in lung function with nadirs occurring at approximately 4 AM. (Adapted from Ref. 17.)

and the nadir around 4 AM (Fig. 2). The changes in lung function can be quite significant, with peak-to-trough swings as great as 50% (17). The nonasthmatic population also experiences this circadian change in lung function, but the peak-to-trough swings are generally 5–8% (17). Cosinor analysis is often used to quantify this circadian change as the best model of the circadian rhythm is approximated by a sine or cosine wave (18). The variables measured include: (1) mesor, the rhythm adjusted mean, a middle value around which a temporal change occurs; (2) amplitude, a measure of the within-rhythm variability equivalent to one-half the peak to trough difference; (3) acrophase, the peak time of the rhythm relative to local midnight; and (4) bathyphase, the trough time of the rhythm relative to local midnight (19) (Fig. 3). Statistical significance is tested by determining if the amplitude differs from zero (20). The large circadian amplitude of bronchial patency is a diagnostic feature of obstructive diseases, particularly asthma (17).

B. Bronchial Hyperresponsiveness

Bronchial responsiveness to inhaled constrictors such as histamine and acetylcholine are markedly increased in asthmatic subjects at night (21), suggesting that airway smooth

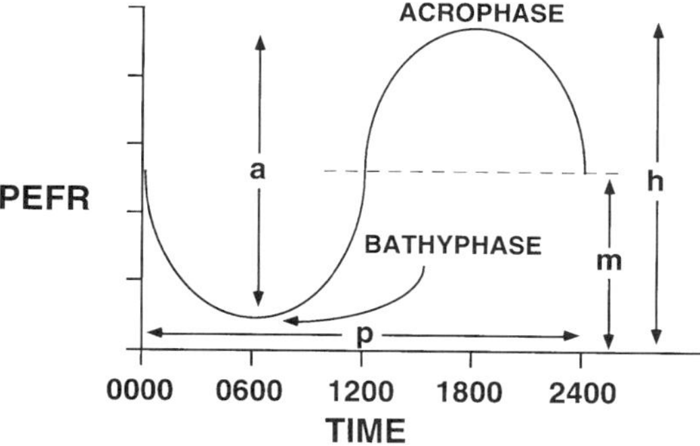

Figure 3 Analysis of the circadian variation of the peak expiratory flow rate: a = amplitude, m = mean or mesor, p = period, h = highest daily reading, acrophase = highest daily value, and bathyphase = lowest daily value. (From Ref. 19, with permission.)

muscle may be more sensitive to constrictor influences at night. deVries et al. found increased airway responsiveness to histamine at night in eleven subjects with asthma (22). Martin et al. demonstrated in 20 subjects with nocturnal asthma that the greater the overnight fall in peak expiratory flow rates, the larger the circadian change in bronchial reactivity (23). The bronchial reactivity was tested at 4 PM and 4 AM with a marked increase in reactivity occurring at 4 AM. Those patients with the greater change in peak flow rates demonstrated such increased bronchial reactivity that their absolute forced expiratory volume in one second (FEV_1) decreased by greater than 20% to inhaled normal saline alone. This effect was not seen at 4 PM. There are some inherent problems with interpretation of changes in bronchial reactivity to methacholine or histamine, and that differences in reactivity may reflect differences only in FEV_1 prior to beginning the challenge (24,25). Others have shown that reactivity does not appear to be related to the FEV_1 in the asthmatic population (26,27). In the study by Martin et al., there was no relationship between the bronchial reactivity and the baseline FEV_1 at 4 PM, but there was a relationship at 4 AM (23). However, in four subjects whose baseline FEV_1 was similar at 4 PM and 4 AM, there was a greater than threefold increase in bronchial reactivity. Thus, the data suggest that there was a true increase in airway reactivity during the night.

C. Airway Cells and Mediators

Now that bronchoscopy with bronchoalveolar lavage (BAL) has become a valuable tool in the study of asthma, examination of airway inflammatory cells, mediators, and their circadian rhythms are now possible. Several studies have shown increased airway eosinophils, neutrophils, superoxide levels, and histamine levels when bronchoscopy with BAL is performed at 4 AM in subjects with nocturnal asthma (28,29). Martin and colleagues performed bronchoscopy and BAL at 4 PM and 4 AM in two groups of asthmatics: those with nocturnal asthma, demonstrating at least a 20% fall in their overnight peak expiratory flow rate (PEFR); and subjects with nonnocturnal asthma, demonstrating an overnight fall in PEFR less than 10% (28).* They demonstrated that airway eosinophils and neutrophils are increased at 4 AM in the lavage fluid from subjects with nocturnal asthma as compared to 4 PM. This change in airway granulocytes was not seen in subjects with nonnocturnal asthma. In addition, the increase in eosinophils and neutrophils correlated with the overnight fall in FEV_1 (Fig. 4). Kraft and colleagues evaluated lung tissue inflammation via bronchoscopy with proximal airway biopsies and distal alveolar tissue biopsies at 4 PM and 4 AM in subjects with nocturnal worsening of asthma (30). They found increased inflammation, particularly eosinophils in the alveolar tissue at night in patients with nocturnal asthma, which also correlated with the overnight fall in FEV_1. Jarjour and colleagues performed bronchoscopy with BAL at 4 PM and 4 AM in subjects with and without nocturnal asthma. They demonstrated spontaneous and stimulated superoxide anion generation by airspace cells were significantly greater at 4 AM compared to 4 PM only in subjects with nocturnal asthma (29). Because oxygen radicals can influence airway function chronically and acutely (31), it is possible than the enhanced release of reactive oxygen compounds is causally associated with airway obstruction in nocturnal asthma.

---

* The percentage fall in PEFR is calculated as follows: bedtime PEFR − AM PEFR/bedtime PEFR.

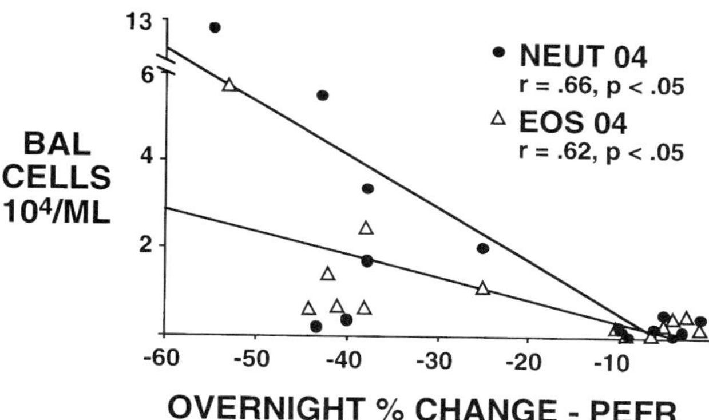

Figure 4 The correlation between the bronchoalveolar lavage (BAL) cell neutrophils (neut) and eosinophils (eos) and the overnight change in peak expiratory flow rate (PEFR) is shown. Neutrophil cell counts are represented by the filled circles, and eosinophil cell counts are represented by the open triangles. (Adapted from Ref. 28.)

III. MECHANISMS ASSOCIATED WITH NOCTURNAL ASTHMA

A. Neurohormonal Changes

Several neurohormones vary in a circadian fashion and are felt to contribute to the overnight fall in lung function. Cortisol is known to vary in a circadian fashion, with peak levels occurring upon awakening, approximately 6–7 AM, and trough levels noted in the early morning hours, approximately 11 PM–12 AM (32). These changes are seen in both asthmatic and nonasthmatic individuals, thus alone they are not felt to be responsible for the overnight fall in PEFR (32). However, the decreased levels at night certainly contribute, because cortisol is felt to exert an anti-inflammatory effect on the chronically inflamed airways of asthmatics.

Epinephrine also varies in a circadian fashion, with peak levels during the afternoon hours, approximately 4 PM, and trough levels during the early morning hours, with the nadir occurring at 4 AM (32). Patients with nocturnal asthma infused with physiologic doses of epinephrine lessened but did not abolish their overnight decline in PEFR (32). Epinephrine relaxes airway smooth muscle and inhibits leakage of histamine and other mediators from sensitized mast cells. Thus, circadian changes in circulating epinephrine promote asthma at night both by reducing bronchodilatation and by contributing to a "permissive" release of spasmogenic mediators from mast cells and other cells, such as eosinophils, that participate in asthma pathogenesis.

B. Cholinergic Tone

There is evidence to suggest that cholinergic or vagal tone is increased at night, thus contributing to the circadian change in airway function (33). Morrison and colleagues (33) administered atropine intravenously to subjects with nocturnal asthma and found improvement in the 4 AM PEFR as compared to placebo. Kallenbach and colleagues studied the heart rate variations induced by deep breathing, Valsalva maneuver, and standing from the recumbent position in asthmatic and nonasthmatic subjects (34). The asthmatic subjects had evidence of enhanced parasympathetic neural drive to the sinoatrial node consistent with increased parasympathetic activity, both during the day and night. The importance to emergency physicians is that ipratropium bromide therefore may be used as a bronchodilator at night, whereas during the day, it may not be as effective.

C. Glucocorticoid and Beta-2 Receptors

In addition to circadian changes in neurohormones and cholinergic tone, the density and function of specific receptors important to asthma also exhibit circadian variation. Szefler and colleagues showed a significant decrease in beta-2 (β_2) receptor number and function during the night as compared to daytime in patients with nocturnal asthma (31). These changes were not noted in asthmatics without nocturnal worsening of symptoms or in normal controls. Although this may be a result of previous β_2-agonist therapy, a reduced density of receptors has also been reported on untreated asthmatics (31). This phenotypic downregulation may be related to a polymorphism within the genetic coding block of the β_2 receptor. Specifically, the placement of amino acid glycine at position 16 (Gly 16) imparts an accelerated downregulation of the receptor as compared to arginine at this position. The frequency of the Gly 16 is 80% in patients with nocturnal asthma as compared to 52% in patients with nonnocturnal asthma (35). This significant over representation of Gly 16 results in an odds ratio of 3.8 for the presence of nocturnal asthma.

Furthermore, Kraft and colleagues showed a reduction in the glucocorticoid receptor binding affinity at night as compared to daytime in patients with nocturnal asthma (36). Thus, the decrements in cortisol and epinephrine along with the loss of function in the respective receptors can potentially allow the inflammatory cascade of asthma to begin and be maintained in the vulnerable individual.

D. Plasma cAMP

Plasma cyclic adenosine monophosphate (cAMP) exhibits a prominent high amplitude circadian rhythm with the highest levels at 4 PM and the lowest at 4 AM corresponding to the time of highest and lowest airway patency (32). The pattern is similar in both asthmatics and nonasthmatics, although the 24-hr mean plasma cAMP level tends to be somewhat greater in nonasthmatics. Changes in plasma cAMP over the day and night probably reflect epinephrine-mediated activation of tissue adenyl cyclase.

E. Plasma Histamine and IgE

Histamine also varies in a circadian fashion with the peak levels coinciding in time with the greatest bronchoconstriction, 4 AM (32). This change is not seen in nonasthmatics. IgE also varies in asthmatics with a fivefold greater mean level as compared with nonallergic controls (37). In asthmatics, highest serum levels occur around midday and the lowest at night and early morning hours. These changes, however, could reflect temporal differences in tissue or cell-bound IgE. That is, the lower the IgE serum level the greater the cell-bound IgE. Cell-bound IgE may play a larger role in mast cell degranulation in the asthmatic airway than circulating IgE.

IV. FACTORS CONTRIBUTING TO THE PRESENTATION OF PATIENTS WITH NOCTURNAL ASTHMA TO THE ED

A. Gastroesophageal Reflux

The relationship between gastroesophageal reflux and nocturnal asthma is controversial. As gastric acid secretion is increased at night (15) and sleep usually takes place in the supine position, it is possible that gastric contents can irritate the esophagus and result in reflex bronchospasm via increased vagal tone. In addition, aspiration of small amounts of gastric contents occurs physiologically with sleep (38,39). This aspiration of gastric contents may result in bronchospasm.

Several surgical reports state that gastroesophageal reflux with possible aspiration is a trigger factor in asthma (40–42). The most important mechanism postulated was an incompetent lower esophageal sphincter with or without an associated hiatal hernia. The medications that asthmatics use, such as bronchodilators and steroids, tend to cause or potentiate the decreased tone in the gastroesophageal sphincter. The cause and effect of reflux asthma was stated to occur in several of these reports (40–42) when asthmatic symptoms were abolished following the surgical restoration of effective lower esophageal sphincter function.

Several nonsurgical studies have been performed to assess the effect of gastroesophageal reflux disease (GERD) on nocturnal asthma. Goodall and colleagues (43) studied 20 patients with nocturnal asthma in a double-blind crossover study using cimetidine. The severity of reflux was graded using a symptom score of heartburn and regurgitation, in addition to objective evaluation of upper gastrointestinal radiograph, fiberoptic endoscopy with biopsy, manometry, pH monitoring of the distal esophagus, and acid infusion testing. Significant improvement was seen in reflux and nighttime symptoms with cimetidine. Fourteen of 18 patients felt that their nocturnal bronchospasm had improved markedly during the period of cimetidine use.

In a similar study, Martin and colleagues (44) studied two groups of asthmatics, one group with esophagitis and the other group without esophagitis based on the results of the Bernstein test. These patients were randomly chosen to receive an infusion of 0.1N hydrochloric acid or saline into the distal third of the esophagus. The respiratory pattern was assessed during sleep using an inductance vest. An inductance vest is a tight fitting vest that measures excursion of the chest wall and abdomen. Saline infusion had no effect on the respiratory pattern. Hydrochloric acid had an effect on the respiratory pattern, but only in those patients with pre-existing esophagitis. They experienced decreased mean expiratory flow, decreased ratio of inspiratory to total breath duration, and decreased inspiratory to expiratory timing. The authors felt that acid in the esophagus alone triggered this altered respiratory pattern and was indirectly indicative of bronchoconstriction. However, other studies have shown only minimal increase in total respiratory resistance or no association between low esophageal pH and worsening of asthma (45–47).

Unfortunately, the above studies supporting a cause and effect for GERD in asthma were inadequate as they lacked reliable, objective, and direct indicators of lower airway bronchoconstriction, such as lower airway resistance measurements, and reliable documentation of esophageal pH. Tan and colleagues addressed these issues by studying nocturnal asthma patients with and without clinical esophagitis using simultaneous and continuous measurements of lower airway resistance and esophageal pH (48). Lower airway

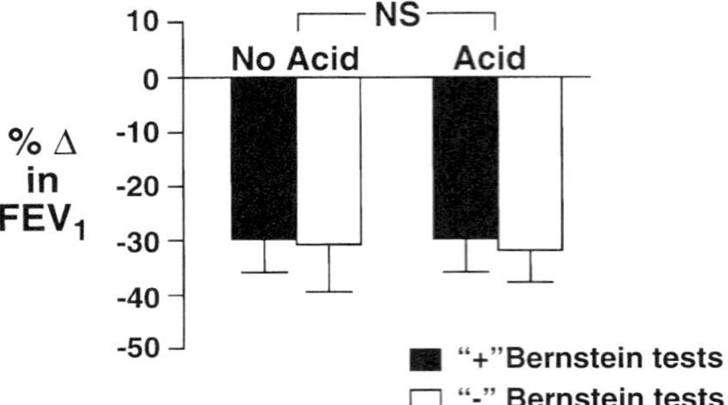

Figure 5 The effect of acid on overnight fall in forced expiratory volume in 1 sec (FEV_1) in 10 patients who had positive Bernstein tests (dark bars) and five patients with negative Bernstein tests (white bars) is shown. There was no difference in percentage fall FEV_1 between the two groups on the two infusion nights. (From Ref. 48, with permission.)

resistance was calculated on a breath-by-breath basis using tidal volume and expiratory flow rates via a tight fitting mask attached to a heated pneumotachygraph and esophageal pressure obtained from an esophageal balloon. All subjects underwent infusion of acid to lower esophageal pH to less than 2 during sleep. In patients with known esophagitis and reflux, the mean lower airway resistance was 2.41 $\pm$ 0.78 cmH_2o/L/sec (normal value for lower airway resistance in nonasthmatics while awake: 1.80 $\pm$ 0.74 cmH_2o/L/sec) (49). This was not significantly different from that obtained during the 30 minutes of acid infusion, 2.24 $\pm$ 0.48 cmH_2o/L/sec. In addition, the increase in lower airway resistance measured during the night was not affected by the presence or absence of acid in the esophagus. The overnight decrement in FEV_1 stayed constant in the presence or absence of esophageal acid in asthmatic patients with and without esophagitis and reflux (Fig. 5). Thus, the study of Tan and colleagues does not support a role for GERD as a direct trigger in asthma. However, aspiration was not evaluated, which could play a role in a subset of asthmatics.

Given the conflicting data, treatment of GERD in nocturnal asthma should be based on symptoms of reflux and not worsening of asthma. However, if the patient complains of a sour taste in their mouth upon arising or has unexplained infiltrates on the chest radiograph, then the possibility of reflux with aspiration should be considered. In this case, treatment includes elevation of the head of the bed with 4–6 in. blocks and a medication such as metoclopramide and propulsid should be given to speed gastric emptying. Protor pump inhibitors and H_2 blockers may also be of benefit in this situation. These treatments can be recommended and carried out in the ED if GERD appears to be an exacerbating factor in nocturnal worsening of asthma (Table 1). If significant aspiration is documented, strong consideration of a Nissen fundoplication is warranted.

B. Obstructive Sleep Apnea

Because sleep apnea occurs in 2–5% of the general population, one would expect to find a subset of patients that have both obstructive apnea and asthma. Although there are concerns about treating an asthmatic patient with nocturnal continuous positive airway pres-

Table 1 Factors Contributing to Nocturnal Asthma

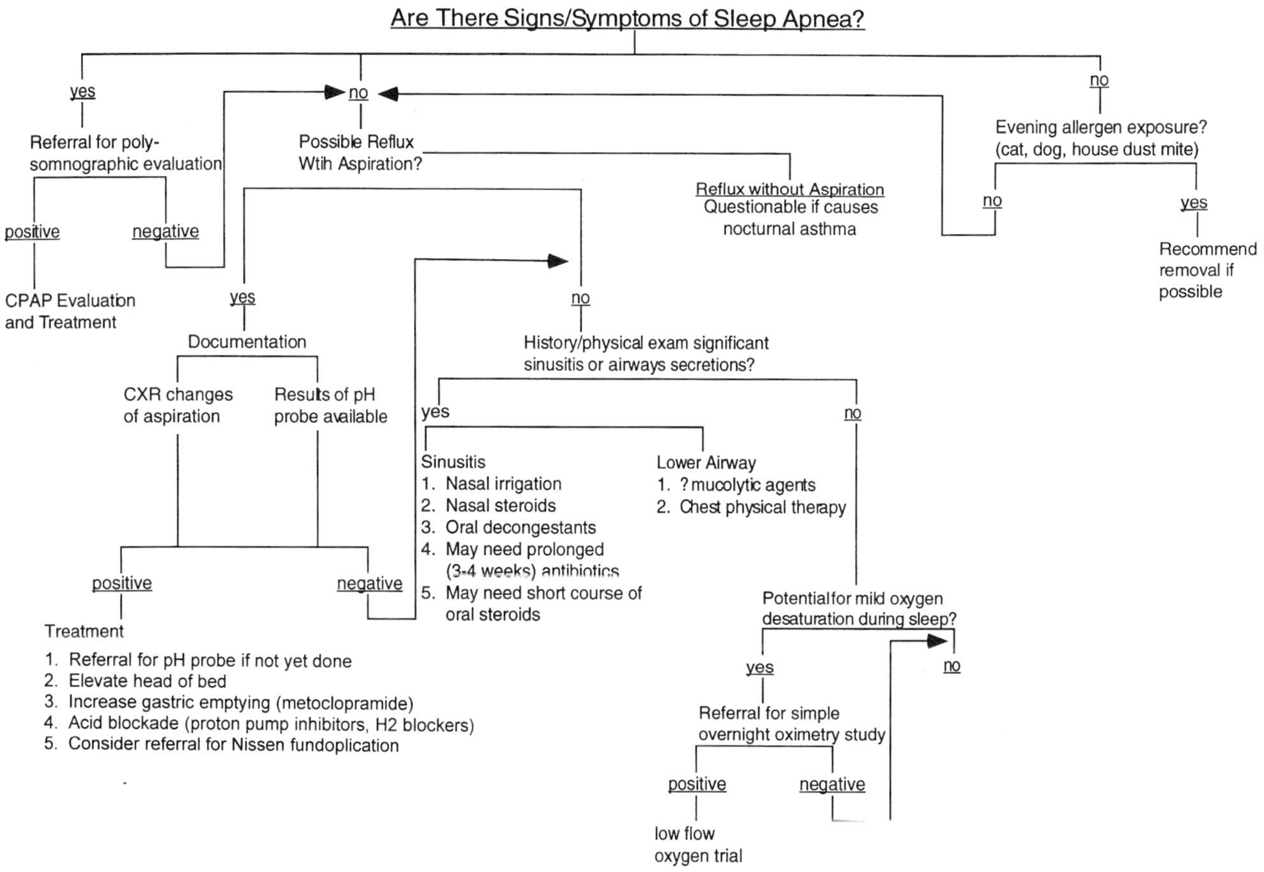

<u>Are There Signs/Symptoms of Sleep Apnea?</u>

<u>yes</u>

Referral for poly-
somnographic evaluation

<u>positive</u>

CPAP Evaluation
and Treatment

<u>negative</u>

<u>no</u>

Possible Reflux
Wtih Aspiration?

<u>yes</u>

Documentation

CXR changes
of aspiration

Results of pH
probe available

<u>positive</u>

Treatment

1. Referral for pH probe if not yet done
2. Elevate head of bed
3. Increase gastric emptying (metoclopramide)
4. Acid blockade (proton pump inhibitors, H2 blockers)
5. Consider referral for Nissen fundoplication

<u>negative</u>

<u>no</u>

History/physical exam significant
sinusitis or airways secretions?

yes

Sinusitis
1. Nasal irrigation
2. Nasal steroids
3. Oral decongestants
4. May need prolonged
(3-4 weeks) antibiotics
5. May need short course of
oral steroids

Lower Airway
1. ? mucolytic agents
2. Chest physical therapy

<u>no</u>

Potential for mild oxygen
desaturation during sleep?

<u>yes</u>

Referral for simple
overnight oximetry study

<u>positive</u>

low flow
oxygen trial

<u>negative</u>

<u>no</u>

<u>Reflux without Aspiration</u>
Questionable if causes
nocturnal asthma

<u>no</u>

Evening allergen exposure?
(cat, dog, house dust mite)

<u>no</u>

<u>yes</u>

Recommend
removal if
possible

sure (CPAP) including airway irritation, reflex mechanisms from the upper airway to the lower airway producing bronchoconstriction, and increased exposure to airborne allergens, Chan and colleagues revealed that it can be quite effective (50). They evaluated nine patients with nocturnal asthma who also had concomitant obstructive sleep apnea. Despite a regimen that included maximal bronchodilator therapy and oral corticosteroids, the frequency and severity of the nocturnal asthma symptoms remained unchanged; three patients had a history of respiratory arrest occurring during the nighttime hours. After the diagnosis of obstructive sleep apnea was made (apnea/hypopnea index between 5 and 67 per hour), these patients were enrolled in a 6-week study, a 2-week baseline evaluation of morning and evening peak expiratory flow rates (PEFR), a nasal CPAP period with PEFR measurements, and then another 2-week period with no nasal CPAP. Nasal CPAP resulted in significant improvement of both the morning and evening PEFR (Fig. 6). Clinically, all patients experienced a marked improvement in nocturnal and daytime asthma symptoms and used their bronchodilators less frequently during both the day and night on nasal CPAP. Actually, only one patient needed nocturnal bronchodilator therapy while on nasal CPAP, a significant improvement from the pretreatment period. Chan and colleagues postulated that the recurrent episodes of upper airway obstruction and snoring act as a chronic irritant that, when eliminated by nasal CPAP therapy, improved the asthma. Neural receptors at the glottic inlet and in the laryngeal region have been shown to have potent bronchoconstrictive reflex activity (51). With repeated stimulation from heavy snoring and apnea of the oropharynx and glottic inlet or laryngeal receptors during the night, a neural reflex arc could be initiated producing bronchoconstriction.

There are other potential mechanisms by which obstructive sleep apnea and snoring could produce nocturnal worsening of asthma. Hypoxia through carotid body stimulation could induce reflex bronchoconstriction (52). Mild daytime hypoxemia in asthmatics has also been shown to increase bronchial reactivity in mild asthmatic patients without sleep apnea (53). Sleep fragmentation seen with sleep apnea may induce mediator release with resulting bronchoconstriction. If this actually occurs, then normalization of the sleep pattern that occurs with nasal CPAP would control the process, thereby stabilizing the airways (54). Finally, vagal tone is increased during obstructive apneas (55). As vagal tone is increased at night, as discussed above, elimination of further marked fluctuation in vagal tone by treating the sleep apnea may reduce the incidence of bronchoconstriction at night.

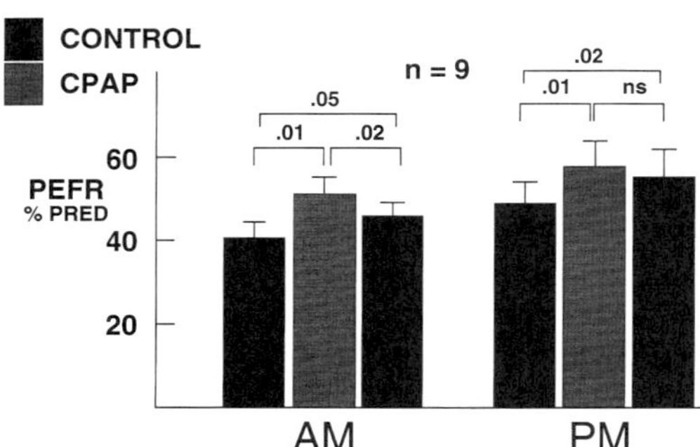

Figure 6 The dark bars represent 2-week periods off nasal CPAP, and the shaded bars represent 2-week periods on nasal CPAP. The prebronchodilator percentage predicted peak expiratory flow rates (PEFR) in the morning and evening, which improve with nasal CPAP. (Adapted from Ref. 50.)

Given the improvement seen in nocturnal asthma if the sleep apnea is treated, does nasal CPAP have a role in the treatment of the nocturnal asthmatic without obstructive sleep apnea? Martin and Pak addressed this issue in nonsnoring, nonapneic asthmatic patients with reproducible nocturnal asthma (56). Several observations emerged from this study. First, each individual had markedly worse sleep when using nasal CPAP. How well the group slept, or sleep efficiency, was 83.1 ± 4.9% on the baseline night and only 66.4 ± 4.3% on the nasal CPAP night. In addition to sleep efficiency, defined as the percentage of hours spent sleeping relative to the total number of hours supine, there was greater rapid eye movement sleep on the baseline night as compared to the nasal CPAP night (14.1 ± 1.5% vs. 3.4% ± 1.3%, respectively). To determine if better adaptation to nasal CPAP would improve the sleep architecture, two patients used nasal CPAP for one week and were restudied. Again, their sleep was poor.

In the above study, the overnight change in lung function with nasal CPAP was variable among patients. Furthermore, the overnight decrement in the FEV_1 for the group was not improved between the baseline and nasal CPAP nights. Using heart rate as an indicator of changes in vagal tone, it appeared in this particular patient population that nasal CPAP did not decrease vagal input, because the mean heart rates were essentially the same on both nights.

Consideration of obstructive sleep apnea should be made with each asthmatic patient so as not to miss an easily treatable factor contributing to nocturnal asthma. If an asthmatic patient has a history of loud snoring, observation by the bed partner of pauses in respiration during sleep, daytime somnolence, restless sleep, morning headaches, or several of the other numerous signs and symptoms of sleep apnea, a full polysomnographic evaluation is warranted (Table 1). Spirometric measurements at bedtime, during the night if the patient awakens, and in the morning at the end of the study should also be performed. Patients in the ED can be observed for these abnormalities, with monitoring of pulse oximetry, electrocardiogram and presence of apneas.

C. Sinusitis/Secretions

Although discussed in more detail elsewhere, sinusitis can contribute nocturnal worsening of asthma in particular. Chronic sinusitis and/or post nasal drip are frequent problems in asthmatics. Not only will daytime symptoms improve as the sinuses are cleared, but nocturnal symptoms can dramatically improve. An example of this process is illustrated by a 52 yr old female who complained of progressive dyspnea and wheezing over a 6-month period. These complaints were associated with postnasal drip and frequent nocturnal awakenings with chest tightness and dyspnea. Her sinus films revealed pansinusitis and her FEV_1 was 50% predicted with the ratio of FEV_1 to FVC of 62%. After a program of inhaled and long-acting oral bronchodilators was initiated, her FEV_1 improved to 79% predicted during the day, but she still experienced poor sleep, with a morning FEV_1 of 50% predicted. She was placed on an intensive program to clear sinus drainage, which included oral decongestants, saline nasal washes, and nasal steroids. Within several days she slept through the night and the morning FEV_1 was 75% predicted.

The mechanisms of sinus disease causing worsening of asthma are not clear. One possibility is a nasal or laryngeal irritation reflex producing bronchoconstriction. Another possibility is the difference between nasal breathing and mouth breathing in asthmatics. Exercise-induced bronchospasm is much greater with mouth breathing than nasal breathing (57). Thus, if nasal congestion is present and the patient is mouth breathing, worsening of nocturnal symptoms may occur. Third, secretions may be aspirated, which can cause direct or reflex mechanisms worsening the asthma. Brugman and colleagues have shown that induced sinus inflammation in an animal model does not produce an increase in pulmonary resistance by itself, but resistance will increase if aspiration of inflammatory components occurs (58).

As an emergency physician assessing patients with nocturnal worsening of asthma, attention to the sinuses as an exacerbating factor is mandatory. Certainly treatment with antibiotics is appropriate if an acute infection of the sinuses is evident, but a program of nasal saline irrigation (once or twice daily) and nasal steroids (1–2 sprays in each nostril once or twice daily depending on preparation) is also a reasonable recommendation (Table 1). Decongestants may also be used, but treatment directed at inflammation is mandatory.

Treatment of the lower airways secretions raises a major problem. Secretions appear to be worse during the sleep-related hours, but very little is known about what treatments will really improve the depressed clearance mechanisms that are present during sleep. Theophylline has been shown to increase ciliary function during the day and may be of some benefit during sleep. It is unclear if some asthmatics would benefit from postural drainage and percussion at bedtime; in certain asthmatics it could worsen lung function (59,60). Mucolytic agents such as acetylcysteine or potassium iodide preparations have a theoretical use, but again it is unknown if any benefit or worsening of lung function would occur from these agents.

There is no doubt that secretions, both intra- and extrathoracic, play a role in asthma and the nocturnal aspect of this syndrome. However, relatively little is known about the problem and, therefore, treatment is limited.

D. Allergic Factors

Exposure to bedding or room allergens, particularly house dust, may be an explanation for nocturnal asthma in some cases, but not for the vast majority (61). The frequency of nocturnal asthma in the hospital environment, which is essentially free of common environmental antigens, does not make an allergic etiology plausible. However, exposure to certain antigens during the day can result in delayed bronchospasm many hours later (62–65). This bronchospasm may occur during the nocturnal hours, depending on the time of exposure.

Mohiuddin and Martin documented that the time of day a patient is exposed to an allergen will determine if a late (delayed) asthmatic response will occur (66) (Fig. 7). Most asthmatic individuals develop an immediate response to an inhaled antigen to which they are sensitive (67). This response is illustrated by a fall in lung function, which is usually measured by the FEV_1. This response occurs within 15–20 min and resolves within an hour. A second or late asthmatic response has been stated to occur in approximately 40% of these patients 3–8 hr after exposure (67). As is usually the case, the testing times have been done only during the day. If an asthmatic is exposed to an allergen during the evening hours as shown by Mohiuddin and Martin, the incidence of the late asthmatic response is significantly increased (Fig. 7). It appears that the time of day that the patient receives the antigen is very important in determining if a late asthmatic response will occur. Therefore, patients who present with nocturnal asthma should be asked about allergies and exposure history. Recommendations to the patient may include avoidance of particular triggers such as animal dander, grasses and pollens, and/or more aggressive treatment of allergies/allergic rhinitis with antihistamines and nasal irrigation. Also, careful attention to the home environment can also be recommended if dust mites and mold

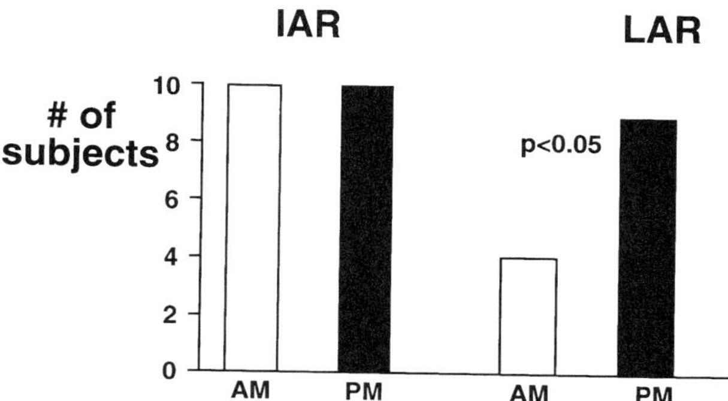

Figure 7 Ten asthmatic patients were challenged with allergen at 8 AM, shown by the white bars (AM), and 8 PM, shown by the dark bars (PM). All patients experienced an immediate asthmatic response (IAR). Four of 10 patients experienced a late asthmatic response (LAR) when challenged at 8 AM, as compared to nine of 10 when challenged at 8 PM. (Reproduced from Ref. 66, with permission.)

are triggers (Table 1) (see Chapter 6 on allergies and asthma). If atopy appears to be a significant trigger of asthma, a discussion with the patients primary care physician is warranted as he or she may need a referral to an allergist.

V. CONCLUSION

Nocturnal worsening of asthma is an important clinical problem that is especially pertinent to the emergency physician. An appreciation of chronobiology and contributing factors will allow the emergency physician to be a more effective clinician. Additionally, he or she may be able to offer particular recommendations, especially in the areas of gastroesophageal reflux disease, obstructive sleep apnea, sinusitis, and allergic factors. Awareness of the importance of nocturnal asthma may also alter discharge plans from the ED. For instance, discharging a patient from the ED at 11 PM who presented with signs and symptoms of acute asthma should result in careful consideration of anti-inflammatory therapy if such therapy was not all ready given. Therapy may consist of methylprednisolone or prednisone prior to discharge. As prevention of nocturnal worsening of asthma is preferred over treatment of an acute event, it is the observations and therapy of the emergency physician that may assist in decreasing the prevalence of this potentially life-threatening aspect of asthma.

REFERENCES

1. Floyer J. A Treatise of the Asthma, London, England: R Witkin and W Inngs, 1698, 7–8.
2. Salter HH. Asthma: Its Pathology and Treatment, Series, 1882, 33.
3. Turner-Warwick M. Epidemiology of nocturnal asthma., Am J Med 1988; 85:6–8
4. Robertson CF, Rubinfeld AR, Bowes G. Deaths from asthma in Victoria; a 12-month survey, Med J Aust 1990; 152:511–517.

5. Cochrane GM, Clark TJH. A survey of asthma mortality in patients between ages 35 and 65 in the greater London hospitals in 1971, Thorax 1975; 30:300–315.
6. Hetzel MR, Clark TJH, Braithwaite MA. Analysis of sudden deaths and ventilatory arrests in hospital., Br Med J 1977; 1:808–811.
7. Bagg LR, Hughes DTD. Diurnal variation in peak expiratory flow in asthmatics, Eur J Respir Dis 1980; 61:298–302.
8. Dethlefsen U, Repgas R. Ein neues therapieprinzip bei nachtilchen asthma, Klin Med 1985; 80:44–47.
9. Storms WW, Bodman SF, Nathan RA, Byer P. Nocturnal asthma symptoms may be more prevalent than we think, J Asthma 1994;31:313–318.
10. Karras DJ, D'Alonzo GE, Heilpern KL. Is circadian variation in asthma severity relevant in the emergency department? Ann Emerg Med 1995; 26:558–562.
11. Smolensky MH, Tatar SE, Bergman SA, et al. Circadian rhythmic aspects of human cardiovascular function: A review by chronobiolgical statistical methods, Chronbiologia 1976; 3:337–371.
12. Goo RH, Moore JG, Greenberg E, et al. Circadian variation in gastric emptying of meals in man, Gastroenterology 1987; 93:515–518.
13. Nicholson PA, Bogie W. Diurnal variation in the symptoms of hay fever; implications for pharmaceutical development, Cur Med Res Opin 1973; 1:395–400.
14. Rocco MB, Barry J, Campbell S, et al. Circadian variation of transient myocardial ischemia in patients with coronary artery disease, Circulation 1987; 75:395–400.
15. Moore JG, Halberg F. Circadian rhythm of gastric acid secretion in men with active duodenal ulcer, Dig Dis Sci 1986; 31:1185–1191.
16. Swannell AJ. Biological rhythms and their effect in the assessment of disease activity in rheumatoid arthritis, Br J Clin Practice 1983; 33:16–19.
17. Hetzel MR, Clark TJH. Comparison of normal and asthmatic circadian rhythms in peak expiratory flow rate, Thorax 1980; 35:732–738.
18. Halberg F, Diffley M, Stein M, Panofsky M, Adkins G. Computer techniques in the study of biological rhythms, Ann NY Acad Sci 1964; 115:695–720.
19. Hetzel MR. The pulmonary clock, Thorax 1981; 36:481–486.
20. Nelson WM, Tong YL, Lee JK. Methods for cosinor rhythmometry, Chronobiologia 1979; 6:305–323.
21. Barnes PJ, Chung KF, Page CP. Inflammatory mediators and asthma, Pharmacol 1988; 40: 49–84.
22. deVries K, Goei JT, Booy-Noord H, et al. Changes during 24 hours in the lung function and histamine hyperactivity of the bronchial tree in asthmatic and bronchitic patients, Arch Allergy Appl Immunol 1962; 20:93–101.
23. Martin RJ, Cicutto LC, Ballard RD. Factors related to the nocturnal worsening of asthma, Am Rev Respir Dis 1990; 141:33–48.
24. Benson MK. Bronchial hyperreactivity, Br J Dis Chest 1975; 69:227–239.
25. Greenspon LW, Morrissey WL. Factors that contribute to inhibition of methacholine-induced bronchoconstriction, Am Rev Respir Dis 1986; 133:735–739.
26. Yan K, Salome CM, Woolcock AJ. Prevalence and nature of bronchial hyperresponsiveness in subjects with chronic obstructive pulmonary disease, Am Rev Respir Dis 1985; 132:25–29.
27. Bhagut RG, Grunstein MM. Comparison of responsiveness to methacholine, histamine, and exercise in subgroups of asthmatic children, Am Rev Respir Dis 1984; 129:221–224.
28. Martin RJ, Cicutto LC, Smith HR, Ballard RD, Szefler SJ. Airways inflammation in nocturnal asthma, Am Rev Respir Dis 1991; 143:351–357.
29. Jarjour NN, Calhoun WJ, Busse WW. Enhanced metabolism of oxygen radicals in nocturnal asthma, Am Rev Respir Dis 1992; 146:905–911.

30. Kraft M, Djukanovic R, Wilson S, Holgate ST, Martin RJ. Alveolar tissue inflammation in asthma, Am J Resp Crit Care Med 1996; 154:1505–1510.
31. Szefler SJ, Ando R, Cicutto LC, Surs W, Hill MR, Martin RJ. Plasma histamine, epinephrine, cortisol and leukocyte beta-adrenergic receptors in nocturnal asthma, Clin Pharmacol and Therapeutics 1991; 49:59–68.
32. Barnes P, FitzGerald G, Brown M, et al. Nocturnal asthma and changes in circulatory epinephrine, histamine and cortisol, N Engl J Med 1980; 303:263–267.
33. Morrison JFJ, Pearson SB, Dean HG. Parasympathetic nervous system in nocturnal asthma, Br Med J 1988; 296:1427–1429.
34. Kallenbach JM, Webste T, Dowdeswell R, et al. Reflex heart rate control in asthma: Evidence of parasympathetic over activity, Chest 1985; 5:644–647.
35. Turki J, Pak J, Martin RJ, Liggett SB. Genetic polymorphisms of the β_2-adrenergic receptor in nocturnal and non-nocturnal asthma, J Clin Invest 1995; 95:1635–1641.
36. Kraft M, Surs W, Vianna EO, Bettinger CM, Leung DYM, Martin RJ. Glucocorticoid receptor binding affinity exhibits circadian variation in nocturnal asthma, Am J Resp Crit Care Med 1996; 153(abstr):A879.
37. Gaultier C, DeMontis G, Reingerg A, et al. Circadian rhythm of serum total immunoglobulin E (IgE) of asthmatic children, Biomed Pharmacother 1987; 41:186–188.
38. Hueley E, Viroslav J, Gray WR, et al. Pharyngeal aspiration in normal adults and patients with depressed consciousness, Am J Med 1978; 64:564–568.
39. Pellegrini CA, De Meester TR, Johnson LF, et al. Gastroesophageal reflux and pulmonary aspiration: incidence, functional abnormality, and results of surgical therapy, Surgery 1979; 86:110–119.
40. Urshel HCJ, Paulson DL. Gastroesophageal reflux and hiatal hernia: Complications and therapy, J Thorac Cardivasc Surg 1967; 53:52.
41. Davis MV. Evolving concepts regarding hiatus hernia and gastroesophageal reflux, Ann Thorac Surg 1969; 7:120–133.
42. Babb RR, Notarangelo J, Smith VM. Wheezing: A clue to gastroesophageal reflux, Am J Gastroenterol 1970; 53:230–233.
43. Goodall RJL, Earis JE, Cooper DN, et al. Relationship between asthma and gastroesophageal reflux, Thorax 1981; 36:116–121.
44. Martin ME, Grunstein MM, Larsen GL. The relationship of gastroesophageal reflux to nocturnal wheezing in children with asthma, Ann Allergy 1982; 49:318–322.
45. Spaulding HSJ, Mansfield LE, Stien MR, Sellner JC, Gremillion DE. Further investigation of the association between gastroesophageal reflux and bronchoconstriction, J Allergy Clin Immunol 1982; 69:516–521.
46. Hughes DM, Spier S, Rivlin J, et al. Gastroesophageal reflux during sleep in asthmatic patients, J Pediatr 1983; 102:666–672.
47. Berquist WE, Rachelefsky GS, Rowhsan N, et al. Quantitative gastroesophageal reflux and pulmonary function in asthmatic children and normal adults receiving placebo, theophylline, and metaproterenol sulfate therapy, J Allergy Clin Immunol 1984; 73:253–258.
48. Tan WC, Martin RJ, Pandey R, et al. Effects of spontaneous and simulated gastroesophageal reflux on sleeping asthmatics, Am Rev Respir Dis 1990; 141:1394–1399.
49. Ballard RD, Tan WC, Kelly PL, Pak J, Pandey R, Martin RJ. Effect of sleep and sleep deprivation on ventilatory response to bronchocontriction, J Appl Physiol 1990; 69:490–497.
50. Chan CS, Woolcock AJ, Sullivan CE. Nocturnal asthma: role of snoring and obstructive sleep apnea, Am Rev Respir Dis 1988; 137:1502–1504.
51. Nadel JA, Widdicombe JG. Reflex effects of upper airway irritation on total lung resistance and blood pressure, J Appl Physiol 1962; 17:861–865.
52. Nadel JA, Widdicombe JG. Effect of changes in blood gas and carotid sinus pressure on tracheal volume and total lung resistance to airflow, J Physiol 1962; 163:13–33.

53. Denjean A, Roux C, Herve P, Bunnoit JP, Comoy E, Durox P, Gaultier C. Mild isocapnic hypoxia enhances the bronchial response to methacholine in asthmatic subjects, Am Rev Respir Dis 1988; 138:789–793.
54. Sullivan CE, Iss FG. Symposium on sleep disorders, In: Obstructive Sleep Apnea, C. E. Sullivan and F. G. Iss, eds., Philadelphia, PA: W.B. Saunders, 1985, 646–648.
55. Tilkian AG, Motta J, Guilleminault C. Sleep apnea syndromes, Cardiac Arrhythmias in Sleep Apnea, A. G. Tilkian, J. Motta and C. Guilleminault, eds., New York: Alan R. Liss, Inc., 1978; 197–210.
56. Martin RJ, Pak J. Nasal CPAP in non-apneic nocturnal asthma, Chest 1991; 100:1024–1027.
57. Shturman-Ellstein R, Zeballos RJ, Buckley JM, et al. The beneficial effect of nasal breathing on exercise-induced bronchoconstriction, Am Rev Respir Dis 1978; 118:65–73.
58. Brugman SM, Larsen GL, Henson PM, Honor J, Irvin CG. Increased lower airways responsiveness associated with sinusitis in a rabbit model, Am Rev Respir Dis 1993; 147:314–320.
59. Darrow G, Anthonisen NR. Physiotherapy in hospitalized medical patients, Am Rev Resp Dis 1980; 122:155–158.
60. Campbell AH, O'Connell JM, Wilson F. The effect of chest physiotherapy upon the FEV1 in chronic bronchitis, Med J Aust 1975; 1:33–146.
61. Gervais P, Reinberg A, Gervais C, et al. Twenty-four hour rhythm in the bronchial hyperreactivity to house dust in asthmatics, J All Clin Immunol 1977; 59:207–213.
62. Davies RJ, Green M, Schofield N. Recurrent nocturnal asthma after exposure to grain dust, Am Rev Resp Dis 1976; 114:1011–1019.
63. Davies RJ, Hendrick DJ, Pepys J. Asthma due to inhaled chemical agents: Ampicillin, benzyl penicillin, 6-amino penicillanic acid and related substances, Clin Allergy 1974; 4:227–247.
64. Gandevia B, Milne J. Occupational asthma and rhinitis due to western red cedar (Thuja plicata), with special reference to bronchial reactivity, Br J Ind Med 1970; 27:235–244.
65. Siracusa A, Curradi F, Abbritti G. Recurrent nocturnal asthma due to toluene diisocyanate: A case report, Clin Allergy 1978; 8:195–201.
66. Mohiuddin AA, Martin RJ. Circadian basis of the late asthmatic response, Am Rev Resp Dis 1990; 142:1153–1157.
67. Booij-Noord H, DeVries K, Sluiter HJ, Orie NGM. Late bronchial obstructive reaction to experimental inhalation of house dust extract, Clin Allergy 1972; 2:43–61.

12

Urban Asthma

Robert Bristow
Columbia-Presbyterian Hospital and Columbia University School of Medicine, New York, New York

Harold H. Osborn
Long Island College Hospital, Brooklyn, New York

I. INTRODUCTION

Despite advances in our understanding and treatment of asthma, the disease is becoming more common, more severe, and more deadly. In the United States, asthma prevalence, morbidity, and mortality are disproportionately higher in large cities, suggesting that factors associated with the urban environment may contribute to the burden of the disease on society (1,2). In New York City, the rate of asthma deaths in children and young adults is three times that of the United States, and in Cook County, Chicago, the rate is twice that of the United States (3). Additionally, in 1986, while New York City housed only 3% of the nation's population, it accounted for 6% of all asthma hospitalizations in the United States (4).

Recent studies demonstrate that the high rates of asthma mortality and hospitalizations are not evenly distributed among urban neighborhoods. Rather they are concentrated in very small "inner-city" areas characterized by extreme poverty. Small-area analysis of mortality in Chicago demonstrated that disproportionate numbers of deaths occurred within a very few inner-city neighborhoods (5). From 1982 to 1987, asthma mortality rates in one very poor New York neighborhood, East Harlem, were nearly 10 times higher than the average U.S. rate (4). Additionally, data collected during 1990–1993 from Lincoln Hospital in NYC's South Bronx serving New York's poorest borough estimate a annual mortality rate roughly eight times the national average (6). When data from all asthma admissions to New York City hospitals were reviewed between 1989 and 1991, Bronx and Manhattan had the highest admissions rates. These areas also contained two zip codes with extremely high rates—East Harlem and the South Bronx (7). Not only does asthma appear to be more deadly in the inner city, but inner-city children have the highest prevalence of asthma and asthma-associated hospitalization rates in the United States (3,8,9). In the Bronx, for example, the prevalence of childhood asthma is twice the national average (9).

Is the phenomenon of urban asthma experienced in U.S. cities other than Chicago and New York? At the present time this question cannot be adequately addressed due to a lack of data. In April of 1996, the Council of State and Territorial Epidemiologists, with assistance from the Center for Disease Control and Prevention, surveyed state and territorial public health departments to determine the status of their asthma surveillance and intervention programs. Of the 51 health departments that responded to the survey, only eight reported that they had implemented an asthma control program within the previous 10 years. Most states were unable to assess the burden of asthma because they lacked data or faced barriers using existing data (10).

Asthma prevalence, morbidity, and mortality are not only on the rise in the United States, but appear to be increasing worldwide, especially in western countries. Over the last decade increases in asthma prevalence and rates of asthma deaths have been reported in Canada, the United Kingdom, New Zealand, Australia, France, Denmark, Sweden, Finland, Germany, Israel, and Japan (11–17). Similarly, asthma hospitalizations among children have increased in England, New Zealand, Australia, and Canada (11). Despite this global trend, some countries are reporting a decrease in asthma mortality. Mortality from asthma in Switzerland during 1969–1993 showed a moderate and steady decline (18), and in Scotland the mortality rate has remained relatively stable over the last two decades (19). Similarly, recent studies are reporting that the rates of death from asthma have decreased sharply in New Zealand and Australia since 1989 (attributed to an overall decrease in the use of β-agonists and greater use of inhaled corticosteroids), despite continued increase in the prevalence of asthma (20). The role the urban environment plays in these international trends requires further investigation. Current information on international trends in asthma is not only limited by a lack of data, but lack of a uniform standard of data collection.

Several recent studies from developing countries like Kenya, Zimbabwe, and Ghana suggest that asthma in children and adolescents is more prevalent in urban areas compared to rural areas (21–23). Similarly, a study from South Australia found asthma prevalence among children ages 5–15 higher in urban versus rural environments (24). The relationship of asthma prevalence to urban status, however, remains somewhat questionable. For example, a postal survey in Sweden found no difference in the prevalence of asthma between urban and rural areas (25). In Finland, the prevalence of asthma was highest in the more rural northern areas of the country (26). Similarly, a recent study found that the prevalence of asthma in Athens, Greece, is rather low compared to similar European cities (27).

Whatever the reasons for the general global increases in asthma prevalence, morbidity, and mortality, it is clear that the urban environment, or particular urban environments, in the United States play a major role in contributing to the trend. It is likely that multiple influences act together to contribute to this ''urban asthma'' phenomenon. These include ethnicity, poverty, family dysfunction, inadequate access to health care and lack of quality health care, overcrowded living conditions, exposures to indoor allergens and outdoor pollutants, and multiple environmental stressors, which may include violence and illicit drug use.

II. ETHNICITY AS A RISK FACTOR FOR ASTHMA

Asthma prevalence, hospitalization, and mortality rates vary by race, being consistently higher in blacks and Hispanics than in whites. This suggests that ethnic background may be a risk factor for asthma. In the U.S. national health surveys, the National Health and Nutrition Examination Survey (NHANES) and the National Health Interview Survey (NHIS), African-American children reported higher rates of asthma than white children (28,29). In 1993, the percent rise in the number of asthma deaths was analyzed using data from the National Center of Health Statistics and compared for African-Americans and Caucasians. The rate of increase for African-Americans in the period 1979–1983 was nearly twice that of Caucasians (30). The U.S. asthma mortality rate in 1987 for black male subjects ages 5–34 years was nearly five times higher than the rate among white patients of both sexes (2). The 1987 hospitalization rate for black children under 5 years old was nearly three times that of white children (31). Similarly, when race and gender differences in asthma prevalence rates were assessed in four U.S. cities, black children had higher rates of asthma than white children. Adjustments for socioeconomic factors, environmental exposures, and body habitus did not significantly reduce the excess respiratory illness prevalence observed among black children (32).

New York City has the highest rate of hospitalization and mortality for childhood asthma of any area in the United States (2,28), and within the city these rates are three to five times higher for African-Americans and Latinos than for the rest of the population. The rate of death from asthma in New York City from 1982 through 1987 among blacks under 35 years of age was 5.5 times higher than for whites in the same age range. The rate among Hispanics was three times that of whites (4). Researchers at the Mount Sinai Hospital in New York City, a 1300-bed tertiary care university hospital located on the border of East Harlem (an inner-city, predominately Hispanic and African-American neighborhood), and Carnegie Hill (an affluent, predominately Caucasian residential area), examined patterns of asthma deaths and near-deaths from 1986 to 1992. They found that all of the asthma deaths and near-deaths except one occurred in low-income African-American and Hispanic patients (33). Another study published in 1992 demonstrated striking differences among asthma hospitalization rates in different New York City neighborhoods. The highest rate, 115 per 10,000 population, occurred in East Harlem, where 93% of the population is Black or Hispanic and where the 1979 median household income was under $11,000. The lowest rate, 7.2 per 10,000, occurred in Greenwich Village/Soho a neighborhood that is 70% white with a 1979 median income that exceeds $19,000 (4). When death certificates were reviewed in Pennsylvania for persons younger than 35 years who had died of asthma during the period 1978–1987, blacks had nearly a sevenfold greater risk of death from asthma than whites. The highest death rates were found among black males and residents of the state's two largest urban areas (34). In Maryland, excess hospitalization rates for black children were observed at all ages and were nearly five times greater in black than in white adolescents (35). When looking at the trends in the prevalence of asthma hospitalizations in the 5- to 14-year-old Michigan Medicaid population during 1980–1986, black race remained a strong predictor for asthma hospitalizations. By contrast, urban residence was only minimally associated with this outcome (36). Patterns of asthma mortality in Philadelphia from 1969 to 1991 reported the highest asthma rates in census tracts with the highest percentage of poor people and minority residents, particularly blacks (1). Out-of-hospital deaths due to asthma in North Carolina during 1980–1988 were higher in rural counties than in urban counties, and were over three times higher for blacks and American Indians than they were for whites (37). A study of childhood asthma that interviewed 9276 mothers during 1993–1994 found that physician-diagnosed asthma as reported by mothers was significantly associated with Hispanic ethnicity, and was not confounded by socioeconomic factors or active smoking in the home (38).

III. BIOLOGICAL DETERMINANTS OF ASTHMA (see Chapter 17)

The inner city in the United States is inhabited by impoverished people who are disproportionately nonwhite. This raises the question as to whether race/ethnicity or socioeconomic status represent the more prominent risk factor in ''urban asthma.'' One study in Philadelphia found that black race was an important risk factor for active diagnosed asthma in those urban children, a relationship not explained by social factors. However, this study drew a distinction between a finding of unexplained persistent wheeze and the diagnosis of asthma. The authors found no association between race and persistent wheeze after adjustment for social factors, suggesting that race was more important to the acquisition of an asthma diagnosis than to the prevalence of the symptoms (39). One possible explanation is that in urban areas physicians treating poor children for attacks of wheezing would tend to be unfamiliar with them because of the episodic nature of their care, and thus would be quicker to label and treat the episode of wheezing as opposed to asthma.

Nonetheless, there is mounting evidence that differences in biological factors among blacks, Hispanics, and whites as well as differences within each ethnic group play a role in asthma risk. For example, all Hispanics do not seem to be equally affected by asthma. Prevalence, morbidity, and mortality rates for asthma have varied among different Hispanic populations from very low among Mexican-Americans and Cuban-Americans to very high among Puerto Ricans (40). One study found that women from Central and South America living in urban environments in the United States may be less at risk for asthma than non-Hispanic white women, while Puerto Rican women appear to be at greater risk (41). Nonasthmatic Mexican-Americans have been reported to have higher expiratory flow rates than non-Hispanics (42) and black subjects have lower expiratory flow rates than white or Mexican-American subjects (43). However, no differences in vital capacity were found among these three groups after adjusting for differences in lung size and sitting heights (44). Spirometry data from the second National Health and Nutrition Survey also demonstrated that black subjects have lower spirometric functions than white persons (45). Lung size, however, was again found to be a factor, because the racial differences all but disappeared when lung size was controlled by forced vital capacity (46).

A survey of 393 Puerto Rican and 354 non-Hispanic pediatric patients revealed a significantly larger percentage of asthmatic subjects among Puerto Ricans, confirming findings of previous studies on adults in New York City (47). Assays of alpha-1 antitrypsin (AAT) concentrations and phenotypes in 61 Puerto Rican asthmatic children revealed a significantly larger number with an S or Z variant in AAT phenotype. Also, a family history of asthma was more common among asthmatics than control subjects and was most common in variant AAT phenotypes among asthmatics and control subjects. The authors speculated that the S or Z variant of AAT affects the inflammatory response in such a way as to predispose to asthma (47). In Michigan, a recent study comparing asthma prevalence among families in a socioeconomically homogeneous, middle class, multiethnic population of schoolchildren found that, after adjusting for sex and maternal education, the prevalence of physician-diagnosed asthma and probable asthma was associated independently with black ethnicity. Since access to medical care and macroenvironmental conditions were similar across this study population, the results were consistent with the hypothesis that differences in biological factors between blacks and whites distinct from socioeconomic factors play a role in asthma (48). Another possible mechanism related to ethnic differences lies in the production of serum IgE, the immunoglobulin that governs the asthmatic response and appears to be related to an individual's likelihood of developing asthma (49,50). In a study of a large white population in Tuscon, Arizona, a strong relationship was found between total serum IgE concentrations and the prevalence of asthma (51). Others have also found a strong correlation between the prevalence and severity of asthma and serum IgE levels at all ages (52). Grundbacher and Massie have shown that blacks at all ages have higher IgE levels than whites (53). It has been suggested that ethnic differences in the production of IgE may contribute to ethnic differences in the prevalence of asthma (48). Further studies are needed to evaluate total serum IgE, ethnicity, and other biological factors controlling for micro-environmental exposures that may influence the risk of asthma.

IV. SOCIOECONOMIC STATUS AND ASTHMA

The precise causal relationships producing racial and ethnic differences in asthma have not been clearly delineated. However, racial and ethnic groups that experience the highest asthma prevalence and morbidity/mortality generally have a lower socioeconomic status (SES), which may be the primary underlying cause of these differences. In fact, in the United States the recent literature suggests a direct relationship between higher asthma prevalence, morbidity, and mortality, and lower SES as opposed to race/ethnicity (3,5,10,11,54–57). However, the states of Mississippi, Louisiana, and West Virginia currently rank highest in proportions of persons in poverty in the United States (58), yet these areas have not been reported as having high asthma mortality or morbidity. In Europe and Canada, the association between asthma and socioeconomic factors is less clear. Most available studies have failed to disclose an association between prevalence of asthma and SES, although some recent studies from Great Britain and Germany have revealed significantly increased severity of asthma among children in families of low socioeconomic status (15,59,60). However, other studies have not found an association between poverty and adverse asthma outcomes among children in Great Britain or Canada (56). These latter findings were thought be due at least in part to differences in health care systems (56). As previously described, asthma mortality in the United States occurs disproportionately in the inner cities of New York City (4), Chicago (5), and Philadelphia (1), suggesting that it is the combination of the urban environment, race/ethnicity, and poverty that constitute the key interaction for asthma mortality in the United States.

Recent efforts to understand the relationship between asthma and SES have focused on the inner city (3). In 1972, one-third of the poor in the United States lived in the central city census tracts with high concentrations of poverty; by 1991, these areas included 60% of the nation's poor (61). Seven out of eight people residing in such areas in 1990 were minority group members, most of them African-American. Indeed, the most rapid growth in concentrated poverty has occurred in African-American neighborhoods (62). During the past decade, the chance of a child being raised in a family with only one parent and limited financial resources has increased (63). In 1987, nearly 50% of black children and 42% of Hispanic children under age six were poor, compared to 10% of white children (64). The same year, 46% of all poor children in the United States lived in central cities (65). From 1975 to 1987 the proportion of poor children living in areas of the central cities where over 20% of the population was poor rose from 54% to 61% (65). Poverty, characterized by unemployment, low income, poor housing, inadequate social support, and little or no access to quality education, is a significant indicator of urban morbidity, mortality, and social malaise

In his recent book, *When Work Disappears: The World of the New Urban Poor* (66), William Julius Wilson notes that urban poverty has become more concentrated because of outmigration of nonpoor African-American families, immigration of poor people, a rise in the number of individuals who became poor while living in these areas, and an exodus of the nonpoor from adjacent and previously mixed-income census tracts. The latter has been a major factor in promoting the growth of concentrated poverty and largely accounts for the geographic expansion of poverty areas in large U.S. cities (62,66). Wilson points out that the nature of concentrated urban U.S. poverty contrasts with Europe, where no city includes areas that are as physically isolated, dilapidated, and prone to violence (66). Residents of American urban poverty areas suffer economic hardship with few legitimate employment opportunities and experience social isolation (5,62,66). Inequalities of professional status, income, housing, and working conditions are reflected in and reinforced by inequalities in health and well-being.

A clear example of the phenomenon described above is New York City's South Bronx. The South Bronx is an area made up of 10 zip codes in the borough of the Bronx. It is a predominately minority area and is characterized by extreme poverty and poor health. The Bronx population in the 1980 census was 1,168,972. Ten years later the population rose to 1,203,789. During that period, the percentage of whites in the area declined from 47.2% to 35.8% and the percentage of blacks and Hispanics increased from 66% to 80.6% (Hispanics are occasionally classified as white and Hispanic) (6). Every community district in the Bronx but one experienced a decrease in their white population during this time. The South Bronx is overwhelmingly minority with 94% of the population being black or Hispanic (6). The total population of the South Bronx was 402,250 in the 1990 census. The median age of people living in the South Bronx is 24.5 years with 50% of the population under 25 years of age and one-third under 18 years of age. One out of four children born in the South Bronx is born to a teenage mother, and one out of three children is born to a mother with late or no prenatal care (6). The median annual income is $7,980 (47% of the New York City median income). Nearly one-half of the population has an income below the poverty line. Only 3% of the population has an income greater that $25,000 a year (6). The epidemiological data for asthma in the South Bronx is quite revealing, indicating a very high prevalence and mortality rate. These rates are much higher than the average for New York City or the nation as a whole.

V. FACTORS RELATED TO SOCIOECONOMIC STATUS AND ASTHMA

Multiple influences that likely act in combination to contribute to poor asthma outcomes in the inner city include family dysfunction, low birthweight, availability of local medical care and health-related resources, quality of health care available, overcrowded living conditions, characteristics of housing, and exposure to indoor allergens and various noxious agents such as noise, stress, pollution, or contaminants. Stress on a personal level is common. The multiple environmental stressors, which may include violence and illicit drug use, can influence care-seeking behavior among residents of urban poverty areas and likely impact upon patterns of therapeutic adherence (3,67–70).

VI. FAMILY AND SOCIAL ENVIRONMENT AND ASTHMA

Family dysfunction has been related to asthma morbidity and mortality (67,71–74). The family is thought to play a central role in recognizing, managing, and preventing asthma symptoms, particularly in children (75). Maladaptive patterns of family interaction have been shown to interfere with adherence to the complicated medical regimes of optimal asthma care (73). Strunk et al. identified family dysfunction as an important risk factor for asthma mortality (67). Others have demonstrated a relationship between pediatric hospitalizations for asthma and the breakdown of family functioning through the lack of early symptom recognition and poor management of episodes (74). Frequent serious family problems were noted among poor families surveyed by Wood et al. (76), including physical and sexual abuse of the mother (41%), drug or alcohol abuse by the mate (39%), drug or alcohol abuse by the mother (21%), and mental illness in the mate (16%) or the mother (8%) in single-parent families. A better understanding of the family environment of the inner-city poor may reveal important factors responsible for asthma morbidity in this population.

An increasingly disproportionate number of families in the inner city are headed by young, single, poorly educated women. In 1987, 20% of all children under age six lived with single mothers (65); the poverty rate (percentage living in poverty) among these children was 61%. Over one-half of all poor young children lived with mothers who were separated, divorced, widowed, or never married. In a 1987 survey of poor Los Angeles families, 62% were headed by single women (76). Single mothers on welfare often have inadequate social support to help them through the stresses of caring for a chronically ill child (77,78). Social support moderates stress and encourages improved coping with illness (79,80). The impact of social support on asthma morbidity through the intervening variables of maternal mental health and family functioning has not been well studied.

The reported prevalence of mental health problems among children exhibits an inverse relationship with SES (81). A recent study found that a low level of social support and high or moderate level of asthma symptoms were associated with behavior problems in children (82). Another study found that when compared to healthy control groups, asthmatic patients had significantly more total anxiety disorders, past school problems, past psychiatric illnesses, and intrafamilial stress (83). There was also more family history of emotional problems in the asthma group (83). Weiss et al. (3) and others suggest that residence in the inner city may amplify the effects of SES and mental health problems disproportionately affecting asthma management behavior.

Family finances are another important aspect of the family environment in the inner city. Several studies highlight the extreme financial burden on poor families in inner cities due to housing costs (76,84). In one study, poor families on average spent more than 60% of their total family income on rent each month, while 25% spent more than 80% of their monthly income on rent (76). These data hint at the disproportionate daily financial stresses on poor families, which may affect their ability to cope with the demands of a family member with a chronic illness such as asthma.

VII. CULTURAL ENVIRONMENT AND ASTHMA

It has also been suggested that the cultural environment of the inner city contributes to its problem with asthma (3). For example, the high proportion of asthma morbidity among the Hispanic population suggests that language, specifically the lack of ability to speak English, may be an important risk factor for poor health status (85) as well as a barrier to care in its own right (86). In one survey, Hispanic subjects reported worse access to care than non-Hispanic whites and a higher proportion reported fair to poor health status (85). Hispanic subjects interviewed in Spanish reported even lower health status and worse access to care. Mansion documented that when compared with Spanish-speaking asthma patients whose physician spoke their language, patients with non-Spanish-speaking physicians were more likely to miss appointments and present to the ED and slightly more likely to omit medication (86). In inner-city areas like East Harlem and the South Bronx in New York City a large percentage of primarily Spanish-speaking residents are being cared for by English-speaking physicians. It is not hard to imagine that communication is a significant barrier to health care and asthma management in busy EDs and outpatient clinics.

VIII. PREMATURITY, LOW BIRTH WEIGHT, AND ASTHMA

Low birth weight has also been associated with asthma. This is, perhaps, because of its association with maternal cigarette smoking (87) or with prematurity and its attendant risk of mechanical ventilation. Survivors of neonatal lung disease, especially its sequelae of bronchopulmonary dysplasia, have been reported to have increased levels of airway obstruction, hyperinflation, and bronchial reactivity in childhood (88). Low birth weight has been associated with decreased flow rates in childhood (89) and with asthma (90). Increased incidence of low birth weight babies has been reported in inner cities in New York and Chicago (6,91). The South Bronx, as previously noted, is an area of extreme poverty within the poorest congressional district in the United States. Many women in this area obtain late or no prenatal care and concomitantly the prevalence of asthma and the number of low birth weight infants are quite high with 13% of all births under 2500 grams (6). In Chicago, a study addressing neighborhood social environments and the distribution of low birth weight babies found that after maternal race and ethnicity, the most substantial risk factor in the model appeared to be the index of economic hardship (92). Based on their findings one can speculate that women in high poverty, high-unemployment communities have fewer material resources and therefore run higher risks for malnutrition, lower quality health care services, and stress resulting in low birth weight babies. Thus the apparently high incidence of low birth weight babies in inner cities may be in part responsible for the higher incidence of asthma in these areas. A recent study looking at pre- and perinatal risk factors in a poor urban area found the following to be strong predictors of asthma in inner city African-American children: lack of prenatal care, history of bronchiolitis, positive pressure ventilation at birth, low maternal weight gain, and maternal smoking during pregnancy (93).

Another consideration is that more low birth weight infants are surviving now due to technological advances in medicine. From 1971 through 1982, U.S. perinatal mortality rates decreased for all birth weights for both black and white babies (94). Are the increasing numbers of surviving premature babies driving up the asthma rates? This is an intriguing possibility that deserves more study.

IX. INADEQUATE ACCESS TO HEALTH CARE AND SEVERE ASTHMA

Decreased accessibility to adequate health care has also been proposed as a cause of the increased severity of asthma in America's inner-city populations. Recent studies have shown that lack of continuing primary care for asthma is associated with increased levels of morbidity in low-income minority children (95). Although effective preventative therapy is available, many African-American and Latino children receive episodic treatment for asthma that does not follow current guidelines (95). Problems such as long waits in the ED, inadequate public transportation, and lack of funds may limit the use of medical facilities in urban areas (96). Additionally, children in urban areas are at high risk for requiring emergency care as a result of both illness and injury. These children inhabit a dangerous environment resulting from the problems of poverty, homelessness, overcrowded living conditions, and drug abuse. They face America's highest rates of violent injury (intentional and unintentional), immunization delays, and preventable infectious diseases such as tuberculosis and measles (97). In addition, they have limited access to quality primary health care and suffer the greatest morbidity rates from chronic diseases such as asthma. In 1985, among children under age six, 30% of the near poor were without health insurance (64). Thirteen percent of those families who were more than 150% above the poverty line were uninsured (64). These poor, uninsured children made 38% fewer visits to a physician than those with insurance (98). One recent study demonstrated that children who lack health insurance are less likely as compared to children with health insurance to receive medical care from a physician when it seems reasonably indicated and are therefore at risk for substantial avoidable morbidity (99). Poor children are also twice as likely to report no regular source of pediatric care and are far more likely to receive their care from overburdened hospital outpatient clinics and EDs rather than individual physicians (3). This makes the management of chronic illness like asthma all the more difficult to achieve.

With the advent of Medicaid, access to medical care for poor children improved considerably. However, many families eligible for Medicaid are not covered, and a growing number of uninsured families do not qualify for Medicaid because their income is above the Medicaid eligibility cutoff (133% to 185% above the poverty line) (65). Between 1979 and 1987, the percentage of asthma hospitalizations for children reporting either Medicaid or self-pay increased (31). Moreover, while Medicaid overcame an important barrier to care for previously uninsured children, it established its own less easily measured barriers such as bureaucratic paper work, long waiting times, and lack of access to office-based physicians. In Maryland, asthma hospitalization rates for children with Medicaid were both higher and slightly more likely to be emergent admissions than those with other forms of health insurance or payment options (35). Recently, two health care professionals from Harvard and Tufts University identified 500 children enrolled in Massachusetts Medicaid and hospitalized for asthma (100). They reviewed their medical claims data for the six-month period after hospitalization. It was found that African-American children had significantly fewer primary care visits than their white counterparts, even after adjusting for potential confounding variables. The authors concluded that racial disparity exists in primary care access among children with asthma. Interventions should be designed to target poor African-American children who suffer disproportionately from this life-threatening yet treatable disease. These reports suggest that at least for asthma, Medicaid may not be providing adequate access to good quality primary health care.

Understanding the differences in the type and quality of health care systems in the inner city may help to elucidate one of the causes of the increased morbidity and mortality of asthma in these areas. In a survey of children attending Baltimore public schools, 40% of whom were receiving public assistance, Mak and co-workers noted that 52% of first graders with asthma reported obtaining their asthma care from the ED (3). In New York City, 42% of physician visits made by the poor and 33% by the nearpoor are made to hospital outpatient departments (ED and clinics), while only 14% of physician visits by the nonpoor are made to those settings (101). In other inner cities, such as the inner city of Indianapolis, the ED use from 1985 to 1992 by residents of inner-city Indianapolis was greater for African-American males than white males. Researchers there concluded that inadequate routine primary care among African-American patients may increase their risk of asthma exacerbation requiring hospitalization (102). Additionally, segments of the population making 60% or more of their physician visits to hospital-based sites include disproportionate numbers of near poor black children aged 5 to 17 and nonpoor Hispanic children aged 5 to 17 (101). Data from the 1988 NHIS on child health identified the following risk factors for ED use as usual source of sick care: black race, single parent, mothers with less than high school education, poor families, urban living, and lack of health insurance (103).

Many recent studies have addressed the adequacy of EDs in managing patients with asthma, particularly with regard to the inner city (104,107). ED care for asthma often does not result in an efficient transition to continuity of care. A cross-sectional survey of adult patients with asthma admitted to the general medical services at the John's Hopkins Medical Institutes in Baltimore, Maryland, found that the outpatient medical therapy was inadequate for these patients (104). This was the first documentation of multiple problems in conforming with the standards of care delineated by the National Asthma Education Project (NAEP) (105) as they relate to the outpatient management of inner-city patients with moderate to severe asthma in the United States. In this population of patients with asthma, management was characterized by underutilization of anti-inflammatory therapy, inability to use inhalation devices properly, inadequate communication between patient and physician of an action plan to be utilized in the event of an acute exacerbation, and inadequate physician intervention during the acute stages of the exacerbation (104). In view of the dramatic underuse of inhaled steroids among urban, minority asthmatic patients, increasing the use of anti-inflammatory agents is an important and basic goal to achieve. The study also documented overutilization of inhaled β-agonists during exacerbations in this population. This is of particular importance since it has been suggested that frequent use of these medications is associated with an increased risk of fatal and near-fatal asthma attacks, even after adjustment for the severity of illness (106). Another recent study involving the EDs of five urban teaching hospitals in the northeast evaluated patient noncompliance with medical advice after the ED visit (107). It found that not having an appointment made before leaving the ED was an independent correlate of missing follow-up appointments. Lack of insurance and dissatisfaction with discharge instructions were independently associated with not filling prescriptions. Finally, a recent prospective survey of patients treated for wheezing in the ED of an academic children's hospital in Pittsburgh identified a subset of patients who were known to have recurrent wheezing but lacked adequate management to avoid expensive hospital services. Of this subset there was a disproportionate number of minority patients from poorer neighborhoods. Very few of these patients were followed by asthma specialist and there was a marked underuse of anti-inflammatory drugs (108).

Some studies suggest that poverty is not in itself an impediment to appropriate care of asthma when adequate health care resources are available. A recent study explored asthma care in an American Indian and Alaskan Native population of children whose level of poverty was similar to that of the inner-city black population (109). Despite similar socioeconomic parameters the morbidity of their asthma were similar to that of the white children. Consistent outpatient care and follow-up of their asthma by the Indian Health Service and the universal coverage provided by this service seem to explain this paradox (109). Similarly, Rea and co-workers looked specifically at ED care of asthmatic patients and its impact upon morbidity (110). ED visits for the treatment of asthma were compared in two large urban hospitals in Auckland, New Zealand, and Toronto, Canada. Forced expiratory volume in 1 sec (FEV_1) and peak expiratory flow rate (PEFR) values seemed to indicate that patients in Auckland had more severe asthma. These Auckland patients used the ED as the primary source of their care, while the Canadian patients were cared for by primary care physicians in addition to the ED. Quality of ED acute care for asthma was not different in the two settings. This overreliance on emergency care with neglect of ongoing preventative care may have led to more severe disease in the New Zealanders. The inner city has a disproportionately high number of patients who use the ED as their primary care physician. This crisis-oriented form of care appears to lead to poor disease control and worsened clinical outcome.

A recent study evaluated the effectiveness of a specialized asthma clinic in reducing asthma morbidity in an inner-city minority population (111). The purpose of the study was to assess whether an outpatient intervention program specifically targeted at a large minority population in East Harlem was successful in reducing asthma morbidity. The outpatient intervention program was successful in reducing asthma morbidity and mortality in this high-risk minority community. Also, those patients enrolled in the specialized asthma clinics made fewer ED and walk-in clinic visits and had fewer hospitalizations.

A similar study was conducted in the New York City Bureau of Child Health clinics and provided continuing, preventative care for asthma to assess whether access, continuity, and quality of care could be improved in pediatric clinics serving low-income children in New York City (112). The authors concluded that the intervention substantially increased the Bureau of Child Health staff's ability to identify children with asthma, involve them in continuing care, and provide them with state-of-the-art care for asthma. A prospective study of asthmatic patients seen in the ED and referred to allergists and general physicians for follow-up care found that six months later those followed by the allergists had significant reductions in nocturnal asthma and ED visits when compared with those followed by general physicians (113). Other studies clearly show that care by an allergist or chest specialist is superior to generalist care in reducing severity of asthma (114,115). Finally, a study of inner-city patients in New Orleans compared the care of asthma in the allergy clinic versus the ED (116). In this study the ED patients were not demographically or socioeconomically different from the allergy clinic group, but the educational level was higher in the patients' caretakers (family member helping patient manage their disease) among the clinic group. This suggests that the ED patients may suffer more severe disease due to a failure to utilize medical resources possibly as a result of the lower level of formal education in their caretakers. This is consistent with studies that show that a lack of formal education is a risk factor for more severe asthma (117,118).

The comprehensive approach to the care of asthma has been shown to be responsible for reduced severity of asthma. This entails the identification of triggers for asthma, identification of sensitizing allergens, and practical methods of allergen elimination, the aggressive use of anti-inflammatory medications, home monitoring of asthma, and written, individualized self-management guidelines. The current state of America's inner cities makes this approach difficult if not impossible for the majority of those residents suffering from asthma. If inner-city asthma patients continue to receive the bulk of their care from overburdened hospital EDs and outpatient clinics as opposed to primary care physicians or allergy–immunology clinics, there is little hope of improving the current morbidity and mortality of inner-city asthma. Even if access and quality of care were improved, this population would still be at risk due to their inability to adhere to current guidelines. Factors such as mental health, family functioning, social support, stress, and personal health behaviors such as smoking and alcohol and drug abuse would compromise their ability to adhere to complicated asthma regimes.

X. DRUG AND ALCOHOL ABUSE AS A RISK FACTOR FOR ASTHMA

Not only does alcohol and drug abuse compromise patients' ability to adhere to complicated asthma regimes, but recent evidence suggests that specific physiological effects of these substances may affect the incidence of asthma and its morbidity and mortality. Cocaine has recently been implicated as a cause of new onset wheezing, asthma exacerbations, pulmonary hemorrhage, pulmonary edema, and numerous other pulmonary abnormalities (119–121). The role that cocaine plays in asthma deaths is uncertain. However, there have been reports of severe asthma exacerbations and death in patients with chronic asthma after smoking cocaine (122,123). Additionally, it has been reported that smoked cocaine causes new onset or recrudescence of asthma in up to 33% of patients (112,123). Smoked cocaine base has been shown to cause acute bronchoconstriction, most probably mediated by local airway irritation (124). This could account for reports of crack-induced wheezing and asthma deaths in nonasthmatic as well as asthmatic individuals (124). The underlying mechanism for increased bronchospasm in asthmatic crack smokers may be multifactorial: bronchial hyperreactivity similar to that caused by other nonspecific irritants (cold air, certain chemicals, stress, exercise), immunologic reactions with specific IgE formation against cocaine or its metabolites, direct liberation of bronchoconstrictor substances, and possible drug interactions between active cocaine metabolites and asthma medications (125). With the high numbers of cocaine users in the inner city, one could postulate a possible association of freebasing cocaine and increasing morbidity and mortality of asthma in this population. A recent study reported that patients with near-fatal asthma had a blunted response to hypoxia and a diminished perception of dyspnea (126). The effects of illicit drugs or alcohol on the central nervous system (CNS) could further reduce the patients' abilities to perceive symptoms, initiate therapy, and obtain the appropriate medical care.

XI. INDOOR AND OUTDOOR IRRITANTS AND ASTHMA IN THE INNER CITY (see Chapter 9)

Many recent studies have looked specifically at the physical environment of the inner city and its impact on asthma. Over the past 20 years there has been a steady strengthening of evidence linking asthma with sensitization to indoor allergens. One theory is that urbanization has increased our exposure to environmental allergens and irritants. Indoor air pollutants show the strongest association with exacerbations of asthma symptoms. Children are sensitized to home allergens early in life, and according to some researchers this may be one reason for increased asthma prevalence (127–129). Exposure to household allergens such as cockroaches (130–132), dust mites (133), fungi (140), and environmental tobacco smoke (134) appear to contribute more to asthma morbidity than outdoor air pollutants (135–137). Building more energy-efficient and tighter homes reduces air exchange rates. By using more carpeting, soft furniture, and central heating and air conditioning, it may be that we are providing the opportunity to concentrate pollutants like cigarette smoke, pathogens responsible for respiratory infections, and allergens such as dust mites and cockroaches. A recent study in Greece supports the theory that modern, urban housing contributes to asthma morbidity (27). Researchers found that the prevalence of asthma and related symptoms in Athens was low when compared with cities of similar size in England, Australia, New Zealand, and the United States. The authors attributed this difference to the fact that, in Greece, wall-to-wall carpets are practically nonexistent, pets in the house are infrequent, and the climate in Athens is very dry and warm so windows are open for most of the year.

Rented housing in the United States and Europe built since 1945 did not benefit from a preliminary consideration of relationship between internal conditions and the wider environment. Shortcomings in the designs of the indoor environment are likely to have implications for health and well-being because people in the Western world are increasingly sedentary and spend the majority of their time inside their homes. This is especially true of older members of the community and children. Outside walls have poor thermal insulation allowing condensation and the growth of fungi. This is of particular importance because recent research suggests a strong association between asthma and living in damp housing (138–141). Patients living in homes with confirmed dampness experienced more airflow obstruction than those living in dry homes. In many high-rise residential buildings with central heating/air conditioning the quality of air cannot be satisfactorily regulated by cross-ventilation, increasing indoor air contaminant concentrations. Additional concerns about inner-city housing result from the deteriorating nature of much of the existing housing stock. Leaks and faulty boilers may lead to increased exposures to indoor air pollution (including any of the known irritant gases) (142), or to aeroallergens such as roaches, mites, cats, and molds. Psychosocial factors like violence, drug abuse, and fear cause inner-city residents to spend even more time indoors, leading to increased exposure to indoor allergens. Overcrowded inner city neighborhoods and homes may lead to increased exposure to both indoor and outdoor pollutants. Finally, overcrowding may also lead to increases in the numbers of pests such as cockroaches, mites, and rodents.

A. Respiratory Infections and Asthma

Weiss and colleagues (3) suggest that crowding, a characteristic of inner-city living, might increase susceptibility to respiratory infections. Respiratory infections (e.g., croup, bronchiolitis, pneumonia), especially before age 2, have been associated with the later development of asthma (143–145). Additionally, these infections are thought to provoke asthma attacks. Persistent abnormalities in pulmonary function and increased bronchospasm have been associated with respiratory syncitial virus infection (146,147). There is extensive evidence that viruses of the picorna group can precipitate acute attacks of asthma (148). Also, researchers have demonstrated the presence of rhinovirus in wheezing children coming into a pediatric ED and have found an association between rhinovirus and episodes of asthma in children followed over a year (149). Finally, it has been shown that rhinovirus infection can upregulate the response of the lungs to allergens (148). In addition, based on seasonal patterns, respiratory infection is the major identifiable risk factor for the large autumnal increase in asthma admissions among children (150). In one study of poor and middle-class pediatric asthma patients in New York City with no difference in reported mean family size, poorer patients resided in fewer rooms (151). Also having older siblings has been postulated to result in more upper respiratory infections at a younger age. Virus transmission is likely to be enhanced when susceptible children are crowded together in poorly ventilated environments.

B. Environmental Tobacco Smoke and Asthma

It is now well established that exposure to environmental tobacco smoke increases the severity of asthma (134,152–157). Available data also reveals that maternal smoking constitutes a clinically significant risk factor for respiratory illness and asthma in children (134,155,158–163) and that younger children are most affected, especially in the first two years of life (134,153,159,164). Maternal smoking has been demonstrated to decrease the expected growth in pulmonary functions (165). Decreased pulmonary functions put an infant at increased risk for wheezing in the first year of life (166). Researchers have noted a relative odds of 2:1 for asthma among children 1–5 years of age in mothers who smoked more than half a pack a day as opposed to mothers who did not smoke (167). The finding that younger children experience the greatest risk from environmental tobacco smoke has major clinical and economic significance insofar as younger children are the most likely to be treated in EDs and require hospitalization (and, indeed, account for a significant portion of the recent increase in asthma hospitalizations) (31,168). A recent study evaluating maternal smoking and medical expenditures for childhood respiratory illness suggested that exposure to passive smoking increases the likelihood that exposed children will experience a respiratory illness for which medical care will be sought, and that the medical expenditures incurred for such children will exceed those for their nonexposed but similarly diagnosed counterparts (167). These findings support the theory that exposure to environmental tobacco smoke increases both the period prevalence and the severity of childhood respiratory conditions. However, data from the National Center for Health Statistics reveal only very minimal reductions in smoking patterns for women aged 18 to 44 between 1987 and 1992 (170). Data from the 1988 child health supplement to the National Health Interview Survey revealed significant differences in smoking exposure by family income, poverty, and total years of maternal education (87). Nearly twice as many children under five in families with the lowest income and with a mother who had not completed high school had been exposed to smoking. Black children were more likely to be exposed to cigarette smoke than white children. A recent study in Washington, D.C., and Baltimore, Maryland, revealed that among urban, minority, asthmatic children, 56% lived with cigarette smoke (171). Risk for exposure to environmental tobacco smoke was higher when parents had no professional education.

Although there has been an overall decline in the proportion of people that are exposed to environmental tobacco smoke, the rate of smoking has remained largely unchanged in some populations, including young women (170). If inner-city women expose their children to environmental tobacco smoke, especially during the perinatal period, this could be associated with an increase in the prevalence of asthma in the urban areas.

C. Cockroaches and Asthma

The domestic cockroach has been identified as an important source of indoor aeroallergens. Because cockroach populations are highest in crowded urban areas, some have suggested that the increased asthma morbidity and mortality rates in inner cities is relate to cockroach allergen exposure (172,173). Recent studies have, in fact, identified cockroach allergy as a significant cause of asthma-related health problems, especially among children in inner-city areas (130–132,175). Young children spend a great deal of time on or near the floor where these allergens are concentrated in dust. The most definitive study, recently published, followed 476 asthmatic children from eight inner-city areas in the United States. The children were evaluated by skin testing for immediate hypersensitivity to cockroach, house dust mite, and cat allergens. Among inner-city children, the highest levels of morbidity due to asthma were associated with the presence of both a positive skin-test response to cockroach allergen and the presence of high levels of cockroach allergen in their bedrooms. This data confirmed earlier reports citing that cockroaches are an important urban source of allergen (132). Similar studies have found cockroach allergen in dust from 37% to 85% of urban homes (130,176). Sensitivity to cockroach allergen has been noted in 23 to 60% of urban residents with asthma (130,131,176–178), and acute asthma has been provoked in allergic persons exposed to cockroach allergen in bronchial-challenge tests (179). Moreover, sensitivity to cockroach allergens was shown to be an important risk factor for more frequent episodes of asthma in case-controlled studies of patients in EDs. A recent stepwise multiple linear regression analysis identified lower socioeconomic status, age greater than 11 years, cockroach exposure, and African-American race as independent risk factors associated with cockroach allergen sensitization (172). They concluded that African-American race and low socioeconomic status were independent risk factors for cockroach allergen. Thus exposure to cockroach allergen has an important role in the increasing morbidity due to asthma among inner-city children.

Cockroaches that infest houses, such as *Blattella germanica* and *Periplaneta americana,* are tropical in origin and require constant warmth. The two determinants of cockroach infestations are continuous heat and food supplies. Overheated and unkempt apartment houses and projects are particularly susceptible. Thus, it is not surprising that in Chicago, Detroit, Philadelphia, New York, and Boston, *B. germanica* may be the major source of indoor allergens associated with inner-city asthma. The problem with cockroaches in low-income areas may be compounded by rules prohibiting pets. Cats, for example, will hunt and eat cockroaches. Cats are an important source of allergens themselves, but recent investigations suggest to keep the cat as allergies to cockroaches are more common than allergies to cats (132). Finally, in the Dominican Republic it was found that sensitization to cockroaches was associated with housing quality. People who lived in concrete homes were at increased risk of hypersensitivity to cockroach antigen when compared to people living in wooden homes (174). Similarly, in Japan recent increases in allergic disease and asthma have been linked to a change in life from wooden homes to concrete buildings (180). This could have important implications when assessing the type and quality of housing in America's inner cities.

D. Dust Mites and Asthma

It is well known that the dust mite allergen is an important causative allergen of bronchial asthma (181–187). House dust mites were ''discovered'' by Fritz Spieksma and Reindert Voorhorst in 1964. Their studies led to widespread use of dust mite extracts in routine skin tests. This was followed by the purification of mite allergens and the development of techniques to measure those allergens in house dust. These measurements have provided good evidence for a dose-response relationship between the mean concentration of each indoor allergen in a community and the prevalence of sensitization to that allergen among children with asthma.

House dust mite allergens play an important role in inducing immunoglobulin E (IgE)-mediated sensitization in susceptible populations and the development of bronchial hyperresponsiveness and asthma (187). Recent data suggest that house dust mite allergens are an important cause of childhood asthma and that reducing exposure to these allergens could have a large public health benefit in terms of asthma prevention (184). As with other allergens concentrated in dust, children who spend a lot of time on or near the floor are at increased risk. In Australia, researchers found that the risk of house dust mite–sensitized children having current asthma doubled with every doubling of dust mite allergen level in the home. In children ages 2–10 years of age living in metropolitan Washington, D.C., 72% were allergic to allergens associated with dust mites (173).

Within the United States, sensitization to dust mites is common in areas of high humidity (the Southeast, the Gulf Coast, and the Pacific Northwest). The primary determinants of mite growth are humidity, temperature, and food supply. Mites flourish in a relative humidity greater than 60% and a temperature over 70° F, and their main food source in houses is thought to be human skin scales. However, it is likely that mold growth on skin scales is essential. Increased indoor temperatures may well have been a major cause of the mite population explosion. In many areas of Europe, Australia, New Zealand, and North America, it used to be unusual to heat bedrooms, even where indoor temperatures could fall below freezing in the winter. Such temperatures kill dust mites and dramatically inhibit growth of populations. In the United States today, and increasingly elsewhere, almost all houses are continuously heated, making the important determinants of mite growth humidity and the presence of suitable nests. Mites are sensitive to transient changes in humidity and maintain hydration by extruding a hygroscopic gel from their joints. They are also photophobic. For both reasons, they require a carpet, chair cushion, mattress, pillow, duvet, or blanket that will retain water during transient fluctuations in ambient humidity. Changes made in many houses over the past 30 years obviously benefitted mites. For example, fitted carpets cannot be thoroughly cleaned or dried. Higher indoor temperatures and decreased ventilation have also helped. In Atlanta, one recent investigation looking at risk factors for asthma in inner-city children showed that 86% of the inner-city houses sampled had significant levels of either mite or cockroach allergen (130). Most children in the study with asthma lived in homes containing levels of allergen previously recognized as high enough to induce sensitization (182,188,189). The high levels of dust mite allergen found are not surprising given the high mean humidity levels in Atlanta, the use of wall-to-wall carpeting in government-subsidized housing, and the lack of a vacuum cleaner in many of these dwellings. Living in substandard housing often constitutes excess exposure to indoor allergens and is probably an important contributing factor of inner-city asthma.

E. Outdoor Air Pollution and Asthma

Outdoor air pollution has been linked to the observation that subjects living in urban and industrialized areas are more likely to have respiratory allergic symptoms and asthma than those living in rural areas (137,190–193). (see Chap. 9). This is of particular concern in inner-city environments. Exposures to inner-city traffic in urban industrial areas may precipitate episodes of wheezing among asthmatic individuals and contribute to inner-city asthma. Hardest hit among the urbanites are those members of low-income minority communities who live near freeways (194). Additionally, many times dump sites, recycling centers, and waste incinerators are often located in inner-city areas characterized by high rates of asthma (195). This is known as environmental racism, defined as the intentional placement of hazardous wastes and polluting industries in low-income, ethnic neighborhood (196). Poor people pay the price for not having the mobility to escape heavily polluted areas.

Our understanding of the health risks posed by air pollution is based on experience with air pollution, occupational health, and controlled human and animal exposures. In the outdoor environment, the most important air pollutants are ozone (O_3), oxides of nitrogen (NO_2), sulfur dioxide (SO_2), acid aerosols, and particulate matter (PM_{10}), in particular diesel exhaust emissions. Also, latex allergens or latex cross-reactive material present in sedimentation and airborne particulate material, derived from tire debris, and generated by heavy urban vehicle traffic could be important in producing latex allergy and asthma symptoms associated with air pollution particles (197). Ambient concentrations of several air pollutants, such as SO_3, suspended particulate matter, NO_2, and O_3, regularly exceed the recommended air-quality guideline concentrations in many large, urban cities (190,197–199). Increased concentrations of ambient photochemical pollution, in particular ozone, are associated with increased ED visits for asthma in many American cities (194). In Sao Paolo, Brazil, mortality due to childhood respiratory disease was influenced by the ambient levels of NO_2 (137). These pollutants, in addition to acting as irritants and causing increased airway hyperreactivity, are thought to modulate the immune response and increase IgE synthesis (193). Atopic states can be upregulated by environmental influences, and some subjects may develop atopic disease in response to these environmental factors. Since airborne allergens and air pollutants are often both increased in the same areas (such as inner cities), potentiation, either in the degree of acquired sensitization or the response to allergens, could explain the increasing frequency of allergic respiratory disease. Studies that examine the quality of both indoor and outdoor air will be important in clarifying the role of air quality in the increasing rate of asthma morbidity and mortality in urban areas.

XII. CONCLUSION

In almost no other field of medicine is the gap between diagnostic and therapeutic knowledge and its general applications so great as it is in asthma. In the United States, asthma prevalence has steadily increased during the past decade. Asthma morbidity, as measured by physician visits and hospitalizations, appears to have increased as well. Since 1988, deaths from asthma in the United States for most ages have stabilized at rates more than 50% higher than those of 1979 (59). However, there is only a suggestion of stabilization of rates at 5–34 years of age. Similarly, available data has documented increasing asthma prevalence, morbidity, and mortality worldwide, particularly in western countries. This has occurred despite substantial advances in our understanding of asthma and the availability of improved pharmacotherapy to treat it.

The reported increase in asthma prevalence may be partially attributed to physicians' increased recognition and diagnosis of the disease. During the past decade, the public and the U.S. medical community have been exposed to the important message that an unexplained wheeze or chronic cough may be asthma, particularly in children. This enhanced diagnostic recognition would clearly affect the self-reported data on asthma prevalence. However, it is unlikely that diagnostic recognition can account for all of the reported increased prevalence.

The true cause of the apparent worldwide epidemic of asthma is not yet clear. However, in the United States, available epidemiological literature is documenting an emerging problem of excess asthma morbidity among racial and ethnic minorities that are both poor and residing in certain urban environments known as the inner city. The children of these minorities are particularly affected. Recent studies have allowed us to create a profile of the asthmatic patient at "high risk" for fatal or nearly fatal asthma. This profile includes African-American race or Hispanic ethnicity combined with poverty and urban area of residence.

Because inner-city populations are disproportionately nonwhite, ethnicity has been proposed as a risk factor for asthma in this population. There is, in fact, mounting evidence that biological differences among blacks, Hispanics, and whites play a role in asthma risk. However, recent literature suggests that lower socioeconomic status is the more important risk factor. Inner-city risk factors for asthma related to poverty include family dysfunction, low birth weight (< 2500g), inadequate access to health care, drug and alcohol abuse, and maternal smoking. Additionally, the crowded, substandard housing of inner cities results in exposure to high concentrations of cockroach and house dust mite allergens in infancy and increased transmission of upper respiratory tract infections among children. The practice of environmental racism (the intentional placement of hazardous wastes and polluting industries in low-income, ethnic neighborhoods) leads to increased exposure to outdoor air pollution within this population. Stress may also intensify when people live in crowded, low-income neighborhoods frequently characterized by high rates of violence and crime. These conditions offer little reason for hope and influence care-seeking behavior and patterns of therapeutic adherence.

The current evidence regarding some of these urban factors and their relationship to asthma is very convincing. More studies, however, are needed to further identify and describe the important urban risk factors for asthma and ways to intervene in the causal pathways toward morbidity and mortality. Research is needed to define regimes effective in reducing exposure to these urban factors. These studies should then be used to carry out controlled trials of avoidance measures. Such investigations should lead to the design and targeted implementation of public health policies and comprehensive clinical interventions that can reduce the disproportionate burden of asthma morbidity and mortality borne by minorities and the poor, particularly in urban populations.

The challenge of urban asthma can be overcome. Changes in asthma mortality should be especially sensitive to changes in quality of management, since most deaths from asthma are avoidable when current guidelines for recognition and treatment are followed. Continued increases in asthma mortality at 5–34 years of age, particularly in inner cities, suggest continued need for education of patients and physicians regarding optimal management and elimination of barriers to care. This should include culturally and linguistically appropriate patient education programs to ensure access to and optimal utilization of asthma care services. Several studies have confirmed that intensive asthma education can improve asthma outcomes in inner-city populations.

In 1900, about 80% of the world population lived in rural areas. By 2000 this will be the proportion living in urban areas. Little has been made of the links between health, urbanization, and the environment, yet it is crucial to acknowledge the importance of the urban environment in connection with such matters such as asthma. Social, urban, and environmental policies should become major components of the domestic agenda in order to promote social cohesion and the quality of life in cities.

In a recent survey of state-level asthma control programs in the United States, only eight of the health departments reported that they had implemented any type of asthma-control project within the previous 10 years (10). The two most important reasons for not having an asthma-control program were lack of funds and shortage of staff. However, 10 of the responding health departments indicated that they did not regard asthma as a public health priority. Starting and maintaining asthma programs may seem costly, yet asthma itself—measured in terms of both direct and indirect costs—represent a large economic burden. The estimated costs associated with asthma were nearly 1% of the total U.S. health care costs in 1985, increasing from $4.5 billion to $6.2 billion between 1985 and 1990 (200). Programs to limit the exposure of people with asthma to allergens and irritants could potentially result in great savings to society.

A national strategy is needed to assure that every person with asthma has access to state-of-the-art case management and appropriate care. Additionally, programs coordinated by state and local public health departments should attempt to eliminate environmental factors that put people with asthma at risk. In the immediate future, the public health sector should focus its limited resources on those at highest risk, namely children living in poverty, especially those in the inner city. With a coordinated approach we should be able to reduce the burden of asthma on people with the disease, on their families, and on the health care system.

REFERENCES

1. Lang DM, Polansky M. Patterns of asthma mortality in Philadelphia: 1969–1991, N Engl J Med 1994; 331:1542–1547.
2. Weiss KB, Wagener DK. Changing patterns of asthma mortality: Identifying populations at high risk. JAMA. 1990; 264:1683–1687.
3. Weiss KB, Gergen PJ, Crain EF. Inner-city asthma: The epidemiology of an emerging U.S. public health concern. Chest 1993; 101:362S–367S.
4. Carr W, Zeitel L, Weiss KB. Variations in asthma hospitalizations and deaths in New York City. Am J Public Health 1992; 82:59–65.
5. Marder D, Targonsky P, Orris P, et al. Effect of racial and socioeconomic factors on asthma mortality in Chicago. Chest 1992; 101:427S–30S.
6. Osborn H, Asthma in the South Bronx. Presentation given at the National Institute of Health, National Heart, Lung, and Blood Institute, Division of Lung Disease Center, 1994.
7. DePalo VA, Mayo PH, Friedman P, et al. Demographic influences on asthma hospital Admission rates in New York City. Chest 1994; 106:447–451.
8. Centers for Disease Control and Prevention (US). Asthma—United States, 1982–1992. MMWR 1995; 43:952–965.
9. Crain EF, Weiss KB, Bijur PE, et al. An estimate of the prevalence of asthma and wheezing among inner-city children. Pediatrics 1994; 94:356–362.
10. Brown CM, Anderson HA, Etzel RA. Asthma—The States'. Public Health Rep 1997; 112: 198–205.
11. Weiss KB, Gergen PJ, Wagener DK. Breathing better or wheezing worse? The changing epidemiology of asthma morbidity and mortality. Ann Rev Publ Health 1993; 14:491–513.
12. Lieberman JS, Kane GC. Asthma mortality: the worldwide response. J R Soc Med 1997; 90:265–267.
13. Buist SA. Reflections on the rise in asthma morbidity and mortality. JAMA 1990; 264:1719–1720.
14. Auerbach I, Springer C, Godfrey S. Total population survey of the frequency and severity of asthma in 17 year old boys in an urban area in Israel. Thorax 1993; 48:139–141.
15. Strachan DP, Anderson HR, Limb ES, et al. A national survey of asthma prevalence, severity, and treatment in Great Britain. Arch Dis Child 1994; 70:174–178.
16. Neukirch F, Pin I, Knani J, et al. Prevalence of asthma and asthma-like symptoms in three French cities. Respir Med 1995; 89:685–692.
17. Abramson M, Kutin J, Czarny D, et al. The prevalence of asthma and respiratory symptoms among young adults: is it increasing in Australia. J Asthma 1996; 33:189–196.
18. LaVecchia C, Levi F, Lucchini F. Trends in mortality from bronchial asthma in Switzerland, 1969–1993. Rev Epidemiol Sante Publique 1996; 44:155–161.
19. Capewell S. Asthma in Scotland: Epidemiology and clinical management. Health Bull (Edinb) 1993; 51:118–127.
20. Wilson JW, Jenkins CR. Asthma mortality: Where is it going? Med J Aust 1996; 164:391–393.
21. Keely DJ, Neil P, Gallivan S. Comparison of the prevalence of reversible airway obstruction in rural and urban Zimbabwean children. Thorax 1991; 46:549–553.
22. Mungai MW, Gicheha CM, Macklem PT. Lung function level among Kenyan school children from rural and urban communities. Abstract from Respiratory Disease Reasearch Unit, Kenya

Medical Research Institute, Nairobi, Kenya & the International Respiratory Disease Research Unit of the IUATLD, McGill University, Montreal, Canada, 1997.
23. Addo Yobo E.O., Custovic A., Taggart S.C. et al. Exercise induced bronchospasm in Ghana: difference in prevalence between urban and rural children. Thorax 1997; 52:161–165.
24. Crockett AJ, Alpers JH. A profile of respiratory symptoms in urban and rural South Australian school children. J Pediatr Child Health 1992; 28:36–42.
25. Lundback B, Nystrom L, Rosenhall L, et al. Obstructive lung disease in northern Sweden: respiratory symptoms assessed in a postal survey. Eur Respir J 1991; 4:257–266.
26. Poysa L, Korppi M, Pietikainen M, et al. Asthma, allergic rhinitis and atopic eczema in Finnish children and adolescents. Allergy 1991; 46:161–165.
27. Papageorgiou N, Gaga M, Marossis C, et al. Prevalence of asthma and asthma-like symptoms in Athens, Greece. Respir Med 1997; 91:83–88.
28. Gergen PJ, Mullally DI, Evans R. National survey of prevalence of asthma among children in the United States. 1976 to 1980. Pediatrics 1988; 81:1–7.
29. Halfon N, Newacheck PW. Childhood asthma and poverty: differential impacts and utilization of health services. Pediatrics 1993; 91:56–61.
30. Malveaux FJ, Houlihan D, Diamond EL. Characteristics of asthma mortality and morbidity in African-Americans. J Asthma 1993; 30: 431–437.
31. Gergen PJ, Weiss KB. Changing patterns of asthma hospitalizations among children: 1979 to 1987. JAMA 1990; 264:1688–1692.
32. Gold DR, Rotnitzky A, Damoosh AI, et al. Race and gender differences in respiratory illness prevalence and their relationship to environmental exposures in children 7 to 14 years of age. Am Rev Respir Dis 1993; 148:10–18.
33. Corn B, Hamrung G, Ellis A, et al. Patterns of asthma death and near-death in an inner-city tertiary care teaching hospital. J Asthma 1995; 32:405–412.
34. Kaplan KM. Epidemiology of deaths from asthma in Pennsylvania, 1978–87. Public Health Rep 1993; 1:66–69.
35. Wissow LS, Gittelsohn A, Szklo M, et al. Poverty, race, and hospitalizations for childhood asthma. Am J Public Health 1988; 78:777–782.
36. Gerstman BB, Bosco LA, Tomita DK. Trends in the prevalence of asthma hospitalizations in the 5- to 14-year-old Michigan Medicaid population, 1980 to 1986. J Allergy Clin Immunol 1993; 91:838–843.
37. Hefflin BJ, Etzel RA. Out-of hospital deaths due to asthma in North Carolina, 1980–1988. Am J Prev Med 1995; 11:66–70.
38. Beckett WS, Belanger K, Gent JF, et al. Asthma among Puerto Rican Hispanics: a multi-ethnic comparison study of risk factors. Am J Respir Crit Care Med 1996; 154:894–899.
39. Cunningham J, Dockery DW, Speizer FE. Race, asthma, and persistent wheeze in Philadelphia Schoolchildren. Am J Public Health 1996; 86:1406–1461.
40. Coutlas DB, Gong H, Grad R, et al. Respiratory diseases in minorities of the United States. Am J R Respir Crit Care Med 1993; 149:S93–S131.
41. David MM, Hanrahan JP, Carey V, et al. Respiratory symptoms in urban Hispanic and non-Hispanic white women. Am J Respir Crit Care Med 1996; 153:1285–1291.
42. Dodge R. A comparison of the respiratory health of Mexican-American and non-Mexican-American white children. Chest 1983; 84:587–592.
43. Hsu KHK, Jenkins DE, His BP, et al. Ventilatory functions of normal children and young adults-Mexican-American, white, and black, II: Wright peak flowmeter. J Pediatr 1979; 95: 192–196.
44. His BP, Hsu KHK, Jenkins DE. Ventilatory functions of normal children and young adults: Mexican-American, white, and black, III; sitting height as a predictor. J Pediatr 1983; 102: 860–869.
45. Schwartz JD, Katz SA, Fegley RW, et al. Analysis of spirometric data from a National sample of healthy 6- to 24- year olds (NHANES II). Am Rev Respir Dis. 1988; 138:1405–1414.

46. Schwartz JD, Katz SA, Fegley RW, et al. Sex and race differences in the development of lung function. Am Rev Respir Dis 1988; 138:1415–1421.
47. Colp C, Pappas J, Moran D, et al. Variants of alpha 1-antitrypsin in Puerto Rican children with asthma. Chest 1993; 103:812–815.
48. Nelson DA, Johnson CC, Divine GW, et al. Ethnic differences in the prevalence of asthma in middle class children. Ann Allergy Asthma Immunol 1997; 78:21–26.
49. Barbee RA, Halonen M, Lebowitz M, et al. Distribution of IgE in a community population sample: correlations with age, sex, and allergen skin test reactivity. J Allergy Clin Immunol 1981; 68:106–111.
50. Grigoreas C, Pappas D, Galatas ID, et al. Serum total IgE levels in a representative sample of a Greek population. I. Correlation with age, sex, and skin reactivity to common aeroallergens. Allergy 1993; 48:142–146.
51. Burrows B, Martinez FD, Halonen M, et al. Association of asthma with serum IgE levels and skin-test reactivity to allergens. N Engl J Med 1989; 320:271–277.
52. Sears MR, Burrows B, Flannery EM, et al. Relation between airway responsiveness and serum IgE in children with asthma and in apparently normal children. N Engl J Med 1991; 325:1067–1071.
53. Grundbacher FJ, Massie FS. Levels of immunoglobulin G,M,A and E at various ages in allergic and non allergic black and white individuals. J Allergy Clin Immunol 1985; 75:651–658.
54. Lang DM. Trends in US asthma mortality: good news and bad news. Ann Allergy Asthma Immunol 1997; 78:333–337.
55. Kington RS, Smith JP. Socioeconomic status and racial and ethnic differences in functional status associated with chronic disease. Am J Public Health 1997; 87:805–810.
56. Gergen P. Social class and asthma-distinguishing between the disease and the diagnosis [editorial]. Am J Public Health 1996; 30:431–437.
57. Anderson RT, Sorlie P, Backlund E, et al. Mortality effects of community socioeconomic status. Epidemiology 1997; 8:42–47.
58. Poverty in the United States-1992. US Bureau of the Census, Current Population Reports, Series P-60-185, US Government Printing Office, Washington DC, 1993.
59. Sly RM, O'Donnell R. Stabilization of asthma mortality. Ann Allergy Asthma Immunol 1997; 78:347–354.
60. Mielck A, Reitmeir P, Wjst M. Severity of childhood asthma by socioeconomic status. Int J Epidemiol 1996; 25:388–393.
61. Kasarda JD. Cities as places where people live and work: Urban change and neighborhood distress In: Interwoven Destinies: Cities and the Nation New York: Norton, 1993; 81–124.
62. Jargowsky PA, Bane MJ. Ghetto poverty in the United States, 1970–1980. In: Jencks C, Perterson P, eds. The Urban Underclass Washington, DC: Brookings Institution, 1991; 235–273.
63. Helmick SA, Zimmerman JD. Trends in the distribution of children among households and families. Child Welfare 1984; 63:401–409.
64. Data Sourcebook: Five Million Children, New York: Columbia University National Center for Children in Poverty, 1990.
65. Five Million Children: A Statistical Profile of our Poorest Young Citizens, New York: Columbia University National Center for Children in Poverty, 1990.
66. Wilson WJ. When Work Disappears: the World of the New Urban Poor. New York: Alfred A. Knopf, 1996.
67. Strunk RC, Mrazek DA, Wolfson-Fuhrman GS. Physiologic and psychologic characteristics associated with death due to asthma in children. JAMA 1985; 254:1193–1198.
68. Greenberger PA, Miller TP, Lifschultz B. Circumstances surrounding deaths from asthma in Cook County (Chicago) Illinois. NER Allergy Proc 1993; 14:321–326.

69. Hartert TV, Windom HH, Peebles RS, et al. Inadequate outpatient medical therapy for patient with asthma admitted to two urban hospitals. Am J Med 1996; 100:386–394.
70. Ford FM, Hunter M, Hensly MJ, et al. Hypertension and asthma: psychological aspects. Soc Sci Med 1989; 29:79–84.
71. Matus I, Bush D. Asthma attack frequency in a pediatric population. Psychosom Med 1979; 14:629–636.
72. Staudenmayer H. Parental anxiety and other psychosocial factors associated with childhood asthma. J Chronic Dis 1981; 34:627–636.
73. Mrazek DA. Childhood asthma: the interplay of psychiatric and physiologic factors. Adv Psychosom Med 1985; 14:16–32.
74. Boxer GH, Carson J, Miller BD. Neglect contributing to tertiary hospitalization in childhood asthma. Child Abuse Negl 1988; 12:491–501.
75. Clark NM, Levinson MJ, Evans D, et al. Communication within low income families and the management of asthma. Patient Education Counsel 1990; 15:191–210.
76. Wood DL, Valdez RB, Hayashi T, et al. Health of homeless children and housed, poor children. Pediatrics 1990; 86:858–866.
77. Haggerty RJ. Life stress, illness and social supports. Dev Med Child Neurol 1980; 22:391–400.
78. McLanahan S, Garfinkel I. Single mothers, the underclass, and social policy. In: Wilson JW, ed., The ghetto underclass: Social science perspectives, Ann Am Acad Polit Soc Sci 1980; 501:92–104.
79. Cobb S. Social support as a moderator of life stress. Psychosom Med 1976; 38:300–314.
80. Ganster DC, Victor B. The impact of social support on mental and physical health. Br J Med Psychol 1988; 61:17–36.
81. Goldberg ID, Roghmann KH, McInerny TK, et al. Mental health problems among children seen in pediatric practice: prevalence and management. Pediatrics 1984; 73:278–293.
82. Butz AM, Malveaux FJ, Eggleston P, et al. Social factors associated with behavioral problems in children with asthma. Clin Pediatr (Phila) 1995; 34:581–590.
83. Bussing R, Burket RC, Kelleher ET. Prevalence of anxiety disorders in a clinic-based sample of pediatric asthma patients. Psychosomatics 1996; 37:108–115.
84. Vance VJ, Taylor WF. The financial cost of chronic childhood asthma. Ann Allergy 1971; 29:455–460.
85. Kirkman-Liff B, Mondragon D. Language of interview: relevance for research of southwest Hispanics. Am J Public Health 1991; 81:1399–1404.
86. Manson A. Language concordance as a determinant of patient compliance and emergency room use in patients with asthma. Med Care 1988; 26:1119–1128.
87. Overpeck MD, Moss AJ. Children's exposure to environmental cigarette smoke before and after birth. Advance data, no. 202, Vital and health statistics of the National Center for Health Statistics, 1991.
88. Blader D, Ramos AD, Lew CD, et al. Childhood sequelae of infant lung disease: exercise and pulmonary function abnormalities after bronchopulmonary dysplasia. J Pediatr 1987; 110:693–699.
89. Chan KN, Noble-Jamieson CM, Elliman A, et al. Lung function in children of low birth weight. Arch Dis Child 1989; 64:1284–1293.
90. McCormick MC, Brooks GU, Workman D. The Health and development status of very low-birth-weight children at school age. JAMA 1992; 267:2204–2208.
91. Collins JW, Herman AA, David RJ. Very-low-birthweight Infants and Income Incongruity among African-American and White Parents in Chicago. Am J Public Health 1997; 87:414–417.
92. Roberts EM. Neighborhood Social Environments and the Distribution of Low Birthweight in Chicago. Am J Public Health 1997; 87:597–603.

93. Oliveti JF, Kercsmar CM, Redline S. Pre- and perinatal risk factors for asthma in inner city African-American children. Am J Epidemiol 1996; 143:570–577.
94. Hoffman HJ, Bergsjo P, Denman DW. Trends in birth weight-specific perinatal mortality rates: 1970–83. In: Proc. of the Int. Collab. Effort on Perinatal and Infant Mortal 1988; 2: 51–71.
95. Evans D, Mellins R, Lobach K, et al. Improving care for minority children with asthma: professional education in public health clinics. Pediatrics 1997; 99:157–164.
96. Evans III R. Asthma among minority children. Chest 1992; 101:368S–371S.
97. Foltin GL. Critical issues in urban emergency medical services for children. Pediatrics 1995; 96:174–179.
98. Parker S, Greer S, Zuckerman B. Double jeopardy: the impact of poverty on early childhood development. Pediatr Clin North Am 1988; 35:1227–1240.
99. Stoddard JJ, St Peter RF, Newacheck PW. Health insurance status and ambulatory care for children. N Engl J Med 1994; 330:1421–1425.
100. Ali S, Osberg JS. Differences in follow-up visits between African American and white medicaid Children hospitalized with asthma. J Health Care for the Poor and Underserved 1997; 8:83–98.
101. Carr W, Cohen S, Schop JA, et al. An unfinished agenda: Reducing the health deficit. In: Krasner MI, ed. Poverty and Health in New York City. United Hospital Fund of New York, 1989.
102. Murray MD, Stang P, Tierney WM. Health care use by inner-city patients with asthma. J Clin Epidemiol 1997; 50:167–174.
103. Halfon PW, Newacheck PW, Wood DL, et al. Routine ED use for sick care by children in the United States. Pediatrics 1996; 98:28–34.
104. Hartert TV, Windom HH, Peebles RS, et al. Inadequate outpatient medical therapy for patients with asthma admitted to two urban hospitals, Am J Med. 1996; 100:386–394.
105. National Heart, Lung, and Blood Institutes. Guidelines for the Diagnosis and Management of Asthma, Bethesda, MD: NIH Publication no. 91-3042, 1991.
106. Spitzer WO, Suissa S, Ernest P, et al. The use of beta-agonist and the risk of death and near death from asthma. N Engl J Med 1992; 326:501–506.
107. Thomas EJ, Burstin HR, O'Neil AC, et al. Patient noncompliance with medical advice after the ED visit. Ann Emerg Med 1996; 27:49–55.
108. Friday GA, Kline H, Lin MS, et al. Profile of children requiring emergency treatment for asthma. Ann Allergy Asthma Immunol 1997; 78:221–224.
109. Hisnanick JJ, Coddington DA, Gergen PJ. Trends in asthma-related admissions among American Indian and Alaskan native Children. Arch Pediatr Adolesc Med 1994; 148:357–363.
110. Rea HH, Garrett JE, Mulder J, et al. Emergency room care of asthmatics: a comparison between Auckland and Toronto. Ann Allergy Asthma Immunol 1991; 66:48–59.
111. Sperber K, Ibrahim H, Hoffman B, et al. Effectiveness of a specialized asthma clinic in reducing asthma morbidity in an inner-city minority population. J Asthma 1995; 32:335–343.
112. Evans D, Mellins R, Lobach K, et al. Improving our public health system's care for children with Asthma: professional education in public health clinics. Pediatrics 1997; 99:157–164.
113. Zeiger RS, Heller S, Mellon MH, et al. Facilitated referral to asthma specialist reduces relapses in asthma emergency room visits. J Allergy Clin Immunol 1991; 87:1160–1168.
114. Freund DA, Stein J, Hurley R, et al. Specialty differences in the treatment of asthma. J Allery Clin Immunol 1989; 84:401–406.
115. Mayo PH, Richman J, Harris HW, et al. Results of a program to reduce admissions for adult asthma, Ann Intern Med 1990; 112:864–871.
116. Moore CM, Ahmed I, Mouallem R, et al. Care of asthma: allergy clinic versus emergency room. Ann Allergy Asthma Immunol 1997; 78:373–380.

117. LeSon S, Gershwin ME. Risk factors for asthmatic patients requiring intubation I. Observations in Children. J Asthma 1995; 32:285–294.
118. Morris RD, Munasinghe RC. Geographic variability in hospital admission rates for respiratory Diseases among elderly in the United States. Chest 1994; 106:1172–1181.
119. Warner EA. Cocaine abuse. Ann Intern Med 1993; 119:226–235.
120. Rebhun J. Association of asthma and freebase cocaine. Ann Allergy 1988; 60:339–342.
121. Levenson T, Greenberger PA, Donoghue ER, et al. Asthma deaths confounded by substance abuse- an assessment of fatal asthma. Chest 1996; 110:604–610.
122. Rubin RB, Neugarten J. Cocaine-associated asthma. Am J Med 1990; 88:438–439.
123. Suhl J, Gorelick DA. Pulmonary function in male freebase cocaine smokers [abstract.] Am Rev Respir Dis 1988; 137:488.
124. Tashkin DP, Kleerup EC, Koyal SN, et al. Acute effects of inhaled and IV cocaine on airway dynamics. Chest 1996; 110:904–910.
125. Roa AN, Polos PG, Walther FA. Crack abuse and asthma: a fatal combination. NY State J Med 1990; 90:511–512.
126. Kikuchi Y, Okabe S, Tamura G, et al. Chemosensetivity and perception of dyspnea in patients with a history of near-fatal asthma. N Engl J Med 1994; 330:1329–1334.
127. Sears MR, Herbison GP, Holdaway MD, et al. The relative risks of sensitivity to grass-pollen, housedust mite and cat dander in the development of childhood asthma. Clin Exp Allergy 1989; 19:419–425.
128. Niemeijer NR, Monchy JG. Age-dependency of sensitization to aero-allergens in asthmatics. Allergy 1992; 47:431–435.
129. Lau S, Falkenhorst G, Weber A, et al. High mite-allergen exposure increases the risk of sensitization in atopic children and young adults. J Allergy Clin Immunol 1989; 84:718–725.
130. Call RS, Smith TF, Morris E, et al. Risk factors for asthma in inner-city children. J Pediatr 1992; 121:862–866.
131. Kang BC, Johnson J, Veres-Thosner C. Atopic profile of inner-city children with a comparative analysis of the cockroach-sensitive and ragweed-sensitive subgroups. J Allergy Clin Immunol 1993; 92:802–811.
132. Rosenstreich DL, Eggleston P, Kattan M, et al. The role of cockroach allergy and exposure to cockroach allergen in causing morbidity among inner-city children with asthma. N Engl J Med 1997; 336:1356–1363.
133. Sporik R, Holgate ST, Platts-Mill TA, et al. Exposure to house-dust mite allergen and the development of asthma in childhood: a prospective study. N Engl J Med 1990; 323:502–507.
134. Martinez FD, Cline M, Burrows B. Increased incidence of asthma in children of smoking mothers. Pediatrics 1992; 89:21–26.
135. Ostro BD, Braxton-Owens H, White MC. Air pollution and asthma: exacerbations among African-American children in Los Angeles. Am J Public Health 1995; 7:711–722.
136. White MC, Etzel RA, Wilcox WD, et al. Exacerbations of childhood asthma and ozone pollution in Atlanta. Envir Res. 1994; 65:56–68.
137. Bascom R. Environmental factors and respiratory hypersensitivity: The Americas. Toxicol Lett 1996; 86:115–130.
138. Williamson IJ, Martin CJ, McGill G, et al. Damp housing and asthma: A case-control study. Thorax 1997; 52:229–234.
139. Brunekreef B, Dockery DW, Speizer FE, et al. Home dampness and respiratory morbidity in children. Am Rev Rerpir Dis 1989; 140:1363–1367.
140. Dales RE, Zwaneburg H, Burnes KR, et al. Respiratory health effects of home dampness and molds among Canadian children. Am J Epidemiol 1991; 134:196–203.
141. Strachen DP. Damp housing and childhood asthma: Validation of reporting of symptoms. Br Med J 1988; 297:1223–1226.

142. Decker C, Dales R, Bartlett S, et al. Childhood asthma and the indoor environment, Chest 1991; 100:922–926.
143. Anderson HR, Bland JM, Patel S, et al. The natural history of asthma in childhood. J Epidemiol Community Health 1986; 40:121–129.
144. Konig P. The relationship between croup and asthma. Ann Allergy 1978; 41:227–231.
145. Pullen CR, Hey EN. Wheezing, asthma, pulmonary dysfunction 10 years after infection with respiratory syncytial virus in infancy. Br Med J 1982; 284:1665–1669.
146. Stokes GM, Milner AD, Hodges ICG, et al. Lung function abnormalities after acute bronchiolitis. J Pediatr 1981; 98:871–874.
147. Sly PD, Hibbert ME. Childhood asthma following hospitalization with acute viral bronchiolitis in infancy. Pediatr Pulmonol 1989; 7:153–158.
148. Gergen PJ, Weiss KB. Epidemiology of asthma. In: Busse W and Holgate S, eds. Asthma and Rhinitis Boston: Blackwell, 1995.
149. Duff AL. Risk factors for acute wheezing in infants and children. Pediatrics 1993; 92:535–540.
150. Dales RE, Schweitzer I, Toogood JH, et al. Respiratory infections and the autum increase in asthma morbidity. Eur Respir J 1996; 9:72–72.
151. Mak H, Johnson P, Abbey H, et al. Prevalence of asthma and health service utilization of asthmatic children in an inner city. J Allergy Clin Immunol 1982; 70:367–372.
152. Fielding JE, Phenow KJ. Health effects of involuntary smoking. N Engl J Med 1988; 319: 1452–1459.
153. Respiratory health effects of passive smoking: Lung cancer and other disorders. Washington, DC: US Environmental Protection Agency; 1992, Publication EPA/600/6-90/006F.
154. Charlton A. Children and passive smoking: A review. J Fam Pract 1994; 3:267–277.
155. Weiss ST, Tager IB, Speizer FE, et al. Persistent wheeze: its relation to respiratory illness, cigarette smoking and level of pulmonary functioning in a population sample of children. Am Rev Respir Dis 1980; 122:697–707.
156. Murray AB, Morrison BJ. Passive smoking by asthmatics: its greater effect on boys than on girls and on older than younger children. Pediatrics 1989; 84:451–459.
157. Murray AB, Morrison BJ. Effect of passive smoking on asthmatic children who have had and who have not had atopic dermatitis. Chest 1992; 101:16-18.
158. DiFranza JR, Lew RA. Morbidity and mortality in children associated with the use of tobacco products by other people. Pediatrics 1996; 97:560–568.
159. Weitzman M, Gortmaker S, Walker DK, et al. Maternal smoking and childhood asthma. Pediatrics 1990; 85:505–511.
160. Gortmaker SL, Walker DK, Jacobs FH, et al. Parental smoking and the risk of childhood asthma. Am J Public Health 1982; 72:574–579.
161. Murray AB, Morrison BJ. The effect of cigarette smoke from the mother on bronchial responsiveness and severity of symptoms in children with asthma. J Allergy Clin Immunol 1986; 77:575–581.
162. Wright AL, Holberg C, Martinez FD, et al. Relationship of parental smoking to wheezing and nonwheezing lower respiratory tract illness in infancy. J Pediatr 1991; 118:207–214.
163. Sears MR, Holdaway MD, Flannery EM, et al. Parental and neonatal risk factors for atopy, airway hyperresponsiveness, and asthma. Arch Dis Child 1996; 75:392–398.
164. Schenker MB, Samet JM, Speizer FE. Risk factors for childhood respiratory disease: the effect of host factors and home environmental exposures. Am Rev Respir Dis 1983; 128: 1038–1043.
165. Speizer FE. Longitudinal study of the effects of maternal smoking on pulmonary function in children. N Engl J Med 1983; 309:699–703.
166. Martinez FD, Morgan WJ, Wright AL, et al. Diminished lung function as a predisposing factor for wheezing in infants. N Engl J Med 1988; 319:1112–1120.

167. Weitzman M, Gortmaker S, Sobol A. Racial, social, and environmental risk factors for childhood asthma. Am J Dis Child 1990; 144:1189–1194.
168. Vollmer WM, Buist AS, Osborne ML. Twenty-year trends in hospital discharges for asthma among members of a health maintaince organization. J Clin Epidemiol 1992; 45:999–1006.
169. Stoddard JJ, Gray B. Maternal smoking and medical expenditures for childhood respiratory illness. Am J Public Health 1997; 87:205–209.
170. National Center for Health Statistics. Health, United States, 1993. Hyattsville, Md.: Public Health Service: 1994.
171. Huss K, Rand CS, Butz AM, et al. Home environmental risk factors in urban minority asthmatic children. Ann Allergy Asthma Immunol 1994; 72:173–177.
172. Sarpong SB, Hamilton RG, Eggleton PA, et al. Socioeconomic status and race as risk factors for cockroach allergen exposure and sensitization in children with asthma. J Allergy Clin Immunol 1996; 97:1393–1401.
173. Malveaux FJ, FletcherVincent SA. Environmental risk factors of childhood asthma in urban centers. Environ Health Perspect 1995; 103:59–62.
174. Barnes KC, Brenner RJ. Quality of housing and allergy to cockroaches in the Dominican Republic. Int Arch Allergy Immunol 1996; 109:68–72.
175. Kang BC, Wu CW, Johnson J. Characteristics and diagnoses of cockroach-sensitive bronchial asthma. Ann Allergy Asthma Immunol 1992; 68:327–344.
176. Gelber LE, Seltzer LH, Bouzoukis JK, et al. Sensitization and exposure to indoor allergens as risk factors for asthma among patients presenting to hospital. Am Rev Respir Dis 1993; 147:573–578.
177. Bernton HS, Brown H. Insect allergy-preliminary studies of the cockroach. J Allergy 1964; 35:506–513.
178. Kang B, Sulit N. A comparative study of prevalence of skin hypersensitivity to cockroach and house dust antigens. Ann Allergy 1978; 41:333–336.
179. Kang B. Study on cockroach antigen as a probable causative agent in bronchial asthma. J Allergy Clin Immunol 1976; 58:357–365.
180. Akiyama K. Environmental allergens and allergic disease. Rinsho Byori 1997; 45:13–18.
181. Newman LJ, Sporik RB, Platts-Mill TAE. The role of house dust mite and other allergens in asthma. In: Busse W and Holgate S, eds. Asthma and Rhinitis Boston: Blackwell Scientific Publications, 1995.
182. Sporik R, et al. Dust mite allergen. N Engl J Med 1990; 323:502–507.
183. Platt-Mills TAE, De Weck AL. Dust mite allergens and asthma: A worldwide problem. J Allergy Clin Immunol 1989; 83:416–427.
184. Peat JK, Tovey E, Toelle BG, et al. House dust mite allergens: a major risk factor for childhood asthma in Australia. Am J Resp Crit Care Med 1996; 153:141–146.
185. Vervloet D, Penaud A, Razzouk H, et al. Altitude and house dust mites. J Allergy Clin Immunol 1982; 69:290–296.
186. Chan-Yeung M, Manfreda J, Dimich-Ward H, et al. Mite and cat allergen levels in homes and severity of asthma. Am J Respir Crit Care Med 1995; 152:1805–1811.
187. Custovic A, Taggart SC, Francis HC, et al. Exposure to house dust mite allergens and the clinical activity of asthma. J Allergy Clin Immunol 1996; 98:64–72.
188. Wood RA, Eggleston PA, Lind P, et al. Antigen analysis of household dust samples. Am Rev Respir Dis 1988; 137:358–363.
189. Smith TF, Kelly LB, Heymann PW, et al. Natural exposure and serum antibodies to house dust mite of mite-allergic children with asthma in Atlanta. J Allergy Clin Immunol 1985; 76:782–788.
190. Bascom R, Bromberg PA, Costa DA, et al. State of the art: health effects of outdoor pollution. Am J Respir Crit Care Med 1996; 153:3–50,477–498.
191. Romieu I, Meneses F, Sienra-Monge JJ, et al. Effects of urban air pollution on emergency visits for childhood asthma in Mexico City. Am J Epidemiol 1995; 141:546–553.

192. Kesten S, Szalai J, and Dzyngel B. Air quality and the frequency of emergency room visits for asthma. Ann Allergy Asthma Immunol 1995; 74:269–273.
193. D'Amato G, Liccardi G, Cazzola M. Environment and development of respiratory allergy. Monaldi Arch Chest Dis 1994; 49:406–411.
194. Humphrey D. It's not easy being green. The New Physician April 1997, 17–20.
195. Nossiter A. Asthma common and on rise in the crowed South Bronx, The New York Times, 5 Sept. 1995:A1.
196. Bullard, R. Overcoming racism in environmental decision-making. Environment 36(4), May.
197. Miquel AG, Cass GR, Weiss J, et al. Latex allergens in tire dust and airborne particles. Environ Health Perspec 1996; 104:1180–1186.
198. World Health Organization. Concern for Europe's tomorrow: Health and the environment in the Who European Region. Who European Centre for Environment and Health. Who-Euro, Stuttgart: Wiss Verl-Ges, 1995.
199. Krzyzanowski M, Methods for assessing the extent of exposure and effects of air pollution. Occup Environ Med 1997; 54:145–151.
200. Weiss KB, Gergen PJ, Hodgson TA. An economic evaluation of asthma in the United States. N Engl J Med 1992; 326:862–866.

13

The Clinical Presentation of Acute Asthma in Adults and Children

Barry E. Brenner and Joseph Adrian Tyndall
The Brooklyn Hospital Center, member of New York–Presbyterian Hospitals, Weill Medical College of Cornell University, Brooklyn, New York

Ellen F. Crain
Albert Einstein College of Medicine and Jacobi Medical Center, Bronx, New York

I. INTRODUCTION

The clinical presentation of an acute asthma exacerbation varies considerably, from the mildest of perceived symptoms with little objective evidence to the dramatic presentation of true "status asthmaticus," which can frighten the most experienced clinician. The severity of the episode may change abruptly even during aggressive treatment, and, although asthma severity is usually classified to formulate appropriate management plans, the clinical course of acute asthma may not be predictable. Patients with occasional symptoms may experience sudden severe life-threatening episodes. The emergency evaluation of a patient presenting with an acute asthma exacerbation, therefore, must be directed towards aggressive and immediate therapy. However brief the initial assessment may be, the preliminary evaluation must be comprehensive enough to diagnose probable asthma and assess the risk of impending respiratory failure and the need for endotracheal intubation.

In the emergency department (ED) the history and physical examination should be rapid, thorough, and focused on the presenting problem. The importance of a directed and specific history and physical examination increases in an acutely dyspneic patient with acute asthma, where time is of the essence and treatment must not be delayed. A brief initial history must be obtained that is limited in scope. A probable diagnosis of acute asthma needs to be established by obtaining what we would term a "primary history" similar to the primary survey in trauma patients. This primary history may be difficult to obtain. The patient may be agitated, apprehensive, and only speak in broken sentences, if at all. The primary history should establish that the patient probably has acute asthma by symptoms of dyspnea or cough and a history of wheezing, use of inhaled β-agonists, or physician-diagnosed asthma in the past. In the older child and the adult, measurement of peak expiratory flow rate (PEFR) or other spirometric readings may document the initial severity and assist in admission/discharge decisions, since some algorithms for admission/

discharge decisions include the initial PEFR. There are disadvantages to performing a PEFR initially on an acutely dyspneic asthmatic, since treatment is delayed while attempting the initial two or three PEFRs. Also, the patient may cough, have increased bronchospasm, and, rarely, even suffer a cardiopulmonary arrest (1). With young children, despite the fact that the parent can give a more detailed history than the young patient, the physician should obtain only a primary history and perform a brief physical examination before initiating therapy. The brief examination focusing on the quality of the breath sounds and I:E ratio is necessary, because young children cannot report that they feel better or perform PEFR monitoring to document improvement.

During an acute exacerbation, abrupt changes in pulmonary function manifest as dyspnea, often accompanied by varying states of anxiety. These abrupt changes in pulmonary function enhance the likelihood of perceiving an exacerbation; however, if these changes occur over a greater period of time (days to weeks), dyspnea may be reduced, leading to an underestimation of severity by the patient and physician (2–6). Subjective symptoms are not helpful in infants and toddlers who may appear alternately playful or irritable despite marked wheezing and tachypnea. School-age children, however, can report breathlessness. Although dyspnea has been consistently associated with spirometric abnormalities, absence of breathlessness does not guarantee that pulmonary function tests are normal (7).

Lougheed et al. (8) elucidated the mechanism for dyspnea in acute asthma. The dynamic hyperinflation of inspiratory muscles affect the function of respiration and contribute to breathlessness during an asthma attack for any given level of bronchoconstriction (8,9). Some asthmatics are more sensitive than others to small changes in lung function (10), and poor perception of asthma symptoms has lead to undertreatment and recognition by both patients and physicians. Patients with diminished perception of airflow obstruction often do not develop dyspnea (11). Dyspnea may be diminished even during hypoxia or hypercapnia; diminished sensitivity of chemoreceptors to these states may be responsible for some cases of near-fatal asthma (12).

Wheezing, although a common manifestation of an exacerbation of asthma, may be minimal, as will be discussed later in this chapter. The patient may, however, report wheezing as part of the history. Symptoms such as exertional dyspnea and coughing may be the only early manifestations (13–16). Cough in asthma essentially presents in three different ways. In ''cough predominant'' asthma the clinical diagnosis of asthma is obvious from common manifestations, such as wheezing, and objective determination of airflow compromise (17). ''Cough variant'' asthma, in which the patient does not have wheezing by history or on physical examination, has been hypothesized as the mildest form, the true diagnosis being made through demonstration of airway hyperresponsiveness (17). The third manifestation of cough in asthma is a persistent chronic dry cough despite optimal maintenance of asthma control and exclusion of other causes (17).

After an initial inhalant treatment, most acute asthmatics can give a clinical history, and a more comprehensive secondary evaluation may be performed. This secondary assessment should include:

1. Risk of relapse, admission to the hospital [ward vs. intensive care unit (ICU)], endotracheal intubation.
2. Medication use, compliance, dose, prior use of glucocorticoids, prior use of β-agonists in the previous 24 hr as well as in the hour before the ED visit.
3. Whether the patient actually has acute asthma or other lung diseases that may

mimic asthma, such as cystic fibrosis, bronchiolitis, sarcoidosis, chronic obstructive pulmonary disease (COPD), or bronchopulmonary dysplasia; foreign body; or nonlung diseases such as vocal cord dysfunction or hyperventilation syndrome; or has ingested a new drug, such as a beta-blocker given for migraine headaches.

4. The presence of associated medical conditions complicating therapy of asthma such as diabetes mellitus, hypertension, or congestive heart failure, in which the gluconeogenic or mineralocorticoid effects of prednisone could be detrimental; pregnancy where epinephrine should be avoided; or psychiatric conditions that mitigate adherence.
5. The duration of the present exacerbation which is associated with the expected response to therapy.
6. Provocative or trigger factors, e.g., upper respiratory infection, allergen exposure, or "running out of medications."

A. Risk

Questions concerning risk of relapse, admission to the hospital (ward vs. ICU), or respiratory failure involve a history of previous endotracheal intubation, the number of previous ED visits or hospitalizations in the past year, lability of asthma, and length of time since last ED visit. It is useful to ask the acute asthmatic about nighttime symptoms, since bronchospasm is often worse at night. Even in the absence of signs of respiratory distress, a report by the patient that "they were profusely diaphoretic and thought they were going to die last night" reflects high risk (see Chapters 11, 17, and 31).

B. Medication Use

A thorough knowledge of the patient's present medications, current adherence, and last dosages is essential. Among adults, sometimes the list of medications may provide an important clue to a diagnosis of asthma in the profoundly dyspneic patient that cannot speak. Medications, such as β-agonist inhalers or theophylline, usually indicate that the dyspneic patient has acute bronchospasm, even with minimal or no wheezing (see Chapter 31). Patients who present to the ED because they have run out of their β-agonist inhaler may not be able to afford the medication. Alternatively, the patient may simply have a less severe form of chronic asthma, i.e., the asthmatic who seldom needs or uses asthma medications may allow himself to run out of medication (18). Running out of prednisone or too rapid a "taper" from glucocorticoids in adults or in children using oral steroids for more than 10 days may result in exacerbations of acute asthma or even adrenal insufficiency.

C. Does the Patient Have Acute Asthma?

Later in this chapter we will discuss the differential diagnosis of acute asthma. Patients with new onset of asthma need a careful evaluation for other etiologies. Among patients with recurrent wheezing, asthma is usually readily controlled with moderate doses of daily glucocorticoids or cromolyn sodium. Poor control of a patient's symptoms, despite adequate doses of glucocorticoids or cromolyn, mandates consideration of other etiologies for the patients' wheezing.

D. Other Medical Conditions

Other medical conditions, apart from simulating acute asthma, may confound treatment. A history of tuberculosis or congestive heart failure may affect discharge medications. Facial pain, postnasal drip, or a productive cough lasting more than one week may require antibiotic therapy for sinusitis. Psychiatric disease in the adolescent or adult patient or the parent of a young patient may impair the patient or caretaker's ability to recognize bronchospasm or adhere to therapy and increases the risk of death from an exacerbation of acute asthma (19,20). Adult asthmatics on antipsychotic medications within the previous 12 months had a 3.2 times greater risk of death or near death from asthma than asthmatic patients who did not use antipsychotics (21). More than 50% of caretakers of inner-city children with asthma studied in the National Cooperative Inner-City Asthma Study reported elevated levels of psychologic symptoms (22).

E. Duration of Present Acute Exacerbation

The length of time that a patient has had symptoms of airway obstruction affects his or her response to therapy. Those symptomatic for less than 12 hr have primarily smooth muscle contraction responsible for airway narrowing and respond well to β-agonists in a brief period of time. Those who have been symptomatic for 2–4 days respond less well to β-agonist inhalers, since the airway narrowing is related more to inflammation than smooth muscle contraction (23). These patients require glucocorticoids for resolution of inflammation and at least 6 hr—but more often days to weeks—for complete resolution of the exacerbation.

F. Provocative or Trigger Factors

Elucidating precipitating factors whenever possible, such as drugs and allergens, is important. The cause of the acute exacerbation does not affect therapeutic decisions in the ED but may change ED admission/discharge decisions, discharge medications, or instructions. The onset of a viral upper respiratory infection is the most common precipitant of acute exacerbations and is a major cause of symptoms of wheezing in both children and adults. Viruses, predominantly rhinoviruses, and mycoplasma, have been shown to be the predominant organisms associated with exacerbations of wheezing (2,24,25). (See Chapters 7 and 8).

Exercise is a relatively common provocative factor in acute asthma, affecting between 50% and 80% of asthmatics (2). McFadden et al. suggest that, given enough intensity, exercise can affect all asthmatics (26). Exercise-induced bronchospasm (EIB) describes the phenomenon of progressive bronchoconstriction typically precipitated 5–10 min after the onset of exertion and lasting for approximately 30 min to 1 hr following termination of the exercise (2). EIB is affected by factors such as the humidity and temperature of the inspired air, and the mechanism of this phenomenon may be independent of airway hyperresponsiveness and inflammation (27).

II. PHYSICAL EXAMINATION

The physical assessment of a patient with asthma begins from the moment of presentation to the ED and continues throughout management. As previously mentioned, the initial portion of the assessment must be rapid and focused on features of the physical examination that affect initial therapy. It must also be comprehensive enough to assist in the diagnosis of probable asthma and assessment of the risk of impending respiratory failure and need for endotracheal intubation. The patient's general physical appearance is indispensable to the initial assessment of the severity of the attack and forms the "primary physical examination" complementary to the "primary history" defined earlier. Older children, adolescents, and adults with severe exacerbations often stand or lean forward ("tripoding") in an effort to improve vital capacity. As the severity of the asthma attack increases, the patient becomes diaphoretic while maintaining the "tripod" position. Infants and young children manifest marked abdominal breathing instead of tripoding. With further deterioration hypercarbia and or hypoxia may ensue. With hypercarbia, the patient becomes lethargic, diaphoretic, and recumbent. With hypoxia, the patient is agitated and cyanotic, and older children and adults may often paradoxically pull off the oxygen mask stating that they can not breathe.

The inability to speak or speech with broken words or incomplete sentences (termed "staccato speech") is also a hallmark of significant distress. In infants this may manifest as a diminished or absent cry with difficulty or inability to feed. Accessory muscle use as well as bilateral wheezing, coughing and obvious decreases in inspiratory/expiratory I:E ratios (> 1:2 or 1:3) are all important in gauging the level of respiratory compromise. Severe distress in an infant may manifest as paradoxic breathing. These findings can all be identified by simply observing the chest and auscultating the lungs of the patient. As part of the primary physical examination, the physician should quickly auscultate the neck for stridor (28) to assess for psychogenic vocal cord dysfunction (VCD), croup, or other causes of upper airway obstruction; palpate the upper chest for subcutaneous emphysema to assess for pneumothorax or pneumomediastinum; and evaluate leg edema to assess for deep vein thrombosis or congestive heart failure. These physical evaluations can assist in quickly excluding other causes of wheezing or dyspnea and complications of acute asthma (see Chapters 26 and 31).

The patient's vital signs are indispensable and correlate well with the degree of severity of an exacerbation. A complete set of vital signs also form an essential part of the primary physical examination. In a large study on adult acute asthma, respiratory rates ranged from 18 to 50 (mean of 31), and the heart rate varied from 64/min to 150/min (mean of 100) (29,30). In adults, pulse rates greater than 130/min are often associated with severe respiratory distress and marked hypoxemia (29,31). Of adult patients with in-hospital complications of asthma, 75% had pulse rates greater than 130/min in the ED, compared to only a 5% incidence of complications if the initial pulse rate was less than 130/min (32). Young children often may have heart rates above 150 with only moderate hypoxemia. Many asthmatics will be tachycardic on presentation. Indeed, toddlers may present with heart rates from 160 to 180, and the physician may be reluctant to give β-agonist therapy for fear of precipitating tachydysrhythmias. But when β-agonists are given, the airway obstruction is relieved, and the heart rate begins to slow, despite the arrhythmogenic effects of β-agonists.

Pulsus paradoxus refers to an exaggerated decrease in systolic blood pressure during inspiration and can be easily obtained depending upon the patient's stability. Approximately 40% of asthmatic patients have an elevated pulsus paradoxus that may range from 15 to 130 mmHg (33). Pulsus paradoxus in asthma is caused by severe hyperinflation of the lungs with mediastinal and pericardial stretching, combined with wide variations in intrapulmonary pressure (33), impairing cardiac output with inspiration. Pulsus paradoxus is normally less than 10 mmHg. If greater than or equal to 15 mmHg, pulsus paradoxus correlates well with a 1-sec forced expiratory volume (FEV_1) of less than 0.9 liters (34,35). In one study, one-third of patients who presented to the ED with pulsus paradoxus of greater than or equal to 15 mmHg did not respond sufficiently to therapy over 12 hr and were admitted to the hospital. Patients admitted to the hospital had an initial elevated pulsus paradoxus that subsequently decreased by only 20% or less after therapy, whereas those discharged from the ED showed an average pulsus paradoxus decrease of 60% (36). Evaluation for pulsus paradoxus may be time consuming, especially in children, and does not add information different from the presence of accessory muscle use or the common spirometric assessments. For these reasons it is rarely part of the routine evaluation of asthma severity.

Clinical hyperinflation of the chest indicates at least moderate asthma (37,38) and is due to persistent intercostal and accessory muscle contraction during exhalation (39). Hyperinflation changes quickly with improvement or exacerbation. Improvement with persistence of hyperinflation may indicate that improvement will be brief.

McFadden et al. (40) studied 22 patients aged 16–45 years with acute bronchial asthma and noted that sternocleidomastoid retraction correlated well with the degree of mechanical impairment of the lung, usually with an FEV_1 of less than 1 liter. The presence of dyspnea, subjective wheezing, and expiratory wheezing was uniformly associated with airway obstruction, but the extent of obstruction could not be determined from these findings with any degree of precision. In fact, although 90% of patients became asymptomatic, 40% were still wheezing. Likewise, Commey and Levison studied 62 children with asthma; pulmonary function measures were worst among the 21 patients with sternocleidomastoid retractions (7).

In evaluating 127 ED visits by 102 acute asthmatics age 15–45 years, Kelsen et al. (41) found that sternocleidomastoid retraction occurred in 40% of episodes. It was more common than hypoxemia ($po_2 < 60$ mmHg) or hypercapnia ($pco_2 > 45$ mmHg), which occurred in 20% and 10% of episodes, respectively. As the severity of the obstruction increased, the incidence of sternocleidomastoid retraction increased. At an FEV_1 of less than 1000 ml, sternocleidomastoid retraction occurred in 50% of cases, whereas hypoxemia and hypercarbia were present in 35% and 15% of episodes respectively. An important implication of these findings is that sternocleidomastoid retraction may signify possible hypoxemia or hypercarbia and reflect the severity of bronchospasm. However, even this reliable clinical sign was absent in half the patients with a severe obstruction.

Wheezing can be heard during any phase of the respiratory cycle. Inspiratory wheezing suggests large airways are narrowed, and expiratory wheezing suggests small airway involvement. Persistent localized wheezing should focus the examiner on other causes of respiratory distress. Exclusive inspiratory wheezing may be due to tumor, foreign body, bronchitis, or stridor misdiagnosed as wheezing. Contrary to traditional thinking, the pitch of the wheeze is not determined by the size of the involved airway (42), but rather by oscillatory characteristics of the mass and elasticity of the bronchial wall. Findings that signify the most severe airway obstruction are mild intensity, high-pitched, inspiratory wheezes without expiratory wheezing with minimal chest wall movement in a patient making enormous efforts to breathe. An urgent finding is the ''silent chest,'' indicating such severe obstruction that flow rates are too low to generate breath sounds. With improvement, wheezing may increase in intensity and become low pitched and coarse as flow rates increase (43,44). Rales are often impossible to hear in asthmatics, because wheezing obscures these sounds. As mentioned earlier, on physical examination the physician should check for subcutaneous emphysema or the presence of a mediastinal crunch (Hamman's sign).

A. The Pediatric Patient

Although we have tried to address the pediatric perspective on all topics discussed in this chapter, the young child who can not provide a history or perform a pulmonary function testing is a special challenge. In young children, rate of breathing is probably the most sensitive observable indicator of lower airway obstruction. This is because infants and young children can effectively increase their minute ventilation only by increasing their respiratory rate, while older children and adolescents are able to increase their tidal volume. As airway obstruction develops, the respiratory rate increases long before hypoxia develops. Despite reports of eupneic hypoxia in children, few children with this condition have been diagnosed with asthma (45).

In many emergency departments, particularly in areas where asthma is prevalent, children are treated in an asthma booth, often sitting on their parent's lap fully clothed. Whenever possible it is helpful to undress young children so that their breathing can be observed from a distance. Most young children will have moderate tachypnea despite little other evidence of airway obstruction. Moreover, although tachypnea is not perfectly correlated with the degree of obstruction, in general, the faster the respiratory rate, the greater the obstruction and V/Q mismatch. The following is a guide to normal respiratory rates in children by age (Table 1). Often guidelines like these (46) are found to be useful in the emergency department asthma treatment area. In infants and children the pulse rate also varies with age. In infants less than 1 year of age, a normal pulse should be less than 160, between 1 and 2 years the pulse should be less than 120, and at 2–8 years of age the pulse should be less than 110. As noted earlier, tachycardia is less ominous in young children than in adults. Tachycardia due to hypoxia, bronchospasm, or anxiety may quickly reverse with the initiation of therapy.

In the physical examination in the pediatric patient, there are important differences between children and adults that must be taken in to account (47). Nasal flaring in the infant and child may be the only sign of respiratory distress, although it usually accompanies tachypnea. The paradoxical movements of portions of the chest and abdominal wall in response to increasing respiratory effort manifest as subcostal and intercostal retractions.

Table 1 Normal Respiratory Rates in Sleeping and Awake Children

	Sleeping			Awake			Mean difference between sleeping and awake
Age	No.	Mean	Range	No.	Mean	Range	
6–12 months	6	27	22–31	3	64	58–75	37
1–2 years	6	19	17–23	4	35	30–40	16
2–4 years	16	19	16–25	15	31	23–42	12
4–6 years	23	18	14–23	22	26	19–36	8
6–8 years	27	17	13–23	28	23	15–30	6

Source: Ref. 199.

These are physical findings suggestive of moderate to severe distress and may also occur with or without tracheosternal retractions and the use of sternocleidomastoid muscles (48). Supraclavicular retractions, referring to the use of the sternocleidomastoid muscles, is a feature of respiratory distress in young asthmatics that seldom occurs without the other physical findings mentioned. Another distinction is that young children become hypercarbic more readily than adolescents and adults.

In normal breathing, the expiratory phase is slightly longer than the inspiratory phase, but it is only briefly audible so that it appears shorter. The ratio of the audible portions of the inspiratory to the expiratory phase of the respiratory cycle, while subjective, has two uses. First, determining the ratio and then monitoring it over time provides a measure of the direction of change in the patient's status. If obstruction increases, the expiratory phase first sounds as long and then longer than the inspiratory phase. The ratio can be characterized as 1:1, 1:2, 1:3, or 1:4 as the expiratory phase lengthens. If β-agonist therapy is successful, the ratio should decrease. The other situation in which the I:E ratio is useful is in evaluating the young child with cough (49). Most young children are not able to cooperate with a request to forcibly exhale, and it is extremely difficult to diagnose mild reactive airway disease in these children in the absence of frank wheezing. In many cases, the only clue on physical examination is a prolonged expiratory phase of the respiratory cycle. Wheezing on auscultation may be absent. Often young children who present to the ED with chronic cough, especially at night or with exertion, but do not appear to be in respiratory distress, may develop audible wheezing following treatment with a β-agonist (50).

B. Asthma Severity

The severity of a given acute exacerbation involves an assessment derived from the history and physical examination, including the patient's general appearance. An objective assessment must, however, be part of the ED evaluation, since physicians as well as patients may underestimate the severity of the exacerbation (41,51). In most patients other than preschool-age children, an examination of PEFR is the most useful objective method of assessing severity (see Chapters 14, 18, and 31), although measurement of oxygen saturation is the simplest and most commonly performed test.

In a study of 49 adult patients, Brenner et al. (52) showed that pulse rate, respiratory rate, and pulsus paradoxus were significantly higher in patients who initially assumed the upright, sitting position on admission to the emergency department; arterial pH, PO_2, and PEFR were significantly lower in the upright patients. All upright patients had sternocleidomastoid retractions. Mean PEFR was 73 liters/min in diaphoretic patients, 134 liters/min in nondiaphoretic, upright patients, and 225 liters/min in recumbent patients ($p < 0.02$). No recumbent, nondiaphoretic patient had a PEFR less than 150 liters/min or PCO_2 higher than 44 mmHg. Therefore, among adults, the position of a patient in the ED and the presence or absence of diaphoresis form a continuum in severity in the initial assessment of acute asthma, with recumbency without diaphoresis being the mildest form, upright position without diaphoresis being more severe, and upright position and diaphoresis being most severe. As is well known among clinicians and exemplified by one patient in this study, recumbent, diaphoretic patients have the most severe bronchospasm and frequently hypoventilate, requiring mechanical assistance to breathe.

C. Hypoxemia, Cyanosis, and Hypercarbia

The most ominous physical findings in acute asthma are those signifying hypoxemia or hypercarbia. Although agitation may be observed in as many as half of patients with asthma, agitation severe enough to halt speech is a sign of severe respiratory distress. In most adult patients with asthma so severe that they are unable to speak, the po_2 is less than 40 mmHg. In some cases thought to be mild, the po_2 is as low as 45 mmHg (29). Physical signs of hypoxia are not observed until hypoxemia is severe. These signs are restlessness, faintness, pallor, and diminished ability to discriminate, which occur at arterial oxygen saturations of less than 75% (53,54). Immediately before unconsciousness due to anoxia, motion of the face and upper body decreases suddenly and the patient seems to be staring. There is amnesia for events preceding the arrest (55).

Hyperventilation, hyperpnea, and tachycardia are all characteristic of hypoxia (54, 56,57). These findings develop when the patients breathe room air, but not when ventilation is controlled, or while hypocarbia is prevented with a CO_2-enriched atmosphere (53).

Severe hypoxemia may be reflected in the development of cyanosis, although most patients with acute asthma do not become cyanotic despite developing hypoxemia. Pulse oximetry has become a common objective method for assessing oxygenation in the patient with acute asthma (see Chapter 16). However, for a multitude of reasons including underestimation of the severity of low oxygen saturation or pulse oximeter malfunction, a discussion of the observation of cyanosis and its limitations is valuable.

Cyanosis is due to the presence of unreduced hemoglobin in dermal papillae and subpapillary venous plexi of the dermis (58). Based on studies of venous blood, Lundsgaard (58,59), showed that 4.5 g to 5.2 g of reduced hemoglobin is needed to exceed the threshold for observing cyanosis. Later Geraci and Wood (60) pointed out that only 3.3 g of reduced hemoglobin was needed to observe cyanosis in white patients. Polycythemia, by providing more hemoglobin for reduction and acidosis by shifting the hemoglobin-oxygen dissociation curve to the right, encourages increased amounts of unreduced hemoglobin and, thereby, enhances the development of cyanosis. Alkalosis will shift the hemoglobin-oxygen dissociation curve to the left, prevent the release of oxygen from hemoglobin, and decrease the amount of reduced hemoglobin. If anemia is so profound that insufficient reduced hemoglobin is present to generate cyanosis, it will prevent the appearance of cyanosis despite severe hypoxemia.

When cyanosis is present, it is important to decide whether it is peripheral or central. Peripheral cyanosis involves the extremities such as nail beds, ear lobes, and nose, and it is caused by slowed circulation resulting from hypoperfusion in states of shock, congestive heart failure, Raynaud's phenomenon, or acidosis, as mentioned earlier. Slowed circulation resulting from stasis is also common in peripheral cyanosis and is evident in cases of polycythemia, superior vena cava obstruction, and venous thrombosis (61). Central cyanosis may be recognized by diffuse patterns involving the lips, tongue, and buccal mucosa. It may be caused by congenital problems such as right to left shunting (Eisenmenger's syndrome), pulmonary arteriovenous anomaly, tetralogy of Fallot, severe acquired pulmonary disease, low levels of inspired oxygen, hemoglobinopathies (e.g., 1.5 g of methemoglobin and 0.5 g of sulfhemoglobin), polycythemia, or marked acidosis (58,62). Intermediate between peripheral and central cyanosis is differential cyanosis, in which only certain regions, such as the upper half of the body, appear cyanotic, as occurs in transposition of the great vessels or coarctation of the aorta.

The presence of cyanosis is unreliable in detecting mild to moderate hypoxemia. In over 3500 observations in white patients made by 12 staff physicians and 12 medical students, Comroe and Botelho (63) noted considerable interobserver variability in the appreciation of cyanosis which emphasized the highly subjective nature of the assessment of this physical finding. Three percent of observers did not note cyanosis when arterial oxygen saturation was 71–75%. Ten percent noted no cyanosis when arterial oxygen saturation ranged from 76% to 80% and 14% of observers noted no cyanosis when saturation ranged from 80% to 84%. Twenty-five percent of observers noted ''slight cyanosis'' despite arterial oxygen saturations of 96–100%. This study showed that most cases of cyanosis (85%) could be diagnosed when arterial oxygen saturation was less than 85%; however, there was a high incidence of false positives.

Geraci and Wood (60) asked observers to evaluate the degree of cyanosis in 1803 white patients. No observers noted cyanosis in patients with arterial saturation averaging 90% (range 69–95%). They observed slight cyanosis at an average arterial saturation of 84% (range 69–95%), definite cyanosis at an average arterial saturation of 80% (range 62–95%), and severe cyanosis at an arterial saturation of 67% (range 56–76%). Overall, although there was marked overlap in the severity of cyanosis observed between patient groups, there was an approximate correlation between the degree of cyanosis and level of arterial oxygen saturation.

In the same study, in 450 observations in black patients, the threshold of arterial oxygen saturation for the appreciation of cyanosis was 3–8% lower than for whites. No black patients were observed with severe cyanosis. Geraci and Wood concurred with Comroe and Botelho that definite cyanosis was seen by all observers where arterial oxygen saturation was less than 75%, but most observers noted cyanosis at less than 85% saturation (60,63,64).

In assessing cyanosis, the choice of the site of observation affected the intraobserver variability in the detection of cyanosis. The presence of cyanosis may be affected by vascularity, pigmentation, and thickness of the skin (58). Lips, tongue, and buccal mucosa are highly reliable sites for the detection of central cyanosis but had a 40% incidence of false positives in one series. If either the lips, tongue, or buccal surfaces were not observed to be cyanotic, it would be rare for arterial oxygen saturation to be less than 75% (65–67). Conjunctivae, ear lobes, and nail beds were poor sites to observe central cyanosis, because these regions were prone to hypoperfusion.

In acute asthma, respiratory failure and hypercarbia may occur and must be diagnosed early. The physical findings of hypercarbia are diaphoresis secondary to increased cutaneous blood flow (68,69), increased cardiac output (69–71), a hyperdynamic cardiovascular system with wide pulse pressure (up to a pco_2 of 90 mmHg) (71,72), elevated blood pressure (69,71,73), and depression of the central nervous system (68). These findings suggest hypercarbia even before the results of the arterial blood gas are known. In children, central nervous system depression, along with decreasing breath sounds, may be the only finding signifying hypercarbia.

Before obtaining the results of arterial blood gases, meaningful information can be obtained from the color of the arterial blood. Morgan-Hughes and Bartlett (74) compared arterial samples with standard samples saturated with oxygen by shaking them for 5 min. All observers noted that blood with less than 85% saturation was darker than the saturated blood. Eighty percent of observers noted that blood with an arterial oxygen saturation of 85–90% was darker than fully saturated blood, and at 90–94% oxygen saturation, 70% of observers noted that the sample was darker than the standard. If the hemoglobin was less than 10g%, then all observers detected which samples were darker at less than 95% arterial oxygen saturation. This technique is superior to the observation of body surfaces in the assessment of cyanosis. For a full discussion of arterial blood gases in acute asthma, see Chapters 15, 26, and Chapter 31.

D. Clinical Scoring Systems for Asthma

Due to the inability of many children to perform PEFR, pediatricians have sought some form of objective criteria by which decisions could be made. To this end, severity indices have been established that attempt to transform subjective criteria in pediatric asthma into an objective index. In some emergency departments, physical signs are combined together into scoring systems to evaluate the patient's response to therapy. One scoring system that is based solely on physical signs is the pulmonary index (PI), developed by Becker et al. (75). It includes the respiratory rate, degree of wheezing, inspiratory-expiratory ratio, and use of accessory muscles (Table 2). Sternocleidomastoid muscle retractions are used to assess accessory muscle use. Each item in the index is scored from 0 to 3, so that the scores can range from 0 to 12. The authors studied 40 children between the ages of 6 and 17 years and compared the pulmonary index to forced vital capacity (FVC), forced expiratory volume in one second, and forced expiratory flow rate from 25% to 75% of the vital capacity. The mean PI before therapy and 30 min after initial therapy correlated significantly with the mean % FEV_1/FVC; six of eight patients with a PI of 6 or more, 30 min after initial treatment in the emergency department, required hospitalization, while no patient with a PI less than 6 required admission.

A well-known scoring system that combines clinical parameters with laboratory criteria is the Wood-Downes-Lecks score (76) (Table 3). This score combines inspiratory breath sounds, accessory muscle use, expiratory wheezing, cerebral function, and arterial carbon dioxide tension or the presence of cyanosis to predict impending respiratory failure from asthma. More recently, the application of the Wood-Downes-Lecks scoring system has been broadened to determination of the severity of an asthma attack and the need for hospitalization (77). The five items are each scored from 0 to 2, and a score of 5 or more is thought to predict respiratory failure. The disadvantage of this scoring system is that it requires an arterial blood gas, though the widespread application of techniques for noninvasive monitoring of oxygen saturation may circumvent this requirement. However, the

Table 2 Clinical Scoring Systems: The Pulmonary Index

Score	RR	Wheeze	I:E ratio	Accessory muscle use
0	<30	None	5/2	0
1	31–45	Terminal expiration with stethoscope	5/3–5/4	±
2	46–60	Entire expiration with stethoscope	1/1	++
3	>60	Inspiration and expiration without stethoscope	<1/1	+++

Source: Adapted from Becker AB, et al. The pulmonary index, Am J Dis Child, 1984; 138:574–576 (Ref. 75).

Table 3 Clinical Scoring Systems: The Wood-Downes-Lecks Score

	0	1	2
Pao_2	>70 in room air	<70 in room air	<70 in 40% FIO_2
Inspiratory breath sounds	Normal	Unequal	Decreased to absent
Accessory muscles used	None	Moderate	Maximal
Expiratory wheezing	None	Moderate	Marked
Cerebral function	Normal	Depressed or agitated	Coma

Source: Adapted from Wood DW, Downes JJ, Lecks HI. A clinical scoring system for diagnosis of respiratory failure. Am J Dis Child 1972; 123:227–228 (Ref. 76).

performance of the score has never been evaluated using pulse oximetry. Baker studied the performance of the Wood-Downes-Lecks scoring system in children with asthma and found that the score was significantly higher for children admitted to the hospital with asthma compared to those discharged home (1.7 vs. 0.5) (77). However, the score was not helpful in identifying children who required prolonged hospitalization or would experience substantial symptoms after discharge including relapse to the emergency department.

E. Formatted or Template Charts

Much of the history and physical examination is similar in patients with acute asthma. This type of repetitive process lends itself to a formatted or template chart. Charts have been developed in which boxes can be checked or numbers circled. Additional information that does not fit or is not appropriate for the template can still be written by hand on the medical record. This type of chart ensures that all questions are prompted and saves time, while maintaining completeness. A formatted chart has been used at the Brooklyn Hospital Center since 1995 for all patients with acute asthma. The data recorded on the chart is subsequently entered into a database (see Appendixes 1 and 2).

F. Differential Diagnosis of Asthma

The diagnosis of asthma is clearly not difficult in patients with a long history of reversible bronchospasm who present with an acute exacerbation. This diagnosis becomes more challenging in older patients with coexisting diseases, and younger patients for whom the differential diagnosis of the most common presenting signs and symptoms can be extensive. Patients who are too dyspneic to give a history or those with their first episode of asthma may present a difficult diagnostic problem.

1. Children

In infants and children, despite an extensive differential diagnosis, most wheezing is secondary to asthma or bronchiolitis (Table 4). In pediatrics, asthma may be difficult to diag-

Table 4 Differential Diagnosis of Acute Asthma in Infants and Children

Upper Airway Obstruction
a. Choanal atresia
b. Tonsillar hypertrophy
c. Laryngotracheal stenosis or laryngeal webs
d. Laryngomalacia, tracheomalacia, or bronchomalacia
e. Vascular rings
f. Foreign bodies
g. Vocal cord paralysis or dysfunction (fixed or psychogenic)
h. Cleft larynx
i. Congenital cysts
j. Retropharyngeal abscess
k. Epiglottitis
l. Laryngotracheal bronchitis (croup)
Middle Airway Obstruction (from the tracheal bifurcation to the larynx)
a. Foreign bodies
b. Tumors
c. Hemangiomas
d. Papillomatous growths and cysts
e. Tracheoesophageal fistulas
f. Tracheomalacia
Lower Airway Obstruction (distal to tracheal bifurcation)
a. Bronchiolitis
b. Cystic fibrosis
c. Bronchopulmonary dysplasia
d. Bronchostenosis
e. Bronchiectasis
f. Congenital lobar emphysema
g. Bronchogenic cysts
Extrapulmonary Conditions
a. Mediastinal masses
b. Right-to-left cardiac shunts
c. Myocarditis
d. Gastroesophageal reflux

Conditions listed in the adult differential diagnosis may also cause wheezing in children.

nose with confidence until the child is more than 3 years old. Allergic diseases, including asthma, rhinitis and sinusitis, secondary to immunoglobulin E (IgE) responses to allergens, rarely present in children until the second or third year of life (80,81). Asthma, however, is most commonly provoked by upper respiratory infections and may be suspected at earlier ages after multiple episodes of wheezing reversed by bronchodilators, especially in the setting of a strong family history of asthma or eczema. Wheezing before the age of 1 yr is likely to be bronchiolitis, most often associated with respiratory syncitial virus during epidemics in the winter to early spring. Other etiologies include influenza and adenovirus, mycoplasma, and chlamydia. Typically there is a prodromal upper respiratory tract infection followed by a cough, wheezing, variable degrees of respiratory distress, and poor feeding. Although wheezing is a fairly consistent finding, rhonchi and coarse rales may also be present. Otitis media may accompany one-half of the cases of bronchiolitis, and fever is variable, but usually low grade.

The association between bronchiolitis and asthma is strong but not well elucidated. Many children who develop asthma had an episode of wheezing associated with a respiratory illness in infancy, but fewer than half of the infants with bronchiolitis go on to develop asthma. At least 60% of children with bronchiolitis and wheezing before the age of 3 will have no further episodes of wheezing after 5 years of age (47,78–81).

The anatomic causes of inspiratory and expiratory airflow abnormalities, include multiple congenital and acquired abnormalities (82), which, while far less common than asthma, are extensive. They include choanal atresia, tonsillar hypertrophy, laryngotracheal stenosis, tracheomalacia, laryngomalacia, brochomalacia (83), laryngeal webs, vascular rings (84), bronchostenosis, tracheoesophageal fistulas, vocal cord paralysis or dysfunction, cleft larynx, congenital lobar emphysema, and bronchogenic cysts (85). With tracheomalacia, which is the most common of these entities, stridor from narrowing of a floppy tracheal segment predominates over expiratory wheezing. The symptoms of coughing or inspiratory noise may also represent infectious upper airway disorders such as laryngotracheal bronchitis or retropharyngeal abscess. The clinical presentation of epiglottitis involves stridor, drooling, fever, and the assumption of the tripod position, and should never be confused with reversible bronchoconstriction (86). Adventitious breath sounds are uncommon. Middle airway obstruction caused commonly by foreign bodies must be considered and ruled out, as well as other less common etiologies of middle airway obstruction including mediastinal masses, such as lymphoma, papillomatous growths, and hemangiomas (see Adult Differential Diagnosis).

Vocal cord dysfunction (VCD) in children and adolescents (87,88) presents a difficult diagnostic and management challenge, especially because of the psychological component, which is most often denied by the patient. VCD can present with symptoms of rapid onset of significant airway obstruction and is predictably resistant to the conventional management of acute asthma. The observation of paradoxic motion of the vocal cords, abduction with inspiration and adduction with exhalation, during direct laryngoscopy is diagnostic. Intervention usually requires psychological evaluation, and speech therapy has been shown to be effective in some cases (see VCD in Differential Diagnosis of Adults).

Infants with a history of prematurity and mechanical ventilation tend to develop bronchopulmonary dysplasia (BPD), which can mimic adult COPD. The manifestations of exacerbations of BPD in this age group are often indistinguishable from asthma, especially because bronchial hyperresponsiveness is often present. Patients with cystic fibrosis may have bronchospasm and bronchiectasis which may be misdiagnosed as acute asthma (89). These children frequently have clubbing of the digits, malabsorption, excessive salt loss, and failure to thrive.

Cardiac asthma may occur in children with left-to-right shunts, anomalous pulmonary venous return, or mitral stenosis or, more commonly, from infectious etiologies such as myocarditis. Other features on physical examination, such as the presence of a murmur, hepatosplenomegaly, or tachycardia, or findings on chest x-ray, such as cardiomegaly or pulmonary congestion, suggest a cardiac etiology for wheezing.

An unusual presentation of acute asthma has been reported in several children involving persistent vomiting as the major symptom. Cough, tachypnea, and wheezing may be minimal or simply masked by this symptom (90–92). A pediatric patient already diagnosed with asthma may develop alternate conditions that may simulate the symptoms of an acute asthma exacerbation. In one case, a child with cardiac asthma secondary to acute myocarditis was initially considered to have had an acute exacerbation of asthma, in part because the child had a history of chronic asthma (93).

2. Adults

The differential diagnosis of asthma in the adult is also extensive (Table 5). The diagnosis of the disease in the elderly is increasing in frequency and presents special challenges to the clinician because it coexists with a daunting number of complicating presentations and underlying diseases (94,95).

COPD is an important differential when dealing with the adult and elderly patient. This disease is often indistinguishable from asthma, and certain components of acute bronchospasm and chronic bronchitis can exist simultaneously. A chronic productive cough usually favors COPD, and there is usually a significant smoking history. Classic physical findings, such as body habitus (barrel chest, pink puffer, blue bloater), clubbing, cyanosis, laboratory evidence of polycythemia and chronic hypercarbia, and radiological hall marks of hyperexpanded lung fields or intrinsic lung disease suggest underlying lung disease (96).

Extrathoracic obstruction refers to common conditions such as head and neck tumors, vocal cord dysfunction, polyps that may present as symptoms of wheezing, or stridor, which may often be mistaken for acute bronchospasm (97) or even an anomalous right aortic arch presenting as exercise-induced bronchospasm (98). Intrathoracic airway obstruction refers to any pathology disease that may cause intermittent airway obstruction and wheezing, such as tracheal or bronchogenic tumors, chronic infections (99), or granulomatous disease (100). A high index of suspicion must always be maintained in such settings to avoid a misdiagnosis or complication. Tracheal, laryngeal, or bronchial tumors (101–106) or inhaled foreign bodies (107–111) may also cause localized inspiratory (large airway, e.g., subglottic) or expiratory (small airway) wheezing or transmitted upper airway sounds erroneously interpreted as wheezing in both adults and children. In adults, mechanical lesions of the airway, such as expiratory collapse of the distal trachea, may present as acute asthma refractory to treatment (112).

Acute bronchitis is both a common condition and frequent discharge diagnosis in the ED. There is frequent wheezing and airway hyperreactivity with postviral bronchitis, which may last up to seven weeks. Due to improvement in symptoms of cough and wheezing and improved expiratory flow rates with β_2-agonists post-viral bronchitis may be confused with new onset asthma (113). Mild hyperreactive airways may even be a normal variant in up to 10% of normal subjects. Whether this represents ''subclinical'' asthma among normal subjects is unclear (114).

Vocal cord dysfunction is a common presentation of refractory acute asthma in adults (115,116). VCD refers to the paradoxical voluntary abduction of the vocal cords during inspiration and/or adduction during exhalation phases of the respiratory cycle and is an important cause of extrathoracic obstruction. As will be discussed in Chapter 7, there is a significant psychological component to this disorder, and some proponents suggest that it is a form of conversion disorder (116–118). The majority of patients presenting with this syndrome are young women, often in medically related fields, between the ages of 20 and 35 (118,119). Some may present with VCD even during vigorous exercise which may be either functional or structural (120–122). The history is one of repeated episodes of highly refractory acute asthma, and the patient is often ingesting relatively large doses of chronic glucocorticoids. In a review of 95 cases of VCD, 53 had an incorrect

Table 5 Differential Diagnosis of Acute Asthma in Adults

1. Cardiac asthma
   a. occult mitral stenosis
   b. myocarditis
   c. cardiogenic pulmonary edema
2. COPD with exacerbation
3. Allergic bronchopulmonary aspergillosis
4. Loeffler's syndrome
5. Chronic eosinophilic pneumonia
6. Occupational asthma
   Organic particle exposure
      a. cotton (byssinosis)
      b. detergent manufacture
      c. red cedar
      d. grains
   Non-organic exposure
      a. toluene diisocyante
      b. metal fumes
      c. colophony
7. Extrinsic allergic alveolitis (e.g., farmer's lung)
8. Chemical irritants
   a. chlorine
   b. sulfur dioxide
   c. smoke inhalation
9. Noncardiogenic pulmonary edema
10. Infectious causes
    a. bronchitis
    b. bronchopneumonia
11. Upper airway obstruction
    a. head and neck tumors
    b. fixed vocal cord dysfunction
    c. laryngeal polyps
    d. subglottic stenosis (post-intubation)
    e. tracheal collapse
12. Psychogenic
    a. hyperventilation syndrome and panic attacks
    b. Munchausen's syndrome
    c. psychogenic vocal cord dysfunction
13. Bronchial tumors
14. Bronchial foreign body or aspiration
15. Pulmonary embolism (4% of cases only wheeze) or foreign body embolism
16. Carcinoid syndrome (20–30% of cases)
17. Invasive worm infestation
    a. Ascaris or Toxocara canis (visceral larva migrans)
    b. hookworm
    c. Strongyloides
    d. filariasis (Wuchereria or Brugia)
18. Allergic angiitis or vasculitis
19. Allergic or anaphylactic reactions
20. Atypical chest pain
21. Angiotensin converting enzyme inhibitor

diagnosis of asthma. VCD had been misdiagnosed as asthma for an average of 5 years. The average daily prednisone dose of those taking prednisone was 30 mg per day. Of those patients diagnosed as asthma, 28% had been intubated in the past. These patients used emergency services often with an average of 10 ED visits and six admissions to the hospital in the previous year (123). Three-fourths of the cases present as acute asthma but occasionally VCD may simulate recurrent anaphylaxis (124). This clinical syndrome is exacerbated by significant psychosocial stressors, and it is not unusual for anxiety and somatoform disorders to present with symptoms suggestive of reversible airway obstruction. Anxiety disorders tend to manifest typically as panic disorders or hyperventilation syndrome, and there is much overlap between VCD, panic disorder, and hyperventilation syndrome (125,126). Some cases of psychogenic asthma have even presented as profound agitation, apprehension and hyperventilation followed by bradycardia, respiratory arrest, and requiring cardiopulmonary resuscitation despite normal arterial blood gas values. One patient self-induced the latter findings with a prolonged Valsalva maneuver. The airway difficulties resolved with sedation (127,128). Terms such as psychogenic upper airway obstruction, Munchausen's stridor, functional laryngeal stridor, factitious asthma, emotional laryngeal wheezing, and psychogenic cough have all been used to describe this mimicry of acute reversible airway obstruction (129,130). Patients most often complain of obstruction of airflow in their upper chest (118). Similar to asthma, the symptoms of VCD may be exacerbated by reflux (131) and upper airway infections. Physical findings that distinguish an acute bronchospastic episode from VCD are derived from careful examination for stridor or "wheezing" more prominent over the neck (28); however, symptoms may be dramatic enough to force the clinician to consider intubation for impending respiratory failure. After intubation, the patient dramatically has no more wheezing and is remarkably easy to mechanically ventilate. Noteworthy in the clinical diagnosis of VCD is that flow volume loops during pulmonary function testing almost never show evidence of expiratory obstruction. Inspiratory abbreviation and flattening of the inspiratory flow volume loop are characteristic of VCD, although it would be unusual for this form of pulmonary function testing to be available in an ED. If there is coexistent asthma plus VCD, even these results may be equivocal (132). The diagnosis is suspected in cases of refractory asthma, especially if a normal pulse oximetry or alveloar-arterial oxygen gradient is present. Occasionally even hypoxia may occur, however (133). Usually the diagnosis is accomplished efficiently with laryngoscopy showing paradoxic motion of the cords with respiration. The emergency physician may notice the paradoxic vocal cord motion during a nonparalyzed intubation and, after the intubation, appreciate that wheezing has disappeared and the patient is easily ventilated with a bag-valve mask. Also Heliox (80% helium and 20% oxygen mixture), a less dense gas, will markedly reduce the degree of stridor and often reassure the patient. Fixed vocal cord defects, such as laryngospasm or bilateral abductor paresis of the vocal cords (134,135), may also be noted at the time of intubation in the ED, and these conditions may simulate acute asthma.

Chest pain as a predominant symptom in the absence of wheezing is an ill-defined presentation of acute asthma. In one study, all patients had an improved clinical response to bronchodilator therapy or a positive methacholine challenge (136,137). There may be much overlap between acute asthma and other causes of chest pain, however. For example, chest pain is common in both hyperventilation syndrome and panic disorder (138,139). In 38 patients that presented with hyperventilation syndrome, 36 had asthma documented subsequently by methacholine challenge (140). Thus, patients that present with chest pain as the main manifestation of acute asthma may have a strong component of anxiety which is responsible for their presentation.

In the adult patient, cardiac asthma, defined as congestive heart failure with wheezing as a predominant manifestation (141,142) may initially seem like bronchial asthma (143). As in COPD there is often evidence of right-sided heart failure in addition to evidence of peripheral edema and compromise of venous return. Both cardiac asthma and COPD with exacerbation must be distinguished from bronchial asthma. In both cardiac asthma and COPD with exacerbation, epinephrine should not be used (143). The distinction is important, since in patients with COPD with exacerbation, high-flow oxygen by nasal cannula may depress the CO_2 respiratory drive and result in respiratory failure. When these patients present in extremis, rapid physical examination, laboratory studies, and chest roentgenograms must be relied on for diagnosis. Cardiac asthma is favored by an absence of leukocytes in the sputum and left ventricular hypertrophy on ECG and chest radiograph. Auscultatory findings other than very loud murmurs are usually obscured by wheezing. Cardiac asthma in a young patient is rare but may result from occult mitral stenosis or myocarditis.

In patients presenting with asthma, pulmonary infiltrates, and peripheral eosinophilia of more than 10%, several major diagnostic possibilities must be considered including allergic bronchopulmonary aspergillosis (APBA). The patient has wheezing, cough, and dyspnea along with pulmonary infiltrates (144). Aspergillus precipitins, positive aspergillus skin tests, and elevated IgE levels may be found in this condition (145,146). IgE levels vary with severity and may be elevated even before clinical complaints are noted (147). The characteristic saccular bronchiectasis of APBA is the most common pulmonary sequela. Patients with APBA usually do respond to bronchodilators, although the cornerstone of treatment involves the use of moderate daily doses of corticosteroids or inhaled corticosteroids (148).

Loeffler's syndrome, parasitic pulmonary diseases (149), and other eosinophilic diseases can also present with peripheral eosinophilia, pulmonary infiltrates, and symptoms of bronchospasm. In Loeffler's syndrome, pulmonary infiltrates with eosinophilia (PIE syndrome) result in minimal symptomatology. The syndrome lasts less than 6 weeks. Chronic eosinophilic pneumonia also may present as asthma, classically in middle-aged women with chronic pulmonary infiltrates simulating the photographic negative of pulmonary edema (150), peripheral eosinophilia, and marked constitutional symptoms (151). These patients respond dramatically to steroids (152,153).

Occupational exposures to allergens and chemical irritants are important to ascertain since prevention results from simple avoidance. Offending agents include cotton fibers in byssinosis, and Actinomyces spores in farmer's lung. Chemicals such as toluene diisocyanate may result in symptoms of chest tightness, dyspnea, and fever (154–156). The diagnosis can often be narrowed by eliciting the pattern of symptoms experienced by the patient. Symptoms usually begin in late afternoons, become worse at night, improve upon awakening, and are usually progressive during the work week with improvement on weekends and holidays (157,158). Colophony fumes (released during soldering) cause bronchospasm, which becomes progressively worse during the week (159).

Other considerations not difficult to distinguish from bronchial asthma are acute chemical injury to the lungs by such agents chlorine or sulfur dioxide (160), smoke inhalation in which carbon monoxide levels may be elevated, and carbonaceous sputum and singed nasal hairs are present (161–164). Other causes of noncardiogenic pulmonary edema with marked or rapidly progressive pulmonary infiltration must be considered. Viral or bacterial pneumonia may precipitate or simulate asthma, but radiographic and sputum findings usually provide rapid distinction.

Pulmonary embolism presenting with sudden wheezing (4% of cases) and hypoxia may be quite difficult to distinguish from acute asthma (165–172). In one case history a young women with frequent ED visits for acute asthma presented with dyspnea, minimal wheezing, a pH of 7.71, a Pco_2 of 9 mmHg, and a Hco_3 of 12 mEq/l (173). She had no tetany and her chest x-ray was normal. Initially she was considered to have acute, severe asthma. With her lack of improvement with β-agonists, however, she was considered to have a psychogenic origin to her dyspnea, but sedation did not improve her symptoms. She was admitted to the intensive care unit, suffered respiratory fatigue, and was intubated. During ventilation her lungs were noted to be particularly compliant and only minimal wheezing was heard. One day later she was extubated. Since she had been on birth control pills, she was evaluated for thromboembolic disease. She had a V/Q scan and an angiogram that documented pulmonary embolism. In this case, the extremely low Pco_2 was a clue to the diagnosis of pulmonary embolism. A history of previous pulmonary embolism, deep vein thrombophlebitis, or strong risk factors (postpartum or recent long bone fracture) may lead directly to a pulmonary angiogram, since ventilation-perfusion scans may be abnormal in acute bronchial asthma (174) as well as in chronic asymptomatic patients (175,176). Septic emboli and foreign body emboli, as may occur with intravenous drug abuse (177), also cause wheezing and bronchospasm and should be aggressively pursued if the appropriate risk factors are present. Inhaled cocaine can also cause bronchospasm (178).

Carcinoid syndrome is associated with wheezing in 20–30% of cases. This syndrome results from the presence of either endobronchial tumor or tracheal or metatstatic disease, usually of gastrointestinal etiology. The symptoms arise from high circulating levels of serotonin and other bronchoconstricting mediators. Often these tumors are treated for years as asthma. Flushing, frequently postprandial, and a murmur of tricuspid stenosis or insufficiency may suggest this diagnosis. Nausea, vomiting, and often explosive diarrhea may also be present. Octreotide improves symptoms both acutely and chronically (179–182).

Invasive phases of worm infestation may mimic a first bout of bronchial asthma. Hookworm, filariasis, *Strongyloides, Ascaris,* or dog round worm [*Toxocara canis* (commonly known as visceral larva migrans)], which may infect 25% of the world's population, are associated with bronchospasm, fever, and eosinophilia from 4 to 16 days after inoculation until years later. The diagnosis may be made definitively by detecting the larvae in the sputum (183–188).

In allergic angiitis (Churg-Strauss Syndrome), described by Churg and Strauss (189,190), and other types of vasculitis, patients may present with intractable bronchial asthma and marked peripheral eosinophilia. Upper respiratory symptoms and abnormalities on chest roentgenograms are frequent. Subsequent development of polyarteritis nodosa or vasculitis in other organs and rapid clinical deterioration is diagnostic; in patients with vasculitis, respiratory disease accounts for 50% of all deaths (191–194).

The mechanisms of an anaphylactic response may result in isolated episodes of severe bronchospasm secondary to exposure to a known or unknown allergen. The clinical diagnosis, as such, is imperative, and intervention must be suitably aggressive. Anaphylaxis with shock and urticaria, sometimes giant urticaria, may occur, and is the hallmark of idiopathic urticaria (195–197).

Patients on angiotensin converting enzyme (ACE) inhibitors often have the side effect of a chronic cough or angioedema. If a history of ACE inhibitor use is not considered, the patient could be misdiagnosed as having either cough variant or acute asthma (198).

The Brooklyn Hospital Center

DEPARTMENT OF EMERGENCY MEDICINE

ADULT ACUTE ASTHMA ASSESSMENT SHEET

PATIENT INFORMATION

Last Name: **First Name:** **Sex:** ❒M ❒F
MR#: **BE#** **Birthdate:**
Address: **Date:**
City: **State:** **Zip:**
Home Phone: **Work Phone:**
Height: **Age:** **Predicted Peak Flow:**

PATIENT HISTORY

Duration of Asthma: <1yr 1-10yrs >10yrs
Steroid use: Never Chronic Intermittent
Last Admission: Floor # months ago < 3 3 -12 >12
times /yr 0 1 2 3 >3
ICU # months ago < 3 3 -12 >12
times /yr 0 1 2 3 >3
Active Smoker: Y N
In last month: Y N
Passive Smoker: Y N
In last month: Y N
Pregnancy: Y N
Drug Allergies: Y N **Name:** ____________
Precipitants:
URI: Y N
Emotions: Y N
Exercise: Y N
Pets: Y N
Food: Y N
ASA: Y N
Paint: Y N
Weather: cold hot wet dry
Other: ____________

H/O Intubation: 0 1 2 >2
Last ED Visit: N < 2wks 2-8 wks 8 wks
No Visits/Yr: 0 1 2 3 >3
PMH HTN DM Heart Lung Disease
Other: ____________
Smoking history: <10pk yrs
10-20pk yrs
>20pk yrs
Medications:
β-agonist inhaler: Y N I D S
β-agonist oral: Y N I D S
Steroid inhaler: Y N I D S
With Spacer: Y N I D S
Prednisone: Y N I D S
Theophylline: Y N I D S
Home nebulizer: Y N I D S
Other new meds: ____________
Home Peak Flow: Y N

Duration of present symptoms: < 1 day 1 day 2 days 3 - 7 days > 1 wk
Fever: Y N
Wheeze: Y N
Chest pain: Y N
Cough: Y N
SOB: Y N
Prehospital treatments: 0 1 2 >2

PHYSICAL EXAM

Accessory Muscles: Y N
Diaphoretic: Y N
Able to Speak: Y N
Staccato Speech: Y N
Cyanotic: Y N
Alert: Y N
JVD: Y N
Edema: Y N
Cardiac: S1 S2 S3 S4 M
SQ Emphysema: Y N
Bilat BS: Y N
Wheeze: Y N
Air Entry: Poor Good
Stridor: Y N

Appendix 1

APPENDIX 1 GLOSSARY

Patient Information, Patient History, Physical Exam: Variable Definitions

Definitions only given for variables that may possibly be unclear.

Patient Information

MR#: Medical record number—this is unique identifier for the *patient.*

BE/CE#: This is the unique identifier for the *visit.* BE is a unique identifier for a Brooklyn Hospital visit. CE# is a unique identifier for a Caledonian Hospital visit (this is the second site for the Brooklyn Hospital Center).

Best peak flow: If the patient has a peak flow meter and uses it *at home,* then his best reading goes here. This is not the patient's best peak flow in the emergency department during previous acute visits.

Predicted peak flow: This value is obtained from a nomogram. We use the one published in the 1991 National Institutes of Health (NIH) guidelines.

Patient History

Left-column variables:

Duration of asthma: Number of years that the patient has asthma. This is not the duration of the patient's present episode of acute asthma.

Oral steroid use (bursts/yr): During an acute asthma exacerbation, many patients are placed on a few days of oral prednisone, sometimes for two weeks. We would term such an administration of prednisone a burst of prednisone. The number of these burst that occur per year is the answer that is put in the blank space. If the patient is on chronic steroids and receives periodic increases in prednisone during an exacerbation, simply list this as chronic under this *oral steroid use variable.*

Last admission: # months ago: This is how long ago was the most recent admission to the hospital. # times per year: This is the number of times in the least year the patient was admitted to the hospital, excluding the present ED visit.

Precipitants: This list running down the page vertically refers to whether these precipitants exacerbate the patient's asthma in general. Running horizontally across the page are *current precipitants.* This is the factor(s) responsible, in the patient's opinion, for the current episode. If the patient has run out of any of his medications for asthma and that is the reason, in the patient's opinion, for this exacerbation, circle 8 under *current precipitants.* If there is no known reason for this exacerbation, write the word *unknown* under #10 of precipitants, and circle 10 under current precipitants. We agree the logic for the "run out of meds" and "unknown" could be improved. It will be improved in the next version.

Duration of present symptoms: This is the duration of the current exacerbation.

Right-column variables:

H/O intubation: Number of times intubated due to asthma exacerbation in the patient's entire life.

Last ED visit: Duration of time since the last ED visit.

No. ED visits/YR: the number of ED visits in the last year related to acute asthma.

PMH: Past medical history with hypertension (Is the patient on a beta blocker exacerbating his asthma?), diabetes mellitus (Is the patient's glucose control a consideration affecting the administration of oral or systemic glucocorticoids?), heart disease (Is this really cardiac asthma, congestive heart failure, or recurrent pulmonary embolism?), or lung disease (Is this really COPD, sarcoid, HIV or pneumocystis, lung CA, pulmonary embolism, or other chronic pulmonary disease simulating asthma). If there is no past medical history, fill in the space with none. Therefore, we would know that there were no other known illnesses , and would not think that the question was left blank or inadvertently missed.

Medications: Note that after each of the medications it states Y, N, I, D, S. This refers to increased usage, decreased usage, or same usage in the three to four days preceding this ED visit. In most cases where the asthmatic is on a medication, the correct answer would require circling Y and circling S (for same usage). After each medication that the patient is currently using, put the name and dosage of the medication. Note the answer *With Spacer* does not require the I, D, S response after it. Under the field *Any New Meds*, circle yes or no and write in the name of this new medication. We are interested in whether the patient may have recently had erythromycin added to theophylline or Hismanole, or whether a beta-blocker was inadvertently instituted.

Borg SOB: This is a visual analogue score of how dyspneic the patient perceives him/herself to be. (See chart—Appendix 3).

Ambulance: Did the patient arrive by ambulance or walk in. After this include the number of prehospital nebulizations received *in the ambulance* in the last hour.

Walk in: Did the patient arrive by ambulance or walk in. After this include the number of pre-hospital nebulizations received *at home* in the last hour.

Signature: *AI* stands for asthma intern. The asthma intern should sign here if they obtained the patient history. This signature must be cosigned by a physician who is attesting to the accuracy of the patient history and signing his physical examination, which follows.

Physical Examination

These variables were derived based on consensus within our faculty in the emergency department at the Brooklyn Hospital Center concerning which of these variables to include and which to exclude for the initial directed physical examination of an asthmatic. We feel that overall this represents a thorough but brief list.

Air Entry: This is scored 0–4 with the scoring system. 0 equals *no problem* and 4 equals *absent/near absent air movement*

The Brooklyn Hospital Center

DEPARTMENT OF EMERGENCY MEDICINE

PEDIATRIC ACUTE ASTHMA ASSESSMENT SHEET

PATIENT INFORMATION

Last Name: **First Name:** **Sex:** ☐ **M** ☐ **F**
MR #: **BE/CE #:** **Birthdate:**
Address: **Date:**
City: **State:** **Zip:**
Parent/Guardian: **Home Phone:** **Work Phone:** **Best Peak Flow:**
Height: **Wt/lb:** **Age:** **Race:** W B H Asian Other: ______ **Predicted Peak Flow:**

PATIENT HISTORY

Duration of Asthma: ______
Oral Steroid Use: Never Chronic Bursts / Yr______
Last Admission: Floor # months ago <3 3-12 >12 Never
times / yr 0 1 2 3 >3
ICU # months ago <3 3-12 >12 Never
times / yr 0 1 2 3 >3

Active Smoker: Y N
In last month: Y N
Passive Smoker: Y N
In last month: Y N
Pregnancy: Y N **LMP:** ______
Drug Allergies: Y N **Specify:** ______

Precipitants:
1. URI: Y N
2. Emotions: Y N
3. Exercise: Y N
4. Pets: Y N ______
5. Food: Y N ______
6. ASA: Y N
7. Paint: Y N
8. Weather: cold hot wet dry windy
9. Ran out of meds Y N
10. Other: ______

Current Precipitants: 1 2 3 4 5 6 7 8 9 10

Duration of present symptoms: < 1 day 1 day 2 days 3-7 days > 1 wk
Fever: Y N
Wheeze: Y N
Chest pain: Y N Pleuritic Y N

H/O Intubation: 0 1 2 >2
Last ED Visit: None <2 wks 2-8 wks 8 wks
No ED Visits/Yr: 0 1 2 3 4 >4
PMH: DM Heart Bronchiolitis Bronchopulmonary Dysplasia
Other: ______

Medications:
β-agonist inhaler: Y N I D S* ______
β-agonist oral: Y N I D S ______
Steroid inhaler: Y N I D S ______
With Spacer: Y N I D S
Prednisone: Y N I D S ______
Theophylline: Y N I D S ______
Home nebulizer: Y N I D S
Other meds:

* I = Increased Usage
D = Decreased Usage
S = Same Usage

Home Peak Flow: Y N
Cough: Y N
Borg SOB: ______ (1 - 10, 10 = Worst)
Ambulance: Y N 0 1 2 3 4**
Walk In: Y N 0 1 2 3 4**

** Number of prehospital nebulizer inhalant treatments in last hour

Signature: ______

M.D. ☐ P.A. ☐
R.N. ☐ M.S. ** ☐
A.I. * ☐

* A.I.: Asthma Intern
** M.S.: Medical Student

PHYSICAL EXAM

Accessory Muscles:	Y N	**Alert:**	Y N	**Bilat BS:**	Y N
Diaphoretic:	Y N	**JVD:**	Y N	**Wheeze:**	Y N
Able to Speak/Cry:	Y N	**Edema:**	Y N	**Nasal Flaring:**	Y N
Staccato Speech/Cry:	Y N	**Cardiac:**	S1 S2 S3 S4 M	**Stridor:**	Y N
Cyanotic:	Y N	**SQ Emphysema:**	Y N	**Air Entry:**	0 1 2 3 4

Appendix 2

APPENDIX 2 GLOSSARY: BROOKLYN HOSPITAL PEDIATRIC ACUTE ASTHMA ASSESSMENT SHEET

Patient Information, Patient History, Physical Exam

I will only note the differences between the adult and the pediatric forms, since they are essentially identical. In the Patient Information area there are two new fields: *Wt/lb* (weight in pounds) and *Parent/Guardian.*

Patient History includes pregnancy and *LMP* since some of the patients are adolescents. Under *PMH* are included two pediatric diagnoses: bronchiolitis and bronchopulmonary dysplasia (the pediatric equivalent of COPD). Physical examination includes *Nasal Flaring*.

APPENDIX 3 MODIFIED BORG SCALE USED TO RATE DEGREE OF DYSPNEA (200)

0	Nothing at all
0.5	Just noticeable
1	Very slight
2	Slight
3	Moderate
4	Somewhat severe
5	Severe
6	Somewhere between 5 and 7
7	Very severe
8	Somewhere between 7 and 9
9	Very, very severe (almost maximal)
10	Maximal

REFERENCES

1. Lemarchand P, Labrune S, Herer B, et al. Cardiorespiratory arrest following peak expiratory flow measurement during attack of asthma. Chest 1991; 100:1168–1169.
2. Turcotte H, Boulet LP. Perception of breathlessness during the early and late asthmatic responses. Am Rev Respir Dis 1993; 148:514–518.
3. Salome CM. Perception of airway narrowing in the general population sample. European Respir J 1997; 10:1052–1058.
4. Daley J, Kopelman R, Comeau E, et al. Practice patterns in the treatment of the acutely ill asthmatic at three teaching hospitals. Variability of resource utilization. Chest 1991; 100: 51–56.
5. Canny GJ, Reisman J, Healy R, et al. Acute asthma: observations regarding the management of a pediatric emergency room. Pediatrics 1989; 83:507–512.
6. O'Holloran SM, Heaf DP. Accident and emergency department attendance by asthmatic children. Thorax 1989; 44:700–705.

7. Commey JOO, Levison H. Physical signs in childhood asthma. Pediatrics 1976; 58:537–541.
8. Lougheed DM. Breathlessness during induced lung hyperinflation in Asthma. Am J Respir Crit Care Med 1995; 152:911–920.
9. Lougheed DM, Lam M, Forkert L, Webb KA, O'Donnell ED. Breathlessness during bronchoconstriction in asthma. Am Rev Respir Dis 1993; 148:1452–1459.
10. Boulet LP, Leblanc P, Turcotte H. Perception scoring of induced bronchoconstriction as an index of awareness of asthma symptoms. Chest 1994; 105:1430–1433.
11. Janson C, Herala M. Dyspnea in acute asthma: relationship with other clinical and physiological variables. Ann Allergy 1993; 70:400–404.
12. Kikuchi Y, Okabe S, Tamura G, et al. Chemosensitivity and perception of dyspnea in patients with a history of near-fatal asthma. N Engl J Med 1994; 330:1329–1334.
13. Corrao WM, Braman SS, Irwin RS. Chronic cough as the sole presenting manifestation of bronchial asthma. N Engl J Med 1979; 300:633–637.
14. McFadden ER Jr. Exertional dyspnea and cough as preludes to acute attacks of bronchial asthma. N Engl J Med 1975; 292:555–559.
15. Li JTC, O'Connell EJ. Clinical evaluation of asthma. Ann Allergy Asthma Immunol 1996; 76:1–14.
16. O'Connell EJ, Li TJ. Chronic Cough. Immunol Allerg Clin North Am. 1996; 16:1–17.
17. Laloo GU, Barnes PJ, Chung KF. Pathophysiology and clinical presentations of cough. J Allergy Clin Immunol 1996; 98:s91–s97.
18. Brenner BE, Leber M, Kohn MS, Camargo C. ED visits for acute asthma by patients who recently ran out of their beta agonist inhaler. Ann Emerg Med 1997; 30:427.
19. Strunk RC. Asthma deaths in childhood: Identification of Patients at risk and intervention. J Allergy Clin Immunol 1987; 80:472–477.
20. Strunk RC, Mrazek DA. Physiologic and psychological characteristics associated with deaths due to asthma in childhood. JAMA 1985; 254:1193–1198.
21. Joseph KS, Blais I, Ernst P, et al. Increased morbidity and mortality to asthma among asthmatic patients who use major tranquillisers. Br Med J. 1996; 312:79–81.
22. Wade S, Weil C, Holden G, et al. Psychosocial characteristics of inner-city with asthma: a description of the NCICAS psychosocial protocol. Pediatr Pulmonol 1997; 24:263–276.
23. Appel D, Karpel JP, Sherman M. Epinephrine improves expiratory flow rates in patients with asthma who do not respond to inhaled metaproterenol sulfate. J Allerg Clin Immunol 1989; 84:90–98
24. Johnston SL, Pattemore PK, Sanderson G, et al. Community Study of the role of viral infections in the exacerbation of asthma in 9–11 year old children. Br Med J 1995; 310:1225–1228.
25. Nicholson KG, Kent J, Hammersley V, Cancio E. Risk factors for lower respiratory complications of rhinovirus infections in elderly people living in the community; prospective cohort study. Br Med J 1996; 313:1119–1123.
26. McFadden ER, Gilbert IA. Exercise induced asthma. N Engl J Med 1994; 330:1362–1367.
27. Jarjour NN, Calhoun WJ. Exercise-induced asthma is not associated with mast cell activation or airway inflammation. J. Allergy Clin Immunol 1992; 89:60–65.
28. Baughman RP, Loudon RG. Stridor: differentiation from asthma or upper airway noise. Am Rev Respir Dis 1989; 139:1407–1409.
29. Rees HA, Millar JS, Donald KW. A study of the clinical course and arterial blood gas tension of patients in status asthmaticus. Q J Med 1980; 37:541–561.
30. Rudolf M, Riordan JF, Grant BJB, et al. Arterial blood gas tensions in acute severe asthma. Eur J Clin Invest 1980; 10:55–62.
31. Ambiavagar M, Jones ES. Resuscitation of the moribund asthmatic: Use of intermittent positive pressure ventilation, bronchial lavage and intravenous infusion. Anaesthesia 1967; 22: 375–391.

32. Cooke NJ, Crompton GK, Grant IWB. Observations on the management of acute bronchial asthma. Br J Dis Chest 1979; 73:157–163.
33. Rebuck AS, Pengelly LD. Development of pulsus paradoxus in the presence of airways obstruction. N Engl J Med 1973; 288:66–69.
34. Knowles GK, Clark TJH. Pulsus paradoxus as valuable sign indicating severity of asthma. Lancet 1973; 2:1356–1358.
35. Rebuck AS, Read J. Assessment and management of severe asthma. Am J Med 1971; 51: 788–798.
36. Gerschke GL, Baker FJ II, Rosen P. Pulsus paradoxus as a parameter in treatment of the asthmatic. J Am Coll Emerg Phys 1977; 6:191–193.
37. Cade JF, Woolcock AJ, Rebuck AS, et al. Lung mechanics during provocation of asthma. Clin Sci 1971; 40:381–391.
38. Woolcock AJ, Read J. The static elastic properties of the lungs in asthma. Am Rev Respir Dis 1968; 98:788–794.
39. Martin J, Powell E, Shore S, et al. The role of respiratory muscles in the hyperinflation of bronchial asthma. Am Rev Respir Dis 1980; 121:441–447.
40. McFadden ER Jr, Kiser R, DeGroot WJ. Acute bronchial asthma: relations between clinical and physiologic manifestations. N Engl J Med 1973; 288:221–225.
41. Kelsen SG, Kelsen DP, Fleegler BF, et al. Emergency room assessment and treatment of patients with acute asthma: adequacy of conventional approach. Am J Med 1978; 64:622–628.
42. Hollingsworth HM. Wheezing and stridor. Clin Chest Med 1987; 8:231–240.
43. Forgacs P. The functional basis of pulmonary sounds. Chest 1978; 73:399–405.
44. McFadden ER Jr, Feldman NT. Asthma: Pathophysiology and clinical correlates. Med Clin North Am 1977; 61:1229–1238.
45. Mower WR, Sachs C, Nidden EL, et al. Pulse oximetry as a fifth vital sign. Pediatrics 1997; 99:681–686.
46. Barone MA, ed. The Harriet Lane Handbook, 14th ed., St Louis, MO: Mosby Yearbook, 1991, p. 444.
47. Martinez FD, Wright AL, Taussig LM. Asthma and wheezing in the first six years of life. N Engl J Med 1995; 332:133–138.
48. Lulla S, Newcomb RW. Emergency management of asthma in children. Pediatrics 1980; 97: 346–350.
49. Parrillo DJ. Cough variant asthma. Pediatr Emerg Care 1986; 2:97–101.
50. Cloutier MM, Loughlin GM. Chronic cough in children: a manifestation of airway hyperreactivity. Pediatrics 1981; 67:6–12.
51. Kendrick AH, Higgs CM, Whitfield MJ, et al. Accuracy of perception of severity of asthma. Br Med J 1993; 307:422–424.
52. Brenner BE, Abraham E, Simon RR. Position and diaphoresis in acute asthma. Am J Med 1983; 74:1005–1009.
53. Brewis RAL. Clinical measurements relevant to the assessment of hypoxia. Br J Anaesthesia 1969; 41:742–750.
54. Blount SG Jr. Cyanosis: Pathophysiology and differential diagnosis. Prog Cardiovasc Dis 1971; 13:595–605.
55. Comroe JH, Botelho S. The unreliability of cyanosis in the recognition of arterial anoxemia. Am J Med Sci 1947; 214:1–6.
56. Lutz BR, Schneider ED. The reactions of the cardiac and respiratory centers to changes in oxygen tension. Am J Physiol 1919; 50:327–341.
57. Richardson DW, Kontos HA, Rapec AJ, et al. Modification by beta-adrenergic blockade of the circulatory responses to acute hypoxia in man. J Clin Invest 1967; 46:77–85.
58. Lundsgaard C. Studies on cyanosis: II. Secondary causes of cyanosis. J Exp Med 1919; 30: 271–293.

59. Lundsgaard C, Van Slyke DD. Cyanosis. Medicine 1923; 2:1–76.
60. Geraci JE, Wood EH. The relationship of arterial oxygen saturation to cyanosis. Med Clin North Am 1951; 35:1185–1202.
61. Barcroft J, Benatt A, Greeson CE, et al. The rate of blood flow through cyanosed skin. J Physiol 1931; 73:344–348.
62. Blount SG Jr. Cyanosis: Pathophysiology and differential diagnosis. Prog Cardiovasc Dis 1971; 13:595–605.
63. Comroe JH, Botelho S. The unreliability of cyanosis in the recognition of arterial anoxemia. Am J Med Sci 1947;214:1–6.
64. Medd WE, French EB, Wyllie VMcA. Cyanosis as a guide to arterial oxygen desaturation. Thorax 1959;14:247–250.
65. Medd WE, French EB, Wyllie VMcCa. Cyanosis as a guide to arterial oxygen desaturation. Thorax 1959; 14:237–250.
66. Goldman HI, Maralit A, Sun S, et al. Neonatal cyanosis and arterial oxygen saturation. J Pediatr 1973; 82:319–324.
67. Kelman GR, Nunn JF. Clinical recognition of hypoxaemia under fluorescent lamps. Lancet 1966; 1:1400–1403.
68. McArdle L, Roddie IC, Sheperd JT, et al. Effect of inhalation of 30 percent carbon dioxide on peripheral circulation of the normal human subject. Br J Pharmacol 1957; 12:293–296.
69. Wendling MG, Eckstein JW, Abboud FM. Cardiovascular responses to carbon dioxide before and after beta-adrenergic blockade. J Appl Physiol 1967; 22:223–226.
70. Barnes PJ, Dollery CT, MacDermot J. Increased pulmonary alpha-adrenergic and reduced beta-adrenergic receptors in experimental asthma. Nature 1980; 285:569–571.
71. Manley ES, Nash CB, Woodbury RA. Cardiovascular responses to severe hypercapnia of short duration. Am J Physiol 1964; 207:634–640.
72. Prys-Roberts C, Smith WD, Nunn JF, et al. Accidental severe hypercapnia during anaesthesia. Br J Anaesth 1967; 39:257–267.
73. Prys-Roberts C, Kelman GR. Haemodynamic influences of graded hypercapnia in anesthetized man. Br J Anaesth 1966; 38:661–662.
74. Morgan-Hughes JO, Bartlett MC. The colour of blood in syringes as a guide to hypoxaemia. Br J Anaesth 1968; 40:310–314.
75. Becker AB, Nelson NA, Simons ER. The pulmonary index: an assessment of a clinical score for asthma. Am J Dis Child 1984; 138:574–576.
76. Wood DW, Downes JJ, Lecks HI. A clinical scoring system for the diagnosis of respiratory failure. Am J Dis Child. 1972; 123:227–228.
77. Baker MD. Pitfalls in the use of clinical scoring. Am J Dis Child 1988; 142:183–185.
78. Boesen I. Asthmatic bronchitis in children: Prognosis for 162 cases observed 6–11 years. Acta Paediatr 1953; 42:87–96.
79. Wittig HJ, Cranford NJ, Glaser J. The relationship between bronchiolitis and childhood asthma. J Allergy 1959; 30:19–23.
80. Sporik R, Holgate ST, Cogswell JJ. Natural history of asthma in childhood—a birth cohort study. Arch Dis Child 1991; 166:1050–1053.
81. Korppi M, Kuikka L, Reijonen T. Bronchial asthma and hyperactivity after early childhood bronchiolitis or pneumonia. Arch Pediatr Adolesc Med 1994; 148:1079–1084.
82. Lesperance MM, Zalzal GH. Assessment and management of laryngotracheal stenosis. Pediatr Clin North Am 1996; 43:1413–1427.
83. Cohn JR. Localized bronchomalacia presenting as worsening asthma. Ann Allergy 1985; 54: 222–223.
84. Loren ML, Cooley RL, Rohr C, et al. Vascular ring presenting as asthma: the value of the flow-volume curve. J Pediatr 1979; 94:610–611.
85. Go RO, Martin TR, Lester MR. A wheezy infant unresponsive to bronchodilators. Ann Allergy Asthma Immunol 1997; 78:449–456.

86. Marcus MG, Semel LJ. An unusual case of epiglottitis in a patient with asthma. Pediatr Emerg Care 1988; 4:124–126.
87. Landwehr LP. Vocal cord dysfunction mimicking exercise induced bronchospasm in adolescents. Pediatrics 1996; 98:971–974.
88. Poirier MP, Pancioli AM, Digiulio GA. Vocal cord dysfunction presenting as acute asthma in a pediatric patient. Pediatr Emerg Care 1996; 12:213–214.
89. Rosenstein BJ, Langbaum TS. Misdiagnosis of cystic fibrosis. Need for continuing follow-up and evaluation. Clin Pediatr 1987; 26:78–82.
90. Schreier L, Cutler RM, Saigal V. Vomiting as a dominant symptom of asthma. Ann Allergy 1987; 58:118–120.
91. Osundwa VM, Dawod ST. Vomiting as the main presenting symptom of acute asthma. Acta Paediatr Scand 1989; 78:968–970.
92. Schreir l, Cutler RM, Saigal V. Vomiting as a dominant symptom of asthma. Ann Allergy 1987; 58:188–120.
93. Singer JI, Isaacman DJ, Bell LM. The wheezer that wasn't. Pediatr Emerg Care 1992; 8: 107–109.
94. Osborne ML. Differential diagnosis of bronchial asthma in the elderly. Immunol Allergy Clin North Am 1997;17: 557–574.
95. Anderson CJ, Bardana EJ. Treatment of asthma and allergic disease in the elderly. Immunol Allergy Clin North Am 1997; 17:587–605.
96. Snider GL. Distinguishing among asthma, chronic bronchitis, and emphysema. Chest 1985; 87 suppl:35s–39s.
97. Tilles SA, Nelson HS. Differential diagnosis of allergic disease: masqueraders of allergy. Immunol Allergy Clin North Am 1996; 16:19–34.
98. Bevelaqua F, Schicchi JS, Haas F, et al. Aortic arch anomaly presenting as exercise-induced asthma. Am Rev Respir Dis 1989; 140:805–808.
99. Caplin I, Haynes JT, Green M. Middle lobe syndrome and intractable asthma. J Asthma Res 1970; 8:57–60.
100. Williams DJ, York EL, Nobert EJ, et al. Endobronchial tuberculosis presenting as asthma. Chest 1988; 93:836–838.
101. Parrish RW, Banks J, Fennerty AG. Tracheal obstruction presenting as asthma. Postgrad Med J 1983; 59:775–776.
102. Skinner EF. All is not asthma that wheezes. So Med J 1964; 57:841–845.
103. Rodriguez LR, DiMaio M, Kidron D, et al. Late presentation of a subglottic hemangioma masquerading as asthma. Clin Pediatr 1992; 31:753–755.
104. Kennedy WP, Milne RM. Endobronchial chondroma presenting as asthma. Br J Dis Chest 1969; 63:227–230.
105. al-Hajjaj MS. Ectopic intratracheal thyroid presenting as bronchial asthma. Respiration 1991; 58:329–331.
106. Klaustermeyer WB. Chondrosarcoma presenting as asthma exacerbation. Ann Allergy 1994; 72:14–17.
107. Aytac A, Yurdakul Y, Ikizler C, et al. Inhalation of foreign bodies in children: report of 500 cases. J Thorac Cardiovasc Surg 1977; 74:145–151.
108. Gay BB, Atkinson GO, Vanderzalm T, et al. Subglottic foreign bodies in pediatric patients. Am J Dis Child 1986; 140:165–168.
109. Jackson C. Overlooked cases of foreign body in the air and food passages. Br Med J 1925; 2:686–693.
110. Storr J, Tranter R, Lenney W. Stridor in childhood asthma. Br J Dis Chest 1988; 82:197–199.
111. Lloyd-Thomas AR, Bush GH. All that wheezes is not asthma. Anaesthesia 1986; 41:181–185.
112. Hunter JH, Stanford W, Smith JM, et al. Expiratory collapse of the trachea presenting as worsening asthma. Chest 1993; 104:633–635.

113. Empey DW, Laitinen LA, Gold WM, et al. Mechanism of bronchial hyperreactivity in normal subjects after upper respiratory tract infection. Am Rev Respir Dis 1976; 113:131–139.
114. Smith L, McFadden ER Jr. Bronchial hyperreactivity revisited. Ann Allergy Asthma Immunol 1995; 74:454–469.
115. Wood RP. Vocal cord dysfunction. J Allergy Clin Immunol 1997; 99 s:773–780.
116. O'Hallaren MT. Dyspnea originating from the larynx. Immunol Allergy Clin North Am 1996; 16:69–76.
117. Tilles SA, Nelson HS. Differential diagnosis of adult asthma. Immunol Allergy Clin North Am 1996; 16:19–34.
118. Martin RJ, Cicutto LC, Smith HR. Airway inflammation in nocturnal asthma. Am Rev Respir Dis 1991; 143:351–357.
119. O'Hollaren MT. Masqueraders in clinical allergy: laryngeal dysfunction causing dyspnea. Ann Allergy 65:351–356.
120. McFadden ER Jr, Zawadski DK. Vocal cord dysfunction masquerading as exercise-induced asthma. A physiologic cause for "choking" during athletic activities. Am J Respir Crit Care Med 1996; 153:942–947.
121. Lakin RC, Metzger WJ, Haughey BH. Upper airway obstruction presenting as exercise-induced asthma. Chest 1984; 86:499–501.
122. Bittleman DB, Smith RJ, Weiler JM. Abnormal movement of the arytenoid region during exercise presenting as exercise-induced asthma in an adolescent athlete. Chest 1994; 106: 615–616.
123. Newman KB, Mason UG 3rd, Schmaling KB. Clinical features of vocal cord dysfunction. Am J Respir Crit Care Med 1995; 152 pt 1:1382–1386.
124. O'Connell MA, Sklarew R, Goodman DL. Spectrum of presentation of paradoxical vocal cord motion in ambulatory patients. Ann Allergy Asthma Immunol 1995; 74:341–344.
125. Gardner WN. The pathophysiology of hyperventilation disorders. Chest 1996; 109:516–534.
126. Schmaling KB, Bell J. Asthma and panic disorder. Arch Fam Med 1997; 6:20–23.
127. Baker CE, Major E. Munchausen's syndrome. A case presenting as asthma requiring ventilation. Anaesthesia 1994; 49:1050–1051.
128. Bernstein JA, Dykewicz MS, Histand P, et al. Potentially fatal asthma and syncope. A new variant of Munchausen's syndrome in sports medicine. Chest 1991; 99:763–765.
129. Gordon FH, Bernstein MJ. Psychiatric mimics of allergic airway[s] disease. Immunol Allergy Clin North Am 1996; 16:199–214.
130. Dailey RH. Pseudoasthma: A new clinical entity. J Am Coll Emerg Phys 1976; 5:192–193.
131. Spechler, SJ. The effects of antireflux therapy on pulmonary function in patients with severe gastroesophageal reflux disease. Am J Gastroenterol 1995; 90:915–918.
132. Elshami AA, Tino G. Coexistent asthma and functional upper airway obstruction. Case reports and review of the literature. Chest 1996; 110:1358–1361.
133. Hayes JP, Nolan MT, Brennan N, et al. Three cases of paradoxical vocal cord adduction followed up over a ten-year period. Chest 1993; 104:678–680.
134. Randolph C, Lapey A, Shannon DC. Bilateral abductor paresis masquerading as asthma. J Allergy Clin Immunol 1988; 81:1122–1125.
135. Chawla SS, Upadhyay BK, MacDonnell KF. Laryngeal spasm mimicking bronchial asthma. Ann Allergy 53:319–321.
136. Whitney EJ, Row JM, Boswell RN. Chest pain variant asthma. Ann Emerg Med 1983; 12: 572–575.
137. Izumi N, Haneda N, Mori C. Methacholine inhalation challenge in children with idiopathic chest pain. Acta Paediatr Jpn 1992; 34:441–446.
138. Betman BD, Basha I, Flaker G, et al. Atypical or nonanginal Chest Pain. Arch Intern Med 1987; 147:1548–1552.
139. Freeman LJ, Nixon PGF. Chest pain and the hyperventilation syndrome-some aetiological considerations. Postgrad Med J 1985; 61:957–961.

140. Demeter SL, Cordasco EM. Hyperventilation syndrome and asthma. Am J Med 1986; 81: 989–994.
141. Pratt JH. Cardiac asthma. JAMA 1926; 87:809–513.
142. Seibert AF, Allison RC, Bryars CH, et al. Normal airway responsiveness to methacholine in cardiac asthma. Am Rev Respir Dis 1989; 140:1805–1806.
143. Fletcher D, Mainardi JL, Brun-Buisson C, et al. Cardiac asthma presenting as status asthmaticus: deleterious effect of epinephrine therapy. Intensive Care Med 1990; 16:466–468.
144. Zhaoming W, Lockey RF. A review of bronchopulmonary aspergillosis. J Investig Allergol Clin Immunol 1996; 6:144–151.
145. Greenberger PA. Diagnosis and managment of allergic bronchopulmonary aspergillosis. Allergy Proc 1994; 15:335–339.
146. Riceson RB 3rd, Stander PE. Allergic bronchopulmonary aspergillosis. Postgrad Med 1990; 88:217–219, 222, 224.
147. Greenberger PA. Allergic bronchopulmonary aspergillosis and fungoses. Clin Chest Med 1988; 9:599–608.
148. Imbeault B, Cormier Y. Usefulness of inhaled high-dose corticosteroids in allergic bronchopulmonary aspergillosis. Chest 1993; 103:1614–1617.
149. Jiva TM. Tropical eosinophilia masquerading as acute bronchial asthma. Respiration 1996; 63:55–58.
150. Gaensler EA, Carrington CB. Peripheral opacities in chronic eosinophilic pneumonia: photographic negative of pulmonary edema. Am J Roentgenol 1977; 128:1–13.
151. Pope-Harmon AL, Davis WB, Allen ED, et al. Acute eosinophilic pneumonia. A summary of 15 cases and review of the literature. Medicine 1996; 75:334–342.
152. Meeker DP. Pulmonary infiltrates and eosinophilia revisited. Cleve Clin J Med 1989; 56: 199–211.
153. Brenner BE, Thorgeirsson G. An association between chronic eosinophilic pneumonia and histiocytic lymphoma. Am J Med Sci 1979; 278:83–88.
154. Venables KM, Chan-Yeung M. Occupational asthma. Lancet 1997; 349:1465–1469.
155. Ho A, Chan H, Tse KS, et al . Occupational asthma due to latex in health care workers. Thorax 1996; 51:1280–1282.
156. Brooks SM, Weiss MA, Bernstein IL. Reactive airways dysfunction syndrome. Case reports of persistent airways hyperreactivity following high-level irritant exposures. J Occup Med 1985; 27:473–476.
157. Bernstein DI. Occupational asthma. Med Clin North Am 1992; 76:917–934.
158. Bernstein JA. Overview of diisocyanate occupational asthma. Toxicology 1996; 111:181–189.
159. Mariano A, Paredes I, Nuti R, et al, Occupational asthma due to colophony in non-industrial environments. Med Lav 1993; 84:459–462.
160. Brooks SM, Weiss MA, Bernstein IL. Reactive airways dysfunction syndrome (RADS). Persistent asthma syndrome after high level irritant exposures. Chest 1985; 88:376–384.
161. Hantson P, Butera R, Clemessy JL, et al. Early complications and value of initial clinical and paraclinical observations in victims of smoke inhalation without burns. Chest 1997; 111: 671–675.
162. Lemiere C, Malo JL, Gautrin D. Nonsensitizing causes of occupational asthma. Med Clin North Am 1996; 80:749–774.
163. DiVincenti FC, Pruitt BA, Reckler JM. Inhalation injuries. J Trauma. 1971; 11:109–117.
164. Paggiaro PL, Vagaggini B, Bacci E, et al. Prognosis of occupational asthma. Eur Respir J 1994; 7:761–767.
165. Boyer NH, Curry JJ. Bronchospasm associated with pulmonary embolism: respiratory failure. Arch Intern Med 1944; 73:403–409.
166. Gurewich V, Thomas D, Stein M, et al. Bronchoconstriction in the presence of pulmonary embolism. Circulation 1963; 27:339–345.

167. Jewett JF. Asthma, emboli and cardiac arrest. N Engl J Med 1973; 288:265–266.
168. Olazabal F Jr, Roman-Irizarry LA, Oms JD, et al. E.J.: Pulmonary embolism masquerading as asthma. N Engl J Med 1968; 278:999–1001.
169. Rebhun J. Pulmonary embolism in asthmatics. Ann Allergy 1970; 28:586–589.
170. The urokinase pulmonary embolism trial: A National co-operative study. Circulation (suppl II) 1973; 47:1–108.
171. Webster JR Jr, Saadeh GB, Eggum PR, et al. Wheezing due to pulmonary embolism: Treatment with heparin. N Engl J Med 1966; 274:931–933.
172. Windebank WJ, Boyd G, Moran F. Pulmonary thromboembolism presenting as asthma. Br Med J 1973; 1:90–94.
173. Clarke RCN, Daly JG, Morrow B. Unusually low P_aco_2 as a sign of pulmonary embolism in acute, severe asthma. Anaesth Intensive Care 1996; 24:617–618.
174. Mishkin FS, Wagner NH, Tow DE. Regional distribution of pulmonary arterial blood flow in acute asthma. JAMA 1968; 203:115–117.
175. Hyde JS, Koch DF, Isenberg PD, et al. Technetium Tc99m macroaggregated albumin lung scans: Use in chronic childhood asthma. JAMA 1976; 235:1125–1130.
176. Wagner PD, Dantzker DR, Iacovoni VE, et al. Ventilation-perfusion inequality in asymptomatic asthma. Am Rev Respir Dis 1978; 118:511–524.
177. Sapira JD. The narcotic addict as a medical patient. Am J Med 1968; 45:555–558.
178. Osborn HH, Tang M, Bradley K, et al. New-onset bronchospasm or recrudescence of asthma associated with cocaine abuse. Acad Emerg Med 1997; 4:689–692.
179. Sjoerdsma A. A clinical, physiologic, and biochemical study of patients with malignant carcinoid. Am J Med 1956; 20:520–532.
180. Melnyk DL. Up-date on carcinoid syndrome. AANAJ 1997; 65:265–270.
181. Pant K, Bhagat R, Chawla R, et al. Primary carcinoid tumor of the trachea. Indian J Dis Chest Allied Sci 1990; 32:193–197.
182. Dipaolo F, Stull MA. Bronchial carcinoid presenting as refractory asthma. Am Fam Physician 1993; 48:785–789.
183. Crofton JW, Livingstone JL, Oswald NC, et al. Pulmonary eosinophilia. Thorax 1952; 7:1–35.
184. Enzenauer RJ, Underwood GH, Ribbing J. Tropical pulmonary eosinophilia. South Med J 1990; 83:69–72.
185. Pansegrouw D. Strongyloides stercoralis infestation masquerading as steroid resistant asthma. Monaldi Arch Dis Chest 1994; 49:399–402.
186. Phills JA, Harrold AJ, Whiteman GV, et al. Pulmonary infiltrates, asthma and eosinophilia due to Ascaris suum infestation in man. N Engl J Med 1972; 286:965–970.
187. Jiva TM, Israel RH, Poe RH. Tropical eosinophilia masquerading as bronchial asthma. Respiration 1996; 63:55–58.
188. Feldman GJ, Parker HW. Visceral larva migrans associated with the hypereosinophilic syndrome and the onset of severe asthma. Ann Intern Med 1992; 116:838–840.
189. Churg J, Strauss L. Allergic granulomatosis, allergic angiitis and periarteritis nodosa. Am J Pathol 1951; 27:277–294.
190. Trittel C. Churg-Strauss Syndrome. A differential diagnosis in chronic polypoid sinusitis. Laryngorhinootologie 1995; 74:577–580.
191. Guillevin L, Le Thi Huong Du, Godeau P, et al. Clinical findings of polyarteritis nodosa and Churg-Strauss angiitis: A study in 165 patients. Br J Rheumatol 1988; 27:258–264.
192. Leatherman JW. The lung in systemic vasculitis. Semin Respir Infect 1988; 3:274–288.
193. Fauci AS, Haynes BF, Katz P. The spectrum of vasculitis: clinical pathologic, immunologic, and therapeutic considerations. Ann Intern Med 1978; 89:660–676.
194. Rose GA, Spencer H. Polyarteritis nodosa. Q J Med 1957; 26:43–81.
195. Krasnick J, Patterson R, Meyers GL. A fatality from idiopathic anaphylaxis. Ann Allerg Asthma Immunol 1996; 76:367–378.

196. Ditto AM, Krasnick J, Greenberger PA, et al. Pediatric idiopathic anaphylaxis: experience with 22 patients. J Allergy Clin Immunol 1997; 100:320–326.
197. Ditto AM, Harris KE, Krasnick J, et al. Idiopathic anaphylaxis: a series of 335 cases. Ann Allergy Asthma Immunol 1996; 77:285–291.
198. Lunde H, Hedner T, Samuelsson O, et al. Dyspnoea, asthma and bronchospasm in relation with angiotensin converting enzymes. Br Med J 1994; 308:18–21.
199. National Asthma Education Program: Guidelines for the diagnosis and management of asthma. Bethesda, MD: National Heart, Lung, and Blood Institute, 1991, NIH Publication No. 91-3042.
200. Borg G. Ratings of perceived exertion and heart rates during short-term cycle exercise and their use in a new cycling strength test. Int J Sports Med 1982; 3:153–158.

14

Pulmonary Function Testing in the Emergency Department

Robert Silverman and Steven M. Scharf
Albert Einstein College of Medicine, Bronx, and Long Island Jewish Medical Center, New Hyde Park, New York

I. INTRODUCTION

Upon arrival to the emergency department (ED), the patient with acute asthma should be assessed for illness severity and treatment should be initiated (1). The continuation of therapy and decision for admission or discharge will in part be based upon response to the initial treatments. If hospitalization is required, the determination to admit to a general medical service or a more closely monitored unit is made in the ED. For patients discharged from the ED, medication and follow-up instructions are given.

To determine illness severity the clinician assesses the patients general appearance, vital signs, degree of breathlessness and wheezing, use of accessory muscles, duration of acute illness, and past asthma and medical history. Even after performing a thorough history and physical examination, the degree of airway obstruction often cannot be accurately determined by the clinician (2–4). Pulmonary function testing with a peak flow meter or spirometer indicates the degree of obstruction in the clinical setting and provides valuable information to the clinician. In this chapter the role of pulmonary function testing in the ED will be discussed.

II. PHYSIOLOGY

There are a number of methods used to assess pulmonary function. Some of these involve the use of maximum voluntary maneuvers, such as forced expiration or the assessment of gas exchange using arterial blood gas tensions, and can be performed in the ED. Other techniques available to assess lung function are more suited for the pulmonary function lab. Included are volume measurement techniques such as helium dilution, nitrogen washout and body plethysmography, various measurements of gas diffusion in the lungs, and exercise or chemical provocation tests to assess airway responsiveness. Since these tests are not practical to perform in the ED, only techniques involving forced expiration will be described here (blood gas measurements are described in Chapter 15). A basic understanding of lung physiology and mechanics provides a foundation for discussing pulmonary function testing and its potential utility in assessing the acutely ill patient.

For the purposes of discussion, the lungs can be viewed as consisting of two areas: (1) the parenchyma, which contains most of the volume of the lungs and is where gas exchange occurs, and (2) the airways that are responsible for conducting flow to the gas exchanging areas. Based on aerodynamic properties and the type of flow regime (turbulent, transitional, and laminar), airways are categorized as being of large, medium, and small size. Pulmonary function is generally assessed in terms of lung volumes, flow rates, and gas exchange. The relationship of flow rates to lung volume provides an evaluation of airway function.

Lung volume is maximized through deep inspiration. Inspiration is caused by contraction of a number of respiratory muscles including the diaphragm, the intercostals, the scalenes, and the sternocleidomastoids. Diaphragmatic contraction will increase lung volume by extending into the abdominal cavity, and the other muscles will increase volume by expanding the lateral and anterior–posterior thoracic diameter. During inspiration the maximal rate of airflow varies directly with the inspiratory effort (5). Expiration is usually passive and is achieved by the relaxation of the respiratory muscles. During times of distress expiration can become dynamic by the contraction of the abdominal as well as the internal intercostal muscles.

Factors that influence maximum airflow during expiration include airways resistance and the elastic recoil of the lung. The smaller the caliber of the airways, the greater the resistance. In airways in which flow is laminar, resistance is proportional to $1/r^4$, where r is the airway radius. Since resistance increases by the inverse of the fourth power of radius, with critical airway narrowing, relatively small changes in airway caliber lead to large changes in airflow resistance. In patients with asthma, airway caliber can be narrowed by contraction of bronchial smooth muscle, edema of the airways due to inflammation, and blockage by mucus.

The driving pressure to maximum airflow is determined in part by alveolar pressure. When alveolar pressure is higher than atmospheric pressure, for example, exhalation can occur. Alveolar pressure is dependent on the muscular effort expended during a forced expiration as well as the elastic recoil of the lungs. At some point however, the driving pressure ceases to be determined by muscular effort and is entirely a function of elastic recoil. The point in a forced expiration at which flow becomes independent of muscular effort is determined by a number of factors, including lung volume and the stiffness of the airways themselves. In practice, in severely obstructed patients the point at which airflow is relatively independent of muscular effort occurs after approximately 30% of the vital capacity has been exhaled (5). For most of the expired maneuver, airflow is therefore independent of the effort applied and is determined by elastic recoil and airways resistance. The higher the initial lung volume, the greater the elastic recoil, and subsequently the greater the flow. The flow-volume loops described below demonstrate the relationship between lung volume and flow (Fig. 1).

A number of lung volumes and capacities can be subdivided from the total lung volume. Total lung capacity (TLC) is defined as the volume of air in the lungs after a maximum inspiratory effort. The total lung capacity is the largest possible volume of gas in the lungs, and residual volume (RV) is the smallest amount of gas possible in the lungs.

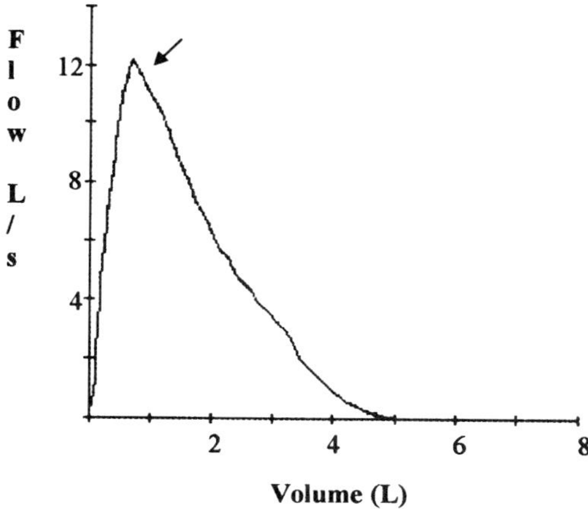

Figure 1 Flow volume loop in a healthy individual. Note that flow is greatest (arrow) after only a small volume of air is exhaled.

The residual volume cannot be measured directly by spirometry as it is the amount of total air left in the lungs after a maximum expiration. The vital capacity (VC) is defined as the difference between total lung capacity and residual volume and is essentially the largest volume that can be exhaled from total lung capacity. The tidal volume (TV) is the amount of air that is moved during normal breathing.

In the ED setting, lung function is generally evaluated using a maximum forced expiration from the total lung capacity. The patient takes a deep inspiration followed by a forced expiration through a mouthpiece connected to a measuring device. A number of measures of airways function based on the forced expiration are available for use in the ED setting, including peak expiratory flow rates, forced expiratory volume over time, and forced vital capacity, as well as other indices of lung function derived from spirometry.

III. SPIROMETRY

A spirometer is a device for measuring the volume of air exhaled over time. The earliest spirometers simply measured volume during the forced exhalation plotted as a function of time, otherwise known as a spirogram or volume-time plot (Fig. 2). A number of useful parameters are obtained from the volume-time plot. The first is the vital capacity. When measured using maximum expiratory force it is called the forced vital capicity (FVC). Normal individuals can exhale their vital capacity almost entirely within a few seconds. However, individuals with substantial obstruction to airflow may take considerably longer to expire their full vital capacity. It is important to recognize that the FVC represents the difference between two lung volumes, and while it is certainly a function of overall lung volume, it does not actually measure the volume of the lungs per se.

The second parameter derived from simple volume-time plots, and the most useful for characterizing severity of obstruction, is the forced expired volume in 1 sec (FEV_1) (Fig. 2). The FEV_1, as the name implies, is measured in the first second of forced expiration and normally accounts for over 75–80% of the total exhaled volume. The FEV_1 is propor-

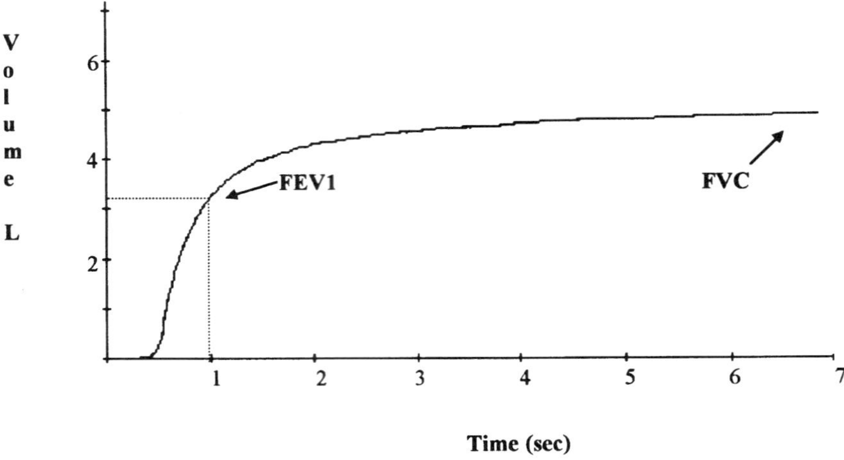

Figure 2 Time-volume plot in a healthy individual. The FEV_1 is the volume forceably exhaled over the first second and the FVC is the maximum amount of air that can be exhaled forceably from the lungs. Both the FEV_1 (3.72 L) and the FVC (4.9 L) are easily identified.

tional to the maximum voluntary ventilation (MVV), which is the maximum air volume that can be ''moved'' by an individual per minute ($FEV_1 \times 35$ is equal to the MVV) (5). The greater the degree of airflow obstruction, the lower the FEV_1. Thus, the FEV_1 is an index of the ventilatory capability of the individual and is used to define the severity of ventilatory compromise.

There are a number of other variables measured from the volume-time plot that are used in routine pulmonary function testing and epidemiological studies. However, these are not considered as useful in the emergency setting and the reader is referred to a text on pulmonary function testing for further discussion.

A. Flow-Volume Loops

Another way of depicting the spirogram is to plot flow directly as a function of volume. It should be emphasized that while there is no more information to be extracted regarding airways function from a flow-volume (FV) plot than from the volume-time plot, flow-volume loops enable easy visualization of lung function and simplify the assessment of adequacy of efforts.

Figure 1 shows a flow-volume loop corresponding to the volume-time plot in Figure 2. The FVC is easily detected. The FEV_1 is not directly measurable from the FV loop since time does not appear as an axis. However, a number of directly measurable flows used to characterize lung function can be taken from the plot. The flow index most often used is the peak expiratory flow rate (PEF), which is the highest flow reached during the FVC maneuver. PEF is sustained for a brief period of time, usually 10 ms. It cannot be read from the volume-time plot, since it is a measure of instantaneous flow, but is clearly seen on the flow-volume loop. The peak flow reflects the caliber of primarily the larger conducting airways such as the lobar bronchi (5). Optimally it occurs very early in expiration and is highly dependent on the strength of the expiratory muscles as well as the effort made by the patient. Like the FEV_1 it is also strongly influenced by lung volume, with the highest peak flows occurring at total lung capacity (5).

B. Reasons for Measuring Lung Function

Studies of pulmonary function are important in assessing degree of airflow obstruction in patients with acute asthma and tests of forced expiration are important surrogates for severity of illness (3,6). This is important because both the patient and clinician's evaluation of illness severity may not correlate well with the actual degree of lung obstruction (2). Some patients may complain of severe symptoms when their lung function is only mildly diminished. Conversely, other patients may delay treatment because of difficulty perceiving their severity of obstruction. Clinicians may either underestimate or overestimate illness severity, which could lead to inappropriate treatment or disposition decisions. Patients with airway obstruction may not manifest wheezing, including those with very severe or very mild respiratory compromise, and this may lead to a missed diagnosis (4). Other patients with asthma may complain primarily of chest discomfort or heaviness, which represent muscle fatigue due to obstructed airways and may be mistaken for other diseases (see Chapter 13). Performing pulmonary function testing may be useful in determining if the complaints are consistent with obstructive airways disease, especially if the complaints resolve and pulmonary function improves with bronchodilator use.

In patients who present to the ED with acute asthma, knowledge of pulmonary function is important for management and disposition decisions. More aggressive or novel therapies, such as higher dose or continuous nebulization of β-agonists, intravenous magnesium, inhaled anticholinergics, or breathing a helium–oxygen mixture have been reported beneficial primarily in patients with severely restricted air movement (7–10). Knowledge of pulmonary function would help to identify those more likely to benefit from these treatments. In addition, the response to initial β-agonist therapy is an important marker for overall ED improvement (11,12). The clinician may modify treatment and disposition decisions based on the progression of pulmonary function values. It has been demonstrated that CO_2 retention, which indicates ventilatory failure, is found more frequently in patients with peak flow values $< 25\%$ predicted (13). In these patients, admission to a monitored unit must be considered. Finally, a number of consensus guidelines have suggested that certain threshold values of pulmonary function should be used to help make a disposition decision (1,14) (see Chapters 31 and 34).

C. Measurement of Pulmonary Function: The Equipment

1. *Spirometer*

A spirometer is a tool that measures the flow and volume of air as it leaves the lungs. There are two basic types of spirometers commonly used: the volume displacing and the flow sensing. Volume-sensing spirometers obtain flow by electronically differentiating change in volume with time. Flow-sensing spirometers obtain volume by electronic integration of flow over time. The flow-sensing spirometers have the advantages of smaller size and portability and are more suitable for ED use. Because they are usually computerized, manual calculations of results are not needed. There are many different models available on the market, ranging in size from hand-held models to laptop-size portable devices

Table 1 Spirometric Values Often Displayed Using Commercially Available Spirometers

FVC	Forced vital capacity
FEV_1	Forced expired volume in 1 sec
FEV_1/FVC	Ratio of FEV_1 to FVC [this is also sometimes called $FEV_1\%$ or $FEV_1\%/VC$ (not to be confused with percent predicted)]
PEF, PEFR	Peak expired flow rate
$FEV_{.5}$	Forced expired volume in first 0.5 sec
$FEV_{2,3}$	Forced expired volume in the second or third second, respectively
FEF_{25-75}	Mean forced expired flow between 25% and 75% of the FVC [also called MMFR (maximum mid-expiratory flow rate)]
$MEFR_{200-1200}$	Maximum expired flow rate between 200 and 1200 mL of the FVC
FEF_{75}	Forced expired flow at 75% of FVC (from FV loop)
FEF_{50}	Forced expired flow at 50% of FVC (from FV loop)
FEF_{25}	Forced expired flow at 25% of FVC (from FV loop)
FET	Forced expiratory time

to larger free-standing units. Most models allow the observer to assess the flow-volume loop in real-time during the actual maneuver, although many hand-held units do not have this capability. Some spirometers will display a variety of information and provide feedback on adequacy of technique, show a programmed interpretation of results, and store information for later retrieval. Many models will have printing capabilities allowing documentation for medical or study records and quality assurance.

The most useful measures obtained by standard spirometry are, as noted above, FVC, FEV_1, FEV_1/FVC, and PEF. Most units also present numerous other indices whose role in the ED setting has not been well-studied or are of questionable value. They are listed in Table 1.

2. Peak Flow Meter

While the PEF can be obtained with a spirometer, hand-held devices such as a Wright or mini-Wright peak flow meter provide the clinician a simpler method of measuring peak flow rates (15). Peak flow measures can also be taken at home, where the patient can use the meter to monitor trends in peak flow measures and initiate therapy as part of a treatment plan. A number of relatively inexpensive devices are commercially available with prices ranging from approximately \$15 to \$35. Results of studies comparing various commercially available meters indicate that while reproducibility is not an issue, the accuracy of different devices can vary, with the reliability of results differing according to flow rates (16–18).

IV. TECHNIQUES FOR PERFORMING TESTS OF PULMONARY FUNCTION

A. Spirometry

1. Background

The American Thoracic Society (ATS) has published recommendations on measurement procedures and acceptability of results for spirometry (19–21). These include end-of-test criteria as well as quality assurance criteria. However, these criteria were not intended for use in the acutely ill patient and some of them, such as the need for the expiratory effort to be at least 6 sec in duration, can be difficult to achieve in the ED. Indeed, given the dependence of spirometric indices on patient cooperation and the difficulty of testing naive subjects who are acutely ill, the performance of lung function testing in the ED presents special challenges.

If the effort appears maximum and is sustained for at least 1 second, the FEV_1 can be used to assess pulmonary function. This is fortuitous since the FEV_1, as noted earlier, is a direct measure of the ability of the patient to ventilate. A strong effort that lasts at least several seconds provides additional assurance that the FEV_1 can be reliably measured. Although the FEV_1 is far less effort dependent than the PEF, the maneuver is more involved than the peak flow measure. The dependence of spirometric values on proper coaching and patient cooperation means that the performance of spirometry in the ED setting should be done only by operators with adequate training in the required techniques and experience doing it in acutely ill patients. Further, the spirometer used should display the flow-volume loop so that the operator can visually assess patient effort. Since expiratory efforts may not be extended long enough to accurately measure the FVC, this measure of lung function has not been used by most in assessing acutely ill asthmatic patients.

2. *Technique*

When testing the asthmatic patient in the ED, the concept of spirometry should be briefly introduced to the patient. The patient should preferably be sitting up with the feet on the floor but in a relaxed position. Occlusive clothing around the neck should be removed. The use of a nose clip, which many acutely ill patients find extremely uncomfortable, can be avoided if nasal exhalation is discouraged. The mouthpiece is placed behind the teeth, the tongue should not occlude the opening and the lips should be sealed tightly. Since the patient may be fatigued and anxious, the instructions should be brief and directed. Explaining the procedure through demonstrable body language is important and examiners may wish to first demonstrate the maneuver on themselves. The patient is instructed to place the mouthpiece into the mouth, take a few normal breaths, and become accustomed to the equipment. When ready to proceed, the patients chest wall must be carefully watched to properly time instructions. The patient is then told to take a deep a breath as possible and ''blast'' the air out as fast and hard as possible and keep on blowing until asked to stop. Encourage at least 3–5 sec of expiration; in many patients a 6 sec or longer expiration is possible, especially if this is a repeat measurement. The clinician should be watching the effort of the real-time screen as well as the patient to determine if the maneuver was adequate. It is possible the flow-volume loop may appear reasonable, but the patient is not giving his or her best effort and the results may still underestimate the patients pulmonary function.

B. Peak Expiratory Flow

As noted earlier, the PEF reflects the interaction between the caliber of the larger airways and the strength of the expiratory effort. Factors that decrease PEF include airways obstruction, weak respiratory muscles, and suboptimal patient cooperation with the maneuver. The ability of the patient to respond to instructions and cooperate with the examiner

Table 2 Summary of Suggested Spirometry Acceptability Criteria

At least three efforts recorded
The two best efforts at each time point are within 10% of each other
Back extrapolation (V extract) less than 5% of the FVC
Expiratory time at least 2–3 sec
A sharp peak flow is present on the flow volume loop
The peak flow occurs less than 120 msec after the exhalation starts, and optimally in less than 85 msec
Lack of glottic closure in the first second, including that due to cough

and the vigilance of the evaluator in obtaining the best effort will strongly influence the peak flow results, more so than the FEV_1.

Patients are asked to take as deep a breath as possible and blow as quickly and hard as they can into the mouthpiece. The expiratory effort is focused and brief with the well-performed peak flow occurring within the first 85–120 msec of expiration. The patient is asked to perform at least three adequate maneuvers and the best is recorded. The patient must be in a comfortable position and adequately coached to ensure the best effort. Patients may be standing or sitting, although subsequent efforts should be measured in the same position, since results may be higher if standing. For practical purposes, acutely ill patients usually have their measures performed while sitting. Flow rates are provided by the hand-held meter in L/min, while the spirometer will typically give results in L/sec.

C. Acceptability Criteria

At present there are no established guidelines for validating adequacy of effort or reliability of either peak flow or FEV_1 values in acutely ill patients. Still, since pulmonary function testing is the best way to measure airway obstruction, and these tests have become an important part of patient assessment, the clinician should have an appreciation of whether the results obtained appear dependable.

Using methods such as back extrapolation, the time to peak flow, and the shape of the flow volume loop, it can be determined if the initial effort was forceful enough to be considered reliable. Anything that interrupts the flow of air during the important first second, such as a cough, may cause the FEV_1 to be underestimated. Any effort less than 1 sec in duration, or where a good effort was not sustained for at least a full second, will not provide valid results. To best approximate the patients pulmonary function while taking into consideration the difficulties of performing pulmonary function tests in the ED, we have used the criteria listed in Table 2. They provide the technician with bedside guidelines for obtaining optimal efforts and allow for quality assurance. The optimal goal is to obtain a minimum of three maneuvers at each time point with at least two ''acceptable'' ratings. Figures 3–7 are examples of spirograms and flow volume curves in acutely ill asthmatics, showing good efforts and some with commonly encountered problems.

The back extrapolated volume (%back extrapolation, or V-extract) is a measure of performance quality and is useful, since many patients do not start their maximum effort as soon as the operator gives the signal. An unsatisfactory start of expiration or air leak may lead to an underestimation of the FEV_1, and this can be identified by calculating the back extrapolated volume. A typical method of calculating this measure is to identify

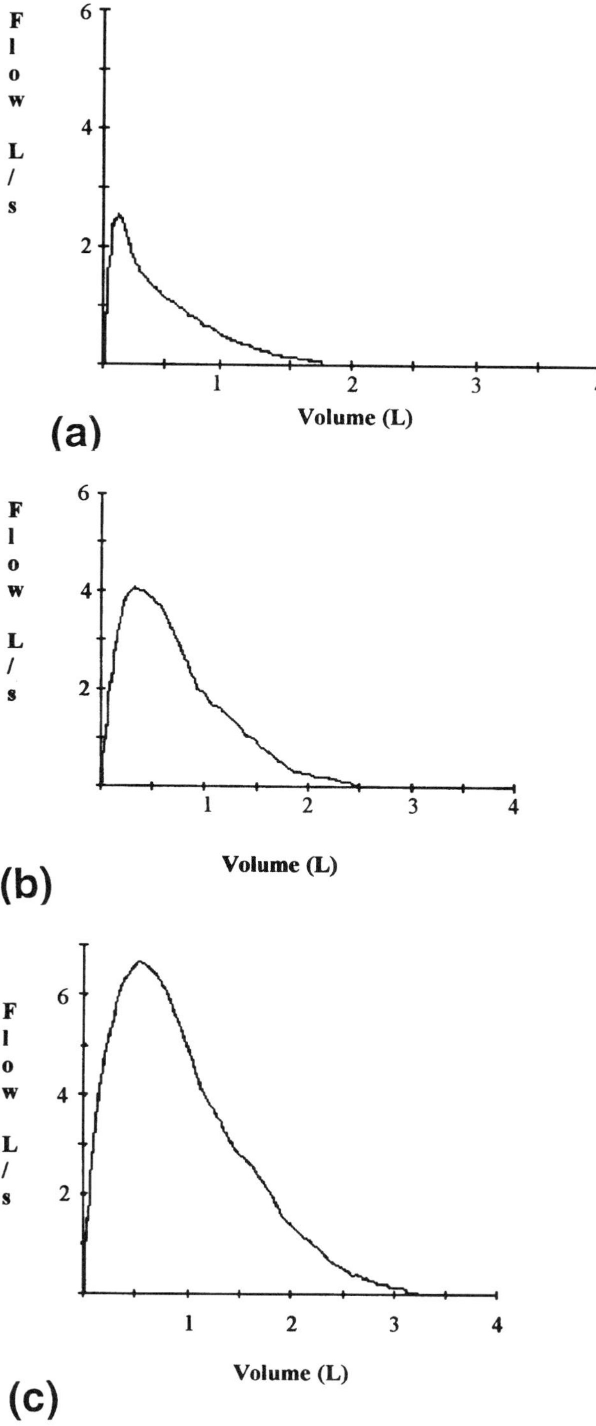

Figure 3 Flow-volume loops in a 27-year-old patient with acute asthma: (a) measure on ED arrival (FEV_1 1.03 L; 30% of predicted); (b) measure after two β_2-agonist treatments (FEV_1 1.7 L; 51% of predicted); (c) measure after 4 hr of therapy (FEV_1 2.42 L; 72% predicted). All of the efforts were considered adequate.

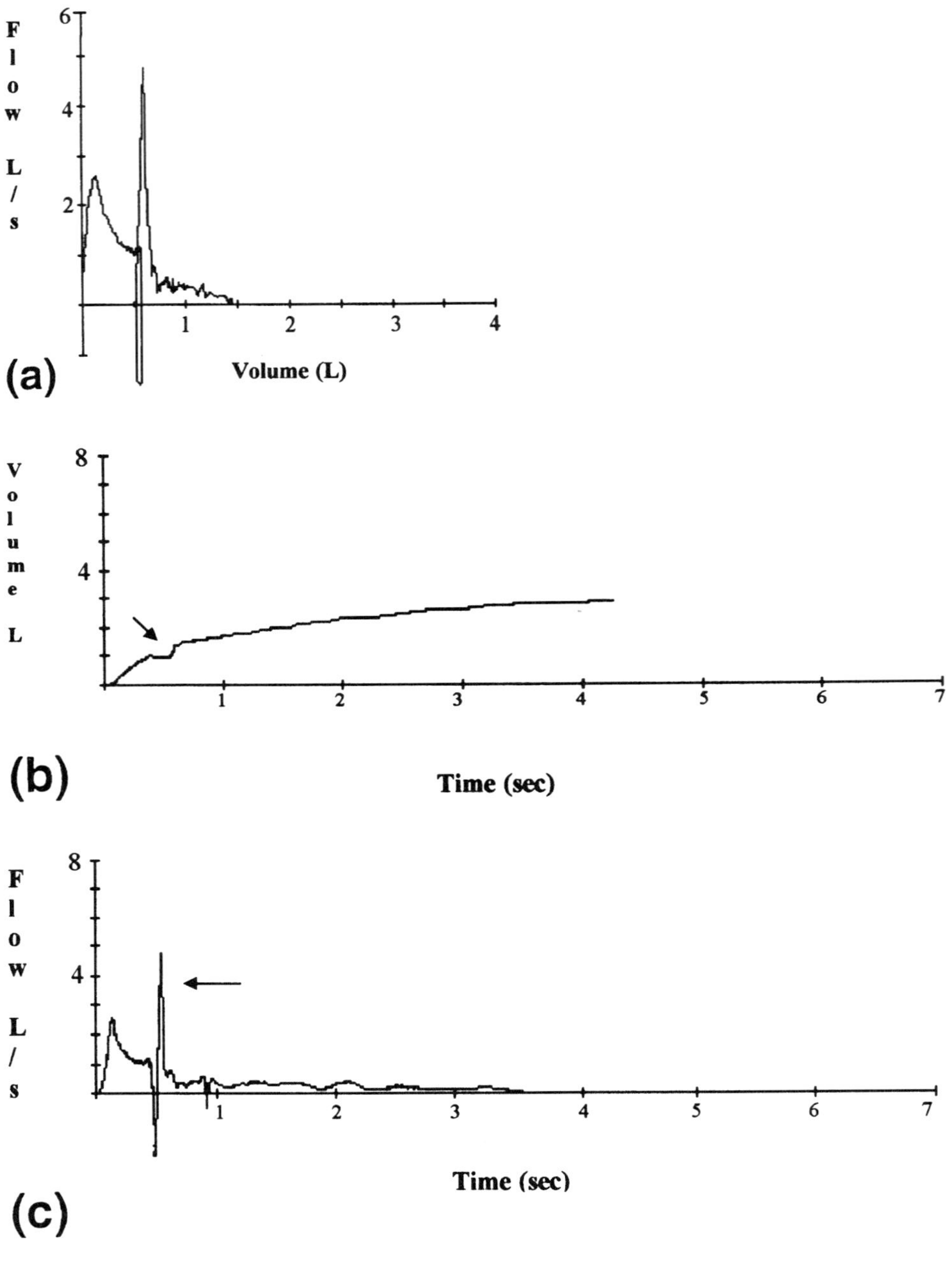

Figure 4 An acutely ill patient who coughed during expiration. Note (a) the glottic closure on the flow-volume loop. By itself, the flow volume loop does not indicate the time at which the cough occurred. The small notch on (b) the time-volume graph indicates the cough occurred during the first second (arrow). This is seen more clearly on (c) the time-flow plot.

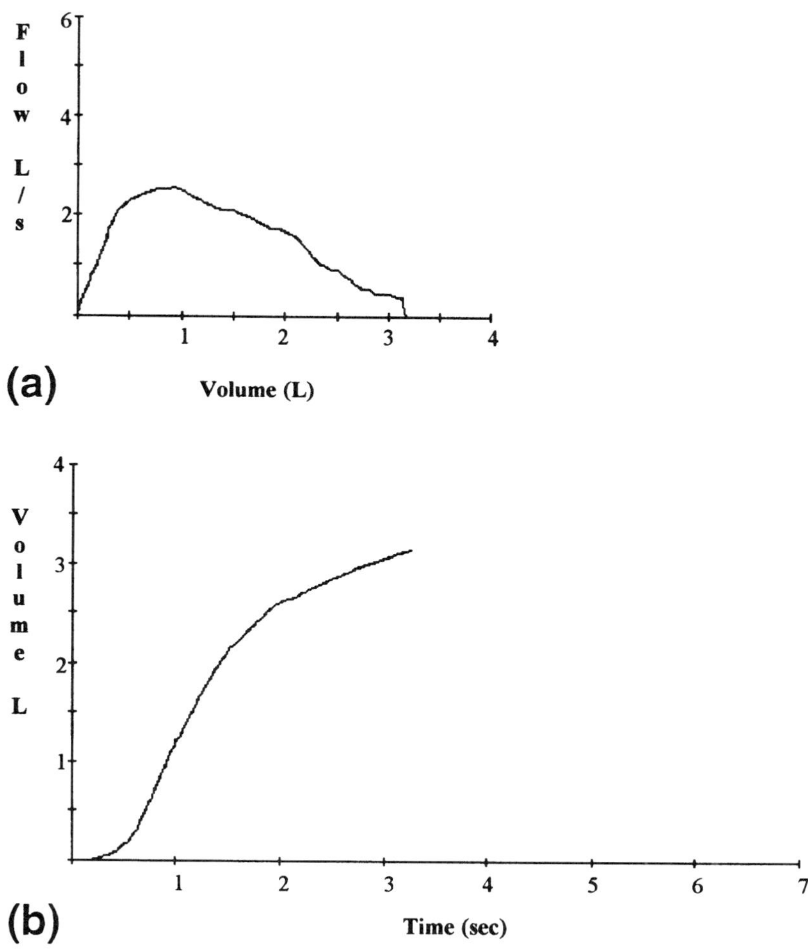

Figure 5 (a) In this poor effort, note the lack of a sharp peak in the flow-volume loop. (b) In the time-volume graph, note that the volume continues to significantly rise after 1 sec, indicating a weak initial effort and therefore the potential to underestimate the FEV_1. FEV_1 = 1.2 L, PEFR = 156 L/min, time to peak = 353 msec, and back extrapolation = 6.7%.

the steepest portion of the spirogram during expiration, and draw a line intersecting the slope with the time axis. This point becomes the ''extrapolated'' or new time 0 value. The volume from the actual start of exhalation up until the new time 0 point is divided by the forced vital capacity, and this is called the back extrapolated volume. If the back extrapolated volume is excessive, for example greater than 5% of the FVC, the maneuver should be repeated with an emphasis on a stronger effort without any initial hesitation (see Fig. 8).

Although acceptability criteria have not been developed for the performance of spirometry in the ED, experience has shown that a properly trained clinician or technician can obtain reproducible results, even in very ill patients. In a recent multicenter study

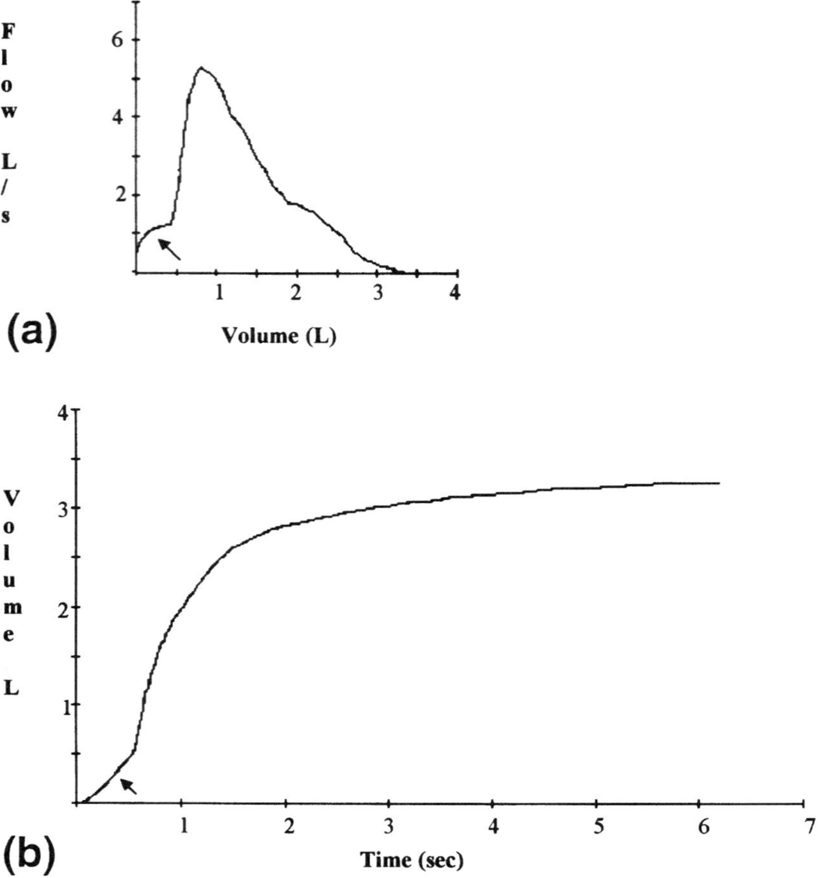

Figure 6 Hesitation at the start of the effort as indicated by the lack of a sharp rise in volume (see arrows). The back extrapolation is 14.7%.

spirometry was performed in patients presenting to the ED to identify those with an FEV_1 < 30% predicted (22). Among these very ill patients enrolled in the protocol, the quality of the data was considered adequate in over 95% of efforts. For study purposes, this meant that for each set of spirograms the two best FEV_1 values were within 10% of each other and the set contained at least one effort that met the other criteria listed in Table 2. For the spirometric assessment of the acute asthmatic on ED arrival, 92% had spirometry that was considered adequate. In this 4-hr protocol that consisted of six sets of assessments, spirometry quality improved greatly over time as patients became more familiar with technique and pulmonary function improved; marked improvement in quality of effort was noted even by the second set of readings at 30 min. For the final 4-hr reading, almost every set of spirograms met criteria for reproduciblity and contained at least one effort that was considered adequate by study standards.

In some patients coughing may occur during the first second and lead to an underesti-

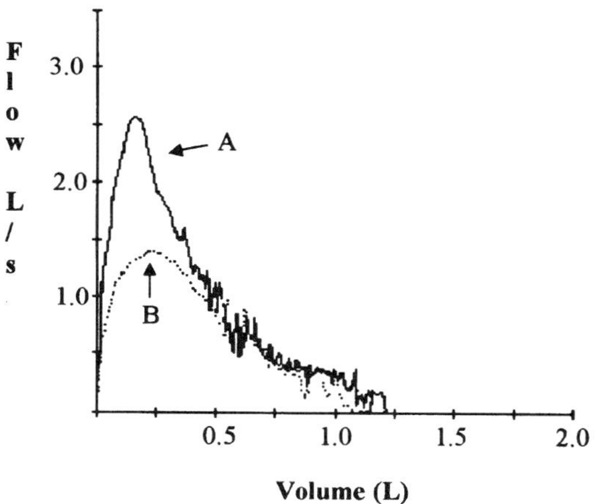

	FEV1	PEF
A	0.88 L, 30% predicted	154 L/min, 42% predicted
B	0.84 L, 29% predicted	84 L/min, 23 % predicted

Figure 7 Flow-volume loops from two efforts in an acute asthmatic 30 min after arrival in the ED. Note the sharp and well-defined peak in effort A (peak flow 154 L/min; 42% of predicted), as compared to the poorly defined peak from the weaker effort B (peak flow 84 L/min; 23% of predicted). Note that although there were large differences in peak flow, the FEV_1 from the two efforts were almost identical (0.88 L, 30% of predicted compared to 0.84 L, 29% of predicted). This is an illustration of the greater effort dependency of the peak flow measurement as compared to the FEV_1. Incidentally, there is also some glottic closure noted in both efforts.

mation of the FEV_1. If coughing is a problem, encourage the patient to give an effort just below the threshold of cough and avoid a lengthy expiration. The clinician must then determine if the efforts are reasonable and the overall quality acceptable.

There are any number of reasons that unreliable spirometry test results will be obtained in the acutely ill patient in the ED setting. This includes inability to obtain full patient cooperation due to acute illness, improperly trained personnel, or poor maintenance of equipment. It can be very difficult to perform a test that requires time and effort in a busy environment. An abbreviated exhalation will not allow measurement of FVC and various other measures related to exhalation. Nonetheless a systematic attempt to improve the quality of pulmonary function testing will lead to results that better approximate the patients severity of airway obstruction and therefore allow the most reliable data to be obtained for clinical and research purposes.

Regarding the performance of peak flow measures with a hand-held peak flow meter, it is difficult to offer any specific guidelines for acceptability and reproducibility. This is in part related to the high variability of peak flow measures seen in patients with acute or uncontrolled asthma as well as the limitations of the instrumentation. Optimally, the results of the two best efforts should be within 10% of each other and the patient should

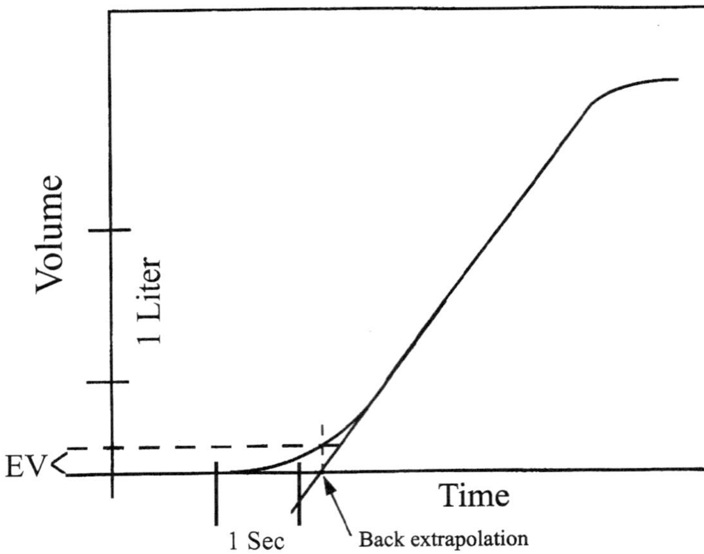

Figure 8 Volume-time graph demonstrating back extrapolation. See text for discussion. EV = extrapolated volume.

appear to be offering a best effort. The clinician can otherwise only rely on the general appearance of patient effort to determine if the maneuvers are adequate and whether the results should be accepted.

V. WHICH TO CHOOSE: FEV_1 OR PEAK FLOW MEASURES?

A. Advantages of FEV_1

There are a number of reasons for obtaining spirometry in the acutely ill asthmatic. The FEV_1 is linearly related to the severity of illness from the range of mild obstruction to life-threatening asthma episodes and is the most reliable measure of pulmonary function available in a clinical setting (3). The FEV_1 measure has much less variability than PEF (23–25). As noted earlier, the FEV_1 is independent of effort once a moderate effort has been made (5). This is important in the ED setting where the patient may be fatigued or unable to fully cooperate. Measuring the FEV_1 also allows assessment of airways smaller than the peak flow measures and overall FEV_1 is a more sensitive indicator of airway obstruction (23).

It should be noted that while excellent correlations between FEV_1 and PEF have been found in both the acute and chronically ill population (23,26–29), these observations must be interpreted with caution. The tight correlations suggest only that as the value of one marker moves in one direction, the value of the other does likewise. This is important information, but it does not mean the PEF and FEV_1% predicted values are equal (30). In fact, in studies of patients with either acute or chronic asthma, the FEV_1% predicted is typically lower than the corresponding PEF% predicted, and relying on the PEF can lead to an underestimation of the severity of airway obstruction. In a study of ED patients with acute asthma, when FEV_1% predicted was plotted against PEF% predicted, the PEF appeared to be higher than the corresponding FEV_1 (27). In a more recent study of patients with acute asthma, the average FEV_1% predicted was 12 percentage points lower than the PEF% predicted before any treatment, and 17 percentage points lower after treatment (28). These differences were present in patients regardless of their degree of airway obstruction. For example, if the mean posttreatment FEV_1 was 35% of predicted, the corresponding PEFR in the same patients was 52% of predicted. If the average FEV_1 was 55% of predicted, the corresponding PEF was approximately 72% of predicted. To complicate matters further, in some patients the FEV_1% predicted was actually higher than the PEF. The precise reasons for all these differences are unclear. Needless to say, they may influence treatment and disposition decisions and the clinician must be aware that the FEV_1 and PEF% predicted values are not equivalent and therefore not interchangeable.

Other reasons for choosing FEV_1 are related to the benefits of certain features of the spirometer, such as the ability to visualize the efforts in real time and identify measures useful for quality assessment. The use of a spirometer allows the clinician to immediately determine adequacy of effort, assess the reliability of the maneuvers and decide if the results are acceptable. If there is poor reproducibility or the tracings suggest poor efforts, the maneuver may be repeated, or the clinician may accept the results with the understanding that they may not best represent the patients ventilatory capability.

B. Limitations of Spirometry

There are a number of obstacles to measuring the FEV_1 in the acute care environment. Performing spirometry requires specialized equipment that must be maintained in good working order. The spirometer generally requires daily calibration. The person performing spirometry needs to be trained on equipment use, performing the maneuver in acutely ill patients, understanding the acceptability criteria, and interpreting results. Some patients will be unable to perform the maneuvers even after adequate instructions and some will refuse to perform the procedure because of added discomfort. Others may be too ill to offer adequate efforts. The clinician may not have the time in the setting of a busy ED to perform spirometry.

C. Advantages of Peak Flow

Since the peak flow device is relatively easy to use by both the staff and patient, peak flow measurements have typically been used in the ED to measure degree of airflow obstruction. The lower costs, less amount of training necessary to use the device, lack of need for specialized equipment, and ease of use by the patient are all advantages the peak flow meter has as compared to the spirometer. Although a peak flow measure at a given point in time may offer limited information, the high correlation between results of PEF and FEV_1 indicate that peak flow rates are very useful in following changes in pulmonary function over time.

D. Limitations of Peak Flow

There are a number of potential limitations to use of the peak flow meter. The results of peak flow measures represent air expulsion from larger airways, although asthma frequently affects smaller airways (31). Therefore the patient can have compromised airways but still present with a relatively normal appearing peak flow rate. A relatively high peak flow measure combined with the lack of wheezing in some patients may also mislead the clinician into believing the airways are normal. The peak flow measure is far more variable than the FEV_1 measure. Results are obtained during a very effort-dependent portion of the expiratory cycle and are therefore highly dependent on patient effort, far more so than FEV_1 (31). This is demonstrated in Figure 7, where a patient with acute asthma gave two efforts, the first better than the second. The two FEV_1 values were relatively close in number, whereas the two peak flow values differed greatly.

Since peak flow meters do not allow graphic visualization of the maneuvers, it may be difficult to gauge the intensity and adequacy of the effort or the accuracy of the recording. Peak flow meters are prone to breakdown over time, and in many departments where the meter is used for extended periods of time the clinician may be unaware of mechanical difficulties. Since there is no graphic recording of the effort, adequate quality control cannot be assured. Finally, the ease of use and accessibility of the device may actually in some ways be a disadvantage. It is possible that inexperienced examiners will obtain unreliable results and this misinformation could lead to inappropriate clinical decisions.

VI. REPORTING OF RESULTS

A. Normal or Predicted Value

Lung function values are not the same for all individuals. The most important factors responsible for variation are sex, size, and age (race is discussed below). The first three factors contribute 30%, 22%, and 8% of the interindivual variability in lung function (32). The large football player clearly will have a larger FVC, FEV_1, and PEF than a smaller individual. In general, spirometric values decrease with a decrease in body size as measured by height. For the same height, women have smaller lungs (hence lower FVC, FEV_1 and PEF) than men. This is probably because the ratio of thorax size to body height is smaller in women, who have relatively longer legs than men. For the same gender and body size, spirometric indices decrease with age, starting around age 20–25 years. Using techniques of multiple regression in studies on large populations of nonsmoking normal individuals, prediction equations have been developed by various investigators that allow for predicting the mean value of a given index of lung function. Among the reference equations more commonly used in the United States are those by the groups of Morris, Crapo, and Knudsen for FEV_1 and Nunn and Gregg for PEFR, and for adults these are based on height, age, and gender (33–36) (see Chapter 18). Other equations also account for body weight, although this may be more relevant in extremely thin or obese subjects (37,38). The indices most often used to assess airway function in the ED, FEV_1, and PEF are generally less dependent on body weight.

There are some adjustments that have been recommended for race or ethnicity as well. Most of the commonly used equations were done on Caucasian populations of European descent. Many other races, however, have relatively smaller lung volumes and FEV_1 values (5). In the African-American, for example, these differences are in part related to the relationship of the thorax size to body height, with blacks on the average having a smaller trunk to leg ratio than whites (39). Regression equations in white subjects typically overestimate FEV_1 predictive values relative to black subjects. Estimates for correcting

FEV_1 and FVC in blacks have ranged widely, although the ATS refers to a 12% correction and OSHA suggests a 15% reduction relative to whites (5,19,39,40,41–43). This single race adjustment, however, may not be accurate for all age, sex, height combinations (37,44) and recently proposed polynomial regression equations may provide better normative values. The need for peak flow correction based on racial and ethnic background has received less attention than FEV_1. Although it is generally accepted that there is some peak flow variation among populations, it appears to be less than for FEV_1, and there is not enough current data available to recommend a correction factor.

B. What Is "Normal"?

Pulmonary function values are generally expressed as percent of the predicted value. For normally distributed values, 95% of the population exists within two standard deviations of the mean. For FVC and FEV_1 this is roughly between 80% and 120% of the predicted values, while the "normal" range for PEF is greater.

The advantage of using percent predicted is that it allows the clinician to have a reference point for comparing illness severity. In the event that patients are not aware of their "best" peak flow values, it allows the clinician to approximate where the patient's pulmonary function falls relative to the population. It gives clinicians the ability to tailor therapy based on severity of illness and to make disposition decisions on the basis of a final pulmonary function. It is again important to point out that FEV_1% predicted is not equivalent to the peak flow% predicted, and the measures should not be substituted for each other.

According to the ATS, for chronic obstructive airways diseases like asthma, FEV_1 greater than 80% of predicted is considered in the normal range (although not necessarily normal for that individual patient), 60–80% of predicted are labeled as "mild" obstruction, 40–60% of predicted are labeled as "moderate" obstruction, and less than 40% of predicted are labeled as "severe" obstruction. FEV_1 values less than 30% of predicted are sometimes labeled as "very severe" obstruction. Importantly, patients with chronic asthma who are considered "under control" may not have a best measure equivalent to 100% of predicted. For some patients their best effort may be far lower and, if available, the best number a patient can achieve would be useful information for the clinician.

VII. CONTRAINDICATIONS AND COMPLICATIONS

Relatively few serious complications have been reported in the literature in patients undergoing pulmonary function testing, with articles generally limited to case reports. One report identifies two patients with asthma who had cardiopulmonary arrests following performance of peak flow maneuvers (45). Other rare complications reported from performance of pulmonary function testing include incarceration of existing inguinal hernia (46) and mediastinal emphysema (47). Syncope has been noted during prolonged expiration. In some patients bronchospasm may occur during performance of spirometry (48). A transient drop in oxygen saturation may occur during pulmonary function testing and caution must be exercised when testing patients with baseline hypoxia. In our ED we will not perform prolonged forced maneuvers in patients with recent surgery or in the later stages of pregnancy. In recent ED studies utilizing spirometry as an outcome variable (22), there have not been any reports of serious complications, although if the procedure becomes more commonly used in the acutely ill asthmatic, it is always possible that complications will be identified.

VIII. SUMMARY: CURRENT USES FOR SPIROMETRY

Pulmonary function testing provides information regarding illness severity that may not be otherwise obtainable in the ED. While the ED is not the optimal environment to perform pulmonary function tests, a thorough understanding of what these tests indicate and how to best perform them will greatly increase their value as surrogate markers of illness. The clinician may choose to use a peak flow meter or a spirometer to assess degree of airway obstruction. The peak flow meter has advantages in ease of use and cost while the benefit of measuring FEV_1 with a spirometer includes better sensitivity and reliability. Still, outcome studies have not been performed in the ED comparing the utility of peak flow to FEV_1 measures and for general clinical purposes one test cannot yet be considered superior to the other. For purposes of clinical research, measuring FEV_1 with a spirometer has significant advantages including reliability and reproducibility, quality control, maintenance of records, and values that are more physiology specific. If the use of a specific treatment or disposition protocol is eventually found to be dependent on a specific FEV_1 value, and this value is found to be a more reliable diagnostic or prognostic index than a peak flow measure, then it may be necessary to use the spirometer more routinely. Until then, clinicians should understand the strengths and limitations of these valuable tools when evaluating acutely ill patients and choose the one that best fits their practice.

REFERENCES

1. Guidelines for the diagnosis and management of asthma: Clinical practice guidelines. National Institutes of Health, National Heart, Lung and Blood Institute, NIH Publication No. 97-4051, April 1997.
2. Shim C, Williams MH Jr. Evaluation of the severity of asthma: Patients versus physicians. Am J Med 1980; 68:11–13.
3. Enright PL, Lebowitz MD, Cockroft DW. Physiologic measures: Pulmonary function tests: Asthma outcome. Am J Respir Crit Care Med 1994; 149:S9–18.
4. Shim CS, Williams MH Jr. Relationship of wheezing to the severity of asthma. Arch Intern Med 1983; 143:890–892.
5. Cotes JE. Structure, expansion and movement of the lung (chapter 5). In: Cotes JE, Lung Function: Assessment and Application in Medicine, Fifth Edition, Blackwell Scientific Publications, Oxford, England 1993.
6. Rubinfeld AR, Pain MCF. Perception of asthma. Lancet 1976; 1:882–884.
7. Bloch H, Silverman R, Mancherje N, et al. Intravenous magnesium sulfate as an adjunct in the treatment of acute asthma. Chest 1995; 107:1576–1581.
8. Rudnitsky GS, Eberlein RS, Schoffstall JM, et al. Comparison of intermittent and continuously nebulized albuterol for treatment of asthma in an emergency department. Ann Emerg Med 1993; 22:1842–1846.
9. Lin RY, Sauter D, Newman T, et al. Continuous versus intermittent albuterol nebulization in the treatment of acute asthma. Ann Emerg Med 1993; 22:1847–1853.
10. Kass JE, Castriotta RJ. Heliox therapy in acute severe asthma. Chest 1995; 107:757–760.

11. Rodrigo C, Rodrigo G. Assessment of the patient with asthma in the emergency department. A factor analytic study. Chest 1993; 104:1325–1328.
12. Rodrigo G, Rodrigo C. A new index for early prediction of hospitalization in patients with acute asthma. Am J Emerg Med 1997; 15:8–13.
13. Martin TG, Elenbaas RM, Pingleton SH. Use of peak expiratory flow rates to eliminate unnecessary arterial blood gases in acute asthma. Ann Emerg Med 1982; 11:70–73.
14. Global Initiative For Asthma. NHLBI/WHO Workshop Report. National Institute of Health Publication Number 95-3659, January 1995.
15. Cross D, Nelson HS. The role of the peak flow meter in the diagnosis and management of asthma. J Allergy Clin Immunol 1991; 87(part 1):120–128.
16. Miller MR, Dickinson SA, Hitchings DJ. The accuracy of portable peak flow meters. Thorax 1992; 47:904–909.
17. Rebuck DA, Hanania NA, D'Urzo AD, et al. The accuracy of a handheld portable spirometer. Chest 1996; 109:152–157.
18. Jackson AC. Accuaracy, reproducibility and variability of portable peak flowmeters. Chest 1995; 107:648–651.
19. American Thoracic Society. Lung Function Testing: Selection of Reference Values and Interpretative Strategies. Am Rev Respir Dis 1991; 144:1202–1218.
20. American Thoracic Society. Standardization of spirometry—1987 update. Am Rev Respir Dis 1987; 136:1285–1298.
21. American Thoracic Society. Standardization of spirometry—1994 update. Am J Respir Crit Care Med 1995; 152:1107–1136.
22. Silverman R, Osborn H, Runge J, et al. Magnesium sulfate as an adjunct to standard therapy in acute severe asthma. Acad Emerg Med 1996; 3(abstrt):467.
23. Vaughan TR, Weber RW, Tipton WR, et al. Comparison of PEFR and FEV1 in patients with varying degree of lung obstruction: Effect of modest altitude. Chest 1989; 95:558–562.
24. McCarthy DS, Craig DB, Cherniack RM. Intraindividual variability in maximum expiratory flow volume and closing volume in asymptomatic subjects. Am Rev Respir Dis 1975; 112: 407–411.
25. Nickerson BG, Lemen RJ, Gerdes CB, et al. Within-subject variability and percent change for significance of spirometry in normal subjects and in patients with cystic fibrosis. Am Rev Respir Dis 1980; 122:859–866.
26. Meltzer AA, Smolensky MH, D'Alonzo GE, et al. An assessment of peak expiratory flow as a surrogate measurement of FEV1 in stable asthmatic children. Chest 1989; 96:329–333.
27. Nowak RM, Pensler MI, Sarkar D, et al. Comparison of peak expiratory flow and FEV1 admission criteria for acute bronchial asthma. Ann Emerg Med 1982; 11:64–69.
28. Silverman R, Gallager EJ, Scharf S. Lack of agreement between FEV1 and PEFR in acute asthma. Am J Respir Crit Care Med. 1996; 153(abstr):A71.
29. Gautrin D, D'Aquino LC, Gagnon G, et al. Comparison between peak expiratory flow rates (PEFR) and FEV_1 in the monitoring of asthmatic subjects at an outpatient clinic. Chest 1994; 106:1419–1426.
30. Bland JM, Altman DG. Statistical methods for assessing agreement between two methods of clinical measurement. Lancet 1986; 1:307–310.
31. Gold WM. Pulmonary function testing. In: Textbook of Respiratory Medicine, Philadelphia, WB Saunders, 1994, p. 798–900.
32. Becklake MR. Concepts of normality applied to the measurements of lung function. Am J Med 1986; 80:1158–1164.
33. Crapo RO, Morris AH, Gardner RM. Reference spirometric values using techniques and equipment that meet ATS recommendations. Am Rev Respir Dis 1981; 123:659–664.
34. Morris JF, Koski A, Johnson LC. Spirometric standards for healthy nonsmoking adults. Am Rev Respir Dis 1971; 103:57–67.

35. Knudsen RJ, Lebowitz MD, Holberg CJ, Burrows B. Changes in the normal expiratory flow volume curve with growth and aging. Am Rev Respir Dis 1983; 127:725–734.
36. Nunn AJ, Gregg I. New regression equations for predicting peak expiratory flow in adults. Br Med J 1989; 298:1068–1070.
37. Schoenberg JB, Beck GJ, Bouhuys A. Growth and decay of pulmonary function in healthy blacks and whites. Respir Physiol 1978; 33:367–393.
38. Dockery DW, Ware JH, Ferris BG Jr, et al. Distribution of forced expiratory volume in one second and forced vital capacity in healthy, white, adult never smokers in six U.S. cities. Am Rev Respir Dis 1985; 131:511-520.
39. van De Wal BW, Erasmus LD, Hechter R. Stem and standing heights in Bantu and white South Africans: Their significance in relation to pulmonary function values. S Afr Med J 1971; 45(suppl):568–570.
40. Rossiter CE, Weill H. Ethnic differences in lung function: evidence for proportional differences. Int J Epidemiol 1974; 3:55–61.
41. Lap NL, Amandus HE, Hall R, et al. Lung volumes and flow rates in black and white subjects. Thorax 1974; 29:185–188.
42. U.S. Department of Labor, Occcupational Safety and Health Administration. Federal Register, June 23, 1978. Occupational Exposure to Cotton Dust. Final Mandatory Occupational Safety and Health Standards, 27418–27463.
43. Damon A. Negro-white differences in pulmonary function (vital capacity, timed vital capacity and expiratory flow rate). Hum Biol 1966; 38:381–393.
44. Glindmeyer HW, Lefante JJ, McColloster C, et al. Blue collar normative spirometric values for Caucasian and African-American men and women aged 18–65. Am J Respir Crit Care Med 1995; 151(2 pt 1):412–422.
45. Lemarchand P, Labrune S, Herer B, et al. Cardiorespiratory arrest following peak expiratory flow measurement during attack of asthma. Chest 1991; 100:1168–1169.
46. Patel V, Raju L, Wollschlager C. Incarceration of existing inguinal hernia as a complication of pulmonary function testing. Chest 1992; 101:876–877.
47. Varkey B, Kory RC. Mediastinal and subcutaneous emphysema following pulmonary function tests. Am Rev Respir Dis 1973; 108:1393–1396.
48. Gimeno F, Berg WC, Sluiter HJ, et al. Spirometry induced bronchial constriction. Am Rev Respir Dis 1972; 105:68–74.

15

Laboratory, Roentgenographic, and EKG Evaluation of Acute Asthma

Rita Kay Cydulka
MetroHealth Medical Center/Case Western Reserve University, Cleveland, Ohio

Mona Shah
Oregon Health Sciences University, Portland, Oregon

I. INTRODUCTION

Patients with acute exacerbation of asthma who present to an emergency department (ED) may vary widely in the degree of airflow obstruction. The assessment of the severity of airway obstruction and its response to treatment is of paramount importance for the emergency physician. The National Asthma Education and Prevention Program (NAEPP) strongly emphasizes the use of objective measures to determine severity and guide therapy (1). This chapter will discuss various laboratory studies available to the emergency physician to assist in the clinical evaluation of patients with acute asthma exacerbation.

II. SPIROMETRY

During severe asthma attacks, patients may manifest certain physical findings that are useful clinical clues to the severity of the attack; however, the severity of airflow obstruction is best assessed by direct measurement using spirometry or peak flow determination (2,3,4).

The NAEPP guidelines, first released in 1991, emphasized the use of objective measures of pulmonary function in the ED management of acute asthma because the physician and the patient tend to underestimate the severity of the abnormalities that contribute to asthma morbidity and mortality (1). The measurement of pulmonary function documents the severity of airway obstruction and response to therapy. Carden et al. (5) demonstrated that clinical parameters, such as pulse rate, respiratory rate, and pulsus paradoxus, are unreliable in predicting the degree of airway obstruction in acute bronchial asthma. Their study revealed that 71% of patients with persistent severe airway obstruction, as defined by posttreatment $FEV_1 < 1.6L$, had no pulsus paradoxus. They found that clinical parame-

Table 1 Baseline Severity of Asthma as Graded by % Predicted FEV_1

FEV_1% predicted	Severity
70–100	Mild
60–69	Moderate
50–59	Moderately severe
35–49	Severe
$<$ 35	Very severe

ters, such as pulse, and respiratory rate, tend to normalize with minimal improvement in airway obstruction (5).

Spirometry is used to measure the volume of air expired in 1 sec from maximum inspiration (FEV_1) and the total volume of air expired as rapidly as possible (FVC) (6). The most important spirometric abnormalities noted in acute asthma are slowing of the expiratory flow rate, reflected in reduction of FEV_1, peak expiratory flow rate (PEFR), and maximal midexpiratory flow rate. Other abnormalities include reduction in vital capacity, increase in functional residual capacity, and, in chronic cases, an increase in total lung capacity (6).

The FEV_1 is the most reproducible pulmonary function parameter and is linearly related to the severity of airway obstruction (7). It is the internationally accepted measure of severity of airway obstruction in countries including Canada, Australia, New Zealand, United Kingdom, and South Africa. The results of spirometry, as roughly correlated to clinical severity based on the guidelines established by the American Thoracic Society (ATS), are defined in Table 1 (8).

The Canadian Thoracic Society Emergency Asthma Management guidelines published in 1994 established pre- and posttreatment criteria using pulmonary function tests (PFTs) or PEFR values to estimate severity of airflow obstruction. During pretreatment assessment, patients were divided into three subgroups: (1) those with impending or actual respiratory arrest; (2) those with severe exacerbation, i.e., FEV_1/PEFR $< 50\%$; and (3) those with FEV_1/PEFR $> 50\%$. Initial treatment is stratified based on clinical assessment and results of PFTs. Posttreatment severity of asthma, as determined by the posttreatment PFTs, is as shown in Table 2.

Nowak et.al. demonstrated the usefulness of pulmonary function tests in predicting the need for hospitalization (9). This study, conducted before the routine use of steroids for the ED treatment of acute asthma exacerbation, revealed that a pretreatment $FEV_1 <$ 0.6 L or a posttreatment $FEV_1 <$ 1.6 L was associated with the need for hospitalization

Table 2 Posttreatment Severity of Asthma as Graded by % Predicted FEV_1/PEFR

FEV_1/PEFR % predicted	Severity
61–100%	Mild
40–60%	Moderate
$<$ 40%	Severe
Exhaustion, cyanosis, confusion	Near-death

or a high relapse rate after discharge from the ED. In fact, 90% of patients with pretreatment $FEV_1 < 0.6$ L and posttreatment $FEV_1 < 1.6$ L required hospitalization. In another study, utilization of PFTs changed ED management in over 20% of patients (10). Emerman and Cydulka (10) demonstrated that physicians tend to underestimate the degree of airway obstruction in patients with acute asthma. Only 39% of the physicians' estimates were found to be within 5.0 percentage points of the actual percentage of predicted PEFR (10). Shim and Williams reported similar findings (13). They found that only 44% of physician estimates of peak flow rates in patients presenting with acute asthma exacerbation were within 20% of measured PEFR (3).

III. PEAK EXPIRATORY FLOW RATE

Peak expiratory flow rate, as measured by the mini-Wright peak flow meter, is the maximum flow rate that can be generated during a forced expiratory maneuver with fully inflated lungs. It is an extremely valuable guide to detect severity of airway obstruction and disposition of the asthmatic patient. The peak flow meter is a simple portable device, easy to use, inexpensive, and reliable. However, it requires good patient cooperation, as its accuracy is effort dependent, and it measures only large airway flow. PEFR does not require full expiration, which may itself provoke bronchoconstriction and worsening of symptoms, and it can be measured repeatedly. Nowak demonstrated good correlation between PEFR and FEV_1 at all stages of treatment with r-values ranging between 0.7370 and 0.8615 (11). Despite its limitations, PEFR is a useful index of airway obstruction.

IV. ARTERIAL BLOOD GAS

Patients with moderately severe bronchospasm, but not in status asthmaticus, only rarely show any significant abnormality of the arterial oxygen saturation or carbon dioxide tension. Most severe attacks of asthma are characterized by mild hypercapnia and hypoxemia.

Arterial blood gas (ABG) determinations help reflect the severity of an acute asthma exacerbation and help elucidate the ventilatory status. Seventy-five percent of patients with acute asthma demonstrate mild to moderate hypoxemia and respiratory alkalosis (12–16). Arterial oxygen tension drops below 55 mmHg in only 5–10% of patients (12,17). The hypoxemia usually results from ventilation-perfusion mismatch, which in turn results from variable degrees of airway obstruction (12). The mismatch improves with therapy, but may paradoxically worsen with administration of bronchodilator treatment, probably secondary to mucous plugging (18–22). Alveolar hyperventilation with respiratory alkalosis is the usual response of the ventilatory control center to acute airflow obstruction, the patient may be unable to maintain the required alveolar ventilation as airway obstruction progresses.

The arterial CO_2 tension rises as respiratory muscles fatigue, as reflected in development of respiratory acidosis. A $Paco_2$ of approximately 40 mmHg in the dyspneic patient with acute asthma, although a normal value, signals impending ventilatory failure (23).

In severe asthma, acidosis may be a result of both ventilatory and metabolic components. Roncoroni et al. described a large group of patients in status asthmaticus who had lactic acidosis (24). Appel et al. (25) reported 12 patients with severe asthma and lactic acidosis. The exact mechanism for the development of lactic acidosis in adults with acute severe asthma remains unknown, although current theories propose that lactic acidosis results from increased respiratory muscle activity causing lactate production, plus lactate underutilization secondary to hypoperfusion of skeletal muscle and liver (25).

ABGs are not routinely indicated if patient responds appropriately to the initial treatment and FEV_1 is > 1 L (26). ABG determination is indicated for patients with persistent respiratory distress, especially if FEV_1 or PEFR is $< 25\%$ predicted (27). PEFR may be used to eliminate unnecessary ABGs (27). Martin et al. demonstrated that patients with a PEFR $> 25\%$ did not require arterial blood gas sampling as no patients with a PEFR $> 25\%$ predicted had a $Paco_2 > 45$mmHg or pH < 7.35 (27).

Oxygen saturation (S_aO_2), as measured by pulse oximeter, is an accurate means of following patient oxygenation noninvasively during treatment (28). However, pulse oximetry is not a substitute for arterial blood gas as one of the primary purposes of the blood gas determination is to assess the adequacy of alveolar ventilation, as reflected by the pco_2. Patients with a pco_2 of approximately 40 mmHg or greater should be admitted to the hospital, and in many cases treated in an intensive care unit (ICU) (16,26).

Hedges et al. (29) evaluated oxygen saturation as measured by pulse oximeter for early identification of patients needing prolonged therapy for acute bronchospasm. They concluded that as isolated variables, S_aO_2 at baseline and at peak drop following bronchodilator therapy were not useful predictors of outcome, although patients with $S_aO_2 < 92\%$ at presentation were not evaluated (29).

Usually arterial sampling is unnecessary in patients with oxygen saturation $> 92\%$, since respiratory failure is unlikely in this group of patients. However ABGs must be pursued if these patients demonstrate FEV_1 or PEFR $< 25\%$ predicted, deterioration, or lack of objective improvement (30).

V. X-RAY

Although chest X-ray is often performed as part of the evaluation of acute asthma managed in the ED, the yield of diagnostically useful information is low (31). The main features on a chest X-ray include pulmonary hyperinflation and peribronchial cuffing, particularly in patients with chronic symptoms. Radiographic findings manifested as complications of asthma and their frequency are as listed in Table 3 (32–39).

In fact, radiographs are normal in most patients (33,40). Zieverink et al. (41) found only 2.2% abnormal radiographs of the 997 X-rays studied over a 4-yr period. Abnormalities included presence of infiltrates, atelectasis, pneumothorax, and/or pneumomediastinum. He concluded that chest X-rays in adults are unnecessary unless the patient was unresponsive to bronchodilators and hospitalized (41). In a retrospective review by Sher-

Table 3 Radiographic Findings on Chest X-ray

Findings	Frequency
Normal	55–82
Hyperinflation	22–12
Infiltrate	1–16
Pneumothorax	0.5–2
Pneumomediastinum	5–10

man et al., only 3% of 135 patients required alteration in treatment due to radiographic abnormalities (42). Petherman et al. found abnormalities that influenced management in 9% of 117 adults with severe acute asthma who were admitted to the hospital (36). Findley and Sahn demonstrated that chest X-ray findings have no significant correlation with need for hospitalization (32). Chest X-rays seem warranted for the following indications: clinical suspicion that one of the complications listed in Table 3 is present and may alter care; ventilatory failure, as defined by a $Paco_2 > 40$mmHg; or persistent hypoxemia, as defined by oxygen saturation $< 92\%$ or $Pao_2 < 60$ mmHg; failure to improve despite aggressive therapy in ED; and, occasionally, newly diagnosed asthma (23). Therefore, most ED patients do not require radiographic evaluation.

On the other hand, White et al. discovered 34% of admission X-rays to be abnormal (34). Abnormalities included focal parenchymal opacities, increased interstitial markings, enlarged cardiac silhouette, pulmonary congestion, pneumothorax, and a new pulmonary nodule. A retrospective review in Great Britain of 1016 admission chest radiographs conducted over a 4-yr period revealed an incidence of 15% of clinically significant radiographic abnormalities, most common being infection and atelectasis. A study from Singapore revealed that of the 116 admission chest radiographs reviewed, 23% were abnormal. In this study, chest radiographs were considered an important investigation tool since most were helpful in detecting complications of asthma or coincidental conditions (44). Although most current literature review supports obtaining an admission chest radiograph, some studies recommend selective ordering of chest X-rays especially in the subgroup with complicated asthma (43–46).

VI. EKG

The most common abnormality noted on an electrocardiogram (EKG) is sinus tachycardia (47–49). As the airway obstruction improves, tachycardia resolves despite the use of sympathomimetics (50). Other EKG findings include p-pulmonale, present in up to 50% of the patients depending on severity of airway obstruction and right axis deviation, which is less common (48). Premature ventricular contractions are observed in a small number of patients. Atrial arrhythmias are very uncommon (47,49). Other reversible EKG changes include right bundle-branch block (RBBB) and right ventricular strain pattern.

VII. BLOOD TESTS

Utilization of complete blood cell count and chemistries is limited and nonspecific. Significant leukocytosis may be present, as a result of stress from repeated injections of epinephrine or corticosteroids (6). Blood eosinophilia $> 4\%$ or 300–400/mm^3 may be noted, regardless of the presence of an associated allergic or atopic component, but its absence does not rule out asthma (51,52). The count generally falls within 24–36 hours after administration of corticosteroids (53). The presence of eosinophils is recognized as a major cellular participant in late-phase allergic airway disease. However, much remains unknown in understanding bronchial inflammation and the role of eosinophils in this process (54). Presence of eosinophila is considered an indication for steroid use, however, in some patients asthma remains severe despite eosinopenia. A more rational approach to management is therefore based on spirometry rather than the eosinophil count.

Serum potassium may be temporarily diminished by 0.6–0.8 mEq/L secondary to the effect of frequent or continuous albuterol aerosols (55–58). Measurement of serum potassium level is appropriate if the patient is on digitalis preparations or arrhythmias are observed.

Serum theophylline level must be monitored in patients exhibiting signs of theophylline toxicity or with recent changes in dosing. Furthermore, some medications for coexisting conditions may affect theophylline elimination and hence serum theophylline level. The target serum concentration should be between 8 and 12 μg/mL and should be monitored routinely, especially in the elderly (51).

VIII. SUMMARY

Clinical evaluation of patients presenting to the ED with acute asthma requires objective measures to determine the degree of airway obstruction. Several studies indicate that physicians vary greatly in their assessment of the severity of asthma and their assessment correlates poorly with lung function (2,3,5,10). Hence, it is essential to determine severity of exacerbation using spirometry or PEFR.

Arterial blood gas determination is most valuable when patients are hypoxemic, i.e., when their O_2 saturation $< 92\%$, they fail to improve, or they rapidly deteriorate after initial treatment.

Initial evaluation of an asthmatic in the ED rarely requires chest X-ray, EKG, and blood tests. Chest X-ray should be considered for all patients requiring hospitalization. Performance of ancillary studies, such as EKG and blood tests, should not be permitted to delay initiation of treatment.

REFERENCES

1. National Asthma Education and Prevention Program: Expert Panel Report II, Guidelines for the diagnosis and management of asthma, DHHS Publication No. 97-4051, 1997.
2. McFadden ER, Kiser R, DeGroot WJ. Acute bronchial asthma: relationships between clinical and physiological manifestations. New Engl J Med 1973; 288:221–225.
3. Shim CS, Williams MH. Evaluation of the severity of asthma: patients versus physicians, Am J Med 1980; 68:11–13.
4. Shim CS, Williams MH. Relationship of wheezing to the severity of obstruction in asthma, Arch Intern Med 1983; 143:890–892.
5. Carden DL, Nowak RM, Sarkar D, Tomlanovich MC. Vital signs including pulsus paradoxus in the assessment of acute bronchial asthma. Ann Emerg Med 1983; 12:80–83.
6. Williams MH, Shim CS. Clinical evaluation, In: E. B. Weiss and M. Stein, eds., Bronchial Asthma: Mechanisms and therapeutics, 3rd ed., Little, Brown & Co., Boston, MA, 1993, p. 447.
7. Enright PL, Lebowitz MD, Cockroft DW. Physiologic measures: PFTs and asthma outcome. Am J Respir Crit Care Med 1994; 149:S9–S18.
8. Becklake M, Crapo RO, Buist AS, et al. Lung function testing: Selection of reference values and interpretative strategies. Official statement of the ATS. Am Rev Respir Dis 1991; 144: 1202–1218.
9. Nowak RM, Gordon KR, Wrobleski DA, Tomlanovich MC, Kvale PA. Spirometric evaluation of acute bronchial asthma. JACEP 1979; 8:9–12.

10. Emerman CL, Cydulka RK. Effect of pulmonary function testing on the management of acute asthma. Arch Intern Med 1995; 155:2225–2228.
11. Nowak RM, Pensler MI, Sarkar DD, Anderson JA, Kvale PA, Ortiz AE, Tomlanovich MC. Comparison of peak expiratory flow and FEV_1 admission criteria for acute bronchial asthma. Ann Emerg Med 1982; 11:64–69.
12. McFadden ER, Lyons HA. Arterial blood gas tensions in asthma. New Engl J Med 1968; 278: 1027–1032.
13. Rees HA, Millar JS, Donald KW. A study of the clinical course and arterial blood gas tensions of patients in status asthmaticus. Q J Med 1968; 37:541–561.
14. Miyamoto T, Mizunok R, Furuya K. Arterial blood gases in bronchial asthma. J Allergy 1970; 45:248–254.
15. Tai E, Read J. Blood gas tension in bronchial asthma, Lancet 1967; 1:644–646.
16. McFadden Jr ER. Management of patients with acute asthma: What do we know? What do we need to know? Ann Allergy 1994; 72:385–389.
17. Kelsen SG, Kelsen DP, Fleegler BF, et al. Emergency room assessment and treatment of patients with acute asthma: Adequacy of the conventional approach. Am J Med 1978; 64: 622–628.
18. Ingram Jr RH, Krumpe PE, Duffell GM, et al. Ventilation-perfusion changes after aerosolized isoproterenol in asthma, Am Rev Respir Dis 1970; 101:364–370.
19. Harris L. Comparison of the effect on blood gases, ventilation and perfusion of isoproterenol-phenylephrine & salbutamol aerosols in chronic bronchitis and asthma, J Allergy Clin Immunol 1972; 49:63–71.
20. Alliott RJ, Lang BD, Rawson DR, et al. Effects of salbutamol and isoprenaline-phenylephrine in reversible airways obstruction, Br Med J 1972; 539–542.
21. Palmer KN, Diament NL. Blood gases and lung function, Lancet 1969; 2:59–60.
22. Tal A, Pasterkamp H, Leahy F. Arterial oxygen desaturation following salbutamol inhalation in acute asthma, Chest 1984; 86:868–869.
23. Fanta CH. Acute asthma, In: Weiss EB and Stein M, eds. Bronchial Asthma: Mechanisms and Therapeutics, Little, Brown, & Co, Boston, MA, 1993, p. 972.
24. Roncoroni AJ, Adrogue HJA, DeObrutsky CW, Marchisio ML, Herrera MR. Metabolic acidosis in status asthmaticus, Respiration 1976; 33:85–94.
25. Appel D, Rubenstein R, Schrager K, et al. Lactic acidosis in severe asthma, Am J Med 1983; 75:580–584.
26. Nowak RM, Tomlanovich MC, Sarkar DD, et al. Arterial blood gas and pulmonary function testing in acute bronchial asthma, JAMA 1983; 249:2043–2046.
27. Martin TG, Elenbaas RM, Pingleton SH. Use of peak expiratory flow rates to eliminate unnecessary arterial blood gases in acute asthma, Ann Emerg Med 1982; 11:70–73.
28. Burki NK, Albert RK. Noninvasive monitoring of arterial blood gases: A report of the ACCP section on respiratory pathophysiology, Chest 1983; 83:666–670.
29. Hedges JR, Amsterdam JT, Cionni DJ, et al. Oxygen saturation as a marker for admission or relapse with acute bronchospasm, Am J Emerg Med 1987; 5:196–200.
30. Carruthers DM, Harrison BDW. Arterial blood gas analysis or oxygen saturation in the assessment of acute asthma? Thorax 1995; 50:186–188.
31. Blair DN, Coppage L, Shaw C. Medical imaging in asthma. J Thorac Imaging 1986; 1:23–35.
32. Findley LJ, Sahn SA. The value of chest roentgenogram in acute asthma in adults, Chest, 1981; 80:535–536.
33. Dalton AM. A review of radiological abnormalities in 135 patients presenting with acute asthma, Arch Emerg Med 1991; 8:36–40.
34. White CS, Lubetsky HW, Austin JH. Acute asthma. Admission chest radiography in hospitalized adult patients, Chest 1991; 100:14–16.
35. Rebuck AS. Radiological aspects of severe asthma, Radiology 1970; 14:262–268.

36. Petheram IS, Kerr IH, Collins JV. Value of chest radiographs in severe acute asthma, Clin Radiol 1981; 32:281–282.
37. Janower ML. Radiography, In: Weiss EB and Stein M, eds. Bronchial Asthma: Mechanisms and Therapeutics, Little, Brown, and Co., Boston, MA, 1993, p. 664.
38. Dattwyler RJ, Goldman MA, Block KG. Pneumomediastinum as a complication of asthma in teenage and young adult patients, J Allergy Clin Immunol 1979; 63:412–416.
39. Burke GJ. Pneumothorax, complicating acute asthma, S Afr Med J 1979; 55:508–510.
40. Gershel JC, Goldman HS, Stein RE, et al, The usefulness of chest radiographs in first asthma attacks, New Engl J Med 1983; 309:336–339.
41. Zieverink SE, Harper AP, Holden RW. Emergency room radiography in asthma: An efficacy study. Radiology 1982; 145:27–29.
42. Sherman S, Skoney JA, Ravikrishnan KP. Routine chest radiographs in exacerbations of chronic obstructive pulmonary disease: diagnostic value, Arch Intern Med 1989; 149:2493–2496.
43. Pickup CM, Nee PA, Randall PE. Radiographic features in 1,016 adults admitted to the hospital with acute asthma, J Accid Emerg Med 1994; 4:234–237.
44. Ismail Y, Loo CS, Zahary MK. The value of routine chest radiographs in acute asthma admissions, Singapore Med J 1994; 35:171–172.
45. Aronson S, Gennis P, Kelly D, et al. The value of routine chest radiographs in adult asthmatics, Ann Emerg Med 1989; 18:1206–1208.
46. Tsai TW, Gallagher EJ, Lombardi G, et al. Guidelines for the selective ordering of admission chest radiography in adult obstructive airway disease, Ann Emerg Med 1993; 22:1854–1858.
47. Rebuck AS, Read J. Assessment and management of severe asthma. Am J Med 1971; 51: 788–798.
48. Gelb AF, Lyons HA, Fairshler RD, Glauser FL, et al. P pulmonale in status asthmaticus. J Allergy Clin Immunol 1979; 64:18–22.
49. Grossman J. The occurrence of arrhythmias in hospitalized asthmatic patients, J Allergy Clin Immunol 1976; 57:310–317.
50. McFadden ER. Clinical physiologic correlates in asthma, J Allergy Clin Immunol 1986; 77(Pt 1):1–5.
51. NAEPP Working Group Report, Considerations for diagnosing and managing asthma in elderly, NIH Publication No. 95-3675, 1996.
52. Horn BR, Robin ED, Theodore J, et al. Total eosinophil counts in the management of bronchial asthma, New Engl J Med 1975; 292:1152–1155.
53. Lowell FC. The total eosinophil count in obstructive pulmonary disease New Engl J Med 1975; 292:1182–1183.
54. Calhoun WJ, Sedgwick J, Busse WW. The role of eosinophils in the pathophysiology of asthma, Ann NY Acad Sci 1991; 629:62–72.
55. Khan MA. Plasma potassium in acute severe asthma before and after treatment, Br J Clin Pract 1989; 43:363–365.
56. Dickens GR, McCoy RA, West R, et al. Effect of nebulized albuterol on serum potassium and cardiac rhythm in patients with asthma or COPD, Pharmacotherapy 1994; 14:729–733.
57. Deenstra M, Haalboom JR, Struyvenberg A. Decrease of plasma potassium due to inhalation of beta-2-agonists: Absence of an additional effect of intravenous theophylline, Eur J Clin Invest 1988; 18:162–165.
58. Küng M, White JR, Burki NK. The effect of subcutaneously administered terbutaline on serum potassium in asymptomatic adult asthmatics, Am Rev Respir Dis 1984; 129:329–332.

16

Noninvasive Monitoring of Asthma

Brian T. Williams and Charles B. Cairns
University of Colorado Health Sciences Center and Colorado Emergency Medicine Research Center, Denver, Colorado

I. INTRODUCTION

The use of objective measures of lung function in asthma is recommended by the National Institutes of Health (NIH) because the patient's report of symptoms and physical examination findings frequently do not correlate with the variability and severity of airflow obstruction (1).

The quantitative assessment of bronchospasm and its use in measuring the effectiveness of therapy is important in the treatment of the acute asthmatic (1). The most commonly used method to assess airflow obstruction in patients with acute asthma is measurement of either the peak expiratory flow rate (PEFR) or the 1-sec forced expiratory volume (FEV_1) technique using spirometry (2). Because both of these techniques require significant effort and cooperation by the patient, these measurements may be highly variable in acute settings (3,4). Additionally, patients who cannot cooperate as a result of age or severity of disease are unable to perform spirometry for measurement of PEFR and FEV_1.

Other noninvasive methods for monitoring the severity of asthma and the reponse to treatment are now available. This chapter will evaluate current and proposed modalities for the objective assessment of asthma.

II. VITAL SIGN MONITORS

A. Heart Rate

Isolated tachycardia is a common, albeit nonspecific, sign of acute asthma. Tachycardia in the patient with acute asthma may be due to numerous factors including fever, dehydration, chest pain, sympathetic discharge, pharmaceuticals (including β-agonists) or hypoxia (2). The mechanism of tachycardia in asthma is thought to involve a central reflex loop responding to hypoxia. It is important to note that a normal heart rate with hypoxemia suggests severe myocardial oxygen deprivation (2).

B. Respiratory Rate

Respiratory rate alone is influenced by multiple factors that may be associated with acute exacerbations of asthma. Some of the factors that influence respiratory rate include hypoxia, hypercarbia, anxiety, fever, sepsis, or metabolic acidosis. Also between patients with acute asthma, there is much intersubject variability (2). However the relationship between respiratory rate and hypoxia is not well established. As shown in Figure 1, respiratory rate does not appear to correlate with arterial oxygen saturation (5). Tachypnea is found with oxygen saturations ranging from poor to normal. Likewise, bradypnea is associated with a wide range of saturations. Because of the independence of the respiratory rate and oxygen saturation, it is likely that two different aspects of the asthma attack are being measured and, as a result, both variables should be independently evaluated (5,6).

Deegan and McNicholas (8) found that as an asthma attack progresses, a patient's chest wall movements first gradually changes from normal concurrent rib cage and abdominal expansion to predominantly abdominal breathing (associated with an inspiratory indrawing of the rib cage and excursion of the abdomen). With further progression, the pattern evolves to predominantly thoracic breathing exhibiting increased rib cage excursion (expansion of the rib cage on inspiration prior to expansion of the abdomen) (8). However, detection of these thoracic movement disorders has not been routinely incorporated into respiratory monitoring.

III. PULSE OXIMETRY

A. Background

In 1935, Matthes and Millikan discovered a technique that enabled them to evaluate oxygen saturation in vivo by transilluminating tissues. This discovery was advanced by Aoyagi in the mid-1970s with the discovery that by analyzing only those light absorbencies

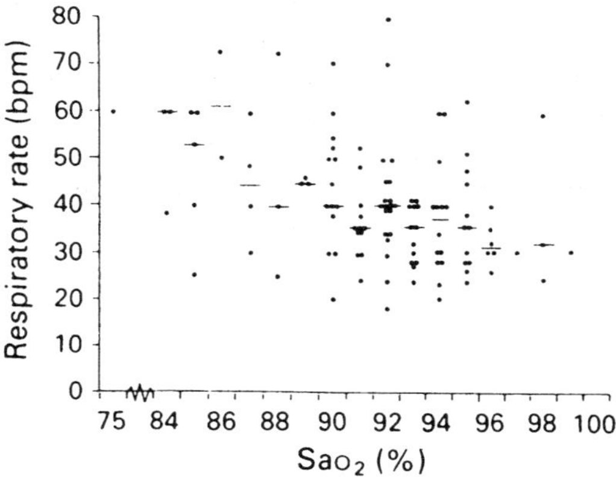

Figure 1 Variability between respiratory rate and Sa_{O_2} in pediatric asthma patients. The respiratory rate is shown along the vertical axis in breaths per minute and the percentage arterial oxygen saturation (Sa_{O_2}) is on the horizontal axis in pediatric patients with asthma. Respiratory rate does not appear to correlate with Sa_{O_2}. (Adapted from Ref. 5.)

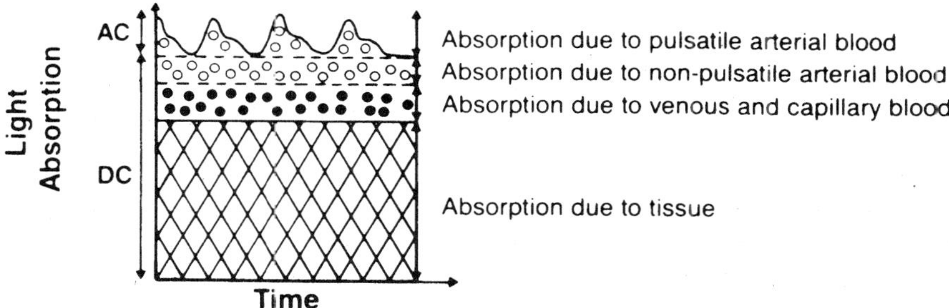

Figure 2 Tissue absorption in pulse oximetry. Pulse oximetry is based upon the changes of light absorption in living tissue during pulsatile flow. The AC signal is due to the pulsatile component of the arterial blood while the DC signal is composed of all the nonpulsatile absorbers in the tissue: nonpulsatile arterial blood, venous and capillary blood, and the other tissues. (Adapted from Ref. 9.)

that were pulsatile (Fig. 2), it was possible to evaluate arterial oxygen saturation quickly and easily. This discovery was refined by Wilber in the late 1970s to incorporate light emitting diodes and photodiodes making pulse oximeters the lightweight and maneuverable equipment currently in widespread use (9).

Pulse oximetry is based on the principle that human blood is made of four components of hemoglobin including oxyhemoglobin (HbO_2), reduced hemoblobin (HbR), methemoglobin (HbMet), and carboxyhemoglobin (HbCO). Each displays unique light absorbencies allowing one to transmit light in the red (680 nm) and infrared (940 nm) ranges through blood and then measure the relative attenuations of the wavelengths to determine the concentrations of each hemoglobin moiety (Fig. 3). This yields a fractional hemoglobin

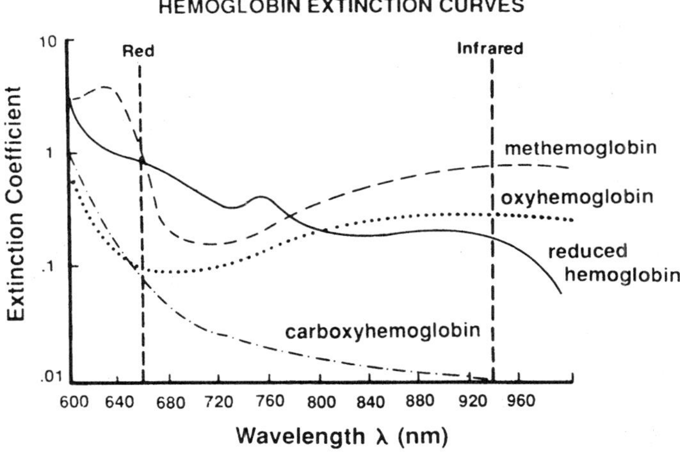

Figure 3 Light absorbance spectra of hemoglobin derivatives. Transmitted light absorbance spectra of four hemoglobin species: oxyhemoglobin, reduced (deoxy-) hemoglobin, carboxyhemoglobin, and methemoglobin. (Adapted from Ref. 9.)

saturation defined as:

$$\text{Fractional Hb Sat}\,(\text{Sa}\text{o}_2) = \frac{\text{HbO}_2}{\text{Total Hb}} \times 100 = \frac{\text{HbO}_2}{\text{HbO}_2 + \text{HbR} + \text{HbMet} + \text{HbCO}} \times 100$$

Most commercially available pulse oximeters evaluate the wavelength absorbencies of only HbO_2 and HbR and thus do not detect HbMet or HbCO, which may potentially erroneously elevate the arterial oxygen saturation (Sao_2) in those situations (i.e, poisonings) in which HbMet or HbCO may be present. In addition, inaccurate readings can be experienced in those conditions in which there is poor light transmission (motion, bright ambient light, intravenous dyes or nail polish) or in low blood-flow states as seen in hypotension (MAP < 35 mmHg), hypothermia $< 35°$C, vascular disease, or vasopressor therapy (9).

B. Clinical Applications

The most common use of pulse oximetry is simply as a tool to detect hypoxemia independent of the cause. The familiar ''beeping'' tone of the pulse oximeter has become ubiquitous in the emergency department (ED), intensive care unit (ICU), and operating rooms. The pulse oximeter alerts physicians and nurses to changes in the heart rate as well as arterial saturation by the rate and pitch of the tone. Additionally, pulse oximetry has been applied to monitor hyperoxia in premature neonates because elevations in Po_2 have been linked to retinopathy and retrolental fibroplasia (9).

C. Clinical Use in Asthma

Since the consequences of asthma should ultimately result in hypoxemia, it stands to reason that pulse oximetry would be a rational and effective manner of evaluation of asthmatics. However, due to the shape of the oxygen dissociation curve (Fig. 4), pulse oximetry does not necessarily reflect desaturation at a Pao_2 greater than 80 mmHg or in the presence of respiratory alkalosis due to hyperventilation (10). As a result, hypoxemia with airway obstruction may not be detectable by pulse oximetry during acute asthma exacerbations. Furthermore, because pulse oximetry is dependent on appropriate light transmission and blood flow, it is recommended by multiple researchers that pulse oximetry only be used in conjunction with clinical assessment and other modalities of evaluation (5,11–13).

Still, several studies support the role of arterial oxygen saturation in the evaluation of acute asthma. Carruthers and Harrison studied 89 adult patients with acute severe asthma admitted to a respiratory care unit and showed that asthmatics with an initial pulse oximeter Sao_2 reading of greater than 92% could be spared arterial blood gas evaluation because respiratory failure in these patients is extremely unlikely (14). However, those asthmatics with a pulse oximeter Sao_2 reading of less than 92% are at significant risk for experiencing respiratory failure and should receive arterial blood gas analysis and close observation (14).

Geelhoed and colleagues (13) studied 52 pediatric patients presenting to the ED with acute asthma. They found that an initial Sao_2 of greater than 91% was able to predict

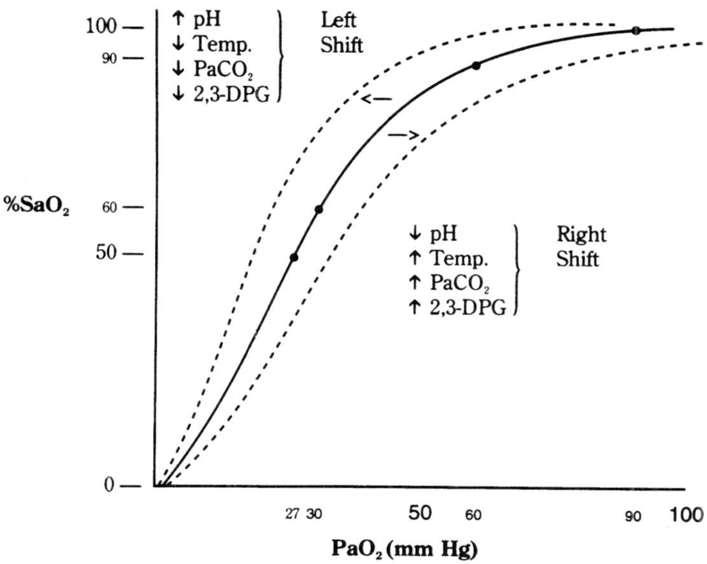

Figure 4 Oxyhemoglobin dissociation curve. The percentage of arterial oxygen saturation (%Sao_2) is shown on the vertical axis and the partial pressure of arterial oxygen (Pao_2) is shown on the horizontal axis in millimeters of mercury pressure (mmHg). A shift of the dissociation curve to the left is associated with a reduction in tissue oxygen availability and is caused by alkalosis (increased pH), hypothermia (decreased temperature), hyperventilation with hypocapnia (decreased $Paco_2$) and reductions in 2,3-diphosphoglycerate (decreased 2,3-DPG). Shift of the dissociation curve to the right is associated with increased tissue oxygen availability and is caused by acidosis (decreased pH), hyperthermia (increased temperature), hypercapnia (increased $Paco_2$), and increases in 2,3-diphosphoglycerate (increased 2,3-DPG).

high parent satisfaction with treatment and low rates of ED recidivism at five days (13). In addition, they demonstrated that the initial saturation is more predictive of outcome than is the overall change in Sao_2 with therapy in the ED (13).

Initial Sao_2 less than 91% has predicted a poor response to first line therapies in 75 pediatric patients admitted for asthma exacerbations (12). While the Sao_2 only weakly correlated with asthma severity score, the Sao_2 was found to be superior to standard clinical assessments in predicting the need for more aggressive interventions (12).

Milhatsch and colleagues (15) found that in 47 patients admitted for acute asthma exacerbations, Sao_2 readings did not recover as rapidly as PEFR measurements. The authors suggest that Sao_2 may better reflect the effects of uneven distribution of airway narrowing caused by inflammation. Interestingly, they also found that children younger than five years tended to recover Sao_2 faster with β-agonist therapy than did older children (15).

Indeed, another study suggests that Sao_2 may be a better predictor of patient outcome than PEFR. Geelhoed et al. found that Sao_2 was superior to PEFR in predicting relapse in pediatric patients discharged home from the ED (16).

IV. CAPNOGRAPHY

A. Background

Capnography, the measurement of respired CO_2, allows one to indirectly detect abnormalities of metabolism, circulation, and ventilation by measuring the output of CO_2 in expired gas (17). Capnography has been used for over 50 years with use of the earliest CO_2 analyzers were on submarines to detect dangerous buildup of CO_2 while on prolonged patrol during World War II (18). Modern developments have allowed capnographs to be adopted as standard monitoring devices during anesthesia.

While the level of CO_2 can be determined using either mass spectrometry or infrared absorption characteristics, infrared capnography is more practical for clinical use. Two forms of infrared capnography are currently in use (Fig. 5). ''Mainstream'' (or ''in-line'') capnography uses a sample chamber setup that is within the breathing circuit with a large diameter tube that allows for response times of < 0.5 sec. ''Sidestream'' infrared capnography uses a diverting system and a small diameter tube that is more prone to obstruction by secretions and water vapor condensation yielding a 2- to 3-sec transit time.

A normal capnogram is demonstrated in Figure 6 (19). The PQ segment represents initial expiration as rapidly exchanging alveolar gases mix with gas in the anatomic deadspace. In the alveolar plateau phase (QR segment), exchange of the remainder of gases slows as expiration concludes, representing predominantly gas exchange from uniformly ventilated alveoli. Finally, the capnogram returns to a baseline CO_2 level of zero during the initial stages of inspiration (RS segment).

B. Clinical Applications

Capnography is currently used in acute care medicine to assess endotracheal tube location and function after intubation (20). An esophageal intubation would yield an abnormally

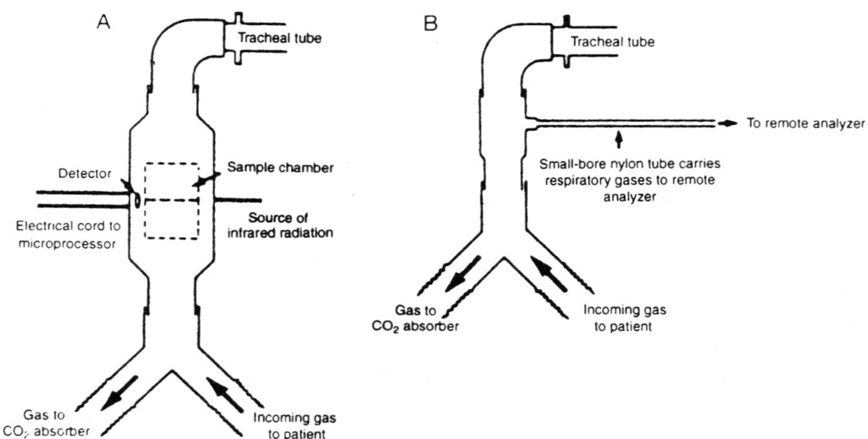

Figure 5 Capnographic analyzers. (A) The mainstream analyzer has the sample chamber within the breathing circuit as close to the patient's airway as possible. Most currently available infrared carbon dioxide (CO_2) analyzers are of this type. (B) The sidestream analyzer has a distant sample chamber. (Adapted from Ref. 20.)

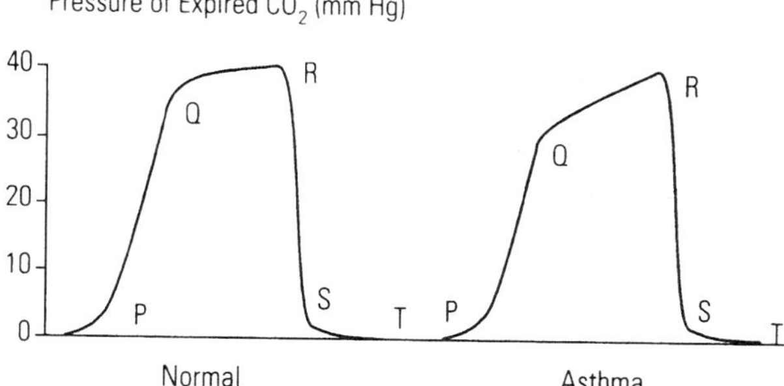

Figure 6 Capnogram of normal and asthmatic patients. The pressure of expired carbon dioxide (CO_2) in millimeters of mercury (mmHg) over time are shown for both normal and asthmatic conditions. P represents the onset of expiration. The PQ segment represents the mixing of dead space and alveolar gases exhibiting a rapid increase in expired CO_2. Segment QR is the plateau phase representing alveolar gas delivery. Point R is the end of expiration. Segment RS represents the beginning of inspiration and point T is the end of inspiration. In the asthmatic, the slope of the plateau phase (QR segment) is decreased when compared to a normal subject due to a prolongation of expiration. (Adapted from Ref. 19.)

low CO_2 output as the gastric space is continuous with ambient air. Kinks, cuff leaks, accidental extubation, and obstruction of the endotracheal tube would also be apparent. Adequacy of mechanical ventilation and weaning can likewise be evaluated. Because blood flow is required for elimination of CO_2, capnography serves as a tool to evaluate blood flow. Hemodynamic parameters can similarly be monitored including assessment of perfusion in cardiopulmonary resuscitation (CPR) and other low-blood-flow states such as shock (21). Finally, capnography is useful in establishing the end-tidal CO_2 (22), a measure of the maximum CO_2 concentration at the end of an expiratory cycle, which is helpful in evaluation of asthma as well as a variety of pulmonary disease states including sleep apnea (23).

C. Clinical Use in Asthma

Recent studies have demonstrated that bronchospasm, much like ARDS and pneumonia, produces a characteristic change in the capnogram (19). The ordinarily near-horizontal alveolar plateau phase (QR segment; Fig. 6) becomes more vertical in response to bronchospasm resulting in an increase in dco_2/dt (slope). This effect is due to more rapid emptying of the normal-resistance hyperventilated airways resulting in lower initial CO_2 concentrations. Bronchospasm then results in a delayed rise in CO_2 as gases from poorly ventilated alveoli empty. As a result, slope and the Q angle are increased (Fig. 6). This capnographic finding has been correlated to both FEV_1 (24) and PEFR (19) and the changes may precede clinical findings of bronchospasm (25).

You and colleagues measured the slope of the QR segment and compared it to usual spirometric measurements (FEV_1) in 21 control and 24 asthmatic pediatric patients. In asthmatic subjects, they found that the slope correlated with FEV_1 ($r = 0.83$) before and after inhalation of β-agonists (24).

Recently, our research group demonstrated that the end-tidal CO_2 correlated with PEFR in adult asthmatic patients in the ED both before and after β-agonist therapy (19).

Obtaining an expiratory capnogram in asthmatics has several advantages over spirometry (19). Capnography is noninvasive and is independent of height, age, and weight. Additionally, capnography is effort-independent. Spirometry requires an awake and cooperative subject and therefore necessitates obtaining the average of three successive trials. Small children and some elderly patients are often unable to understand or appropriately operate spirometric equipment. These patients, as well as individuals on mechanical ventilation can be evaluated using capnography, but not spirometry.

V. NEAR-INFRARED SPECTROSCOPY

A. Background

In 1977, Jobsis first described a near-infrared instrument capable of measuring oxyhemoglobin, reduced hemoglobin, and cytochrome a,a_3 redox state (26). Near-infrared spectroscopy (NIRS) offers the potential for noninvasive, continuous monitoring of tissue oxygen delivery and oxygen utilization (27–29). Similar to pulse oximetry and mixed venous oxygen saturation monitors, NIRS utilizes differences in light transmission and absorbance between oxyhemoglobin (HbO_2) and deoxyhemoglobin (HbR) to gauge the concentrations of those moieties (29). NIRS directs light of wavelengths 700–1000 nm into tissue via fiberoptic cable and the amount of reflected light is quantified. Trends in HbO_2, HbR, total hemoglobin (HbO_2 + HbR), tissue saturation of oxygen (StO_2) and the cytochrome a,a_3 are then determined. Thus, NIRS can be used as a direct monitor of tissue oxygen delivery. Because near-infrared wavelengths are longer than those of visible light, NIRS is well-transmitted through bone, muscle, and other tissue, allowing it to be utilized in evaluation of deeper visceral organs and cerebral blood flow (26).

In addition, NIRS can be used to detect the redox state of mitochondrial cytochrome a,a_3 (also known as cytochrome c oxidase). The cytochrome a,a_3 redox action accounts for over 90% of all cellular oxygen utilization (26). Normally, the a,a_3 redox state closely follows oxygen availability. With falling tissue oxygen tensions, the redox state reduces, and as oxygen tensions rise, the redox state oxidizes (30).

However, the redox state is also dependent upon the availability of high energy electrons within the electron transport chain (30,31). Almost all cellular substrates are converted by dehydrogenases to the high energy electron carriers, NADH and $FADH_2$, which are transported within the mitochondria to the electron transport chain (30). If electron transport is inhibited proximal to cytochrome a,a_3, then the redox state becomes oxidized. This decoupling of the redox state from oxygen availability may result in anomalous electron transport and could potentially lead to free radical formation and damage (32).

Direct NIRS monitoring of the coupling relationship between tissue oxygen availability and mitochondrial oxygen utilization may provide more direct insight into pathophysiological states and treatment strategies (31,33,34).

B. Clinical Applications

Potential clinical applications for NIRS are vast. At the present time, studies are underway to determine exactly for which conditions NIRS is best suited. Previous studies have used

NIRS to evaluated tissue oxygenation in the setting of ischemia of various anatomic structures, cerebral blood flow in the preterm infant, blood flow in peripheral musculature, and blood flow during cardiac bypass (35). Likewise, NIRS has been used to predict multiple organ failure in severely injured trauma patients (36,37). It has been further hypothesized that NIRS may be useful in delineating anatomical injury, for instance in intracerebral bleeds, and multiple recent studies have utilized NIRS in the evaluation of intracerebral blood flow in both adults and neonates.

C. Clinical Use in Asthma

Although further studies need to be performed, recent data suggest that NIRS may have practical applications to asthma. Recently, our research group has demonstrated that in nocturnal asthmatics, oxygen saturation has been demonstrated to drop in conjunction with a reduction in cytochrome a,a_3 redox state during an attack, suggesting that reductions in peripheral tissue oxygen delivery and cellular oxidation are both associated with bronchospasm (38). These peripheral changes were independent of changes in Sao_2 measured by pulse oximetry.

VI. OTHER TECHNOLOGIES

A. Transcutaneous ABG

When heated to a temperature between 40 and 45°C, the structural characteristics of the stratum corneum are modified, thus allowing oxygen to readily diffuse. Based upon this principle, transcutaneous oxygen monitors are able to approximate peripheral tissue Po_2 which follows the trend established by P_ao_2 and is a more representative measure of end-organ oxygenation than arterial Sao_2 (Fig. 4). As a flow-dependent parameter, transcutaneous Po_2 ($Ptco_2$) may be more useful than Pao_2 in the evaluation of tissue oxygenation (39).

Uses of $Ptco_2$ have included neonatal ICU monitoring of hyperoxia, multiorgan failure, anesthesia, and in-shock states (39). In the asthmatic, $Ptco_2$ has been found to correlate well with arterial oxygen values under a variety of conditions, most importantly assessing the efficacy of bronchodilator therapy (40). In addition, falls in $Ptco_2$ have been found to closely follow the deterioration found in obstructive airway disease in young children (41). To date, the bulk of the data on transcutaneous monitoring has involved neonates and very young children, therefore the generalizability to older populations is unknown.

B. Optodes

Optodes, or optical gas electrodes, provide continuous pH, Po_2, and Pco_2 measurements through the use of a fluorescent dye at the tip of an optical fiber (42). This fiber is connected to a light source that activates electrons to a higher energy state and measures decay as the electrons return to baseline. The photons emitted from these activated electrons from the dye are increased by CO_2 and H^+ and are decreased by O_2 via competitive inhibition (43). Since the photons are absorbed by the CO_2, H^+, and O_2 molecules, the dyes will emit fewer photons when higher quantities of those molecules are present (42). The primary advantage of optodes over conventional arterial blood gas (ABG) laboratory evaluation is cost and elimination of blood loss in repeated evaluation.

Potential uses of optodes include extracorporeal monitoring during acute resuscitations, surgery, ICU monitoring of mechanical or borderline ventilation, and other situations in which ABGs might be obtained repeatedly. Benefits and risks of invasive serial ABG analysis in the asthmatic patient is discussed elsewhere in this book (see Chapter 15). Repeated ABGs are more useful than single values in the evaluation of the asthmatic (2) and a noninvasive method of ABG analysis may prove useful in monitoring acute asthma attacks. This may be especially true in the younger asthmatic in which arterial needle sticks may be anxiety-provoking and could potentially lead to deterioration of the clinical state (2).

C. Conjunctival Po_2

Conjunctival monitoring of Po_2 ($Pcjo_2$) involves the attachment of a miniature Clark electrode to the inner surface of the palpebral conjunctiva. Unlike the transcutaneous Po_2 monitor, the conjunctival unit does not require the tissue to be heated to 40–45°C due to the small number of cells between the capillaries and the surface probe (29). Like $Ptco_2$ monitors, the $Pcjo_2$ monitor is related to cardiac output and reflects changes in regional blood flow from the carotid artery (29). It may prove useful as a minimally invasive measure of central organ oxygen delivery in patients with asthma.

VII. CONCLUSIONS

No single clinical or laboratory finding alone is predictive of the degree of obstruction that an asthmatic experiences (44). Thus, noninvasive assessment modalities must be used in combination with clinical signs and symptoms in order to evaluate and effectively treat patients with acute asthma. The noninvasive modalities discussed in this chapter may provide unique physiological information that could guide the therapeutic response in acute asthma (45).

REFERENCES

1. National Asthma Education Program. Guidelines for the Diagnosis and Mangement of Asthma. NIH publication No. 91-3042, Bethesda, MD, 1991.
2. Gayle MO, Kissoon N. Assessment of respiratory distress in the asthmatic child: When should we be concerned?, Pediatr Ann 1996; 25:128–135.
3. American Thoracic Society, Standardization of spirometry. Am Rev Respir Dis 1987; 136: 1285–1298.
4. Nowak RM, Pensler MI, Sarkar DD, et al. Comparison of peak expiratory flow and FEV_1 admission criteria for acute bronchial asthma, Ann Emerg Med 1982; 111:64–69.
5. O'Keefe PT. Pulse oximetry in acute asthma [letter], Arch Dis Child 1992; 67:567.
6. Bishop J, Nolan T. Pulse oximetry in acute asthma [comment], Arch Dis Child 1992; 67:567.
7. Martell JA, Lopez JG, Harker JE. Pulsus paradoxus in acute asthma in children, J Asthma 1992; 29:349–352.
8. Deegan PC, McNicholas WT. Continuous non-invasive monitoring of evolving acute severe asthma during sleep, Thorax 1994; 49:613–614.
9. Tremper KK, Barker SJ. Pulse oximetry, Anesthesiology 1989; 70:98–108.

10. American College of Surgeons Committee on Trauma, Shock, Advanced Trauma Life Support, Chicago, IL: American College of Surgeons, 1993, p. 106.
11. Bishop J, Nolan T. Pulse oximetry in acute asthma, Arch Dis Child 1991; 66:724–725.
12. Connett GJ, Lenney W. Use of pulse oximetry in the hospital management of acute asthma in childhood, Pediatr Pulmonol 1993; 15:345–349.
13. Geelhoed GC, Landau LI, LeSouef PN. Predictive value of oxygen saturation in emergency evaluation of asthmatic children, Br Med J 1988; 297:395–396.
14. Carruthers DM, Harrison BD. Arterial blood gas analysis or oxygen saturation in the assessment of acute asthma?, Thorax 1995; 50:186–188.
15. Mihatsch W, Geelhoed GC, Landau LI, LeSouef PN. Time course of change in oxygen saturation and peak expiratory flow in children admitted to hospital with acute asthma, Thorax 1990; 45:438–441.
16. Geelhoed GC, Landau LI, LeSouef PN. Oximetry and peak expiratory flow in assessment of acute childhood asthma, J Pediatr 1990; 117:907–909.
17. Tremper KK. Non invasive monitoring of oxygenation and ventilation. 40 years in development, West J Med 1992; 156:662–663.
18. Mogue LR, Rantalta B. Capnometers, J Clin Monit 1988; 4:115–121.
19. Yaron M, Padyk P, Hutsinpiller M, Cairns CB. Utility of the expiratory capnogram in the assessment of bronchospasm, Ann Emerg Med 1996; 28:403–407.
20. Stock MC. Capnography for adults. Crit Care Clin 1995; 1:219–232.
21. Szarflarski NL, Cohen NH. Use of capnography in critically ill adults, Heart Lung 1991; 20: 363–372.
22. Trillo G, von Planta M, Kette F. $ETCO_2$ monitoring during low flow states: clinical aims and limits, Resuscitation 1994; 27:1–8.
23. Magnan A, Philip-Joet F, Rey M, Reynaud M, Porri F, Arnaud A. End-tidal CO_2 analysis in sleep apnea syndrome, Chest 1993; 103:129–131.
24. You B, Mayeus D, Rkiek B, et al. Expiratory capnography in asthma: Perspectives in the use and monitoring in children, Rev Mal Respir 1992; 9:547–52.
25. Mayeux D, Vesppignani H, Kohler C, et al. Relations between sleep stages and asthma crisis: Continuous study of electroencephalography and capnography (letter), Presse Med 1988; 16: 697–698.
26. Jobsis FF. Noninvasive infrared monitoring of cerebral and myocardial oxygen sufficiency and circulatory parameters, Science 1977; 198:1264–1270.
27. Proctor HJ, Cairns C, Fillipo D, Jobsis FF. Near infrared spectrophotometry: potential role during intracranial pressure. Adv Exp Med Biol 1985; 191:863–71.
28. Wahr JA, Tremper KK, Samra S, et al. Near-infrared spectroscopy: theory and applications, J Cardiothorac Vasc Anesth 1996; 10:406–418.
29. Wahr JA, Tremper KK. Non invasive oxygen monitoring techniques. Crit Care Clin 1995; 11:199–217.
30. Chance B, Williams GR. The respiratory chain and oxidative phosphorylation, Adv Enzymol 1956; 17:65–134.
31. Cairns CB, Fillipo D, Palladino GW, Proctor HJ. Direct noninvasive assessment of brain metabolism during increased intracranial pressure: Potential therapeutic vistas. J Trauma 1986; 26:863–868.
32. Cairns CB, Wang J, Walther JM, Harken AH, Banerjee A. Ischemic preconditioning prevents cytochrome a,a_3 induced cellular oxidation during global ischemia, Circulation. 1996; 94(suppl)(8) 8:I-362–I-363.
33. Proctor HJ, Palladino GW, Cairns CB, Jobsis FF. An evaluation of perfluorochemical resuscitation after hypoxic hypotension, J Trauma 1983; 23:79–83.
34. Cairns CB, Fillipo D, Proctor HJ. A noninvasive method for monitoring the effects of increased intracranial pressure with near infrared spectrophotometry. Surg Gynecol Obstet 1985; 161: 145–148.

35. MacNab AJ, Gagnon RE. Near-infrared spectrophotometry data collection faults due to fiberoptic failure, Biomed Instrum Technol 1995; 29:405–409.
36. Moore FA, Haenel JB, Moore EE, Gallea BL, Ortner JP, Rose SJ, Cairns CB. Evidence for early supply independent mitochondrial dysfunction in patients developing multiple organ failure after trauma, J Trauma 1997; 42:532–536.
37. Moore FA, Haenel JB, Moore EE, Gallea BL, Ortner JP, Cairns CB. Early impaired oxygen consumption due to supply-independent mitochondrial dysfunction occurs in patients who develop MOF, Surg Forum 1995; 46:74–76.
38. Williams BT, Bell GR, Walther JM, Pak J, Martin RJ, Kraft M, Cairns CB. Nocturnal asthmatic patients show evidence of inflammation-induced decoupling of micochondrial oxidative metabolism. Academic Emerg Med 1998; 5:422.
39. Tremper KK, Barker SJ. Transcutaneous oxygen measurement: experimental studies and adult applications, Int Anesthesiol Clin 1987; 25:67–96.
40. Holmgren D, Sixt R. Transcutaneous and arterial blood gas monitoring during acute asthmatic symptoms in older children, Pediatr Pulmonol 1992; 14:80–84.
41. Wennergren G, Engstrom I, Bjure J. Transcutaneous oxygen and carbon dioxide levels and a clinical symptom scale for monitoring the acute asthmatic state in infants and young children, Acta Paediatr Scand 1986; 75:465–469.
42. Tremper KK, Barker SJ. The optode: next generation in blood gas measurement [editorial], Crit Care Med 1989; 17:481–482.
43. Shapiro BA. Intra-arterial and extra-arterial pH, PCO_2 and PO_2 monitors. Acta Anaesthesiol Scand 1995; 39:69–74.
44. Kelsen SG, Kelsen DP, Fleeger BF, Jones RC, Rodman T. Emergency room assessment and treatment of patients with acute asthma. Adequacy of the conventional approach, Am J Med 1978; 64:622–628.
45. Nowak RM, Hurd SS, Skobeloff EM, Taggart VS. Asthma research: future directions for emergency medicine. The NHLBI Asthma Working Group, Ann Emerg Med 1996; 27:244–249.

17

Fatal Asthma

Kim Guishard
The Brooklyn Hospital Center, member of New York–Presbyterian Hospitals, Weill Medical College of Cornell University, Brooklyn, and New York University School of Medicine, New York, New York

I. INTRODUCTION

We understand the disease process: near fatal and fatal asthma are now problems of physician communication and patient compliance.

A. Definitions

Fatal asthma: Patients that have succumbed to acute asthma.

Rapidly fatal asthma: Patients that have succumbed to acute asthma within three hours of the onset of symptoms.

Slowly fatal asthma: Patients that succumbed to acute asthma greater than 3 hr after the onset of symptoms.

Near fatal asthma: An acute asthma attack that results with respiratory arrest or $Paco_2$ greater than 50 mmHg (6.7 pka).

B. History

At the turn of the century, nearly fatal and fatal asthma were felt not to exist (1). A common belief was that fatal asthma was a real but rare occurrence (2). There has been a steady increase in mortal asthma since its nadir in 1977 (3,4). Despite better knowledge of the pathophysiology of acute asthma, mortality incidence continues to increase (5). A greater understanding of the multiple processes involved in patients with near fatal asthma is needed. Environmental (6), socioeconomical (7), and other risk factors (8), as well as access to health care all have a role in the anatomy of fatal asthma (9). The most sobering and disturbing fact is that most deaths from asthma are preventable (10). Asthma mortality is frequently the result of patient noncompliance and not failure of therapy. If improvement can be made in patient compliance with medication and the physician's ability to communicate with their patients, then asthma mortality should decrease. Subsequently, effective therapeutic modalities for asthma will be discussed. Unfortunately, suboptimal implementation of these regimens has had significant impact on the increase in asthma mortality.

II. INCIDENCE

Fatal asthma affects African-Americans more commonly than Hispanics, who are affected more frequently than Caucasians (11). African-Americans predilection for fatal asthma may be explained by increased genetic atopy, which is the strongest marker for asthma. A more plausible explanation for the increased incidents found in African-Americans can be better explained in socioeconomic terms. The less-affluent have higher incidences of asthma (12). Their access to health care is limited and exposure to antigens is higher. A larger number of women die from asthma than men. This might be attributable to diurnal hormonal variation. Skobeloff et al. (13) found women to be more susceptible to asthma just prior to and during menses. The exact mechanism that progesterone and estrogen have in near fatal asthma remains to be clarified.

Fatal asthma in children, up to 14 years old had the greatest increase in incidence from 1980 to 1989 than any other age group (5). Greater allergen exposure might be a plausible explanation for the increase in mortality found in this young age group. O'Hallaren et al. (14) found young asthmatics that tested positive for *Alternaria alternata*, a commonly found spore, had a 200-fold increase in respiratory arrest when compared to asthmatics that tested negative. Deaths from the spores were seasonal, occurring mostly in June to November. In New York City, deaths occur most frequently in the winter months. Death from asthma seems to be an urban problem (see Chapter 12). New York City and Chicago account for 21% of the national death rate from asthma (3). City air pollution could be the cause of the increase in urban fatal asthma; this, however, does not seem to be the case. Lang and Polansky (7) showed decreasing concentrations of the outdoor air pollutants, ozone, carbon monoxide, nitrogen dioxide, particulate matter, and sulfur dioxide in Philadelphia from 1965 to 1990 despite a steady increase in asthma mortality. The outdoor air pollutants that Lang and Polansky studied are probably not the cause of the increased incidents of near-fatal asthma. Indoor pollutants seem to be associated with near-fatal asthma (15). Within the indoor environment can be cockroaches and/or tiny insects termed bed mites. Increased concentration of mites in the midwest (16) and cockroach allergens in the northeast (17,18) have been noted to cause asthma.

A. Who Are the Patients That Develop Near-Fatal Asthma?

Most patients that succumb to asthma are outside or en route to the hospital. Death from acute asthma tends to occur at night and within 24 hr of the onset of symptoms. Mortality from asthma is more frequent among urban residents (Table 1). In 1952, 76 cases of fatal

Table 1 Fatal Asthma

Who	Black	$>$	Hispanic	$>$	Whites
Where	Inner City	$>$	Suburbs		
When	Night	$>$	Day		
Mortality rate	15–34	$>$	35 $>$		

asthma were recorded nationally (19). In 1991, 5102 deaths from asthma were reported (3). The increase in asthma fatality has prompted studies to identify patients that are at risk for fatal asthma. Many of these patients had prior episodes of near-fatal asthma.

B. Slow vs. Rapid Onset Asthma

Recently, patients have been grouped into two categories; slow and rapid near-fatal asthma (20). Patients with slow near-fatal asthma are more refractory to treatment. Their deaths are more avoidable than patients with rapid near-fatal asthma. In slow near-fatal asthma, symptoms occur over days, whereas in rapid near-fatal asthmatics, severe symptoms develop within hours.

Kesten et al. (21) studied patients with near-fatal asthma. He found no difference between patients with near-fatal asthma and hospitalized patients with less severe asthma. Others have found real differences between patients with near fatal asthma and mild asthmatics (22–23). Patients with potentially fatal asthma are 300 times more likely to die from asthma than asthmatics with less severe disease (24). Death rates among hospitalized patients with near-fatal asthma varied from 0 to 16.5% during their hospitalization (25). Hospitals' death rate from acute asthma vary. The wide range in death rates between hospitals is probably attributable to the varying degree of asthma severity in the patient population that they serve. There is also interhospital variation in the level of care of an acute asthmatic. These differences may also contribute to the wide range in death rates for patients hospitalized with acute asthma. Out-of-hospital death rates of patients with nearly fatal asthma over a study period of 6 yr were as high as 41% (26).

III. PATHOPHYSIOLOGY

A. Fatal Asthma

The pathology of near-fatal and fatal asthma are the same. With the progression of the attack, inflammation and mucous plugging become more prominent. There are three major components involved in asthma: airway hyperreactivity, bronchial obstruction, and inflammation (27–29). Airway hyperreactivity and bronchospasm occurred early on in the course of acute asthma. The early asthma response (EAR) is easily reversed by β_2-agonists. As patients progress from bronchospasm to inflammation, response to therapy with β_2-agonists and other treatments becomes blunted. Early pharmacological interventions will help to stop the cascade of cellular events, which progress from EAR to late asthma response (LAR). Patients with rapid-onset asthma die from asphyxiation. Sur et al. (30,31) found patients with rapidly fatal asthma (died within 2.5 hr) to be distinctively different from patients that died greater than 2.5 hr after manifestation of their symptoms. Autopsy showed patients with rapidly fatal asthma had a neutrophil cellular predominance. Patients with slow onset had eosinophil predominance. These latter patients died from mucous plugging, resulting in suffocation. These data might suggest the existence of two distinct entities, or more plausibly, that we are viewing the same process during different stages of the cellular and molecular cascade of events.

B. Near-Fatal Asthma

Wasserfallen et al. (20) studied rapid near-fatal asthma in patients whose attacks lasted less than 3 hr before endotracheal intubation. They were more hypercapnic on presentation than the slow-onset near-fatal asthmatic. The patients' duration on mechanical ventilation was reduced and their hypercapnia was more readily reversed in rapid-onset asthma. Kallenbach et al. (32) also found a positive correlation between the duration of the acute attack and the duration of mechanical ventilation. The more acute attacks had higher risks of a near fatality but were more readily reversed into stable asthma (Fig. 1). No serious cardiac arrhythmias were found during the resuscitation. Therefore, deaths from early and late onset asthma were not due to medication induced arrhythmias (32). Asthmatics die from suffocation and asphyxiation. Deaths are more avoidable in slow-onset asthma possibly because the patient has more time to seek medical intervention.

C. Nocturnal Asthma

Deaths from asthma occur mostly at night. The pathophysiological mechanism for nocturnal asthma has been elucidated (33) (see Chapter 11). Endogenous steroids and catecholamines are at their lowest point during the evening and early morning hours. The vagal influences have maximal activities during these hours. Low levels of endogenous steroids and catecholamines, increased airway hyperresponsiveness, and vagal activity are ideal conditions to facilitate bronchospasm and nocturnal asthma.

IV. RISK FACTORS

There are five major categories in which risk factors can be placed. They include the patient's past medical history, behavioral dysfunction, economic status, physician factors, and the milieu in which the patient lives (Fig. 2).

A. Past Medical History

Past medical history can help physicians recognize some of the patients at risk for fatal asthma. Two of the best indicators that a patient has suffered near-fatal asthma and is at risk for fatal asthma are (1) their history of prior endotracheal intubations and (2) admissions to the hospital within the previous 12 months (34). More accurate methods of identifying patients that are in risk for fatal asthma are needed. Emergency physicians can easily and

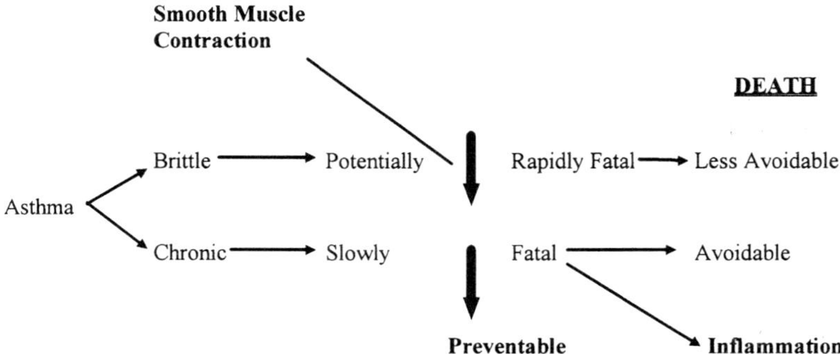

Figure 1 Fatal asthma.

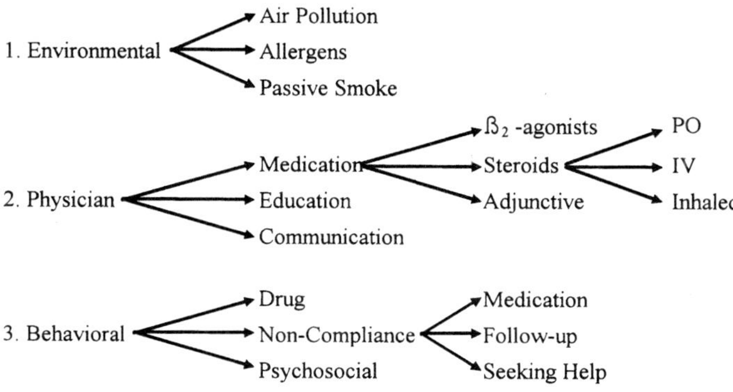

Figure 2 Near-fatal/fatal asthma: risk factors.

quickly identify some of the patients that are at an increased risk of dying from asthma by just obtaining the aforementioned two historical facts. Other risk factors, active smoking, history of atopy, and low economic status are less predictive of near-fatal asthma (discussed below) (35).

B. Behavior

Profound emotional upsets and psychosocial problems have been linked to fatal asthma (36). Levenson et al. (37) also found that on autopsy 31% of the patients dying from asthma in Chicago had traces of recreational drugs. The most common substance of abuse was alcohol.

Many patients overly rely on their medication, which can result in delays in seeking medical attention. Other patients may understand the instructions on how to use their medication, but they may not believe that the medication actually helped to improve their wheezing. A salient reason that patients do not use steroid inhalers is that these inhalers do not provide immediate relief from their breathlessness, so the inhaler is perceived as ineffective. Some patients are habitually noncompliant. Clearly, if an asthmatic has lost, refuses, or minimizes use of the β_2 inhaler, then severe bronchospasm and even death may ensue. Treating patients with potentially fatal asthma is complicated by many problems that are not reconcilable by merely manipulating medications.

C. Socioeconomics

Low socioeconomic status may be more of a risk factor for near-fatal and fatal asthma than ethnicity (38). Less-affluent patients are exposed to more allergens, have less access to health care, and are less likely to be seen by the same physician on a regular basis.

D. The Physician

The physician's ability to communicate with a patient is more important in the outpatient setting than during the patients' inpatient stays. During hospitalization, the physician's orders are acted upon by the nurse and are less patient dependent. In an outpatient, setting the physician's orders become only recommendations that are now made to the patients. Compliance is now entirely patient dependent. The patient's level of compliance is affected, in part, by the physicians' ability to communicate with them concerning the ''when and why'' of the medications they are supposed to use.

Most of the care given to the asthmatics is in an outpatient setting. Some of the most important changes in their regimens occur in the acute outpatient setting of the emergency department (ED). During this time, it is important for the emergency physician to communicate with the patient so that the patient can understand the changes in their medication regimen that are being recommended because of their acute presentation with bronchospasm. Making arrangements for follow-up care is a necessity. Ninety-one percent of relapses occur even before the patients see their primary care physician (39).

E. Environment

Outdoor (6), indoor (40), and occupational pollutants all have had a causative link to fatal asthma. Outdoor pollutants have seasonal variations that can be attributed to multiple allergens and pollen. Seasonal and weather changes can precipitate acute asthma attacks. Deaths in patients less than 35 yr occur between June and August, the time period that ED visits for acute asthma are lowest. In the elderly, mortality is most frequent from December through February (5). Indoor pollutants, cigarette smoke, and mite and cockroach allergens have also contributed to fatal-asthma death rates.

V. MEDICATION

A. β_2-Agonists

β_2-agonists are the rescue medications of choice for acute asthma. There has been much debate as to whether these medications were the treatment or the cause of fatal asthma (41,42). Greater use of β_2-agonists are associated with asthma fatalities, because the patients that use them have more severe asthma. Whitelow (43) aptly stated that we give more medications to the most acutely ill patient, not less. Purported mechanisms by which β_2-agonists could exert their direct toxic effects include malignant arrythmias (44), paradoxic bronchospasm (45), and possible inhibition of anti-inflammatory (46) effects. Wanner (47) and Sears (48) have presented excellent arguments concerning the use of scheduled versus PRN β_2-agonist use. β_2-agonists were once thought to be the cause of increasing asthma mortality. The patients that died from asthma were found to use a more potent β_2-agonist, e.g., fenoterol; the larger dosages were also thought to have a causal relationship with asthma deaths. The general consensus presently is that sicker asthmatics use β_2 agonist inhalers more frequently and that the greater use of β_2-agonist inhalers is not causing fatal asthma but only a manifestation of the severity of the patient's disease.

It is possible that there is a small subset of patients with fatal and near-fatal asthma that are sensitive to β_2-agonists. Robin and Lewiston (49) described healthy patients that died in seconds to minutes after using β_2-agonists prior to being apparently well. Thus there seemed to be a small subset of asthmatics that were at risk for β_2-agonist–induced sudden death. This group might be identified by electrocardiographic screening for β_2-agonist induced QT prolongation (50). Screening the 10 million asthmatics for QT prolongation would be costly. β_2-agonist toxicity alone cannot explain the increased incidence of asthma mortality since the nadir in 1977. In New Zealand during the 1980s, asthma mortality fell as β_2-agonist metered dose inhaler (MDI) consumption increased. In England, prescription usage of MDI tripled without a corresponding increase in mortality (51). No correlation has been found between inhaled β_2-agonists and mortality in the United States.

The increase in asthma mortality cannot be solely or partially explained by β_2-agonist toxicity. Perhaps some of these patients that succumbed to asthma after apparent wellness died from rapidly fatal asthma, which is primarily a respiratory event.

B. Steroids

Steroids are recognized as the most important medication in treating airway inflammation in asthmatics. The earliest beneficial effect takes 6 hr (52). In the ED, steroids should be given immediately to expedite the onset of therapeutic effects. The efficacy of inhaled corticosteroids in treating newly detected (53), stable, and mild asthma (54) has been proven. Ernest et al. (55) found patients that were dispensed one or more steroid inhalers had a statistically significant decrease in near-fatal and fatal asthma. Littenberg et al. (56) showed a 60% reduction in admission for patients given 125 mg of intravenous methylprednisolone. Interestingly, there was no statistical difference in objective data, such as peak expiratory flow rate (PEFR), between the groups of patients that did and those that did not receive the steroids. Nevertheless, the current standard of care in emergency medicine is to give 125 mg of methylprednisolone to acute asthmatics (see Chapter 22). The cardinal feature of late asthma response is inflammation. Deaths due to late asthma are caused by suffocation that is secondary to mucous plugging. The mucous plugs are cellular debris caused by the inflammatory reaction. Decreasing the inflammatory response will help to abate plug formation. The remaining plugs are coughed up by the patient, phagocytized and reabsorbed. Glucocorticoids need to be prescribed to all ED presentations of near-fatal asthma, providing that there is no contraindication to their use.

C. Magnesium

Magnesium, a bronchodilator, is involved in over 350 enzymatic reactions. Magnesium is effective in treating children (57) and severe asthmatics, as defined by an FEV_1 of $< 25\%$ of predicted on presentation to the ED (58) (see Chapter 24). The risk–benefit ratio is low, in that there are no side effects to using magnesium in the therapeutic dose of 2 g over 30 min. Intravenous magnesium may be useful in aborting fatal asthma, converting it to near-fatal asthma.

VI. EDUCATION

Question: When are the best and worst asthma treatment regimens equal? When is the medication regimen prescribed by the best physician equal to that prescribed by the worst physician?

Answer: When the ''rate-limiting step'' for the cascade of events leading to successful treatment is the noncompliance of the patient, especially when this noncompliance is due to a lack of knowledge of their disease and medications.

The above exchange illustrates that the medication prescribed by physicians can only be effective if the patient takes the medication. Increasing patient adherence is of critical importance, especially in the near fatal asthmatic whose nonadherence may result in death. Many therapeutic protocols to treat the asthmatic patient have been developed (59,60). What remains elusive is improving the communication between the physician and the asthmatic patient. Nonadherence to these therapeutic protocols have been commonplace. Noncompliance both behaviorally and with medication regimens has ranged from 30 to 70% (61,62). Behaviorally noncompliant patients may use recreational substances that further exacerbate delays in their seeking health care. Other patients may believe their medications have no effect on their disease. Noncompliance with medication can vary from nonusage, to delays in taking them, to a lack of knowledge about how to modify and vary therapeutic regimens (63). The noncompliant patient increases health care expenditures. In the last 10 years there has been a marked change in both our knowledge of asthma and the medical armamentarium that can be used to combat the disease. With the many changes, one principle has remained the same and in fact become more apparent. The physician/patient relationship is of paramount importance. There are levels of achievement that patients have to reach in order to really understand their disease. The first level must be physician/patient communication. Emergency physicians must be good communicators. The episodic patient encounter in the ED requires a physician to develop rapid rapport with patients. The patient needs to understand the instructions concerning how and when to take each medication and their disease process. Asthmatics also need general information concerning their disease; the nature of bronchospasm and inflammation needs explanation for the lay person. Doctors should ensure that the patient not only comprehends the instructions but retains them and understands how to implement the self-evaluation and treatment protocols (Fig. 3). Over 50% of asthmatics use the ED as their source of primary care when they have a problem with their asthma. For acute asthma, emergency physicians have been thrust into the role of a primary care physician (PCP). All PCPs should be excellent communicators to engender an excellent relationship between the physician and the patient (see Chapter 5).

VII. LOCATION

Deaths from asthma occur in two settings: hospitalized and nonhospitalized (Fig. 4).

A. In the Hospital

Slightly less than 50% of all deaths from asthma occurred in the hospital (64).

1. *Peak Expiratory Flow Rate*

Hetzel et al. (65) published an interesting study in which consecutive asthma hospital admissions were reviewed. The more severe asthmatics were managed in a special care area. The mild asthmatics were admitted to the wards. Nine of the patients admitted to the wards suffered respiratory arrest; three of them died. One patient in the special care unit required ventilatory support. The patients admitted to the wards did not have severe asthma (as defined by PEFR $>$ 100 L/min, pulse rate $<$ 120, and pulsus paradoxus $<$ 20 mmHg). They found that the risk of respiratory arrest and sudden deaths was not related to the severity of the initial attack but related more to the presence of excessive diurnal

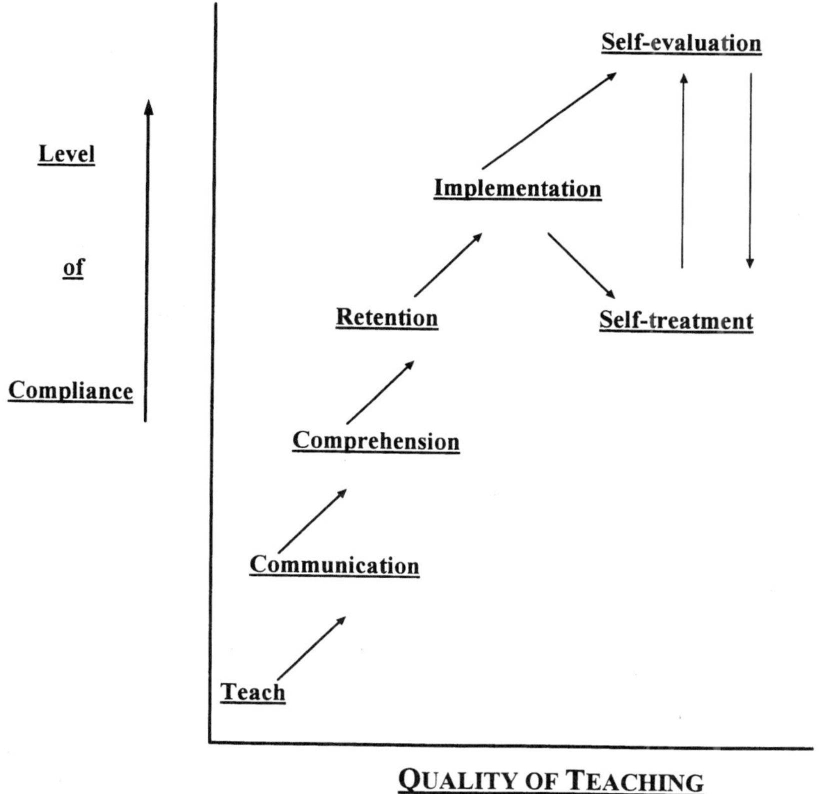

Figure 3 Compliance equation.

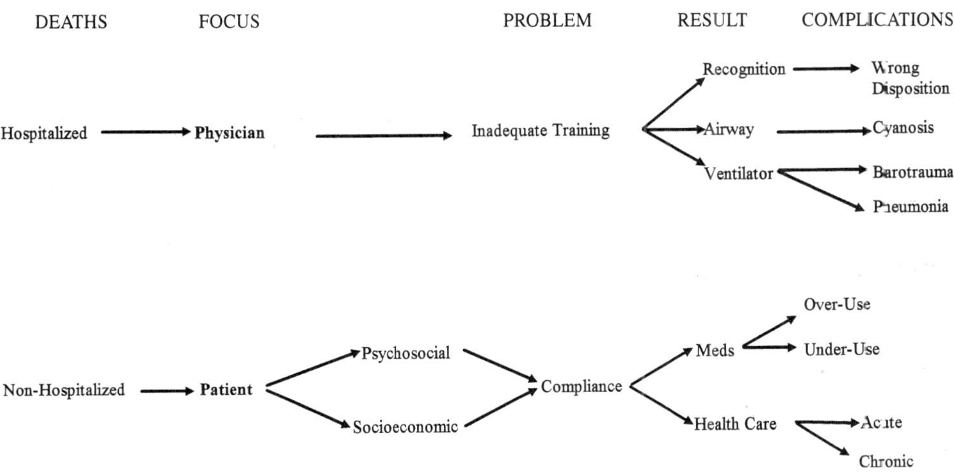

Figure 4 Problem identification schematic for fatal asthma.

variations in PEFR. Measurements of PEFR variations might help to reduce hospital asthma death rates. Some asthmatic deaths result from the physician's failure to recognize the severity of the attack, complications from ventilatory support, or an inability to secure the patient's airway (66,67) (see Chapters 26 and 30).

2. Physician Training

Asthma morbidity and mortality could be significantly decreased by training physicians to reduce errors of commission and omission. Severe asthmatics should be placed in monitored settings, so that any deterioration in their respiratory status could be rapidly recognized and treated (see Chapter 31). Barotrauma can be avoided by hypoventilating patients on mechanical ventilation (25). Prompt use of antibiotics should be encouraged if pneumonia is present.

B. Nonhospital

The majority of deaths from asthma occur in a nonhospital setting. These deaths can be decreased by better educating the patient about acute asthma. Socioeconomic status has been documented as a risk factor for fatal asthma. Psychological characteristics have also been found. Psychological disturbances in children that have been identified are depression, adjustment problems, disregard for symptoms of asthma and suicidal ideation (68). The manifestations of psychological disturbances in the adults varies. One example is recreational drug use (37). There are many barriers that are obstacles to the patients' understanding what the physician is trying to communicate. They can range from language barriers, the patient's inability to understand the physician's medical terminology; the patient's nonretention of information, and the physician's time constraints limiting the physicians' ability to educate the patient. Emphasis must be placed on training physicians to better communicate with their patients. "It is difficult to avoid the conclusion that improved education of both patients and physicians is needed" (68) (Table 2).

VIII. PREVENTION

The more things change the more they stay the same.

Our knowledge base about asthma is constantly changing and growing. With this growth in knowledge, important aspects of asthmatics care have remained unchanged. In the late 1950s, the adverse effects of overly aggressive use of sedatives became apparent. In England and Wales during the 1960s, an increased incidence of fatal asthma was noted (69). At that time, it was felt to be caused by excessive use of β_2-agonists. In the early 1980s, Sly (70) and Paulozzi et al. (71) found asthma deaths to be increasing. Some be-

Table 2 Barriers to Patient Communication

Patient	Physician
1. Lack of comprehension	1. Time constraints
2. Lack of retention	2. Teaching skills
3. Language barrier (natural tongue)	3. Language barrier (terminology)

lieved the increased death might be caused by overuse of asthma medication. β_2-agonists again were thought to increase deaths by the arrhythmogenic effects. In the 1990s, Kallenbach et al. (32) helped to disprove the hypothesis that β_2-agonists induced cardiac arrhythmias. Now it is believed that β_2-agonists increase fatal asthma by their indirect effect of "lulling" the patient into a false sense of security, thereby delaying when the asthmatic would seek medical attention.

Today the medications that are debated have changed—we now are focusing on the therapeutic effects of glucocorticoids—but the debate is the same: is the medication, in this instance steroids being under- or overutilized? In the 1980s, the primacy and importance of the inflammatory response found in asthma was reported, and by the early 1990s the underutilization of glucocorticoids was publicized and increased usage advocated. Presently the debate on overutilization of steroids has begun (72). Over the last 40 years, discussion of asthma mortality and morbidity has concerned excessive utilization of sedatives and β_2-agonists to glucocorticoids. But one feature has remained constant and is becoming more apparent: preventive measures are of great importance. The merits of prevention were never in doubt, but the emphasis placed on increasing prevention has been suboptimal. We have gone full circle and rediscovered what we all ready knew, that "the focus should remain on prevention" (73). We should not concentrate our efforts in treating but instead on preventing the asthma attack by educating the patient about their disease. In the ED the focus at the time of discharge should be more education of the patient rather than manipulating their medications.

IX. THE FUTURE

A. Therapeutics

Steroids should be used liberally, especially in patients that have experienced near-fatal asthma. The emergency physician must be aggressive in prescribing steroids to the patients that are being discharged. Hartert and colleagues' hospital-based study showed that monitoring and use of steroids was suboptimal.

1. Age Specific. Some treatments might be better suited for different age groups. Ipratropium might be more efficaciously used in older patients.

2. Hospital Specific. Slightly less than half of the patients who succumb to asthma are in a hospital environment. Each hospital must analyze how they can improve health care delivery to their asthmatic patients (75). Deaths from asthma are preventable and hospital-specific policies, such as community education, timely and "physician-specific" prompt referrals, will bring about a greater reduction in asthma fatalities. Continuous nebulization might be beneficial in EDs, where health care providers are not readily available to give nebulization treatments in a timely fashion.

B. Delivery

1. Age Specific. The adolescent has specific problems that should be addressed; adjustment reactions and difficulties with the family unit are but a few. Adults specifically should have the problem of recreational drug use addressed. Smoking cessation programs for the asthmatic smoker should be beneficial.

2. Hospital Specific. Hospital-specific policies will be effective in decreasing inpatient and outpatient hospital fatalities. For example, some hospitals might find it more

cost effective to dispense prednisone rather than giving prescriptions that the patient might not have filled.

3. Patient Recognition. The patient at risk for fatal asthma should be identified and every attempt should be made to avoid the occurrence of a mortal event. A comprehensive program to increase communication, retention, and implementation of treatment modalities should be instituted in all fatally prone patients.

There is no one cure that will singularly decrease asthma fatalities. A concerned attempt to address the multifactorial processes that are involved in near-fatal and fatal asthma should be undertaken. Improvement physician communication, patient education, allergen avoidance, and therapeutic protocols and a more aggressive use of steroids should be undertaken to bring about a decrease in asthma.

X. SUMMARY

Fatal asthma has evolved from a nonexistent occurrence to an uncommon event. There is no single cause that can be attributed to the increase in asthma mortality, but instead multiple causal relationships that are interwoven. Patient behavior, social milieu, airborne pollutants, and the physician's communication skills and ability to evaluate the patient form complex relationships that can potentiate or attenuate the risks for both fatal and near-fatal asthma. Emphasis should be placed on encouraging the generous use of both inhaled and oral steroids. The efficacy of glucocorticoids in reducing asthma mortality has been proven. Magnesium used on the pediatric population is especially effective (57), its utility in the severe asthmatic adult with $FEV_1 < 25\%$ predicted has been established (58). β_2-agonists have not increased the incidence of fatal asthma. They should be used as needed and not on a regular set time basis. Future emphasis will shift from stressing the manipulation of therapeutic modalities to concerted efforts to make the physicians better able to communicate with their patients and to enhance patient understanding and increase compliance of the medication regimen. The emphasis should be focused more on the *patients* than on their *medications!*

REFERENCES

1. Osler W. The Principles And Practice Of Medicine, 4th Ed., Edinburgh, Scotland: Pentland, 1901.
2. Wobig EK, Rosen P. Death from asthma: rare but real. J Emerg Med 1996; 14:233–240.
3. Robin ED. Risk benefit analysis in chest medicine. Chest 1988; 93:614–618.
4. Asthma: United States, 1982–1992. MMWR 1995; 43:952–955.
5. Weiss KB. Seasonal trends in US asthma hospitalizations and mortality. JAMA 1991; 263: 2323–2328.
6. Population at risk from air pollution. United States 1991. MMWR 1993; 42:301–304.
7. Lang DM, Polansky M. Patterns of asthma mortality in Philadelphia from 1968 to 1991. N Engl J Med 1994; 331:1542–1546.
8. Strunk RC. Identification of the fatality-prone subject with asthma. J Allergy Clin Immunol 1989; 83:477–485.
9. McFadden ER Jr. Fatal and near-fatal asthma. N Engl J Med 1991; 324:409–410.
10. British Thoracic Association. Death from asthma in two regions in England. Br Med J 1982; 285:1251–1255.

11. Carr W, Zeitel L, Weiss K. Variations in asthma hospitalization and deaths in New York City. Am J Public Health 1994; 82:59–69.
12. Pappas G, Queen S, Hadden W, Fisher G. The increasing disparity in mortality between socio-economic groups in the United States, 1960 and 1986. N Engl J Med 1993; 329:103–109.
13. Skobeloff EM, Spivey WH, Silverman R, et al. The effect of menstrual cycle in asthma presentations in the emergency department. Arch Int Med 1996; 156:1837–1840.
14. O'Hollaren MT, Yunginer JW, Offord KP, et al. Exposure to an aeroallergen as a possible precipitating factor in respiratory arrest in young patients with asthma. N Engl J Med 1991; 324:285–288.
15. Gelber LE, Setter LH, Bouzoukis JK, et al. Sensitization and exposure to indoor allergens as risks factors for asthma among patients presenting to hospital. Am Rev Res Dis 1993; 147: 573–578.
16. Platts-Mills TA. Dust and mite allergens and asthma—a world wide problem. J Allergy Clin Immun 1989; 83:416–427.
17. Calls RS, Smith TF, Morris E, et al. Risk factors for asthma in inner city children. J Pediatr 1992; 121:862–866.
18. Kang BC, Wu CW, Johnson J. Characteristics and diagnosis of cockroach sensitive bronchial asthma. Ann Allergy 1992; 68:237–244.
19. Bullen SS Sr. Correlation of clinical and autopsy findings in 176 cases of asthma. J Allergy 1952; 23:193–203.
20. Wasserfallen J, Schaller M, Feihl F, et al. Sudden asphyxic asthma: A Distinct Entity? Am Rev Respir Dis 1990; 142:108–111.
21. Kesten S, Chew R, Hanania NA. Health-care utilization after near-fatal asthma. Chest 1995; 107:1564–1569.
22. Molfino NA, Nannini AN, Matelli A, et al. Respiratory arrest in near-fatal asthma. N Engl J Med 1991; 99:358–362.
23. Barriot P, Riou B. Prevention of Fatal Asthma. Chest 1987; 92:460–466.
24. Vital statistics of the United States, U.S. Departments of Health, Education and Welfare, National Center for Health Statistics, Public Health Services, Hyattsville, Maryland, 1974–1991.
25. Pacht ER, Lingo S, St. John RC. Clinical features, management, and outcome of patients with severe asthma admitted to the intensive care unit. J Asthma 1995; 32:375–377.
26. Marquette CH, Saulvier F, Leroy O, et al. Long-term Prognosis of Near-Fatal Asthma: A 6-Year Follow-Up Study of 145 Asthmatic Patients Who Underwent Mechanical Ventilation for a Near-fatal Attack of Asthma. Am Rev Respir Dis 1992; 146:76–81.
27. Kamp D. Physiologic evaluation of asthma. Chest 1992; 101:396S–399S.
28. Jagoda A, Shepard SM, Spevitz A, et al. Refractory asthma, part 1: epidemiology, pathophysiology, pharmacological interventions. Ann Emerg Med 1997; 29:262–271.
29. Reid LM. The presence or absence of bronchial mucus in fatal asthma. J Allergy Clin Immunol 1987; 80(part 2):415–416.
30. Sur S, Crotty TB, Kephard GM, et al. Sudden-onset fatal asthma: A distinct entity with few eosinophils and relatively more neutrophils in the airway submucosa. Am Rev Respir Dis 1993; 148:713–719.
31. Azzawi M, Johnston PW, Majumdar S, et al. T Lymphocytes and activated eosinophils in airway mucosa in fatal asthma and cystic fibrosis. Am Rev Respir Dis 1992; 145:1477–1482.
32. Kallenbach JM, Frankel AH, Lapinsky SE, et al. Determinants of near fatality in acute severe asthma. Am J Med 1993; 95:265–272.
33. Barnes PJ, FitzGerald G, Brown M, et al. Nocturnal asthma and changes in circulating epinephrine, histamine, and cortisol. N Engl J Med 1980; 303:263–267.
34. Crane J, Pearce N, Burgess C, et al. Markers of risk of re-admission in the 12 months following a hospital admission for asthma. Int J Epidemiol 1992; 21:737–744.
35. Leson S, Gershwin ME. Risk factors for asthmatic patients requiring intubation. III. Observations in young adults. J Asthma 1996; 33:27–35.

36. Tough CS, Green FY, Paul JE, et al. Sudden death from asthma in 108 children and young adults. J Asthma 1996; 33:179–188.
37. Levenson T, Greenberger PA, Donoghue ER., et al. Asthma deaths confounded by substance abuse. An assessment of fatal asthma. Chest 1996; 110:604–610.
38. Schwartz E, Kotia VY, Rivo M, et al. Black/white comparison of deaths preventable by medical intervention. United States and the District of Columbia 1980-1985. Int J Epidemiol 1990; 19:591–598.
39. Emerman CL, Cydulka RK. Factors associated with relapse after emergency department treatment for acute asthma. Ann Emerg Med 1995; 26:6–11.
40. Gold DR. Indoor air pollution. Clinics in Chest Med 1992; 12:215–229.
41. Suissa S, Ernst P, Boivin JF, et al. A cohort analysis of excess mortality in asthma and the use of inhaled β-agonists. Am J Respir Crit Care Med 1994; 149:604–610.
42. Spitzer WO, Suissa S, Ernst P, et al. The use of β_2-agonists and the risk of death and near death from asthma. N Engl Med 1992; 326:501–506.
43. Whitelow WA. Asthma deaths. Chest 1991; 99:1507–1510.
44. Nicklas RA, Whitehurst VE, Donohoe RF. Combined use of beta-adrenergic agonists and methylxanthines. J Allergy Clin Immunol 1984; 73:20–24.
45. Nicklas RA. Paradoxical bronchospasm associated with the use of β_2 agonists. J Allergy Clin Immunol 1990; 85:959–964.
46. Page CP. One explanation of asthma paradox: inhibition of natural anti-inflammatory mechanism by β_2-agonists. Lancet 1991; 337:717–720.
47. Wanner A. Is the routine use of inhaled β-adrenergic agonists appropriate in asthma treatment? Am J Respir Crit Care Med 1995; 151:597–599.
48. Sears MR. Is the routine use of inhaled β-adrenergic agonists appropriate in asthma treatment? Am J Respir Crit Care Med 1995; 151:600–601.
49. Robin ED, Lewiston N. Unexpected, unexplained sudden death in young asthmatic subjects. Chest 1989; 96:790–793.
50. Robin ED, McCauley R. Sudden cardiac death in bronchial asthma and inhaled β-adrenergic agonists. Chest 1992; 101:1699–1702.
51. Ziment I. Infrequent cardiac deaths occur in bronchial asthma. Chest 1992; 101:1703–1705.
52. Fanta CH, Rossing TH, McFaddin ER, Jr. Glucocorticoid in acute asthma. A critical controlled Trial. Am J Med 1993; 74:845–851.
53. Juniper EF, Vanzieleghem A, Ramsdale EH, et al. Effect of long term treatment with an inhaled corticosteroid (budesonide) on airway hyperresponsiveness and clinical asthma in non-steroid dependent asthmatics. AM Rev Respir Dis 1990; 142:832–836.
54. Haahtela T, Jarvinen M, Kava T, et al. Effects of reducing or discontinuing inhaled budesonide in patients with mild asthma. N Engl J Med 1994; 331:700–705.
55. Ernest P, Spitzec WO, Suissa S, et al. Risk of fatal and near fatal asthma in relation to inhaled corticosteroids use. JAMA 1992; 268:3462–3464.
56. Littenberg B, Gluck E. A controlled trial of methylprednisolone in the emergency treatment of acute asthma. N Engl J Med 1986; 314:150–152.
57. Ciarallo L, Sauer AH, Shannon MW. Intravenous magnesium therapy for moderate to severe pediatric asthma. J Pediatr 1996; 129:809–814.
58. Bloch H, Silverman R, Mancherja N. Intravenous magnesium sulfate as an adjunct in the treatment of acute asthma. Chest 1995; 107:1576–1581.
59. McFadden ER Jr, Elsanadi N, Dixon L, et al. Protocol therapy for acute asthma therapeutic benefits and cost savings. Am J Med 1995; 99:651–661.
60. Rand CS, Wisa RA. Measuring adherence to asthma medications regimens. Am J Respir Crit Care Med 1994; 149:S69–S76.
61. Baum D, Creer TL. Medication compliance in children with asthma. J Asthma 1986; 23:49–59.
62. Smith M. The cost of noncompliance and the capacity of improved compliance to reduce

health care expenditures. In: Improving Medication Compliance, Washington, DC: National Pharmaceutical Council, 1985; 35–42.

63. Kolbe J, Vamos M, Fergusson W, et al. Differential influences on asthma self-management knowledge, and self-management behavior in acute severe asthma. Chest 1996; 110:1463–1468.
64. McFadden ER, Warren E. Observations on asthma mortality. Ann Intern Med 1997; 127:142–147.
65. Hetzel MR, Clark TJH, Branthwaite MA. Asthma: Analysis of sudden deaths and ventilatory arrests in hospitals. Br Med J 1977; 808–811.
66. Rothwell RP, Rea HH, Sears MR, et al. Lesson from the national asthma mortality study: circumstances surrounding death. NZ Med J 1987; 100:10–13.
67. Rea HH, Sears MR, Beaglehole R. Lesson from the national asthma mortality study: circumstances surrounding death. NZ Med J 1987; 100:199–202.
68. Strunk RC, Mrazek DA, Fuhrman GS, et al. Physiologic and psychological characteristics associated with deaths due to asthma in childhood. A Case-Controlled Study. JAMA 1985; 254:1193–1198.
69. Benatar SR. Fatal asthma. N Engl J Med 1986; 314:423–429.
70. Sly RM. Increases in deaths from asthma. Ann Allergy 1984; 53:20–25.
71. Speizer FE, Noll R, Heaf P. Observation on recent increase in mortality from asthma. Br Med J 1968; 1:335–339.
72. Paulozzi LS, Coleman JJ, Buist AS. A recent increase in asthma mortality in the northwestern states. Ann Allergy 1986; 56:392–395.
73. Strunk RC. Death due to asthma: New insights into sudden unexpected deaths, but the focus remains on prevention. Am Rev Respir Dis 1993; 148:550–552.
74. Hartert TV, Windom HH, Peeples RS, et al. Inadequate outpatient medical therapy for patients with asthma admitted to two urban hospitals. Am J Med 1996; 100:386–394.
75. Patterson R, DeSwarte RD, Grammer LC, et al. Evolution of patient care education and research in asthma by one academic team of investigators over 35 years. Allergy Proc 1994; 15:169–178.

18

National and International Guidelines for the Emergency Management of Adult Asthma

Richard M. Nowak
Henry Ford Health Systems, Detroit, Michigan

Many have felt that the education of health care professionals, public health officials, and patients themselves will result in better management strategies for asthma with the hope of reducing the morbidity and mortality associated with this disease. As part of this effort to educate, many guidelines for asthma management have been developed, both internationally and by individual countries. There have been, to date, approximately 21 separate published asthma management protocols. The input to the development of these guidelines has generally been quite broad with an attempt to incorporate as many appropriate individuals, organizations, and government officials as possible to insure their accuracy and applicability. A major focus of these guidelines has been to recommend appropriate approaches to prevention and control of the disease. In the United States, there have been further guidelines developed that address specific aspects of management of the disease. These include reports on managing asthma during pregnancy (1), in the elderly (2), and in minority children (3), and others that have outlined specific roles for individuals such as pharmacists (4) or institutions such as schools (5,6). Most of the asthma management guidelines have documented information on the nature and extent of the disease and have recommended appropriate approaches to its prevention and control. A few have outlined the management of the acute attack in the emergency department (ED).

I. EMERGENCY MEDICINE–SPECIFIC GUIDELINES

In 1995, the National Institutes of Health (NIH) published the ''Global Strategy for Asthma Management and Prevention NHLBI/WHO Workshop Report'' (7). This global initiative for asthma was the product of workshops convened by the National Heart, Lung and Blood Institute (NHLBI) and the World Health Organization (WHO). Twenty-one workshop participants from 17 countries met three times to generate this report, which was additionally reviewed by consultant contributors and reviewers and international organizations. The summary figure for the ''Management of Exacerbation of Asthma: Hospital-Based Care'' is detailed in Figure 1. It describes treatment in the ED for the patient with acute asthma. It is the same algorithm that was published in the ''International Consensus Report on the Diagnosis and Management of Asthma,'' published by the NHLBI in June 1992 (8). This latter international report was the result of a working group of 18 physicians and scientists representing 11 nationalities committed specifically to develop an international consensus statement on the diagnosis and management of this disease.

The second guideline to be presented is the algorithm for the ''Management of Asthma Exacerbations: Emergency Department and Hospital-Based Care'' that is contained in the 1997 National Asthma Education and Prevention Program (NAEPP) Expert Panel Report on ''The Guidelines for the Diagnosis and Management of Asthma'' (9). This is an NIH initiative that was first published in 1991 (10) and subsequently updated by a second expert panel in 1996. The 1997 document was generated by an expert panel representing many disciplines and points of view, including that of emergency medicine. It has been reviewed by over 25 experts and organizations with the intent of presenting a broad consensus on the diagnosis and management of this disease including the emergency assessment and therapy of acute exacerbations. The specific guideline recommended for the assessment and care of acute asthma in the ED is found in the algorithm in Figure 2.

The third guideline to be reviewed is that produced by the Canadian Association of Emergency Physicians and the Canadian Thoracic Society Asthma Advisory Committee and endorsed by the Canadian Association of Emergency Physicians, the Canadian Thoracic Society, and the Association des Médecins d'Urgance du Québec. These ''Guidelines for Emergency Management of Adult Asthma'' have recently been published in the *Canadian Medical Association Journal* (11) but have for a few years been distributed in poster format (12) for EDs throughout Canada (Fig. 3). It is this latter format that has been reproduced in this chapter as it provides specific recommendations concerning assessment and treatment that is relevant for emergency medicine.

The Thoracic Society of Australia and New Zealand published the ''Asthma Management Plan, 1989'' in the Medical Journal of Australia (13). This plan was widely promoted through the National Asthma Campaign in those countries, but did not have specific recommendations for the assessment and management of acute exacerbations in the ED. However, in 1992, in the *Thoracic Society News,* the Australasian College of Emergency Medicine published the national asthma campaign, ''Acute Asthma Management'' (14). The initial management component is shown in Table 1 in this chapter.

In 1990, the *British Medical Journal* published guidelines for the management of asthma in adults, which were the result of initiatives by the British Thoracic Society, the Research Unit of the Royal College of Physicians, the King's Fund center, and the National Asthma Campaign (15). They were the first national guidelines for the management of a specific condition in the United Kingdom and they were intended to be reviewed and revised after two years. The revision of these guidelines, published in 1993 in the *British Medical Journal* (16) and *Thorax* (17), have benefited from the input of the British Association for Accident and Emergency Medicine, the Royal College of Practitioners, and the General Practitioners in Asthma Group. The summary chart that is relevant to emergency

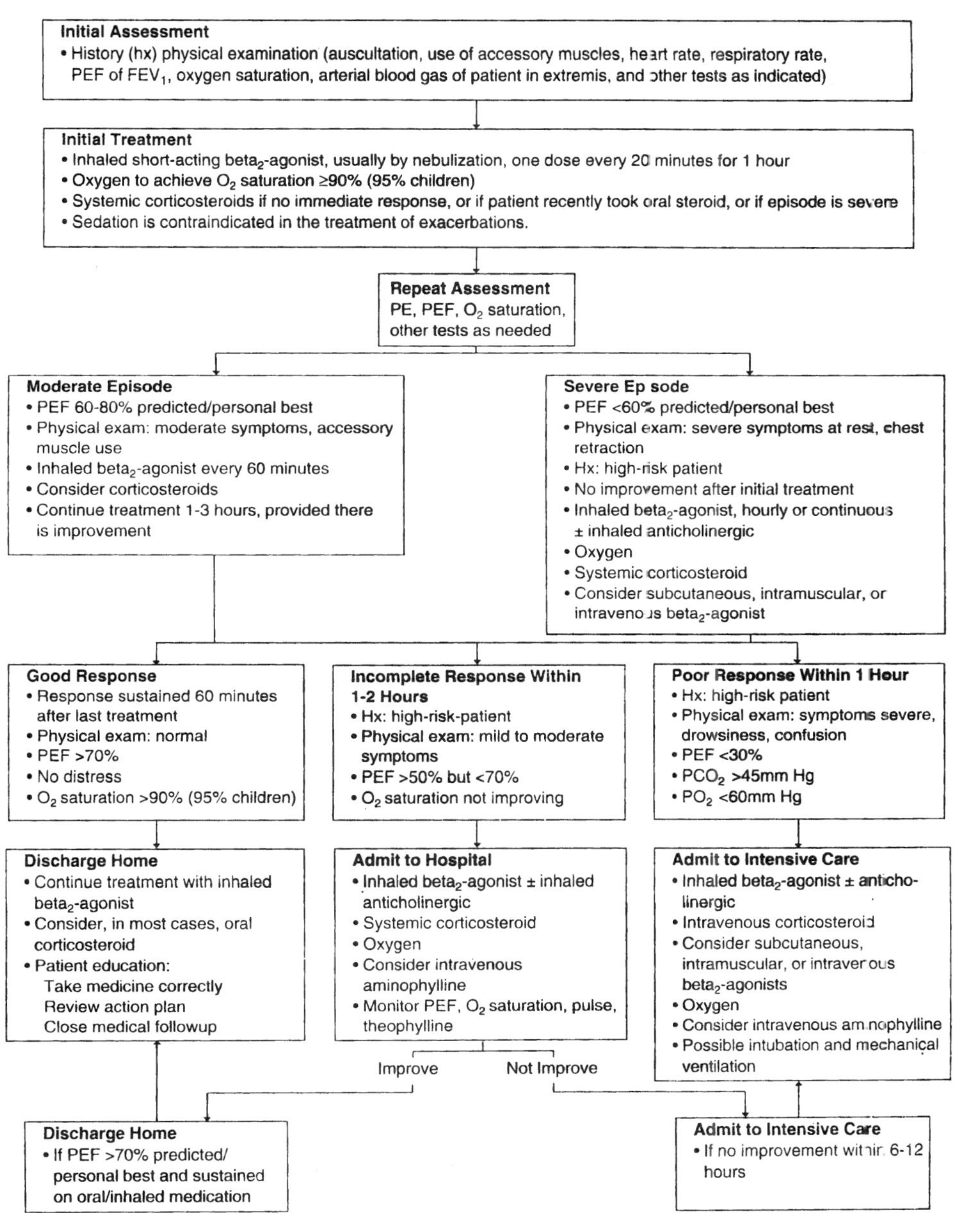

Figure 1 Management of exacerbation of asthma: hospital-based care. (From Ref. 8.)

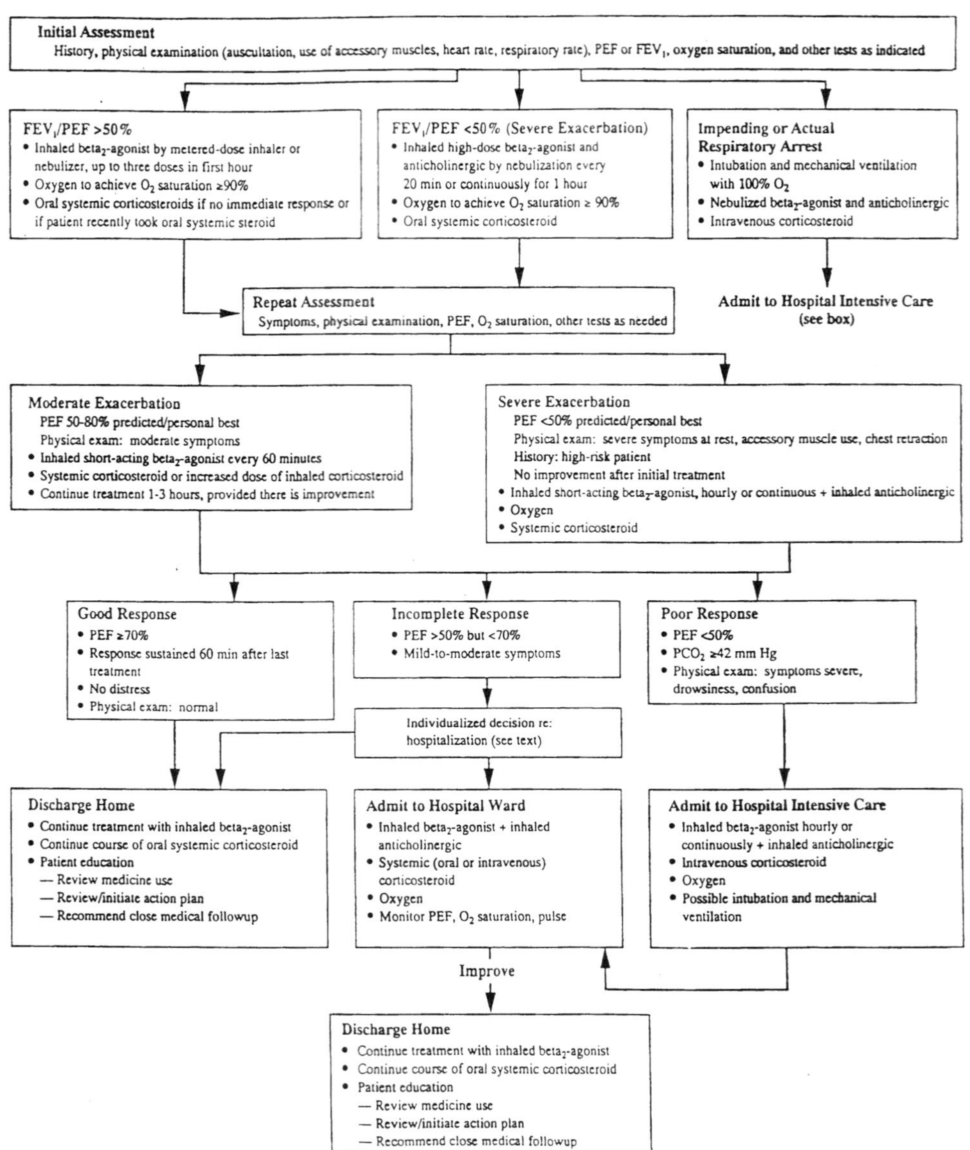

Figure 2 Management of asthma exacerbations: emergency department and hospital-based care. (From Ref. 9.)

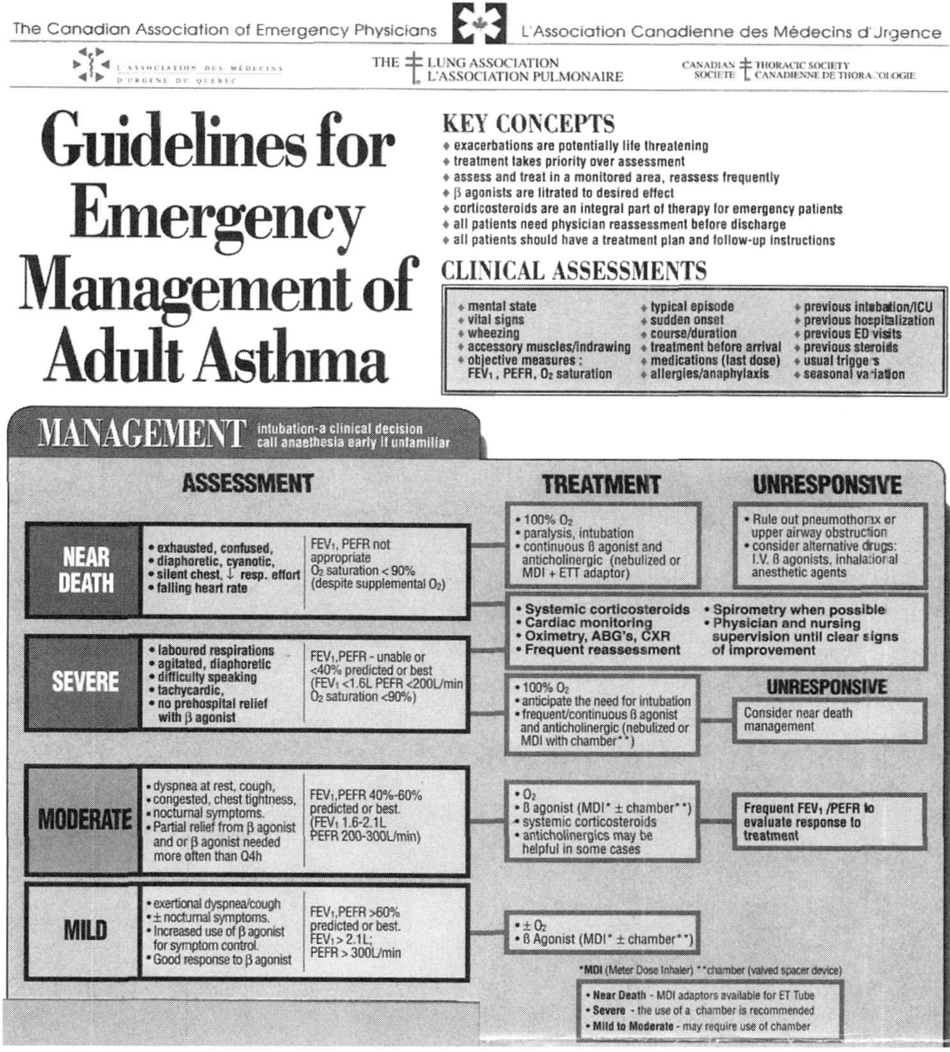

Figure 3 Guidelines for emergency management of adult asthma. (From Ref. 12.)

medicine is reproduced in Figure 4 and is entitled ''Asthma in Accident and Emergency Departments.''

Lastly, a working group of the South African Pulmonology Society has published guidelines (18) for the care of acute asthma to encourage a uniform approach to the management of exacerbations, whether of rapid or gradual onset, mild or severe. The summation document, entitled ''Management of Exacerbation of Asthma in Practice Rooms, Clinics and Hospitals,'' is shown in Figure 5.

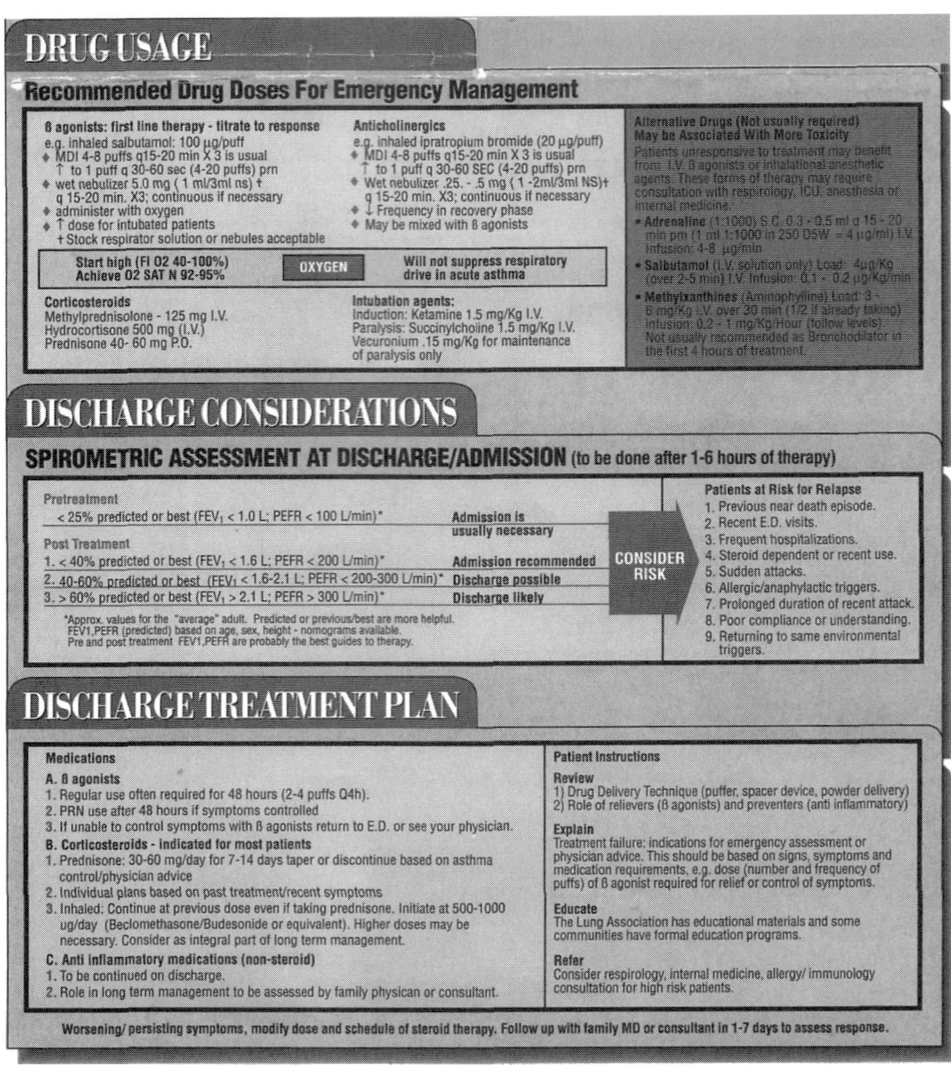

DRUG USAGE

Recommended Drug Doses For Emergency Management

β agonists: first line therapy - titrate to response
e.g. inhaled salbutamol: 100 μg/puff
- MDI 4-8 puffs q15-20 min X 3 is usual
  ↑ to 1 puff q 30-60 sec (4-20 puffs) prn
- wet nebulizer 5.0 mg (1 ml/3ml ns) †
  q 15-20 min. X3; continuous if necessary
- administer with oxygen
- ↑ dose for intubated patients
  † Stock respirator solution or nebules acceptable

Anticholinergics
e.g. inhaled ipratropium bromide (20 μg/puff)
- MDI 4-8 puffs q15-20 min X 3 is usual
  ↑ to 1 puff q 30-60 SEC (4-20 puffs) prn
- Wet nebulizer .25. - .5 mg (1 -2ml/3ml NS)†
  q 15-20 min. X3; continuous if necessary
- ↓ Frequency in recovery phase
- May be mixed with β agonists

Start high (FI 02 40-100%)
Achieve 02 SAT N 92-95%
OXYGEN
Will not suppress respiratory drive in acute asthma

Corticosteroids
Methylprednisolone - 125 mg I.V.
Hydrocortisone 500 mg (I.V.)
Prednisone 40- 60 mg P.O.

Intubation agents:
Induction: Ketamine 1.5 mg/Kg I.V.
Paralysis: Succinylcholine 1.5 mg/Kg I.V.
Vecuronium .15 mg/Kg for maintenance of paralysis only

Alternative Drugs (Not usually required)
May be Associated With More Toxicity
Patients unresponsive to treatment may benefit from: I.V. β agonists or inhalational anesthetic agents. These forms of therapy may require consultation with respirology, ICU, anesthesia or internal medicine.
- **Adrenaline** (1:1000) S.C. 0.3 - 0.5 ml q 15 - 20 min prn (1 ml 1:1000 in 250 D5W = 4 μg/ml) I.V. Infusion: 4-8 μg/min
- **Salbutamol** (I.V. solution only) Load: 4μg/Kg (over 2-5 min) I.V. Infusion: 0.1 - 0.2 μg/Kg/min
- **Methylxanthines** (Aminophylline) Load: 3 - 6 mg/Kg I.V. over 30 min (1/2 if already taking) infusion: 0.2 - 1 mg/Kg/Hour (follow levels). Not usually recommended as Bronchodilator in the first 4 hours of treatment.

DISCHARGE CONSIDERATIONS

SPIROMETRIC ASSESSMENT AT DISCHARGE/ADMISSION (to be done after 1-6 hours of therapy)

Pretreatment
< 25% predicted or best (FEV_1 < 1.0 L; PEFR < 100 L/min)* — **Admission is usually necessary**

Post Treatment
1. < 40% predicted or best (FEV_1 < 1.6 L; PEFR < 200 L/min)* — **Admission recommended**
2. 40-60% predicted or best (FEV_1 < 1.6-2.1 L; PEFR < 200-300 L/min)* — **Discharge possible**
3. > 60% predicted or best (FEV_1 > 2.1 L; PEFR > 300 L/min)* — **Discharge likely**

*Approx. values for the "average" adult. Predicted or previous/best are more helpful.
FEV1,PEFR (predicted) based on age, sex, height - nomograms available.
Pre and post treatment FEV1,PEFR are probably the best guides to therapy.

CONSIDER RISK

Patients at Risk for Relapse
1. Previous near death episode.
2. Recent E.D. visits.
3. Frequent hospitalizations.
4. Steroid dependent or recent use.
5. Sudden attacks.
6. Allergic/anaphylactic triggers.
7. Prolonged duration of recent attack.
8. Poor compliance or understanding.
9. Returning to same environmental triggers.

DISCHARGE TREATMENT PLAN

Medications

A. β agonists
1. Regular use often required for 48 hours (2-4 puffs Q4h).
2. PRN use after 48 hours if symptoms controlled
3. If unable to control symptoms with β agonists return to E.D. or see your physician.

B. Corticosteroids - indicated for most patients
1. Prednisone: 30-60 mg/day for 7-14 days taper or discontinue based on asthma control/physician advice
2. Individual plans based on past treatment/recent symptoms
3. Inhaled: Continue at previous dose even if taking prednisone. Initiate at 500-1000 ug/day (Beclomethasone/Budesonide or equivalent). Higher doses may be necessary. Consider as integral part of long term management.

C. Anti inflammatory medications (non-steroid)
1. To be continued on discharge.
2. Role in long term management to be assessed by family physican or consultant.

Patient Instructions

Review
1) Drug Delivery Technique (puffer, spacer device, powder delivery)
2) Role of relievers (β agonists) and preventers (anti inflammatory)

Explain
Treatment failure: indications for emergency assessment or physician advice. This should be based on signs, symptoms and medication requirements, e.g. dose (number and frequency of puffs) of β agonist required for relief or control of symptoms.

Educate
The Lung Association has educational materials and some communities have formal education programs.

Refer
Consider respirology, internal medicine, allergy/ immunology consultation for high risk patients.

Worsening/ persisting symptoms, modify dose and schedule of steroid therapy. Follow up with family MD or consultant in 1-7 days to assess response.

The generous financial support for this project by GLAXO, ASTRA and FISONS pharmaceutical companies is gratefully acknowledged.

Figure 3 Continued

II. COMPARISONS BETWEEN EMERGENCY MEDICINE–RELATED GUIDELINES

Overall, there are some common themes that run through all of these guidelines. The initial assessment is very brief and treatment is instituted as soon as is possible after arrival in the ED. Adequate oxygenation is reflected by ensuring, when appropriate, supplemental oxygen to maintain a pulse oximetry oxygen saturation of greater than 90%. In the absence of pulse oximetry, the recommendations suggest supplemental oxygen be used in all cases.

Virtually all guidelines have as an integral part of the assessment of severity of disease and response to therapy, objective measurements of airflow (FEV_1, PEFR). This reflects the underlying belief that more subjective assessments of airflow obstruction by either the patient or the physician are inadequate and often underestimate the severity of the exacerbation.

It is also clear that inhalation of β_2-agonist bronchodilators, in dosages proportionate to the severity of the obstruction, are the agents to be used initially. Their continued use in terms of both dosage and frequency is driven by the response or lack thereof to therapy. Systemic corticosteroid medications are recommended for virtually all acute exacerbations of the disease reflecting the belief that the uncontrolled nature of the exacerbation reflects increasing airways inflammation. Lastly, the guidelines reflect the need for some attempts at educating patients regarding their disease and to provide a discharge plan that includes continuing aggressive therapy and close outpatient supervision by the ongoing care practitioner.

The comparative differences in the guidelines presented in this chapter are summarized in Table 2. It is of interest to comment on some of the differences in approaches. First, four of the six determine aggressiveness of therapy on the presenting pulmonary function testing (PFT) while the remaining two treat all patients the same initially, regardless of PFT, and determine aggressiveness of therapy on the response or lack thereof to initial treatment. Which approach is better is currently unclear as there are no clinical studies addressing this issue.

Although all guidelines recommend the use of PFTs, only two give absolute flow recommendations while all recommend the use of predicted or personal best values. Only one gives predicted values within the pictorial display of the guideline. The uniform inclusion of predicted values all guidelines would increase the likelihood of practicing emergency physicians to utilize them in the decision-making process. The actual values given to define a severe attack or when patients can be discharged home vary somewhat from guideline to guideline. There is clearly the need for clinical studies to better define these parameters.

β-agonist therapy tends to be aggressive in all the approaches in terms of dosage and frequency. However, there is generally a preference for use of nebulization to deliver these agents, especially in severe cases. Use of a metered dose inhaler (MDI) with spacer seems to be increasingly popular, especially in mild to moderate exacerbations. For life-threatening exacerbations of acute asthma, five of the six guidelines recommend the use of intravenous β_2 agonists, especially salbutamol (albuterol). The U.S. guidelines uniquely do not recommend use of intravenous therapy because of a lack of studies showing benefit when compared to aggressive inhalation treatment and a concern for toxicity. More studies are needed to better define the type, dose, and route of administration of β_2 agonists for varying degrees of acute airways obstruction.

All guidelines recommend β_2 agonists to be combined with anticholinergics (ipratropium bromide) in severe cases with the understanding that the benefit varies from patient to patient and is generally small. Yet dose and frequency of administration remains varied.

Although all guidelines recommend very liberal use of systemic corticosteroids for exacerbations, the type, frequency, and route of administration varies in the six approaches. This necessitates further study, especially in more severe cases where undermedication could be a potential problem.

In general there is agreement that aminophylline therapy is not a helpful in most

Table 1 Initial Management of Acute Asthma in Adults

Treatment	Mild	Moderate	Severe and life threatening
Admission necessary	Probably not	Probably	Yes—consider ICU
Oxygen	High flow of at least 8 L/min to achieve an inspired oxygen concentration of about 50%. Monitor effect by oximetry. If oxygen saturation remains abnormal, use a nonrebreathing mask with a reservoir bag with 15 L O_2/min.		
Nebulized B_2 agonist, e.g., salbutamol or terbutaline, with 8 L/min O_2	1 mL 0.5% salbutamol + 3 mL saline	2 ml 0.5% salbutamol + 2 mL saline 1 to 4 hourly	2 mL 0.5% salbutamol + 2 mL saline every 15–30 min. Give IV when no response to aerosol, e.g., 250 μg IV bolus and then 10 μg/kg/hr.
Nebulized ipratropium bromide	Not necessary	Optional	2 mL 0.025% ipratropium bromide with β_2 agonist hourly
Oral corticosteroids, e.g., prednisone	Yes (consider)	Yes	Yes, 30–60 mg/day initially, or IV
Intravenous steroids, e.g., hydrocortisone (or equivalent)	Not necessary	200 mg stat	200 mg 6 hourly for 24 hr, then review

Theophylline/aminophylline	Uncertainty exists regarding the benefits of this drug: reserve for those unresponsive to maximal doses of β_2 agonist.		
			IV aminophyline 5 mg/kg then 0.5 mg/kg/hr IV. Use up to half of this loading dose of aminophylline if the patient is maintained on regular oral theophylline.
Adrenaline	Not indicated	Not indicated	Adrenaline 0.5 mg IM for anaphylaxis or IV (diluted to 10 mL with saline) for cardio-respiratory arrest.
Chest X-ray	Not necessary unless focal signs present	Not necessary unless focal signs present	Necessary if no response to initial therapy or suspect pneumothorax.
Observations	Regular	Continuous	Continuous
Other investigations	Not required	Not required	Check for hypokalemia.

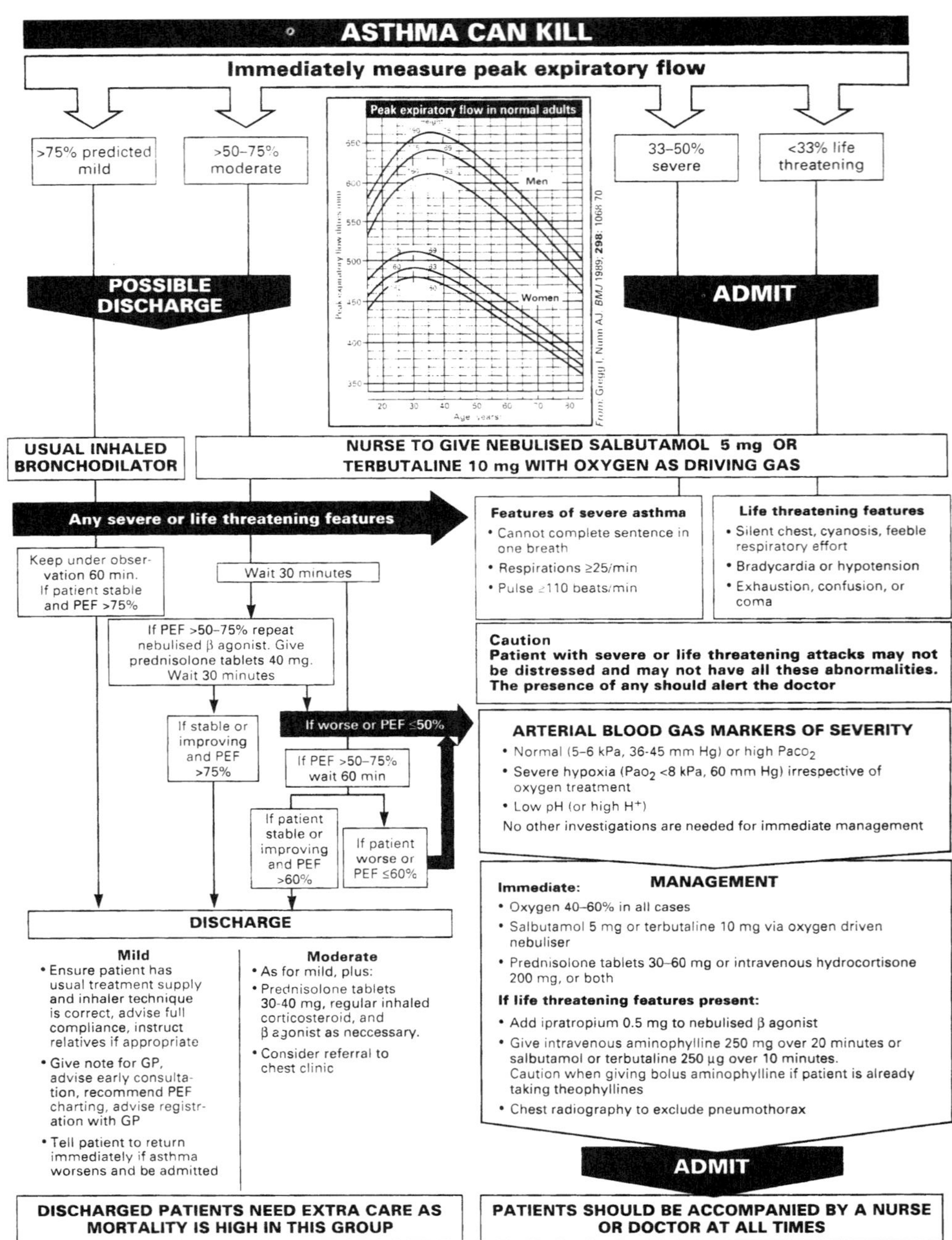

Figure 4 Asthma in accident and emergency departments.

MANAGEMENT OF EXACERBATION OF ASTHMA IN PRACTICE ROOMS, CLINICS AND HOSPITALS

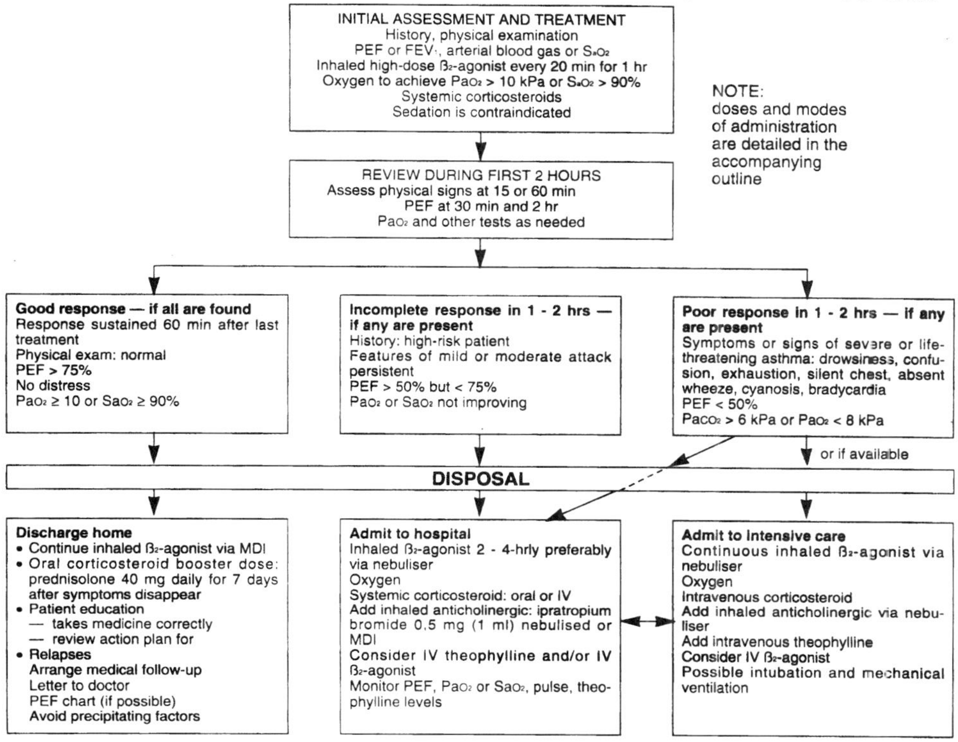

INITIAL ASSESSMENT AND TREATMENT
History, physical examination
PEF or FEV_1, arterial blood gas or S_aO_2
Inhaled high-dose β_2-agonist every 20 min for 1 hr
Oxygen to achieve Pa_{O_2} > 10 kPa or S_aO_2 > 90%
Systemic corticosteroids
Sedation is contraindicated

NOTE:
doses and modes of administration are detailed in the accompanying outline

↓

REVIEW DURING FIRST 2 HOURS
Assess physical signs at 15 or 60 min
PEF at 30 min and 2 hr
Pa_{O_2} and other tests as needed

↓

Good response — if all are found
Response sustained 60 min after last treatment
Physical exam: normal
PEF > 75%
No distress
Pa_{O_2} ≥ 10 or Sa_{O_2} ≥ 90%

Incomplete response in 1 - 2 hrs — if any are present
History: high-risk patient
Features of mild or moderate attack persistent
PEF > 50% but < 75%
Pa_{O_2} or Sa_{O_2} not improving

Poor response in 1 - 2 hrs — if any are present
Symptoms or signs of severe or life-threatening asthma: drowsiness, confusion, exhaustion, silent chest, absent wheeze, cyanosis, bradycardia
PEF < 50%
Pa_{CO_2} > 6 kPa or Pa_{O_2} < 8 kPa

or if available

DISPOSAL

Discharge home
- Continue inhaled β_2-agonist via MDI
- Oral corticosteroid booster dose: prednisolone 40 mg daily for 7 days after symptoms disappear
- Patient education
  - — takes medicine correctly
  - — review action plan for
- Relapses
  Arrange medical follow-up
  Letter to doctor
  PEF chart (if possible)
  Avoid precipitating factors

Admit to hospital
Inhaled β_2-agonist 2 - 4-hrly preferably via nebuliser
Oxygen
Systemic corticosteroid: oral or IV
Add inhaled anticholinergic: ipratropium bromide 0.5 mg (1 ml) nebulised or MDI
Consider IV theophylline and/or IV β_2-agonist
Monitor PEF, Pa_{O_2} or Sa_{O_2}, pulse, theophylline levels

Admit to intensive care
Continuous inhaled β_2-agonist via nebuliser
Oxygen
Intravenous corticosteroid
Add inhaled anticholinergic via nebuliser
Add intravenous theophylline
Consider IV β_2-agonist
Possible intubation and mechanical ventilation

SYNOPSIS OF DRUGS AND DOSES IN ACUTE ASTHMA

OXYGEN
Use highest concentration mask (60% or higher)

BETA-2-AGONISTS — INHALED
Via NEBULISER (preferably oxygen-driven)
dose: fenoterol 1 mg — 1 ml in 4 ml sterile normal saline
hexoprenaline 0,25 mg
salbutamol 5 mg
frequency: initially every 20 minutes for 1 hour
2 - 4-hourly while in hospital/surgery
Via MDI and SPACER
dose: fenoterol 100 μg/puff; hexoprenaline 100 μg/puff; salbutamol 100 μg/puff; terbutaline 250 μg/puff — several deep breaths from spacer after each 2 puffs to total of 20 to 50 puffs
frequency: initially every 20 minutes for 1 hour
2 - 4-hourly while in hospital
spacers: minimum volume 500 ml
Volumatic (Allen & Hanbury)
Nebuhaler (Astra)
plastic bottle with base removed to fit snugly onto face

CORTICOSTEROIDS
Initial dose: prednisone, methylprednisolone or prednisolone 30 mg oral
or hydrocortisone 200 mg IV
or methylprednisolone 125 mg IV
further doses:
Initial good response: continue daily oral dose for 7 days after complete recovery. No tapering necessary unless on long-term oral dose
Partial response: continue daily oral dose or hydrocortisone 200 mg IV 4 - 6-hourly or methylprednisolone 125 mg IV twice daily
Poor response: continue IV doses

IPRATROPIUM BROMIDE
Via NEBULISER (preferably oxygen-driven)
dose: 0,5 mg (2 ml in 3 ml sterile normal saline)
frequency: 4-hourly
Via MDI and SPACER
dose: 20 μg/puff; up to 20 puffs
frequency: 4-hourly

AMINOPHYLLINE — INTRAVENOUS
loading dose: 6 mg/kg over 30 minutes
(10 ml ampoule = 250 mg)
Withhold or give only half to patients on oral theophyllines
maintenance dose: 0,6 mg/kg/hour (± 1 000 mg/24 hours)
Increase by one-third (0,9 mg/kg/hour) in smokers and patients taking phenytoin
Decrease by one-third in congestive cardiac failure, elderly, liver disease, treatment with macrolide antibiotics, ciprofloxacin or cimetidine.
monitor: blood levels daily and adjust dose

BETA-2-AGONISTS — INTRAVENOUS
Initial dose: salbutamol 0,25 mg IV slowly
maintenance dose: salbutamol 3 - 20 μg/minute (5 mg diluted in 500 ml dextrose water or normal saline)
duration: until sustained improvement (usually less than 24 hours)
monitor: serum K^+ daily

Figure 5 Guidelines to management of asthma exacerbations and synopsis of drugs and doses used to treat acute asthma.

Table 2 Comparative Analysis of Six Different National and International Guidelines for the Management of Exacerbations of Adult Asthma

	NHLBI/WHO global initiative	United States NHLBI	Canada	Australia/ New Zealand	United Kingdom	South Africa
Supplemental oxygen guidelines	O_2 sat ≥90%	O_2 sat ≥90%	O_2 sat ≥92%	Monitor O_2 sat by oximetry	Oxygen 40–60% in all cases	O_2 sat >90%
Pulmonary function testing (PFT)	PEFR or FEV_1	PEFR or FEV_1	PEFR or FEV_1	PEFR or FEV_1	PEFR	PEFR or FEV_1
Predicted values provided?	No	No	No	No	Yes	No
Initial therapy strategy	Same for all	Stratified by PFT and assessment.	Stratified by PFT and assessment.	Stratified by PFT and assessment.	Stratified by PFT and assessment.	Same for all.
Severe attack (P/PB) by PFT	PFT < 60% P/PB after initial therapy.	PFT < 50% P/PB on arrival or after initial therapy.	PFT < 40% P/PB, or PEFR < 200 L/min or FEV_1 < 1.6 L on arrival.	PFT < 40% predicted, or PEFR < 100 L/min or FEV_1 < 1.0 L on arrival.	PEFR < 50% P/PB on arrival (<33% P/PB is life-threatening).	PEFR < 50% P/PB after initial therapy.
Initial β_2-agonist therapy	One dose q 20 min x's 3 (dose unspecified). Nebulization preferred over MDI.	Inhaled high-dose (albuterol 5 mg) by nebulization q 20 min or continuously for 1 hr for severe. Inhaled by MDL (per protocol) or nebulization (albuterol 2–5 mg) up to 3 doses in the first hour for nonsevere.	Nebulized salbutamol 5 mg q 15–20 min x's 3 for severe, continuous if necessary, MDI with or without spacer for all but preferred for mild to moderate attacks (multiple-dose protocol).	Nebulized salbutamol 5 mg q 15–20 min as needed.	Nebulized salbutamol 5 mg or terbutaline 10 mg q 15–30 min as needed.	Nebulized preferred, fenoterol 1 mg or hexoprenaline 0.25 mg or salbutamol 5 mg q 20 min x's 3. MDI with large spacer (multidose protocol) if nebulizer not available.

Intravenous β_2 agonists for life-threatening asthma	Parenteral delivery if no response to nebulized (type and dose not specified).	Not recommended.	Salbutamol 4 μg/kg load over 2–5 min, then 0.1–0.2 μg/kg/min infusion. Adrenaline 4–8 μg/min infusion.	Salbutamol 250 mcg bolus, then 10 mcg/kg/hr.	Salbutamol or terbutaline 250 μg over 10 min.	Salbutamol 0.25 mg load slowly, then 3–20 μg/min infusion.
Anticholinergic therapy	Add to β_2 agonist for severe cases. Type and dose not specified.	Add on for severe cases. Nebulized ipratropium 0.5 mg q 30 min x's 3, then q 2–4 hr as needed.	Add for severe, consider for moderate. Nebulized ipratropium 0.25–0.5 mg q 15–20 min x's 3. MDI with spacer (multiple-dose protocol).	Add on for severe cases. Nebulized ipratropium .5 mg q 2 hr.	Add on for life-threatening. Nebulized ipratropium 0.5 mg q 6 hr.	Add on for severe cases. Nebulized ipratropium 0.5 mg q 4 hrs or by MDI with spacer (multiple-dose protocol).
Corticosteroids	If no immediate response, severe episode, recently on steroids. Oral (preferred) or intravenous route. Dose and type unspecified.	If no immediate response, severe episode, recently on steroids. Oral (preferred) or intravenous. Prednisone, methylprednisolone, or prednisolone 120–180 mg/day in 3–4 divided doses.	For all but mild attacks. Methylprednisolone 125 mg IV or hydrocortisone 500 mg IV or prednisone 40–60 mg p.o.	Prednisone orally for all but mildest, use 30–60 mg. For moderate or severe use intravenous equivalent of hydrocortisone 200 mg.	For all but mildest, use prednisolone orally 30–60 mg or intravenous hydrocortisone 200 mg, or both if very ill.	For all cases. Oral prednisone, methylprednisolone, or prednisolone, 30 mg. Intravenous hydrocortisone 200 mg or methylprednisolone 125 mg, for severe attacks.

Table 2 Continued

	NHLBI/WHO global initiative	United States NHLBI	Canada	Australia/ New Zealand	United Kingdom	South Africa
Aminophylline therapy	Not recommended in first 4 hr. May have role if admitted.	Not recommended in ED. Role in admitted is controversial.	Not recommended in first 4 hr.	For those not responsive to maximal β_2-agonists. Give 5 mg/kg, then 0.5 mg/kg/hr IV (If not taking oral theophylline).	For life-threatening, give 250 mg IV over 20 min followed by infusion of 750 mg/24 hr if small and 1500 mg/24 hr if large. No bolus if on oral theophylline.	Consider for severe cases. Give 6 mg/kg over 30 mins, if not taking, then .6 mg/kg/hr (adjust accordingly).
Intubation and mechanical ventilation	Indication only	Indications and ventilator strategy (permissive hypercapnia)	Indications and intubation agents	Manage in ICU in most cases	Indications, manage in ICU in most cases	Indications, manage in ICU in most cases
PFT discharge from ED criteria	PFT > 70%, predicted and sustained.	PFT ≥ 70% P/PB or >50% but <70% P/PB without high risk factors	PFT > 60% P/PB or > 40% but < 60% P/PB without high risk factors.	Mild cases (>60%), generally home, moderate cases (40–60%) generally admitted.	PEFR > 75% P/PB or > 60% P/PB after more prolonged therapy.	PFT > 75% P/PB or > 50% but < 75% P/PB without high risk factors.
Discharge planning	Instructions, education, and follow-up described.	Instructions, education, and follow-up described.	Instructions, education, and follow-up described.	Minimal discussion of instructions, education, and follow-up.	Instructions, education, and follow-up discussed.	Instructions, education, and follow-up discussed.
Evidence-based	No	No	Yes	No	No	No
Cost analysis	No	No	No	No	No	No

P/PB = predicted/personal best.

cases of acute asthma, yet three of the six guidelines recommend considering its use in severe nonresponding cases. Whether aminophylline therapy in severe acute asthma is truly beneficial needs further study.

For the management of the asthmatic patient who requires intubation and mechanical ventilation, the guidelines are uniformly disappointing. Although all give indications for this intervention, only one discusses the pharmacological agents to be used and another discusses ventilator strategies. Three imply that this intervention should be accomplished in the intensive care unit whenever possible. It seems that deteriorating asthmatics should be managed/stabilized in the ED according to all the guidelines. An expanded discussion of this management should be included in all future guidelines. The specific role of the intensivist and the interface between the ED and the intensive care unit (ICU) in these cases should be clearly addressed.

Only the Canadian guidelines can claim to be evidence based. They were developed using the evidence-based approach recommended by the Canadian Medical Association (19). Thus these recommendations are graded A through C based on the strength of the clinical trials (levels 1 to 3) referenced or whether a recommendation was simply a consensus opinion. Some have expressed concerns about the impartiality of the other guidelines and whether they have been able to improve clinical practice (20,21). A critical appraisal of published asthma management guidelines using criteria based on clinical decision making has shown major deficiencies with the assembly of evidence that formed the basis of the guidelines (22). Future guidelines should systematically evaluate the evidence, grade the strength of this evidence by the tools of clinical epidemiology, and include these analyses in the guidelines (22).

While specific drug therapies are suggested, there is no report on the magnitude of expected benefits or any potential side effects of treatment. None of the guidelines has evaluated the cost implications of their recommendations. Although there are difficult issues to address, in today's cost-conscious health care environment, attempts must be made to incorporate the cost/benefit of instituting therapy based on guidelines (23).

III. DISSEMINATION/UTILIZATION OF EMERGENCY MEDICINE GUIDELINES

In general the dissemination of the guidelines has been through mailings to EDs and emergency physicians (24), publications in relevant journals or periodicals, discussions and debates at national and international meetings, and general public educational opportunities. What is the best way to disseminate guidelines is unclear. In a recent survey of emergency physicians in the United States, only 33% of respondents reported receiving information regarding asthma management from the NHLBI/NAEPP guidelines (25). Why this number is so low requires further study (25).

Some studies have been completed to assess the success of guidelines in different countries. In the United States, Emerman has reported that emergency physicians use β_2 agonists and steroids at least as often as the guidelines suggest but a majority do not use PFTs in the recommended manner (25). Two studies in the United Kingdom have shown high (97%, 82%) (27,28) compliance with the emergency use of PFTs but much poorer compliance with the suggested use of nebulized bronchodilators and corticosteroids (57%). In two studies in New Zealand and Australia, compliance with the use of PFTs in the ED was better (79%, 95%) (29,30) than the compliance with the use of corticosteroids (22%). Thus different countries seem to have different acceptances by emergency personnel of different aspects of their guidelines.

Is the deficient utilization of the guidelines related to inadequate or ineffective dissemination? Do emergency physicians disagree with the suggestions in the guidelines because of limited evidence to support them? Is the fact that there is little evidence to support improved ED outcome by following the guidelines a reason not to incorporate them into practice? All of these questions need to be answered by clinical studies if overall improvement in guidelines' utilization and outcomes is the goal.

IV. SUMMARY

Guidelines for medical care, including emergency medicine assessments and treatments, will continue to be part of health care as we attempt to more standardize our therapies based on the strongest scientific data available. Evidence-based guidelines should minimize the discrepancies among different countries and allow greater acceptance by the practicing physician. In addition, outcome changes based on the guidelines will need to be proven to reinforce the importance of these guidelines. This chapter has reviewed the current status of the available guidelines for the emergency care of the acute exacerbation of asthma in adults.

REFERENCES

1. National Asthma Education Program: Management of asthma during pregnancy. Bethesda, MD: National Heart, Lung, and Blood Institute, 1993, NIH Publication No. 93-3279.
2. National Asthma Education and Prevention Program: Considerations for diagnosing and managing asthma in the elderly. Bethesda, MD: National Heart, Lung, and Blood Institute, 1996, NIH Publication No. 95-3675.
3. National Asthma Education and Prevention Program: Asthma management in minority children. Bethesda, MD: National Heart, Lung, and Blood Institute, 1995, NIH Publication No. 95-3675.
4. National Asthma Education and Prevention Program: The role of the pharmacists in improving asthma care. Bethesda, MD: National Heart, Lung, and Blood Institute, 1995, NIH Publication No. 95-3280.
5. National Asthma Education Program: Managing asthma: A guide for schools. Bethesda, MD: National Heart, Lung, and Blood Institute, 1991, NIH Publication No. 91-2650.
6. National Asthma Education Program: Asthma awareness: Curriculum for the elementary classroom. Bethesda, MD: Heart, Lung, and Blood Institute, 1993, NIH Publication No. 93-2894.
7. National Institutes of Health: Global strategy for asthma management and prevention, NHLBI/WHO Workshop Report. Bethesda, MD: National Heart, Lung, and Blood Institute, 1995, NIH Publication No. 95-3659.
8. National Institutes of Health: International consensus report on diagnosis and treatment of asthma. Bethesda, MD: National Heart, Lung, and Blood Institute, 1992, NIH Publication No. 92-3091.
9. National Asthma Education and Prevention Program: Guidelines for the diagnosis and management of asthma. Bethesda, MD: National Heart, Lung, and Blood Institute, 1997, NIH Publication No. 97-4051.
10. National Asthma Education Program: Guidelines for the diagnosis and management of asthma.

Bethesda, MD: National Heart, Lung, and Blood Institute, 1991, NIH Publication No. 91-3042.
11. Beveridge RC, Grunfeld AF, Hodder RV, Verbeek PR, for the CAEP/CTS Asthma Advisory Committee. Guidelines for the emergency department management of asthma in adults. Can Med Assoc J 1996; 155:25–37.
12. Canadian Association of Emergency Physicians, Lung Association, and Thoracic Society. Guidelines for the emergency management of adult asthma, emergency department poster, 1992.
13. Woolcock A, Rubenfeld AR, Seale JP, Landau LL, Antic R, Mitchell C, Rea HH, Zimmerman P. Asthma management plan, 1989. Med J Austr 1989; 151:650–653.
14. Australasian College of Emergency Medicine. National asthma campaign, acute asthma management. Thoracic Soc News 1992; 35: June.
15. British Thoracic Society, Research Unit of the Royal College of Physicians of London, King's Fund Center, and National Asthma Campaign. Guidelines for management of asthma in adults: II—acute severe asthma. Brit Med J 1990; 301:797–800.
16. British Thoracic Society and Others. Guidelines for the management of asthma: A summary, Brit Med J 1993; 306:776–782.
17. British Thoracic Society and Others. Guidelines for the management of asthma. Thorax 1993; S18–S24.
18. Statement by a Working Group of the South African Pulmonology Society. Guidelines for the management of asthma in adults in South Africa. Part II. Acute asthma. South Afr Med J 1994; 84:332–338.
19. Guidelines for Canadian Clinical Practice Guidelines. Canadian Medical Association, Ottawa, Canada, 1994.
20. Haines A, Feder G. Guidance on guidelines. Brit Med J 1992; 305:785–786.
21. Sheldon TA, Smith GD. Consensus conference as drug promotion. Lancet 1993; 341:100–102.
22. Gibson P. Asthma based guidelines and evidence-based medicine. Lancet 1993; 342:1305.
23. Fitzmourice DA, Bradley CP, Salter R, Slater AE. Evidence used to formulate guidelines on managing asthma did not include costs. Brit Med J 1996; 313:113–114.
24. National Asthma Education and Prevention Program. Asthma management kit for emergency departments. Bethesda, MD: National Heart, Lung, and Blood Institute, 1994, NIH Publication No. 94-2992.
25. Emerman CL, Cydulka RK, Skobeloff E. Survey of asthma practice among emergency physicians. Chest 1996; 109:708–712.
26. Sarwar A. Guidelines in need of guidance. Chest 1996; 109:594–595.
27. Bell D, Layton AM, Grabbay J. Use of a guideline based questionnaire to adult hospital care of acute asthma. Brit Med J 1991; 302:1440–1443.
28. Neville RG, Clark PC, Hoskins G, Smith B. For General Practitioners in Asthma Group, National asthma attack audit 1991–2. Brit Med J 1993; 306:559–562.
29. Epton MJ, Skidmore C, O'Hagen JJ, et al. An audit and international comparison of asthma management in the emergency department. NZ Med J 1994; 107:26–29.
30. Gibson PG, Talbot PI, Hancock J, Hensley MJ. A prospective audit of asthma management following emergency asthma treatment at a teaching hospital. Med J Aust 1993; 158:775–778.

19

Management with Inhaled β_2-Agonists

Theodore J. Gaeta
New York Methodist Hospital, member of New York–Presbyterian Hospitals, Weill Medical College of Cornell University, Brooklyn, New York

I. INTRODUCTION

Bronchodilator therapy with adrenergic agents continues to be the mainstay of the symptomatic treatment of acute asthma. Although recent guidelines have stressed the importance of anti-inflammatory medications, bronchodilators are still an essential component of all phases of asthma care (1). Beta-adrenergic agonists have an established advantage over both methylxanthines and anticholinergics for the treatment of acute, severe asthma (2–4). More specifically, short-acting β_2-receptor agonists are critical in the treatment of acute asthma and for providing the most immediate improvement in airflow dynamics. While controversy exists regarding their chronic use, β_2-agonists remain the most necessary part of the emergency department (ED) armamentarium.

The following chapter will provide a brief overview of the history and evolution of β-agonist therapy and highlight the physiological actions and pharmacodynamics of the β-receptor. A summary of routes of administration, dosing, and adverse/toxic effects and a discussion of areas of controversy follows. Special considerations for the use of β-agonists in children, pregnancy, and the elderly patient, as well as the use of intravenous beta agonists is provided elsewhere (see Chapters 25, 27, and 28).

II. HISTORY AND EVOLUTION

In the early 1900s, adrenaline (epinephrine) was extracted and synthesized and quickly replaced anticholinergic agents for the acute management of bronchospasm (see Chapter 1). Unfortunately, while considered extremely valuable, in its native form epinephrine produced many undesirable cardiovascular effects. Manipulation of epinephrine's chemical structure [replacement of the terminal methyl group with an isopropyl group unveiled isoprenaline (isoproterenol)] led to the development of agents that had less vasodilatation and less pressor effects (5). In fact, the concept of dual alpha and beta-adrenergic receptors was established as a result of this research (6).

It was not until 1967 that Lands proposed the theory of distinct β_1- and β_2-receptor subtypes (the former primarily present in the heart and the latter in the bronchi, vasculature, and uterus) (7). Attempts at synthesizing compounds with longer half-lives and selected β_2 activity were fraught with difficulty. The compound orciprenaline (metaproterenol) was one of the first agents to achieve a prolongation of action, and despite its weak or nonexistent β_2 selectivity, this agent became one of the widely used bronchodilators throughout the 1970s and 1980s. β_2 selectivity was attained with the creation of the following three compounds: salbutamol (albuterol), terbutaline, and fenoterol. All three are highly potent β_2-agonists with somewhat limited activity at the β_1-receptor.

III. PHYSIOLOGICAL ACTIONS

An understanding of the physiological changes related to acute, severe asthma and the pharmacology of the bronchodilators will help explain the efficacy of beta-adrenergic agonists. The changes that occur with asthma are primarily the result of inflammatory events within the airway. These events include cellular infiltration and release of inflammatory mediators (such as histamine; prostaglandins D2 and F2a; thromboxane; leukotrienes C4, D4, and E4; platelet activating factor; bradykinin; adenosine; substance P; neurokinin A; and serotonin) (8). These substances all produce bronchoconstriction. Many of these mediators produce their effect by directly acting on bronchial smooth muscle, while some produce at least part of their bronchoconstriction through stimulation of afferent cholinergic receptors (9). β-agonists are functional antagonists of bronchoconstricting mediators in that they reverse smooth muscle contraction regardless of the stimulus (3).

In general, stimulation of the β_2-adrenergic receptors produces relaxation of bronchial, vascular, and uterine smooth muscle. Additional actions include enhancement of water output from bronchial mucous glands and improvement of mucociliary clearance (10). Evidence supporting an anti-inflammatory effect produced by the use of β-agonists continues to grow (11–14). The most likely mechanism whereby β_2-agonists exert anti-inflammatory effects appear to be inhibition of discharge of mediators from sensitized mast cells and reduction in inflammatory mediated microvascular permeability. In vitro, β_2 stimulation causes inhibition of histamine release from mast cells, antibody production by lymphocytes, and enzyme release from polymophonuclear leukocytes (15). Clinically, it is presumed that these actions augment the actions of inhaled or systemic corticosteroids.

On the cellular level, stimulation of the β_2-adrenergic receptor activates the enzyme adenyl cyclase, which converts intracellular adenosine triphosphate (ATP) to cyclic adenosine monophosphate (cAMP). Through phosphorylation, cAMP activates several intracellular proteins (16). Relaxation is thought to be caused by a reduction in myoplasmic calcium due to the effects of increased cAMP on binding of intracellular calcium to the cell membrane and endoplastic reticulum (17).

Beta-adrenergic receptor agonists have a wide spectrum of physiological effects (Table 1). Despite their beneficial effects on the airways, in large doses even β_2-agonists carry some risk for adverse metabolic and cardiac events. A detailed description of potential adverse effects, as well as a description of potential areas of controversy, will be discussed in a later section.

Table 1 Therapeutic Actions of β_2-Agonists

Pulmonary effects	Bronchial smooth muscle relaxation
	Inhibition of cholinergic transmission through airway ganglia
	Reduction in bronchial edema
	Improved mucociliary clearance
Cardiovascular effects	Cardioacceleration
	Vascular smooth muscle relaxation
	Reduction of pulmonary hypertension
	Improvement of right ventricular ejection fraction
Musculoskeletal effects	Uterine smooth muscle relaxation
	Improvement in diaphragmatic contractility
Immune effects	Inhibition of cell mediator release
	Decreased capillary permeability

IV. PHARMACODYNAMICS

A. Choice of Agents: Nonselective vs. Selective β_2-Agonists

The choice of aerosol β-agonist agents may be considered academic. A review of the literature comparing nonselective and selective β_2-agonist aerosol administration concluded that the selective β_2-agonists produce less cardiac stimulation than do nonselective agents (18). Unfortunately, despite selectivity, in sufficient doses even these medications may cause cardioacceleration (19). The two mechanisms proposed for cardioacceleration are response to a fall in systemic vascular resistance and stimulation of β_2-receptors in the sinoatrial (SA) node and right atrium.

In addition, airway obstruction and the resulting hypoxemia causes excessive cardiac stimulation. It is not uncommon to have a resulting tachycardia with or without atrial and ventricular premature contractions (20). Relief of the underlying pathophysiology often results in a decrease in heart rate and an improvement in the patients cardiac rhythm.

However, with equivalent success of bronchodilation and evidence of less risk of cardiac stimulation, many physicians err on the side of caution and treat empirically with selective β_2-agonists.

B. Administration of Beta-Adrenergic Agonists

There are currently four classes of beta-adrenergic agonists available for use in the Unites States: catecholamines (epinephrine, isoetharine, isoproterenol), resorcinols (metaproterenol, terbutaline), saligenins (albuterol), and a prodrug (bitolterol).

In general, medications used for the treatment of asthma can be administered directly (by the inhaled route), or indirectly (by the oral, subcutaneous, intramuscular, intravenous route). Controversies exist concerning the most efficacious and safest means of administration of these agents. Chapters 20 and 25 discuss the risks and benefits of subcutaneous and intravenous β-agonists, respectively. The following section will critically concentrate on the inhaled route.

1. *Inhaled Administration*

Historically, many clinicians felt that parenteral administration of bronchodilators was the preferred route initially in the management of severe lung obstruction. This was primarily based on the concerns about adequacy of delivery of aerosolized medication to the airways in the face of severe obstruction. However, ED-based clinical trials in the late 1970s and early 1980s clearly demonstrated that the aerosol route was as effective as systemic administration and often produced less toxicity (21–32).

Although it is difficult to compare individual studies due to differences in drug doses, dosage intervals, delivery systems, and patient populations, the evidence overwhelmingly implies that aerosol administration produces as effective bronchodilatation as parenteral with fewer adverse events.

Pharmacokinetics

Inhalation has the clear advantage of delivering the drug directly into the lungs. Higher concentrations can be delivered more effectively to the airways and the systemic side effects can be minimized (33). A variety of devices are available for the delivery of inhaled medications, or aerosols, to the lung. There is a growing pool of literature discussing the safety (34), efficacy (35–38), and patient satisfaction/compliance (39) associated with the various devices.

Particle size is an important characteristic of inhalation therapy. Aerosol deposition is dependent upon the size of the droplets, which varies according to the delivery device (40). Particles too large do not reach the lower respiratory tract, whereas particles too small (< 1 micron) are subject to Brownian motion and tend to be exhaled without being deposited. Droplets between 1 and 5 microns in diameter are ideal for penetration to the small airways. In contrast, droplets in the range of 5–10 microns deposit primarily in the central airways, as well as the oropharynx (41). Studies suggest that adrenergic receptors are present in high concentrations in the small conducting airways and that cholinergic receptors are present predominantly in the larger airways (42). It is therefore therapeutically advantageous to target β-agonists to their principle site of action. Although both larger and smaller particles may have clinical benefit, the acceptable range for particle size has been suggested to be between 1 and 5 microns for inhaled β-agonist therapy.

Updraft Nebulization. Updraft nebulization is used for inhalation therapy in many EDs throughout the United States. Nebulizers are used for delivery of relatively large (or continuous) doses of bronchodilator drugs (43), for patients who cannot coordinate the use of metered-dose inhalers (MDIs) (44), and for delivery of drugs that cannot conveniently be given by MDIs.

Important characteristics of nebulizer systems for clinical applications include the drug output, the aerosol particle size generated, and the amount of drug delivered to the patient. Nebulizer function is also affected by diluent volume, flow rate of the driving gas, the nebulization time, and nebulizer brand (45). Increasing the diluent volume (3–5 mL) decreases the amount of the drug trapped in the unit (dead volume), increases the nebulization time, and increases the amount of drug delivered to the patient. The clinical efficacy of the nebulized aerosol is dependent on the amount of aerosol in the respirable range that is available to the patient for their defined breathing pattern. Differences in drug availability varied fourfold depending on nebulizer, medication, or flow rate (46). Hess et al. suggest that a flow rate between 8 and 10 L/min increases the mass of particles at the respirable range of 1–5 microns and decreases the nebulization time (offsetting the effect of a larger diluent) (45).

Although further work is needed to evaluate the effect of different breathing patterns, when patient performance is suspect and high doses are required, nebulized β-agonists have a clear advantage over other delivery systems.

Intermittent Positive Pressure Breathing. Intermittent positive pressure breathing (IPPB) can be used as a technique for the administration of aerosolized pharmacological agents. In fact, in the 1970s and early 1980s, it was most common for patients with acute asthma exacerbations to be treated in the ED with aerosol therapy driven by IPPB (47–49). With the risk of barotrauma in mind, IPPB had fallen out of favor because a number of studies had failed to demonstrate any substantial, reproducible benefit from its use compared to passive nebulization (50–52).

Metered Dose Inhalers (with Spacer). Authors have suggested that a metered dose inhaler attached to a spacer device is an acceptable alternative to updraft nebulization for the delivery of β_2-agonists in acute, severe asthma (53). Conventional updraft nebulizers have inherent inefficiencies; the most dramatic is the loss of medication to the surrounding atmosphere during exhalation. Metered dose inhalers with the addition of a spacer have been proposed to help overcome the deficiencies of nebulization. Spacing devices by design eliminate the need for hand-breath coordination and reduce the deposition of large particles in the upper airway. A review of the literature comparing nebulizers and MDIs in the acute setting of the ED reveal contrasting results (54). A wide range of efficacious doses and dosing frequencies have been described. Even with this in mind, the data strongly suggest that in the acute care setting MDIs are as effective as nebulizers in the treatment of acute asthma (55–59).

Alternative Drug Delivery Systems

Nasal Bilevel Positive Airway Pressure Circuit (see Chapter 25). Noninvasive inspiratory ventilatory support has been used with limited success in patients with acute bronchospasm (60,61). The combination of inspiratory pressure and continuous positive airway pressure, as is delivered with nasal bilevel positive airway pressure (BiPAP) circuit, has been shown to be effective in the treatment of acute bronchospastic exacerbations of obstructive pulmonary disease (62,63). In 1995, Pollack et al. performed the first clinical trial comparing the efficacy of β-agonist aerosol delivered by BiPAP to jet nebulization (64). In their study, patients treated with BiPAP improved faster and were well tolerated in the ED. Further investigation is warranted (see Chapter 25).

Heliox. Heliox is a blend of helium and oxygen with a gas density less than that of air. Several studies have shown that this mixture decreases airway resistance in patients with upper, as well as lower airway disease (65,66). In one study, Heliox led to significant increase in peak expiratory flow rates when compared to placebo (air) (67). This study found both a decrease in inspiratory and expiratory airway resistance in those treated with Heliox. It is suggested that Heliox improves laminar flow in the most turbulent airways. Flow dynamics and particle deposition parameters suggest improved delivery of particle to the lower airway of asthmatics when the solution is aerosolized with a helium-oxygen mixture (68). Clinical trials evaluating the efficacy of Heliox as a driving gas for β-agonist nebulization are in progress (see Chapter 25).

Optimal Dose and Frequency

In acute asthmatic exacerbations, the optimal dose and frequency of administration of inhaled β-agonists is poorly defined. Few studies have compared different dosing intervals while total dose administered was maintained constant. It is suspected that the duration of effect following inhaled β-agonists is considerably shorter during the acute attack than it is in chronic stable asthma. The question of dosing frequency was first raised by Robertson et al., who showed that, after an initial dose of nebulized β-agonist, patients responded better to dosing every 20 min than every 60 min using the same total dose (69). In fact, after each 60 min dose, there was a peak response followed by a decline, suggesting that under conditions of severe bronchospasm rapid dissipation of drug from the site resulted in more spasm and less access to the next dose.

In the ED, β-agonists can be given with a frequency dictated in part by the severity of the symptoms. Routinely, this schedule involves nebulization treatments every 20–30 min during the first hour and hourly thereafter while the patient remains in the ED. If a standard dose of medication is used with each treatment (2.5 mg albuterol in 3 mL diluent), side effects are generally acceptable and serious complications are few (70).

Dose Response and Continuous Nebulization. The response to a given dose of inhaled β-agonist is unpredictable. There appears to be great individual variability (71), yet there is a correlation between total dose administered and the response for the group as a whole. Schuh et al. showed that, in children, 0.15 mg/kg of albuterol delivered every 20 min for six doses produced a more rapid response than 0.05 mg/kg per dose (72). Considerable variability of plasma levels were noted, reflecting interindividual differences in absorption and hence drug delivery to the lung.

Both the intensity and duration of action of aerosolized β_2-agonists are dose-dependent. An increased contractile stimulus will not only shift the bronchodilitation curve but will result in a shorter duration of action (73). Thus, aerosolized β_2-agonists should be given in higher doses more frequently for optimal results in acute severe asthma.

Studies evaluating continuous nebulization using a continuous flow nebulizer in line with a face mask system have revealed results that have been generally been comparable to those achieved with frequent repeated nebulizer administration when equivalent doses of β-agonists were given. However, there is some evidence (on post-hoc analysis) that the advantage to continuous nebulization is in the most severely ill asthmatic patients. In the subgroup analysis of patients with PEFR < 200 L/min or $FEV_1 < 50\%$ of predicted, continuous nebulization appeared to be more effective in relieving airflow obstruction, decreasing admission rate, and shortening respiratory therapy time and hospital stay (58,74,75). It is speculated that continuous nebulization is more effective than intermittent nebulization because it provides sustained stimulation of pulmonary β_2-receptors, thereby preventing the potential rebound bronchospasm that can occur when aerosols are delivered intermittently. In a busy ED, administration of β_2-agonists every 20 min by inhalation may be desirable, but in actuality it may not occur. Continuous nebulization offers a more reliable medication delivery system.

There are few potential disadvantages to continuous nebulization, including the possibility of tachyphylaxis and facial skin irritation underneath the center points of the mask needed to provide this mode of delivery. Hence, it appears that continuous nebulization should be considered for the patients with severe obstruction if the proper nebulizer setup is available and close follow-up and monitoring of the patients is provided.

Metered Dose Inhalers. In discussing dosing and frequency of administration one must consider the alternative methods of delivery of inhaled β-agonists, specifically, metered dose inhalers. Clinical trials involving MDIs together with spacers have yielded impressive results. Despite the much smaller dose of medication per treatment (i.e., 2–4 mg of metaproterenol by MDI vs. 15 mg by updraft nebulizer), the bronchodilitation achieved with the two delivery systems were equivalent (54,76–79). A variety of doses and dose schedules have been utilized, with anywhere from 3 to 8 inhalations from the MDI being considered equivalent to one nebulizer treatment. The dose of albuterol contained in a single activation of an MDI is 0.09 mg (1/25th the dose given via nebulization).

There are only a few groups of patients in which MDIs cannot be used effectively. Patients who cannot generate a sufficient inspiratory flow to achieve proper deposition of the medication (i.e., infants, very small children and the severely dyspneic or fatigued) are unlikely to benefit from pressurized MDIs with or without spacers.

The choice of a specific delivery method should be determined on an individual basis, taking into account the issues of cost, timeliness of administration, and personnel availability. When an MDI is used patient performance is a major determinant of aerosol delivery. With the updraft nebulizer, it appears that the performance of the nebulizer is the major determinant of aerosol delivery.

Whether given by interrupted or continuous nebulization, or by MDI, the optimal total dose of inhaled β_2-agonist for acute asthma is poorly defined. It is uncertain where on the bronchodilitation dose-response curve the currently recommended dose (i.e., albuterol 7.5 mg by nebulizer during the initial 60–90 min) is positioned. Additional studies are needed to define more clearly the optimal dose of β_2-agonists as well as to assess interindividual variability in responsiveness.

V. TOXICITY/ADVERSE EFFECTS

A. Systemic Effects/Side Effects

Oral and parenteral routes of administration of beta-adrenoreceptor agonists produce the greatest adverse consequences. Inhalation of these drugs seldom present a clinical problem.

When large doses of β-agonists are used to treat status asthmaticus even selective β_2-agonists carry some risk for adverse metabolic and cardiac events. Systemic events such as tachycardia, hypokalemia, and hypoxia may occur during intensive therapy.

As mentioned earlier, even β_2-selective-agonists can produce a rise in heart rate. The tachycardia is generally mild and easily monitored in the ED setting. The greatest degree of tachycardia generally occurs in the first 60–80 min of therapy and then diminishes despite continued administration (80). This probably reflects cardiac β_2-receptor downregulation as well as improvement in airways obstruction.

Hypokalemia, hyperglycemia, and worsening hypoxemia are common β-agonist effects, but the degree of change is small and usually clinically insignificant with the inhaled route of delivery. Stimulation of the sodium-potassium pump on cell membranes causes intracellular shift in potassium and a decrease in serum potassium. With inhaled β-agonists the average fall in serum potassium is approximately 0.4 mEq/L (81). Stimulation of the β-receptors in the pancreas leads to inhibition of insulin release and a resultant rise in blood glucose. Although poorly quantified, the resultant hyperglycemia is also thought to be transient and clinically insignificant.

The vasodilator properties of β_2-agonists may increase ventilation-perfusion mismatching, producing or worsening hypoxemia. However, this has not been a consistent finding or proved to be a significant effect. Using oxygen as the driving gas for the nebulizer seems to obviate any potential problem (82).

Careful monitoring and reasonable prophylactic measures can prevent most of the potential adverse effects to high-dose inhaled β_2-agonists. In general it is prudent to use the smallest therapeutic dose in older, compromised patients but inhaled β_2-agonists can be administered safely in the elderly and persons with known coronary disease (9).

B. Mortality and Shadows of Doubt (see Chapter 17)

Recent published epidemiological studies have suggested that regular use of β_2-receptor agonists may actually worsen asthma and are a risk factor for near death from asthma. The long running controversy of β-agonists and asthma deaths stretches back to the 1960s. In 1968, reports from the United Kingdom strongly indicated a connection between β-agonist sales (specifically, isoprenaline) and an increase in mortality from asthma in the 5–35 years of age group (83,84). Further investigations revealed that epidemics in asthma deaths only occurred in the six countries where isoprenaline forte had been sold (85).

In the late 1970s, there was new epidemic of asthma deaths in New Zealand. The high mortality rate was correlated specifically to inhaled treatment with fenoterol in several epidemiological studies (86–89). Fenoterol was introduced in New Zealand in 1976. The increase in death rate started at about the same time and continued as the market share for inhaled fenoterol increased. One study revealed that the odds ratio for death for patients using fenoterol was 2.7 compared to 0.5 for salbutamol. These data, along with the temporal relationship between death rates and the introduction of fenoterol in New Zealand, strengthened the association between fenoterol and asthma mortality.

Epidemic increases in asthma deaths were observed in the 1960s and 1970s; a tangible increase in death rate was correlated with the introduction of more potent asthma inhalers. This has been attributed to the lack of effect in reducing inflammation, masking of ongoing deterioration in lung function by relieving symptoms almost continuously, and possibly an increase in exposure to allergens and environmental toxins. With widespread publicity an alarm was raised and education and treatment of patients improved. There was an elimination of nonprescription β_2-agonists, earlier admission to the hospital, more general prescription of corticosteroids, and a decrease in the mortality rate (90,91).

The Saskatchewan Asthma Epidemiology Project (1992) was developed in order to validate or refute the earlier findings (92). The authors began by examining the computerized files of the Saskatchewan Prescription Drug Plan, which held prescriptions for drugs for asthma listed in the Saskatchewan formulary that had been dispensed to eligible residents of the province aged 5–54 years during 1980–1987. The Canadian study found increased odds ratio for death and near-death events for most drugs used in asthma treatment. This effect was most impressive for inhaled fenoterol, but was also obvious for inhaled salbutamol. A dose-response effect on the odds ratio for fatal events was found with both drugs. However, unlike the earlier studies, there was not an increase in asthma death rate in Canada when these agents were first introduced. In fact, the asthma death rate was very low in that region during the study years. The authors also investigated the possibility that the association of fenoterol with asthma death was due to confounding by severity (selective prescribing of fenoterol to patients with more severe asthma). It was determined that there was little evidence in their study group linking selective prescribing and the association of fenoterol with asthma deaths (93).

A more recent publication by the Saskatchewan group reported that the increase in death rate in the earlier study was restricted to patients who used more than 150–200 inhalations per month (94). This usage may reflect scheduled administration of β_2-agonists (e.g., two puffs fours times per day equals 240 puffs per month) or a marker of undertreatment of asthma. Clearly the more severe asthmatics have a higher mortality risk. Since the severe asthmatics have more bronchospasm than mild ones, their use of inhaled β-agonists would likewise also be higher. The question concerns whether excessive β-agonist use is an independent risk factor for fatal asthma, especially in individuals who would be sensitive to inhaled beta agonists (see Chapter 17).

Many authors feel that the media coverage following the Spitzer's original report was misguiding and misleading. An analysis of six case-control studies of β_2-agonists and asthma deaths failed to reveal an obvious relationship between life-threatening asthma and either oral or inhaled β-agonists by metered dose inhaler (95). This study did find an association between nebulized β_2-agonist use and increased mortality.

It appears that there is no convincing study showing any relationship between inhaled β_2-adrenoreceptor agonists (except nebulized and high-dose fenoterol) in currently recommended doses and increase in asthma death. Confirmation and reproduction of the findings with respect to nebulized β-agonists may play an important role in the choice of route of administration of these agents.

VI. CONCLUSION: THE FUTURE

With the increased emphasis on anti-inflammatory therapy of asthma, bronchodilators are assuming a subsidiary role as "mop-up" operation. However, there is no substitute for their vigorous use in the acute attack, nor in the management of residual bronchospasm. Constricted airways still kill patients. Understanding and identification of airway receptor phenotypes and receptor pharmacology may lead us towards a better understanding of the role of the present classes of β_2-agonists. We can anticipate more developments in the mode of delivery, the philosophy of their use and their combinations, and an increased understanding of their adverse effects.

REFERENCES

1. NHBLI National Asthma Education Program. Expert panel report guidelines for the diagnosis and management of asthma. Bethsesda, MD: U.S. Department of Health and Human Services, Publication No. 97-4051, 1997.
2. McFadden ER. Therapy of acute asthma. J Allergy Clin Immunol 1989; 84:151–158.
3. Kelly HW. Controversies in asthma therapy with theophylline and beta-2 adrenergic agonists. Clin Pharmacol 1984; 3:386–395.
4. Kelly HW, Murphy S. Should anticholinergics be used in acute, severe asthma? DICP Ann Pharmacother 1990; 24:409–416.
5. O'Donnell SR. The development of beta receptor agonist drugs. In: Beasley R, Pearce NE, eds., The Role of Beta Receptor Agonist Therapy in Asthma Mortality. Boca Raton, FL: CRC Press, 1993, 4–26.
6. Ahlquist RP. A study of adrenotropic receptors. Am J Physiol 1948; 153:586–600.
7. Lands AM, Arnold A, McAuliff JP, et al. Differentiation of receptor systems activated by sympathomimetic amines. Nature 1967; 214:597–598.
8. Barnes PJ. New concepts in the pathogenesis of bronchial hyperresponsiveness and asthma. J Allergy Clin Immunol 1989; 83:1013–1026.
9. Kelly HW, Murphy S. Beta adrenergic agonists for acute, severe asthma. Ann Pharmacother 1992; 26:81–91.
10. Nelson HS. Adrenergic therapy of bronchial asthma. J Allergy Clin Immunol 1987; 77:771.
11. Tewntyman OP, Finnerty JP, Holgate ST, et al. The inhibitory effect of nebulized albuterol on the early and late asthmatic reactions and increase in airway responsiveness provoked by inhaled allergen in asthma. Am Rev Respir Dis 1991; 14:782–787.
12. Tewntyman OP, Finnerty JP, Harris A, et al. Protection against allergen-induced asthma by salmeterol. Lancet 1990; 336:1338–1342.

13. Palmqvist M, Balder B, Lowhagen D, et al. Late asthmatic reaction decreased after treatment with salbutamol and formoterol, a new long-acting beta-2 agonist. J Allergy Clin Immunol 1992; 89:844–849.
14. Butchers PR, Vardey CJ, Johnson M. Salmeterol: a potent and long-acting inhibitor of inflammatory mediator release from human lung. Br J Pharmacol 1991; 104:672–676.
15. Nelson JS. Beta adenergic agonists. Chest 1982; 82:33s.
16. Maddens M, Sowers J. Catecholamines in critical care. Crit Care Clin 1987; 5:871–877.
17. Schneid CR, Honeyman TW, Fay FS. Mechanisms of beta-adrenergic relaxation of smooth muscle. Nature 1979; 277:32–36.
18. Reed MT, Kelly HW. Sympathomimetics for acute severe asthma: should only beta-2 selective agonists be used? DICP Ann Pharmacother 1990; 24:868–873.
19. Kaumann AJ. Is there a third heart beta-adrenoceptor? Trends Pharmacol Sci 1989; 10:316–320.
20. Chapman KR, D'Urzo AD, Druck MN, Rebuck AS. Cardiovascular response to acute airway obstruction and hypoxemia. Am Rev Respir Dis 1989; 140:1222–1227.
21. Rossing TH, Fanta CH, Goldstein DH, et al. Emergency therapy for asthma: comparison of the acute effects of parenteral and inhaled sympathomimetics and infused aminophylline. Am Rev Respir Dis 1980; 122:365–371.
22. Lawford P, Jones BJM, Milledge JS. Comparison of intravenous and nebulized salbuterol in the initial treatment of severe asthma. Br Med J 1978; 1:84.
23. Pliss LB, Gallagher EJ. Aerosol vs. injected epinephrine in acute asthma. Ann Emerg Med 1981; 10:353–355.
24. Schwartz AL, Lipton JM, Warburton D, et al. Management of acute asthma in childhood: a randomized evaluation of beta-adrenergic agents. Am J Dis Child 1980; 134:474–478.
25. Rossing TH, Fanta CH, McFadden ER. A controlled trial of the use of single versus combined drug therapy in the treatment of acute episodes of asthma. Am Rev Respir Dis 1981; 123: 190–194.
26. Pancorbo S, Fifield G, Davies S, et al. Subcutaneous epinephrine versus nebulized terbutaline in the emergency department treatment of asthma. Clin Pharmacol 1983; 2:45–48.
27. Tinkelman DG, Vanderpool GE, Carroll MS, et al. Comparison of nebulized terbutaline and subcutaneous epinephrine in the treatment of acute asthma. Ann Allergy 1983; 50:398–401.
28. Baughman RP, Ploysongsang Y, James W. A comparative study of aerosolized terbutaline and subcutaneously administered epinephrine in the treatment of acute bronchial asthma. Ann Allergy 1984; 53:131–134.
29. Uden DL, Goets DR, Kohen DP, et al. Comparison of nebulized terbutaline and subcutaneous epinephrine in the treatment of acute asthma. Ann Emerg Med 1985; 14:229–232.
30. Elenbaas RM, Frost GL, Robinson WA, et al. Subcutaneous epinephrine vs. nebulized metaproterenol in acute asthma. Drug Intell Clin Pharmacol 1985; 19:567–571.
31. Naspitz CK, Sole D, Wandalsen N. Treatment of acute attacks of bronchial asthma. A comparative study of epinephrine (subcutaneous) and fenoterol (inhalation). Ann Allergy 1987; 59: 21–24.
32. Appel D, Karpel JP, Sherman M. Epinephrine improves expiratory flow rates in patients with asthma who do not respond to inhaled metaproterenol sulfate. J Allergy Clin Immunol 1989; 84:90–98.
33. Newhouse MT, Dolovich MB. Control of asthma by aerosols. N Engl J Med 1986; 315:870–874.
34. Higgins RM, Cookson W, Lane DJ, et al. Cardiac arrhythmias caused by nebulized beta-agonist therapy. Lancet 1987; 2:863–864.
35. Crompton G, Duncan J. Clinical assessment of a new breath-actuated inhaler. Practitioner 1989; 233:268–269.
36. Everard ML, Clark AR, Milner AD. Drug delivery from holding chambers with attached facemask. Arch Dis Child 1992; 67:580–585.

37. Fuglsang G, Pedersen S. Comparison of Nebuhaler and nebulizer treatment of acute severe asthma in children. Eur J Respir Dis 1986; 69:109–113.
38. Goren A, Noviski N, Avital A, et al. Assessment of the ability of young children to use a powder inhaler device (Turbuhaler). Pediatr Pulmonol 1994; 18:77–80.
39. Ahrens R, Lux C, Bahl T, Ham SH. Choosing the meter-dose inhaler spacer of holding chamber that matches the patient's need: Evidence that the specific drug being delivered is an important consideration. J Allergy Clin Immunol 1995; 96:288–294.
40. Johnson MA, Newman SP, Bloom R, et al. Delivery of albuterol and ipratroprium bromide from two nebulizer systems in chronic stable asthma: efficacy and pulmonary deposition. Chest 1989; 96:4–10.
41. Gerrity TR, Lee PS, Hass FJ, et al. Calculated deposition of inhaled particles in the airway generations of normal subjects. J Appl Physiol 1979; 47:867–873.
42. Barnes PJ, Basbaum CB, Nadel JA, et al. Localization of beta-adrenoreceptors in the mammalian lung by light microscopic autoradiography. Nature 1982; 229:444–447.
43. Blake KV, Hoppe M, Harmon E, et al. Relative amount of albuterol delivered to lung receptors from a metered-dose inhaler and nebulizer solution: bioassay by histamine bronchoprovocation. Chest 1992; 101:309–315.
44. Kacmarek RM, Hess D. The interface between patient and aerosol generator. Respir Care 1991; 36:952–976.
45. Hess D, Fisher BS, Williams P, et al. Medication nebulizer performance: effects of diluent volume, nebulizer flow, and nebulizer brand. Chest 1996; 110:498–505.
46. MacNeish CF, Meisner D, Thibert R, et al. A comparison of pulmonary availability between Ventolin (albuterol) nebules and Ventolin (albuterol) respirator solution. Chest 1997; 111: 204–208.
47. Bloomfield P, Carmichael J, Petrie GR, et al. Comparison of salbutamol given intravenously and by intermittent positive pressure breathing in life threatening asthma. Br Med J 1979; 1: 848–850.
48. Choo-Kang YFJ, Grant IWB. Comparison of two methods of administrating bronchodilator aerosol to asthmatic patients. Br Med J 1975; 1:119–120.
49. Light RW, Taylor RW, George RB. Albuterol and isoproterenol in bronchial asthma: efficacy and toxicity of drugs administered via intermittent positive pressure breathing. Arch Intern Med 1979; 139:639–643.
50. Campbell IA, Hill A, Middleton H, et al. Intermittent positive pressure breathing. Br Med J 1978; 1:1186.
51. Fergusson RJ, Carmichael J, Rafferty P, et al. Nebulized salbutamol in life-threatening asthma: is IPPB necessary? Br J Dis Chest 1983; 77:255–261.
52. IPPB Study Group. Intermittent positive pressure breathing therapy of chronic obstructive pulmonary disease: a clinical trial. Ann Intern Med 1983; 99:612–620.
53. Benton G, Thomas RC, Nickerson BG, et al. Experience with a metered-dose inhaler with a spacer in the pediatric emergency department. Am J Dis Chil 1989; 143:678–681.
54. Kisch GL, Paloucek FP. Metered-dose inhalers and nebulizers in the acute setting. Ann Pharmacother 1992; 26:92–95.
55. Salzman GA, Steele MT, Pribble JP, et al. Aerosolized metaproterenol in the treatment of asthmatics with severe airflow obstruction. Chest 1989; 95:1017–1120.
56. Levitt MA, Gambrioli EF, Fink JB. Comparative trial of continuous nebulization versus metered-dose inhaler in the treatment of acute bronchospasm. Ann Emerg Med 1995; 26:273–277.
57. Idris AH, McDermott MF, Raucci JL, et al. Emergency department treatment of asthma: metered-dose inhaler plus holding chamber is equivalent in effectiveness to nebulizer. Chest 1993; 103:665–672.
58. Chou KJ. Metered-dose inhalers with spacers vs. nebulizers for pediatric asthma. Arch Ped Adol Med 1995; 149:201–205.

59. Rudnitsky GS, Eberlein RS, Schoffstall JM. Comparison of intermittent and continuously nebulized albuterol for treatment of asthma in an urban emergency department. Ann Emerg Med 1993; 22:1842–1846.
60. Bochard L, Isabey D, Piquet J, et al. Reversal of acute exacerbation of chronic obstructive lung disease by inspiratory assistance with a face mask. N Engl J Med 1990; 323:1523–1530.
61. Bott J, Carroll MP, Conway JH, et al. Randomized controlled trial of nasal ventilation in acute ventilatory failure due to chronic obstructive airways disease. Lancet 1993; 341:1555–1557.
62. Ambrosino N, Nava S, Bertone P, et al. Physiologic evaluation of pressure support ventilation by nasal mask in patients with stable COPD. Chest 1992; 101:385–391.
63. Appendii L, Patessio A, Zanaboni S, et al. Physiologic effects of positive end-expiratory pressure and mask pressure support during exacerbations of chronic obstructive pulmonary disease. Am J Respir Crit Care Med 1994; 149:1069–1076.
64. Pollack, CV, Fleisch KB, Dowsey K. Treatment of acute bronchospasm with beta adrenergic agonist aerosols delivered by a nasal bilevel positive airway pressure circuit. Ann Emerg Med 1995; 26:552–557.
65. Tobias JD. Heliox in children with airway obstruction. Ped Emerg Care 1997; 13:29–32.
66. Kass JE, Castriotta RJ. Heliox therapy in acute severe asthma. Chest 1995; 107:597–598.
67. Manthous JM, Hall JB, Caputo MA, et al. Heliox improves pulsus paradoxus and peak expiratory flow in nonintubated patients with severe asthma. Am J Respir Crit Care Med 1995; 151: 310–314.
68. Anderson M, Svartengren M, Bylin G, et al. Deposition in asthmatics of particles inhaled in air or in helium-oxygen. Am Rev Respir Dis 1993; 147:524–528.
69. Robwertson CF, Smith F, Beck R, Levison H. Response to frequent low doses of nebulized salbutamol in acute asthma. J Pediatr 1985; 106:672–674.
70. Moan MJ, Fanta CH. Bronchodilator therapy in the management of acute asthma. Comp Ther 1995; 21:421–427.
71. Mitchell CA, Armstrong JG, Bartholomew MA, Scicchitano R. Nebulized fenoterol in severe asthma: determinants of dose response. Eur J Respir Dis 1983; 64:229–233.
72. Schuh S. High versus low-dose frequently administered nebulized albuterol in children with severe, acute asthma. Pediatrics 1989; 83:513–518.
73. Jenne JW, Arhens RC. Pharmacokinetics of beta-adrenergic compounds. In: Jenne JW, Murphy S, eds. Drug therapy for asthma: Research and clinical practice. New York: Marcel Dekker, Inc., 1987, 213–258.
74. Lin RY, Sauter D, Newman T, et al. Continuous versus intermittent albuterol nebulization in the treatment of acute asthma. Ann Emerg Med 1993; 22:1847–1853.
75. Colacone A, Walhove N, Stern E, et al. Continuous nebulization of albuterol in acute asthma. Chest 1990; 97:693–697.
76. Papo MC, Frank J, Thomson AE, et al. A prospective, randomized study of continuous versus intermittent nebulized albuterol for severe status asthmaticus in children, Crit Care Med 1993; 21:479–486.
77. Turner JR, Corkery KJ, Eckman D, et al. Equivalence of continuous flow nebulizer and metered-dose inhaler with reservoir bag for treatment of acute airflow obstruction. Chest 1988; 93:476–481.
78. Tarala RA, Madsen BW, Paterson JW. Comparative efficacy of salbutamol by pressurized aerosol and wet nebulizer in acute asthma. Br J Clin Pharmacol 1980; 10:393–397.
79. Prendergast J, Hopkins J, Timms B, et al. Comparative efficacy of terbutaline administered by nebuhaler and by nebulizer in young children with acute asthma. Med J Aust 1989; 151: 406–408.
80. Schuh S, Reider MJ, Canny G, et al. Nebulized albuterol in acute childhood asthma: comparison of two doses. Pediatrics 1990; 86:509–513.
81. Wong CS, Pavord ID, Williams J, et al. Bronchodilator, cardiovascular, and hypokalemic effects of fenoterol, salbutamol, and terbutaline in asthma. Lancet 1990; 336:1396–1399.

82. Douglas JG, Rafferty P, Fergusson RJ, et al. Nebulized salbutamol without oxygen in severe acute asthma: how effective and how safe? Thorax 1985; 45:180–183.
83. Speizer FE, Doll R, Heaf P. Observations on recent increase in mortality from asthma. Brit Med J 1968; 1:335–339.
84. Speizer FE, Doll R, Heaf P, Strang B. Investigation in the use of drugs preceding death from asthma. Brit Med J 1968; 1:339–342.
85. Stolley PD. Why the United Stated was spared an epidemic of death due to asthma. Amer Rev Respir Dis 1972; 105:883–890.
86. Burgess C, Pearce R, Thiruchelvam, et al. Prescribed drug therapy and near-fatal asthma attacks. Eur Respir J 1994; 7:498–503.
87. Crane J, Flatt A, Jackson R, et al. Prescribed fenoterol and death from asthma in New Zealand, 1981-1983, case control study. Lancet 1989; I:917–922.
88. Grainger J, Woodman K, Pearce N, et al. Prescribed fenoterol and death from asthma in New Zealand, 1981-1987: a further case control study. Thorax 1995; 46:105–111.
89. Pearce N, Grainger J, Atkinson M, et al. Case control study of prescribed fenoterol and death from asthma in New Zealand, 1977–81. Thorax 1990; 45:170–175.
90. Garret J, Kilbe J, Richards G, et al. Major reduction in asthma morbidity and continued reduction in asthma mortality in New Zealand: what lessons have we learnt? Thorax 1995; 50:303–311.
91. Pearce N, Beasley R, Crane J, et al. End of the New Zealand asthma mortality epidemic. Lancet 1995; 345:41–45.
92. Spitzer WO, Suissia S, Ernst P, et al. The use of B-agonists and the risk of death and near death from asthma. New Engl J Med 1992; 326:501–506.
93. Ernst P, Habbick B, Suissa S, et al. Is the association between inhaled beta-agonist use and life-treatening asthma because of confounding by severity? Am Rev Respir Dis 1993; 148: 75–79.
94. Suissa S, Ernst P, Boivin JF, et al. A cohort analysis of excess mortality in asthma and the use of inhaled β-agonists. Amer J Resp Crit Care Med 1994; 149:604–610.
95. Mullen ML, Mullen B, Carey M. The association between β-agonist use and death from asthma: a meta-analytic integration of case-controlled studies. JAMA 1993; 270:1842–1845.

20

Epinephrine

Barry E. Brenner
The Brooklyn Hospital Center, member of New York–Presbyterian Hospitals, Weill Medical College of Cornell University, Brooklyn, New York

In the doses used to treat asthma, it is possible to categorize the effects of epinephrine into three major clinical actions: α-adrenergic vasoconstriction; β_1-inotropic, chronotropic, and increased speed of atrioventricular conduction; and β_2-bronchial smooth muscle relaxation (see Chapter 19) (1–3). The effects of epinephrine vary with the dose (4). Subcutaneous or intravenous injection of low doses of epinephrine causes tachycardia, increases systolic pressure, and usually decreases diastolic pressure, mean arterial pressure, and peripheral vascular resistance. High doses, however, will induce a marked peripheral vasoconstriction and will elevate blood pressure and peripheral resistance (3,5). Physiologic doses of epinephrine, but not norepinephrine, are effective in ameliorating bronchospasm (6,7). In adults with asthma, epinephrine traditionally has been injected at a dose of 0.3–0.5 mL of a 1 : 1000 solution subcutaneously every 20–30 min for three doses. In children, the dose is 0.01 mL/kg (8,9). Although the dose is typically given in three subcutaneous injections, if the patient does respond, the response would occur within two injections in the vast majority of children (10). Epinephrine in these doses and schedules is clearly effective in acute asthma (11–15). In 484 children presenting with acute asthma, 61 were well enough to be sent home after a single dose of epinephrine, 101 after two injections, and 166 after three injections (0.01 mL/kg to a maximum of 0.3 mL of 1 : 1000 aqueous epinephrine at 20-min intervals). Therefore, 328 (76%) of children with acute asthma improved progressively and sufficiently with each injection of epinephrine to be discharged from the emergency department (ED) after only epinephrine therapy. No information was available on the number of patients whose symptoms recurred during the immediate follow-up period or ED relapse (16).

However, epinephrine has clearly waned in popularity for the treatment of acute asthma due to the fact that β_2-agonist inhalants have been equally effective and not invasive; this latter fact was much appreciated by the children, their parents, and the nurses who would have to administer the subcutaneous epinephrine injections (17,18). In fact, nausea, vomiting, headache, and pallor occurred exclusively in 50% of the children receiving the injections of epinephrine and none in the children receiving the β_2-agonist inhalants (17). Long-acting slow-release preparations of epinephrine (Sus-phrine®) were standard in the 1970s to the mid-1980s at the time of discharge from the ED in children. But these injections were shown also to be equally effective as β_2-agonist inhalants (19) and their use also has virtually disappeared.

Epinephrine is considered a nonselective β-agonist with potential for producing arrhythmias. As the dose of epinephrine is increased from 0.1 to 0.5 mg, there is a progressive response in the degree of bronchodilation with either insignificant or small degrees of tachycardia even at the 0.5 mg dose. No dysrhythmias were noted in these studies, although Holter monitoring was not utilized (11–16,20). When patients receiving both epinephrine and intravenous aminophylline received Holter monitoring during therapy of an acute asthmatic episode, complex dysrhythmias were noted, especially in the patients older than 40 years of age (21). Thus 40 was considered the age above which epinephrine was contraindicated. Others have found no difference in the incidence of ventricular arrhythmias by Holter monitoring between epinephrine, aminophylline, or their combination. However, the risk of giving these medications to an acute asthmatic with occult heart disease remains unclear (22). In view of the side effects, the possible adverse consequences of epinephrine in the treatment of asthma will be reviewed.

I. ARRHYTHMOGENIC EFFECTS

Epinephrine is one of the most potent arrhythmogenic drugs, perhaps second only to isoproterenol. During a continuous intravenous infusion of 2 μg/kg/min of epinephrine in dogs, a large decrease in the threshold for ventricular fibrillation is observed during the first 1–5 min. The more rapid the infusion, the greater the lowering of the threshold for ventricular fibrillation (23,24). This effect is related to the β-agonist effects of epinephrine (25–27). During this infusion an inhomogeneous distribution of epinephrine in adjacent myocardial cells occurs, termed increased ''temporal dispersion,'' and the cells are no longer excited in a programmed, orderly sequence. Therefore, a normally conducted beat meets an inhomogeneous myocardium, where some fibers are excitable and other fibers remain in the refractory state. Ventricular re-entry rhythms may occur, bringing about ventricular fibrillation (28,29). Such mechanisms may be involved in cardiac arrests due to the administration of epinephrine through a central intravenous catheter or rapid administration of large doses of epinephrine (30–35).

This effect of epinephrine on the threshold for ventricular fibrillation is independent of an initial elevation in systolic blood pressure. Verrier et al. (36) carefully studied the effects of phenylephrine or aortic occlusion, which elevate blood pressure, on the threshold for ventricular fibrillation with epinephrine. They could not obtain a decrease in the threshold for ventricular fibrillation with either method (36). Similar results were noted by Papp and Szekeres who further demonstrated that only in the presence of heart failure does an elevation in blood pressure lower the threshold for ventricular fibrillation by epinephrine (37).

Opie et al. (38,39) have reviewed the probable mechanisms for the arrhythmogenic action of epinephrine, of which three are most likely to account for the lowered threshold for ventricular fibrillation observed during early infusions of epinephrine. The first is catecholamine stimulation, especially in the presence of hypoxia which, may cause a localized inhomogeneous distribution of potassium secondary to leakage of potassium from myocardial cells. If the local hyperkalemia is severe, phase 0 sodium entry into myocardial cells is blocked, and the calcium-mediated slow channel inward current predominates, which results in asynchrony and re-entrant rhythms. The second is that catecholamines shorten the duration of the action potential, and, if inhomogeneous, may result in re-entrant rhythms. Finally, catecholamines increase the activity of spontaneous pacemakers by causing a more rapid outward current of potassium and, therefore, increasing the rate of spontaneous diastolic depolarization (phase 4) and encouraging ectopic pacemaker rhythms (38–40).

These effects of epinephrine may be mediated by cyclic adenosine monophosphate (cAMP). In the perfused heart, cAMP levels, either added exogenously to the perfusate or generated by the addition of theophylline or epinephrine, correlate closely with a low threshold for ventricular fibrillation. Furthermore, this correlation is much closer with cAMP than with levels of potassium or high energy phosphates (41,42). In a different study, intramyocardial cAMP concentration correlated well with the presence of ventricular fibrillation produced by sympathomimetics (43).

In the presence of severe asthma, epinephrine may precipitate arrhythmias. Severe acute respiratory disorders predispose to arrhythmias (44) and severe asthma is characterized by hypoxemia and respiratory acidosis. Respiratory acidosis with hypoxemia lowers the threshold for ventricular fibrillation. Respiratory acidosis alone or hypoxemia alone does not lower the threshold in normal hearts. Furthermore, metabolic acidosis produced either by lactic acid or by hydrochloric acid infusion lowers the threshold for ventricular fibrillation once bicarbonate values of 10 mEq/L are attained; this lowered threshold in metabolic acidosis is unaffected by normalization of the low serum pH by hyperventilation (45–47). In other studies, respiratory acidosis alone with a pH of 7.15 diminished the threshold for ventricular fibrillation (48). Also, the threshold for ventricular fibrillation was lowered dramatically with severe degrees of hypoxia with an arterial saturation of 40–50% (49–51). More severe hypoxia produces T-flattening and inversion, hypotension (52–54), and slowing of cardiac rate with idionodal and idioventricular pacemakers dominating (55–57). Ectopic beats, asystole, and ventricular fibrillation are well known in terminal electrocardiograms in patients with asphyxia (58).

Therefore, asthmatics in severe respiratory distress have a tendency to develop unstable cardiac rhythms. Epinephrine may accelerate this process. The survival of dogs that were rendered hypoxic by breathing a mixture of 9% oxygen in nitrogen was shortened from 93 min to 43 min by the administration of epinephrine. Furthermore, hypoxic dogs survived a significant 111 min when treated with propranolol (59,60). Other β-adrenergic agonists also potentiate the arrhythmogenicity of hypoxia (60). In hypoxic dogs with a Po_2 of 40 mmHg, cardiac toxicity was produced to doses of isoproterenol that in dogs breathing room air produced only normal responses (61). In addition, acute asthmatics with hypercapnia have markedly elevated increase in endogenous plasma epinephrine levels; however, this elevation in epinephrine levels strikingly does not occur in the usual cases of acute asthma (62–65). Therefore, the addition of exogenous epinephrine may predispose to severe arrhythmias in acute asthmatics with respiratory failure.

Epinephrine, in doses used for asthma, may cause arrhythmias and many cases of sudden death have been reported (66–75). In presumably healthy hearts, β agonists have produced myocardial necrosis or ischemia under clinical (68,76–79) and experimental (80,81) conditions. Novey and Meleyco reviewed much of this literature on epinephrine toxicity (82) and noted that syncope and arrhythmias, at times fatal, occur in children as well as adults (67,83). In view of the potentiation of arrhythmias by hypoxia or respiratory acidosis with epinephrine, this drug is probably too arrhythmogenic to use under these conditions even in patients with normal hearts. In patients with heart disease, especially masquerading as cardiac asthma, epinephrine may produce arrhythmias (71,84–87), angina (88–90), or cardiomyopathy with cardiogenic shock (91). Patients over age 40 may be particularly predisposed to develop arrhythmias with epinephrine (21). Based on 39 patients over the age of 40 that received three doses of subcutaneous epinephrine, Cydulka et al. concluded that arrhythmias did not occur more in the older than younger age groups (92). In fact in the older age group, blood pressure, heart rate, and respiratory rates decreased more in the over 40 group than in the under 40 group. These findings are in contrast with the numerous case reports of cardiac difficulties with epinephrine cited earlier. The discrepancies between the case reports and the series by Cydulka et al. may arise from different routes and doses of epinephrine as well as the fact that the study by Cydulka et al. may not have had sufficient power to detect the deleterious effects noted above. Relative contraindications to the administration of epinephrine include hyperthyroidism and pheochromocytoma that may predispose to arrhythmias after the administration of epinephrine (83). Patients given tricyclic or monoamine oxidase inhibitor antidepressants may develop hypertensive crisis with epinephrine, best treated with α-adrenergic blocking agents (84,93). Epinephrine and anesthetics, for example, halothane, cyclopropane, and methoxyflurane, interact to produce severe arrhythmias (94).

II. EFFECT OF pH

Metabolic or respiratory acidosis with arterial pH of 7.1–72 inhibit the chronotropic and inotropic responses to epinephrine (95–107) and other sympathomimetics (108,109). This inhibition varies with the dose and choice of sympathomimetic; although in extremis with severe acidosis, irreversible hypotension and arrhythmias invariably ensue (58). Acidosis also inhibits the bronchodilator effects of epinephrine and other β agonists (110,111). These effects have led to the recommendation for the administration of 1–2 mEq/kg of sodium bicarbonate to be given over 3–5 min to asthmatics in respiratory failure. Bicarbonate may be useful to counterbalance the necessary respiratory acidosis from permissive hypercapnia (see Chapter 30). This dose of bicarbonate should increase serum bicarbonate at most 5 mEq/L and should increase sensitivity to the bronchodilator effects of β agonists (112,113). During bicarbonate therapy, the ventilation-perfusion defect increases as a result of an increase in blood flow to regions that are poorly ventilated, bringing about a decrease in Po_2 as much as 10 mmHg (114). Similar decreases of Po_2 and increases in ventilation-perfusion mismatch have been observed with epinephrine, aminophylline, isoproterenol, and other inhaled β agonists (115–119).

III. SIDE EFFECTS

Besides arrhythmias, many problems unique to the administration of epinephrine are the result of α-adrenergic effects of epinephrine. The decongestant α-adrenergic effect of epinephrine may be desirable with bronchial mucosal edema, especially in children and in anaphylaxis, but most α-adrenergic receptor stimulation is undesirable. Alpha receptors cause bronchoconstriction in vitro and in vivo in human subjects (120,121). This effect is magnified several thousand times by bacterial endotoxins, perhaps explaining the aggravation of bronchospasm by infections (122). Alpha-adrenergic stimulation also enhances the effects of histamine and plays a role in exercise-induced asthma, and the α effect offer no advantages clinically (124). Alpha-adrenergic agents increases the release of cytokines (see Chapters 3 and 4). Epinephrine (0.3 mg) also causes hypokalemia of about 0.6 mEq/L and hyperglycemia of 25 mg/dL (125). Even lactic acidosis has been described in young patients with acute asthma receiving parenteral or subcutaneous epinephrine (126).

In the initial therapy of the acute asthmatic, subcutaneous epinephrine was the gold standard but has waned in favor of the noninvasive β_2-inhalant bronchodilators which have different and more selective sites of action (127–131). In the First Multicenter Research Collaboration during the fall of 1996, epinephrine was used in only 0.9% of 585 ED visits for acute asthma (personal communication, C. Camargo, M.D., 1997). Epinephrine therapy has diminished due to concerns about (1) arrhythmias; (2) β_2-receptor defects found after injection of epinephrine; and (3) toxicities associated with the alpha receptor effects of epinephrine. The onset of action did not favor one agent over the other. In all studies the onset of action of both subcutaneous epinephrine and inhaled β agonists demonstrate identical onset of action in 2–5 min (127,131). This ''third class status'' of epinephrine we feel is undeserved, and emergency physicians have been shelving a medication for acute asthma which has been efficacious and familiar after over 70 years of use.

Appel et al. (132) have well-demonstrated certain advantages of epinephrine. They studied 100 patients with severe acute asthma, all presenting with peak expiratory flow rate (PEFR) less than 150 L/min. Patients gave consent, were untreated for the first 10 min, and divided into two groups. One group received inhaled metaproterenol and subcutaneous placebo (at both 30 and 60 min) and the other group received inhaled placebo and subcutaneous epinephrine (both agents at 30 and 60 min). At 120 min the groups were crossed, each group then treated with the missing active agent and corresponding placebo to each group (both agents at 120, 150, and 180 min). Lack of initial improvement was defined as failure to improve $\geq 20\%$ above baseline and PEFR >120 L/min. This initial improvement was measured at 120 min. Lack of crossover improvement was defined as failure to improve $\geq 20\%$ above baseline and PEFR >120 L/min. This crossover improvement was measured at 240 min. The final PEFR at 240 minutes was considered their maximum improvement during the study period. The percent maximum improvement that was achieved was calculated as:

$$\frac{\text{Observed flow rate} - \text{baseline flow rate}}{\text{Maximum flow rate} - \text{baseline flow rate}}$$

As has been shown in other studies (see Chapter 19), there was no difference between the two groups (β-agonist vs. epinephrine) in PEFR, either initially or at crossover, throughout the 240 min duration of the study. The noteworthy findings are that 89% of the patients responded to epinephrine compared to 61% with metaproterenol ($p < 0.01$). Also during the crossover treatment phase, of the six patients that failed to respond to epinephrine, only one improved with metaproterenol, whereas of the 18 patients who failed to respond to metaproterenol, 13 improved after epinephrine. Changes in flow rates during the first 2 hr of treatment were calculated for each patient as the percent of their maximum improvement. Patients who did not improve after initial metaproterenol therapy had symptoms for a significantly longer duration of time than patients who did improve after initial metaproterenol therapy. The bronchodilator response to epinephrine among the metaproterenol patients that did not respond was less than responses of the metaproterenol and epinephrine groups that did respond to their respective treatments. Patients who did improve with metaproterenol had more bronchospasm than the nonresponders who had more bronchial edema, inflammation, and mucous plugging impairing the response to metaproterenol. Significantly higher percentages of improvement occurred in the group during treatment with epinephrine ($p < 0.05$). Tremor, nervousness, and sensation of palpitations occurred more frequently in the epinephrine group, but arrhthymias (all minor) occurred with equal frequency between metaproterenol and epinephrine groups. This study has demonstrated that although PEFRs between the two groups were not different, three times as many patients failed to improve after inhaled metaproterenol than after epinephrine and almost 75% of the metaproterenol patients that failed to improve did improve after treatment with epinephrine. Changes in PEFR were more rapid in the patients treated with epinephrine as compared to the metaproterenol-treated patients. Since admission and discharge criteria are dependent on how much time the physician is allowed before being obligated to decide (see Chapters 31 and 33), a more rapid improvement in PEFR would reduce admissions to the hospital by separating the patients who could readily respond to bronchodilators from those who will need several days of inpatient therapy. The decline in epinephrine therapy for acute asthma may be a factor in the increased hospitalization of those patients over the last 15 years.

In Chapter 19 on β agonists, the effects of epinephrine, terbutaline, and aminophylline were contrasted in their roles as the initial therapy of the acute asthmatic.

IV. HEMATOLOGICAL EFFECTS

Epinephrine affects the white cell count and differential. Leukocytosis of approximately 200% occurs after epinephrine administration in a biphasic fashion with onset at 5 min and a maximum effect at 20 min for phase I. During this phase, neutrophils increase 45%, lymphocytes 130%, and eosinophils 50%. These values return to normal and are followed by phase II, in which there is an increase in leukocytes of 50% with an 85% increase in neutrophils, 3–6% increase in band cells, and reduction in lymphocytes and eosinophils of 15% and 40% respectively with maximum effect at 1.5–2 hr (133–136). Since these effects have been observed in splenectomized patients, the spleen plays no essential role in response to epinephrine (137); if the spleen is intact, however, there is an efflux of granulocytes from the spleen in human subjects during epinephrine infusion (138). The lymphocytosis of phase I can be reproduced with either an α- or β-adrenergic agent (139). The lymphocytosis is not due to an increase in lymphocytes entering the venous system from the lymph nodes (140). The increase in neutrophils has been shown to be due to release of marginated neutrophils (141) from the lungs (142). These changes in the marginated neutrophils cannot be explained simply as the α and β effects of epinephrine. The α- but not the β-adrenergic stimulants cause the increase in neutrophils (139). However, both α and β blockers singly do not impede the increase in neutrophils in response to epinephrine. But when α and β blockers are administered together, no increase in neutrophils is observed (143,144).

Long-term administration of β agonists decreases the number and responsiveness of β-agonist receptors termed "downregulation" (145). Physical exercise or stressful calculations increases the β-agonist receptor number and responsiveness of β-agonist receptors (146,147). This increase in β-agonist receptors is demonstrated by infusion of β epinephrine and not norepinephrine (148,149) and is blocked by propranolol (150). This increase in density of β-agonist receptors is caused by release of lymphocytes from the spleen or exchange between the spleen and the circulation (149). This provides some of the mechanisms behind "tachyphylaxis" to β agonists, particularly epinephrine, and mechanisms for augmenting β-agonist responsiveness.

Epinephrine is an effective drug in acute asthma, but is no longer the first line agent. It is useful in acute asthmatics that have not responded to inhaled β_2 agonists and may respond quite well to subcutaneous epinephrine. Its parenteral use in acute asthmatics in extremis carries significant potential risks.

REFERENCES

1. Ahlquist RP. A study of the adrenotropic receptors. Am J Physiol 1948; 153:586–600.
2. Lands AM, Arnold A, McAuliff JP, et al. Differentiation of receptor systems activated by sympathomimetic amines. Nature 1967; 214:597–598.
3. Lands AM. The pharmacological activity of epinephrine and related dihydroxyphenylalkylamines. Pharmacol Rev 1949; 1:279–309.
4. Wilkie D. The relation between concentration and action of adrenaline. J Pharmacy Exp Ther 1928; 34:1–14.
5. Allwood MJ, Keck EW, Marshall RJ, et al. Correlation of hemodynamic events during infusion of epinephrine in man. J Appl Physiol 1962; 17:71–74.
6. Berkin KE, Inglis GC, Ball SG, et al. Effect of low dose adrenaline and noradrenaline infusions on airway calibre in asthmatic patients. Clin Sci 1986; 70:347–352.
7. Knox AJ, Campos-Gongora H, Wisniewski A, et al. Modification of bronchial reactivity by physiological concentrations of epinephrine. J Appl Physiol 1992; 73:1004–1007.
8. Bresnick E, Beakey JF, Levinson L, et al. Evaluation of therapeutic substances employed for the relief of bronchospasm. V. Adrenergic agents. J Clin Invest 1949; 28:1182–1189.
9. Karetzky MS. Acute asthma: The use of subcutaneous epinephrine in therapy. Ann Allergy 1980; 44:12–14.
10. Lewis JE, Richards W, Church JA, et al. Therapy of acute asthma: I. Evaluation of successive bronchodilator treatments. Ann Allergy 1985; 55:472–475.
11. Karetzky MS, Brandstetter RD, Meyer RC, et al. Acute asthma. Part I: A comparison of the immediate effects of six different modes of therapy. Am J Med Sci 1974; 267:213–224.
12. Karetzky MD. Acute asthma. Part II: The effects of therapy on heart rate and blood pressure. Am J Med Sci 1978; 275:319–357.
13. Lindholm B, Helander E. The effect on the pulmonary ventilation of different theophylline derivatives compared to adrenalin and isoprenaline. Acta Allergol 1966; 21:299–306.
14. Rossing TH, Fanta CH, Goldstein, et al. Emergency therapy of asthma: Comparison of the acute effects of parenteral and inhaled sympathomimetics and infused aminophylline. Am Rev Respir Dis 1980; 122:365–371.
15. Schwartz AL, Lipton JM, Warburton D, et al. Management of acute asthma in childhood: A randomized evaluation of β-adrenergic agents. Am J Dis Child 1980; 134:474–478.
16. O'Brien SR, Hein EW, Sly RM. Treatment of acute asthmatic attacks in a holding unit of a pediatric emergency room. Ann Allergy 1980; 45:159–162.
17. Becker AB, Nelson NA, Simon FER. Inhaled salbutamol (albuterol) vs. injected epinephrine in the treatment of acute asthma in children. J Pediatr 1983; 102:465–469.
18. Uden DL, Goetz DR, Kohen DP, et al. Comparison of nebulized terbutaline and subcutaneous epinephrine in the treatment of acute asthma. Ann Emerg Med 1985: 14:229–232.
19. Kornberg AE, Zuckerman S, Welliver JR, et al. Effect of long-acting epinephrine in addition to aerosolized albuterol in the treatment of acute asthma in children. Pediatr Emerg Care 1991; 7:1–3.

20. Brandstetter RD, Gotz VP, Mar DD. Optimal dosing of epinephrine in acute asthma. Am J Hosp Pharmacy 1980; 37:1326–1329.
21. Josephson GW, Kennedy HL, MacKenzie EJ, et al. Cardiac dysrhythmias during the treatment of acute asthma. A comparison of two treatment regimens by a double blind protocol. Chest 1980; 78:429–435.
22. Emerman CL, Crafford WA, Vrobel T. Ventricular arrhthymias during treatment for acute asthma. Ann Emerg Med 1986; 15:699–702.
23. Hoffman BF, Siebens AA, Cranefield PE, et al. The effect of epinephrine and norepinephrine on ventricular vulnerability. Circ Res 1955; 3:140–146.
24. Siebens AA, Hoffman BF, Enson Y, et al. Effects of I-epinephrine and I nor-epinephrine on cardiac excitability. Am J Physiol 1953; 175:1–7.
25. Murnaghan MF. The effect of sympathomimetic amines on the ventricular fibrillation threshold in the rabbit isolated heart. Br J Pharmacy 1975; 53:3–9.
26. Papp JG, Szekeres L. Analysis of the mechanism of adrenergic actions on ventricular vulnerability. Eur J Pharmacy 1968; 3:15–26.
27. Papp JG, Szekeres L. The arrhythmogenic action of sympathomimetic amines. Eur J Pharmacy 1968; 3:4–14.
28. Cranefield PF. Ventricular fibrillation. N Engl J Med 1973; 289:732–736.
29. Moore EN, Spear JF. Ventricular fibrillation threshold. Its physiological and pharmacological importance. Arch Intern Med 1975; 135:446–453.
30. Camarata SJ, Weil MH, Hanashiro PK, et al. Cardiac arrest in the clinically ill. I. A study of predisposing causes in 132 patients. Circulation 1971; 44:688–695.
31. Death after adrenaline injection. Br Med J 1958; 1:716.
32. Freedman BJ. Accidental adrenaline overdosage and its treatment with piperoxan. Lancet 1955; 2:575–578.
33. Johnson HRM, Chir B. Therapeutic accidents: Adrenaline poisoning. J Forens Med 1960; 7:198–205.
34. McGinty AP, Baer LS. Effect on the heart of an overdose of epinephrine, report of a case. Am Heart J 1947; 33:102–106.
35. Piscatelli RL, Fox LM. Myocardial injury from epinephrine overdosage. Am J Cardiol 1968; 21:735–737.
36. Verrier R, Calvert A, Lown B, et al. Effect of acute blood pressure elevation on the ventricular fibrillation threshold. Am J Physiol 1974; 226;893–897.
37. Papp G, Szekeres L. Influence of stretch and dynamic functional state of the myocardium or tendency of the heart to arrhythmia. Acta Physiol Acad Sci Hung 1967; 32:163–174.
38. Opie LH, Muller CA, Lubbe WF. Cyclic A.M.P. and arrhythmias revisited. Lancet 1978; 2: 921–923.
39. Opie LH, Nathan D, Lubbe WF. Biochemical aspects of arrhythmogenesis and ventricular fibrillation. Am J Cardiol 1979; 43:131–148.
40. Wit AL, Hoffman BF, Rosen MR. Electrophysiology and pharmacology of cardiac arrhythmias. IX. Cardiac electrophysiologic effects of β-adrenergic receptor stimulation and blockade. Part A. Am Heart J 1975; 90:521–533.
41. Lubbe WF, Podzuweit T, Daries PS, et al. The role of cyclic adenosine monophosphate in adrenergic effects on ventricular vulnerability to fibrillation in the isolated perfused rat heart. J Clin Invest 1978; 61:1260–1269.
42. Ueda I, Loehning RW, Ueyama H. Relationship between sympathomimetic amines and methylxanthines inducing cardiac arrhythmias. Anesthesiology 1961; 22:926–932.
43. Sugiura M, Ogawa K, Yamazaki N. Concentration of myocardial cyclic AMP and ventricular fibrillation induced by aminophylline. Jpn Heart J 1979; 20:177–182.
44. Ayres SM, Grace WJ. Inappropriate ventilation and hypoxemia as causes of cardiac arrhythmias. Am J Med 1969; 46:495–505.

45. Dong E Jr, Stinson EB, Shumway NF. The ventricular fibrillation threshold in respiratory acidosis and alkalosis. Surgery 1967; 61:602–607.
46. Gerst PH, Fleming WH, Malm JR. Increased susceptibility of the heart to ventricular fibrillation during metabolic acidosis. Circ Res 1966; 19:63–70.
47. Rogers RM, Spear JF, Moore EN, et al. Vulnerability of canine ventricle to fibrillation during hypoxia and respiratory acidosis. Chest 1973; 63:986–994.
48. Turnbull AD, Dobell ARC. The effect of pH change on the ventricular fibrillation threshold. Surgery 1966; 60:1040–1043.
49. Burn JH, Hukovic S. Anoxia and ventricular fibrillation with a summary of evidence on the cause of fibrillation. Br J Pharmacol 1960; 15:67–70.
50. Szekeres L, Papp G. Effect of arterial hypoxia on the susceptibility to arrhythmia of the heart. Acta Physiol Acad Sci Hung 1967; 32:143–162.
51. Turnbull AD, MacLean LD, Dobell ARC, et al. The influence of hyperbaric oxygen and of hypoxia on the ventricular fibrillation threshold. J Thor Cardiovasc Surg 1965; 50:842–868.
52. May SH. Electrocardiographic response to gradually induced oxygen deficiency. Am Heart J 1939; 17:655–658.
53. Randall WC. Electrocardiographic changes of relation to tolerance of sustained anoxemic anoxia in dogs. Am Heart J 1944; 27:234–245.
54. Sands J, DeGraff AC. The effects of progressive anoxemia on the heart and circulation. Am J Physiol 1925; 74:416–435.
55. Greene CW, Gilbert NC. Studies on the responses of the circulation to low oxygen tension. III. Changes in the pacemaker and in conduction during extreme oxygen want as shown in the human electrocardiogram. Arch Intern Med 1921; 27:517–557.
56. Greene CW, Gilbert NC. Studies on the response of the circulation to low oxygen tension. V. Stages in the loss of function of the rhythm producing and the conducting tissue of the human heart during anoxemia. Am J Physiol 1921; 56:475–480.
57. Harris AS. Terminal electrocardiographic patterns in experimental anoxia, coronary occlusion and hemorrhagic shock. Am Heart J 1948; 35:895–909.
58. Kristoffersen MB, Rattenborg CC, Holaday DA. Asphyxial death: The roles of acute anoxia, hypercarbia and acidosis. Anesthesiology 1967; 28:488–497.
59. Cain SM. Survival time of hypoxic dogs given epinephrine or propranolol. Am J Physiol 1973; 225:1405–1410.
60. Gauduel Y, Karagueuzian HS, deLeiris J. Deleterious effects of endogenous catecholamines on hypoxic myocardial cells following reoxygenation. J Molec Cell Cardiol 1979; 11:717–731.
61. Collins JM, McDevitt DG, Shanks RG, et al. The cardiotoxicity of isoprenaline during hypoxia. Br J Pharmacy 1969; 31:35–45.
62. Larsson K, Carlens P, Bevegard S, et al. Sympathoadrenal responses to bronchoconstriction in asthma: an invasive and kinetic study of plasma catecholamines. Clin Sci 1995; 88:439–446.
63. Parke TR, Steedman DJ, Robertson CE, et al. Plasma catecholamine responses in acute severe asthma. Arch Emerg Med 1992; 9:157–161.
64. Emerman CL and Cydulka R. Changes in serum catecholamine levels during acute bronchospasm. Ann Emerg Med 1993; 22:1836–1841.
65. Ind PW, Causon RC, Brown MJ, et al. Circulating catecholamines in acute asthma. Br Med J 1985; 290:267–269.
66. Pratt JH. Cardiac asthma. JAMA 1926; 87:809–813.
67. Buranakul B, Washington J, Hilman B, et al. Causes of death during acute asthma in children. Am J Child 1974; 128:343–350.
68. Collins-Williams C, Nizami R, Lamenza C. The use of isoproterenol in the treatment of the acute asthmatic attack with report of case. J Asthma Res 1969; 7:17–24.
69. Dworetzsky M, Plulson AD. Review of asthmatic patients hospitalized in the pavilion service

of the New York Hospital from 1948 to 1963 with emphasis on mortality rate. J Allergy 1968; 41:181–194.
70. Earle BV. Fatal bronchial asthma: A series of fifteen cases with a review of the literature. Thorax 1953; 8:195–213.
71. Flaherty GN. Deaths amongst asthmatics in Tasmania. Med J Aust 1970; 1:1083–1086.
72. Ghannam RD, Schreier L, Vanselow NA. Fatal bronchial asthma: An analysis of terminal treatment in twenty cases. Ann Allergy 1968; 26:194–204.
73. Greenberg MJ. Isoprenaline in myocardial failure. Lancet 1965; 2:442–443.
74. Lund E. Pluselig dod hos asthmapatienter. 14 secerede tilfaelde. Ugeskr Laeg 1966; 128: 297–300.
75. McManis AG. Adrenaline and isoprenaline: A warning. Med J Aust 1964; 2:76.
76. Kurland G, Williams J, Lewiston NJ. Fatal myocardial toxicity during continuous infusion intravenous isoproterenol therapy of asthma. J Allergy Clin Immunol 1979; 63:407–411.
77. Lepeschkin E, Marchet H, Schroeder G, et al. Effect of epinephrine and norepinephrine on the electrocardiogram of 100 normal subjects. Am J Cardiol 1960; 5:594–603.
78. Matson JR, Loughlin GM, Strunk RC. Myocardial ischemia complicating the use of isoproterenol in asthmatic children. J Pediatr 1978; 92:776–778.
79. Rhatigan RM, de la Torre A. Myocardial necrosis and bronchial asthma. Ann Allergy 1970; 28:434–438.
80. Kahn DS, Rona G, Chappel CI. Isoproterenol-induced cardiac necrosis. Ann NY Acad Sci 1969; 156:285–293.
81. Rosenblum I, Wohl A, Stein AA. Studies in cardiac necrosis. 1. Production of cardiac lesions with sympathomimetic amines. Toxic Appl Pharmacy 1965; 7:1–8.
82. Novey HS, Meleyco LN. Alarming reaction after intravenous administration of 30ml of epinephrine. JAMA 1969; 207:2435–2436.
83. Speer F, Tapay NJ. Syncope in children following epinephrine. Ann Allergy 1970; 28:50–54.
84. Adverse interactions of drugs. Med Lett Drug Ther 1979; 21:5–12.
85. Clough HD. Studies on epinephrine. III. Effect of epinephrine on the electrocardiograms of patients with "irritable heart." Arch Intern Med 1919; 24:284–294.
86. Lockett MF. Dangerous effects of isoprenaline in myocardial failure. Lancet 1965; 2:104–106.
87. Maling HM, Morgan NC. Ventricular arrhythmias induced by sympathomimetic amines in dogs following coronary artery occlusion. Circ Res 1957; 5:409–413.
88. Cottrell JE, Wood FC. The effect of epinephrin in angina pectoris; with report of a case. Am J Med Sci 1931; 181:36–39.
89. Katz LN, Hamburger WW, Lev M. The diagnostic value of epinephrine in angina pectoris. Am Heart J 1932; 7:371–379.
90. Levine SA, Ernstene AC, Jocobsan BM. The use of epinephrine as a diagnostic test for angina pectoris: With observations on the electrocardiographic changes following injections of epinephrine into normal subjects and into patients with angina pectoris. Arch Intern Med 1930; 45:191–200.
91. Fletcher D, Mainardi JL, Brun-Buisson C, et al. Cardiac asthma presenting as status asthmaticus: deleterious effect of epinephrine therapy. Intens Care Med 1990; 16:466–468.
92. Cydulka R, Davison R, Grammer L, et al. The use of epinephrine in the treatment of older adult asthmatics. Ann Emerg Med 1988; 17:322–326.
93. Boakes AJ, Laurence DR, Teoh PC, et al. Interactions between sympathomimetic amines and antidepressant agents in man. Br Med J 1973; 1:311–315.
94. Katz RL, Bigger JT Jr. Cardiac arrhythmias during anesthesia and operation. Anesthesiology 1970; 33:193–213.
95. Burget GE, Visscher MB. Variations of the pH of the blood and the response of the vascular system to adrenaline. Am J Physiol 1927; 81:113–123.

96. Campbell GS, Houle DB, Crisp NW Jr, et al. Depressed response to intravenous sympathicomimetic agents in humans during acidosis. Dis Chest 1958; 33:18–22.
97. Darby TD, Aldinger EE, Gadsen RH, et al. Effects of metabolic acidosis on ventricular isometric systolic tension and the response to epinephrine and levarterenol. Circ Res 1960; 8: 1242–1253.
98. Houle DB, Weil MH, Brown EB Jr, et al. Influence of respiratory acidosis on ECG and pressor responses to epinephrine, norepinephrine and metaraminol. Proc Soc Exp Biol Med 1957; 94:561–564.
99. Keith HB, Snyder DD, Campbell GS. Effect of metabolic acidosis on cardiac output and pressor responses to epinephrine. Trans Am Soc Artif Intern Organs 1960; 6:275–279.
100. Kirimli B, Harris LC, Safar P. Evaluation of sodium bicarbonate and epinephrine in cardiopulmonary resuscitation. Anesth Analg (Cleve) 1969; 48:649–657.
101. Pearson JW, Redding JS. The role of epinephrine in cardiac resuscitation. Anesth Analg (Cleve) 1963; 42:599–606.
102. Redding JS, Pearson JW. Evaluation of drugs for cardiac resuscitation. Anesthesiology 1963; 24:203–207.
103. Redding JS, Pearson JW. Resuscitation from ventricular fibrillation: Drug Therapy. JAMA 1968; 203:255–260.
104. Schaer H. Influence of respiratory and metabolic acidosis on epinephrine inotropic effect in isolated guinea pig atria. Pflugers Arch 1974; 347:297–307.
105. Thrower WB, Darhy TD, Aidinger EE. Acid-base derangements and myocardial contractility: Effects as a complication of shock. Arch Surg 1961; 82:56–65.
106. Weil MH, Houle DB, Brown EB Jr, et al. Vasopressor agents: Influence of acidosis on cardiac and vascular responsiveness. Calif Med 1958; 88:437–440.
107. Wood WB, Manley ES Jr, Woodbury RA. The effects of $C0_2$-induced respiratory acidosis on the depressor and pressor components of the dog's blood pressure response to epinephrine. J Pharmacy Exp Ther 1963; 139:238–247.
108. Downing SE, Talner NS, Gardner TH. Cardiovascular responses metabolic acidosis. Am J Physiol 1965; 208:237–242.
109. Ford GD, Cline WH, Fleming WW. Influence of lactic acidosis on cardiovascular response to sympathomimetic amines. Am J Physiol 1968; 215:1123–1129.
110. Blumenthal JS, Blumenthal MN, Brown EB, et al. Effect of changes in arterial pH on the action of adrenalin in acute adrenalin-fast asthmatics. Dis Chest 1961; 39:516–522.
111. Blumenthal MN. The importance of metabolic changes in the treatment status asthmaticus. Univ Michigan Med Center J 1968; 34:22–26.
112. Mithoefer JC, Porter WF, Karetzky MS. Indications for the use of sodium bicarbonate in the treatment of intractable asthma. Respiration 1968; 25:201–215.
113. Mithoefer JC, Runser RH, Karetzky MS. The use of sodium bicarbonate in the treatment of acute bronchial asthma. N Engl J Med 1965; 272:1200–1203.
114. Milledge IS, Benjamin S. Arterial desaturation after sodium bicarbonate therapy in bronchial asthma. Am Rev Respir Dis 1972; 105:126–128.
115. Hales CA, Kazemi H. Hypoxic vascular response of the lung: effect of aminophylline and epinephrine. Am Rev Respir Dis 1974; 110:126–132.
116. Knudson RJ, Constantine HP. An effect of isoproterenol on ventilation-perfusion in asthmatic versus normal subjects. J Appl Physiol 1967; 22:402–406.
117. Palmer KNV. Effect of broncho-dilator drugs on arterial blood gas tensions in bronchial asthma. Postgrad Med J 1971 (suppl); 47:75–77.
118. Rees HA, Borthwick RC, Millar JS, et al. Aminophylline in bronchial asthma. Lancet 1967; 2:1167–1169.
119. Rees HA, Millar JS, Donald KW. Adrenaline in bronchial asthma. Lancet 1967; 2:1164–1167.
120. Patel KR, Kerr JW. The airways response to phenylephrine after blockade of alpha and beta receptors in extrinsic bronchial asthma. Clin Allergy 1973; 3:439–448.

121. Snashall PD, Boother FA, Sterling GM. The effect of alpha-adrenoreceptor stimulation on the airways of normal and asthmatic man. Clin Sci Mol Med 1978; 54:283–289.
122. Simonsson BG, Svedmyr N, Skoogh B-E, et al. In vivo and in vitro studies on alpha-receptors in human airways. Potentiation with bacterial endotoxin. Scand J Respir Dis 1972; 53:227–236.
123. Gross GN, Souhrada JF, Farr RS. The long-term treatment of an asthmatic patient using phentolamine. Chest 1974; 66:397–401.
124. Baldwin DR, Sivardeen Z, Pavord ID, et al. the effect of adrenaline on airway smooth muscle contractility in vitro and on bronchial reactivity in vivo. Thorax. 1994; 49:1103–1108.
125. Rohr AS, Spector S, Rachelefsky GS, et al. Efficacy of parenteral albuterol in the treatment of asthma. Comparison of its metabolic side effects with subcutaneous epinephrine. Chest 1986; 89:348–351.
126. Murphy F, Manown T, Knutson SW, et al. Epinephrine-induced lactic acidosis in the setting of status asthmaticus. South Med J 1995; 577–578.
127. Pancorbo S, Fifield G, Davies S, et al. Subcutaneous epinephrine versus nebulized terbutaline in the emergency treatment of asthma. Clin Pharm 1983; 2:45–48.
128. Aviado DM. Adrenergic agents in bronchial asthma, emphasizing undesirable reactions. In Weiss, EB (ed). Status Asthmaticus. Baltimore: University Park Press, 1978:215.
129. Reed CE. Adrenergic bronchodilators: pharmacology and toxicology. J Allergy Clin Immunol. 1985; 76 (pt 2) 2:335–341.
130. Baughman RP, Ploysongsang Y, James W. A comparative study of aerosolized terbutaline and subcutaneously administered epinephrine in the treatment of acute bronchial asthma. Ann Allergy. 1984; 53:131–134.
131. Lin YZ, Hsieh KH, Chang LF, et al. Terbutaline nebulization and epinephrine injection in treating acute asthmatic children. Pediatr Allergy Immunol 1996; 7:95–99.
132. Appel D, Karpel JP, Sherman M. Epinephrine improves expiratory flow rates in patients with asthma who do not respond to inhaled metaproterenol sulfate. J Allergy Clin Immunol 1989; 84:90–98.
133. Enberg R, McCullough J, Ownby D. Epinephrine-induced leukocytosis in acute asthma. Ann Allergy 1986; 57:337–339.
134. Martin HE. Physiological leucocytosis: The variation in the leucocyte count during rest and exercise, and after the hypodermic injection of adrenaline. J Physiol 1932; 75:113–129.
135. Samuels Al. Primary and secondary leucocyte changes following the intramuscular injection of epinephrine hydrochloride. J Clin Invest 1951; 30:941–947.
136. White C, Ling TH, Klein AM. The effect of administration of epinephrine on leukocyte count of normal subjects. Blood 1950; 5:723–731.
137. Patek AJ, Doland GA. The effect of adrenaline injection on the blood of patients with and without spleens. Am J Med Sci 1935; 190:14–22.
138. Toft P, Hansen-Helbo HS, Tonnesen E, et al. Redistribution of granulocytes during adrenaline infusion and following administration of cortisol in healthy volunteers. Acta Anaesthesiol Scand 1994; 38:254–258.
139. Gader AMA, Cash JD. The effect of adrenaline, noradrenaline, isoprenaline and salbutamol on the resting levels of white blood cells in man. Scand J Haematol 1975; 14:5–10.
140. French EB, Steel CM, Aitchinson WRC. Studies on adrenaline-induced leucocytosis in normal man: The role of the spleen and of the thoracic duct. Br J Haematol 1971; 21:413–421.
141. Athens JW, Raeb SO, Haab OP, et al. Leukokinetic studies. III. The distribution of granulocytes in the blood of normal subjects. J Clin Invest 1961; 40:159–164.
142. Bierman HR, Kelly KH, Cordes FL, et al. The release of leukocytes and platelets from the pulmonary circulation by epinephrine. Blood 1952; 7:683–692.
143. French EB, Steel CM, Aitchinson WRC. Studies on adrenaline-induced leucocytosis in normal man. Il. The effect of α and β adrenergic blocking agents. Br J Haematol 1971; 21: 423–428.

144. Gader AMA. The effect of β-adrenergic blockade on the responses of leucocyte counts to intravenous epinephrine in man. Scand J Haematol 1974; 13:11–16.
145. Brodde O-E, Brinkmann M, Schemuth R, et al. Terbutaline-induced desensitization of human lymphocyte β_2-adrenoreceptors. Accelerated restoration of β-adrenoreceptor responsiveness by prednisone and ketotifen. J Clin Invest 1985; 76:1096–1101.
146. Butler J, Kelly JG, O'Malley K, et al. β adrenoreceptor adaption to acute exercise. J Physiol Lond 1983; 344:113–118.
147. Graafsma SJ, Van Tits B, Westerhof B, et al. Adrenoreceptor density on human blood cells and plasma catecholamines after mental arithmetic in normotensive volunteers. J Cardiovasc Pharmacy 1987; 10(suppl 4):S107–S109.
148. Brodde O-E, Daul A, Wellstein A, et al. Differentiation of β1 and β2-adrenoceptor mediated effects in humans Am J Physiol 1988; 254:H199–H206.
149. Van Tits, LJH, Michel MC, Grosse-Wilde H, et al. Catecholamines increase lymphocyte β2-adrenergic receptors via a β2-adrenergic, spleen dependent process. Am J Physiol 258(1pt1): E191–E202.
150. Brodde O-E, Daul A, Wang XL, et al. Dynamic exercise induced increase in lymphocyte beta2 adrenoreceptors: abnormality in essential hypertension and its correction by antihypertensives. Clin Pharmacy Ther 1987; 41:371–379.

21

Aminophylline

Charles L. Emerman
MetroHealth Medical Center/Cleveland Clinic Foundation, Cleveland, Ohio

Mary H. Stewart
MetroHealth Medical Center, Cleveland, and Allen Memorial Hospital, Oberlin, Ohio

I. INTRODUCTION

Aminophylline has been used for many disorders since the beginning of the 20th century. It has been advocated for use in congestive heart failure, sleep disordered breathing, neonatal apnea, and cerebral infarction, and as a nonspecific analeptic (1). The use of aminophylline for the management of acute asthma has been advocated for almost 60 years (2,3). Although its role in this setting has been eclipsed in recent years by the popularity of the selective β-agonists, it still has a role in selected patients. The emergency physician needs to be familiar with this medication since a number of patients still use it. The precise indications for the use of aminophylline in acute asthma remain controversial in spite of numerous studies. Because of the narrow therapeutic index and potential for drug interactions, caution should be used when employing this agent.

Successful use of aminophylline in the treatment of status asthmaticus began in the 1930s, although the lack of convenient methods to monitor theophylline levels complicated its use (4–8). The role of aminophylline in the treatment of patients with status asthmaticus came into question with reports of significant morbidity and even death, particularly following injection of the agent over short periods of time (9,10). A series of studies in the 1980s called into question the use of aminophylline in the emergency department (ED) treatment of asthma. Many of these studies were limited by small sample size and their relevance to modern therapy may be questioned in light of the changes in accepted treatment of acute asthma since that time.

II. PHARMACODYNAMICS

Theophylline is a methylated xanthine derivative found in plants widely distributed throughout the world (11). Chemically, theophylline is a 1,3-dimethylxanthine (12). Methylxanthine solubility is low and greatly enhanced by the formation of complexes with numerous compounds. For example, aminophylline is the 1:1 complex of theophylline and ethylenediamine (11). These complexes dissociate to yield the parent form in aqueous solutions.

The methylxanthines are rapidly absorbed after parenteral or oral administration of uncoated tablets (13,14). Rectal solutions are completely absorbed; rectal suppositories are often erratically and incompletely absorbed. Enteric coated and slow release formulations can result in incomplete or unpredictable absorption (13,15). Food generally slows the rate of absorption of theophylline, but not the completeness (11,13). TheoDur, UniDur, and SloBid are completely absorbed in the presence or absence of food (15,16). Some formulations, such as Theo24 and Uniphyl, have increased absorption in the presence of food (13).

Once absorbed, theophylline is approximately 40% protein bound, the remaining free drug distributes in the extracellular water (11,15). The volume of distribution (V) is a measure of the apparent space in the body available to contain the drug (V = amount of drug in body/concentration of drug in blood). The volume of distribution for theophylline averages 0.5 L/kg in both adults and children. The peak serum concentration after a single loading dose is that dose divided by the volume of distribution; therefore, 1 mg/kg will increase the serum concentration by roughly 2 μg/mL (17). Theophylline freely crosses the placenta and is found in breast milk but no major adverse reactions have been reported in infants receiving the drug in this manner (11).

Theophylline is eliminated from the body via several pathways. The kidney excretes 10–20% of administered drug unchanged in the urine. The majority is eliminated as metabolites formed by the hepatic cytochrome P-450 isoenzymes (18). Genetic factors, environmental factors, and other drugs alter the activity of these isoenzymes and thus the elimination of the drug. Theophylline clearance, the ability of the body to eliminate the drug, in otherwise healthy adults averages 0.04 L/h/kg (18). There is marked interindividual and intraindividual variation in the rate of elimination of theophylline necessitating close monitoring of serum levels and specific formulations during treatment (15,18,19).

The elimination half-life of theophylline varies in individuals based on age, genetic, and environmental factors. The range varies from approximately 24 hr in neonates to 2–10 hours (mean 4 hr) in 1–9 year olds (15). In adults, the average half-life is 8–9 hr (11). Children therefore require weight-adjusted doses that may be significantly higher than adult doses (per/kg). There is some recent evidence that theophylline clearance rates are lower than those previously reported, implying that daily dosage needs are 25% lower than some published guidelines (20).

Because absorption of theophylline can be influenced by individual variation, those products with complete and consistent absorption are preferred. Predicted fluctuations in serum concentration for patients with defined rates of metabolism must be considered when choosing a drug and dosing regimen. The initial dosing should allow tolerance to develop to the minor side effects of therapy (caffeine-like symptoms). This can be accomplished by the utilization of low initial doses with slow clinical titration over 1–2 weeks to achieve the final therapeutic dose. Once the final dose is established, there is generally little change in dosage requirements unless environmental or clinical changes occur affecting absorption or elimination. Final dosage should be guided by serum levels drawn at peak concentration time, 3–7 hr post dose, when the dosage has been reliably maintained for at least 48 hr (11,12,15,18).

III. PHARMACOLOGICAL EFFECTS

Theophylline has a number of potentially beneficial properties for the patient with acute asthma. In the 1960s, the action of theophylline inhibiting cyclic adenosine monophosphate (cAMP) phosphodiesterase was first discussed (21,22). The inhibition of the cAMP phosphodiesterase leads to an elevation of cAMP with subsequent bronchodilation. This proposed mechanism of clinical activity was questioned by the demonstration by Polson that therapeutic doses are insufficient to significantly inhibit phosphodiesterase (23,24). Alternatively, some have proposed that theophylline blocks adenosine receptors (25). Adenosine acts as a bronchoconstrictor, probably by decreasing cAMP levels. Adenosine administration, however, does not antagonize the action of theophylline in smooth muscles. Furthermore, clinically active theophylline analogs such as enprophylline do not demonstrate adenosine inhibitory activity (26). Other theories have suggested that theophylline acts by augmenting the activity of β-adrenergic receptors (27), blocks the inflammatory response (28), modifies immune activity (29), and reduces airway response to bronchoconstriction (29).

Low-dose theophylline has been demonstrated to reduce activated eosinophils during chronic treatment in asthmatic patients (30). Theophylline has been shown to have a serum concentration–related effect on leukotriene by levels associated with nocturnal asthma (31). Clinical studies have demonstrated an effect on T-lymphocyte activation (32,33). Even at subtherapeutic doses, theophylline appears to modulate the late asthmatic response with effects on CD4 and CD8 counts (34). All of these effects may serve to modulate the inflammatory cascade in asthmatic patients (see Chapter 4).

Clinically, aminophylline clearly leads to bronchodilation both in patients with acute and stable asthma. Mitenko and Ogilvie demonstrated a log dose relationship between serum theophylline levels and improvement in the FEV_1 (35). Although the therapeutic range for theophylline is typically given as 10–20 μg/mL, data indicate that bronchodilation begins to occur at around 5 μg/mL (36). In 1995, the Food and Drug Administration (FDA) altered the labeling guidelines for theophylline products. The new guidelines state that physicians may wish to consider a decrease in the dosage in patients with a theophylline level of 15–20 μg/mL in order to provide a wider margin of safety (37). Continued augmentation of bronchodilation occurs even as the level rises above the ''toxic'' level of 20 μg/mL.

Both theophylline and other methylxanthines, such as caffeine, improve respiratory muscle strength. Theophylline improves the pressure generated by the human diaphragm by roughly 15% (38). Theophylline also improves the recovery from respiratory muscle fatigue. Similar effects have been demonstrated in patients with chronic obstructive pulmonary disease (39).

Theophylline has effects on cardiac function. Theophylline increases cardiac contractility and increases heart rate (40). In addition, as is the case with other β-adrenergic agents, theophylline leads to a reduction in pulmonary vascular resistance (41,42). These affects account for the beneficial use of theophylline in patients with acute decompensated congestive heart failure. Theophylline may be beneficial in patients with chronic obstructive pulmonary disease (COPD) who may have concomitant cardiac disease or right ventricular failure. The same effects however, are also partly responsible for theophylline toxicity.

Theophylline has a proven clinical efficacy in patients with stable asthma. Theophylline has been demonstrated to protect against histamine-induced bronchoconstriction (29). There is a dose-response relationship between the serum theophylline concentration and the dose of histamine or methacholine required to induce bronchospasm. Theophylline has been demonstrated to inhibit exercise induced bronchospasm, even at subtherapeutic levels (43). Some studies, however, have not found theophylline useful in protecting against exercise-induced asthma (44).

Theophylline may be particularly useful in the management of patients with nocturnal asthma. Several studies have found that once daily administration of sustained release theophylline can decrease the signs and symptoms of nocturnal asthma (45–47). Studies of preparations with moderate or prolonged duration of action have also shown this benefit.

The use of theophylline for the management of patients with chronic asthma has been demonstrated in a number of studies (48,49). Theophylline has been shown to provide greater control of asthma than cromolyn (50). Theophylline may also be useful in patients requiring steroids for maintenance of their asthma (51). On the other hand, it is clear that the β-adrenergic agents have a much greater bronchodilator effect than theophylline, with a lower risk of side effects. A number of studies have demonstrated that the combination of theophylline and β-adrenergic agents provides additive bronchodilation (52–54). Some studies demonstrate an advantage to oral theophylline over oral albuterol therapy for asthma management in children (55).

IV. THEOPHYLLINE IN ACUTE ASTHMA

The indications and uses of theophylline in acute asthma is not well defined. A series of studies by McFadden and colleagues in the early 1980s questioned the use of theophylline in acute asthma (4,5,56). In the earliest study, 48 patients were followed for 60 min after receiving either subcutaneous epinephrine, inhaled isoproterenol, or an infusion of aminophylline (5). Treatment with the two adrenergic agents provided threefold greater improvement in FEV_1 than did the treatment with aminophylline alone. In the next study, 89 patients were again followed for 60 min after receiving either subcutaneous epinephrine alone, epinephrine with an infusion of aminophylline, or aerosolized isoproterenol plus aminophylline (56). The patients treated with either combination had greater improvement in FEV_1 than those treated with epinephrine alone. This effect was most marked in those patients with an initial FEV_1 less than 1 L. In the last study in the series, 102 patients were followed for 60 min after receiving inhaled isoproterenol, inhaled isoproterenol with intravenous aminophylline, or inhaled isoproterenol with theophylline elixir (4). There was no significant advantage to the administration of the combination of agents. A reasonable interpretation of these results is that inhaled sympathomimetics are as or more effective than injected agents, and that the addition of aminophylline to these more potent agents does not offer any significant advantage.

Other studies have been performed, evaluating the effects of the combination of aminophylline with either epinephrine or inhaled β-agonist. Josephson found no advantage to adding aminophylline to a group of patients who received between 0.3 and 0.5 mL of subcutaneous epinephrine every 30 min for a total of three doses (6). A companion article found that the combination treatment increased the incidence of arrhythmia, generously defined as any extraventricular beats over the course of 30 min. Similarly, Appel et al. followed 37 patients over the course of 1 hr treated with either epinephrine, aminophylline or the combination of the two agents (7). Again, no significant advantage to the combination of aminophylline and epinephrine was found. Epinephrine either alone, or in combination with aminophylline, produced significantly greater improvement in pulmonary function compared to patients treated with aminophylline alone. Siegel et al. (8) evaluated 40 patients treated initially with inhaled metaproterenol and then given additional doses of metaproterenol either with or without aminophylline infusion. Some patients in this study received steroids (8). Once again, there was no significant advantage to the combination treatment although there was a marked increase in theophylline side effects. More recently, Carter et al. evaluated the advantage of adding theophylline to nebulized albuterol and methylprednisolone in children hospitalized with severe asthma (57). No significant advantage to the addition of aminophylline was found over the course of 36 hr. Other studies of both adult and pediatric patients treated either in the ED or as inpatients have failed to demonstrate a beneficial effect with combination treatment (58–62).

An advantage to aminophylline treatment has been suggested by several other studies. A study in children evaluated the use of intravenous aminophylline in children who had failed treatment with epinephrine (63). These children additionally received intravenous fluids, corticosteroids, oxygen, and treatment with nebulized phenylephrine and intravenous isoproterenol. There was a significant advantage to administration of aminophylline both at one hour and at 24 hr. More recently, Huang et al. (64) evaluated the effects of intravenous aminophylline in hospitalized adults who were treated additionally with nebulized albuterol and methylprednisolone. There was a significant improvement in FEV_1 at 3 hours which persisted to 48 hr (64). Finally, Wrenn et al. evaluated 133 adult patients treated with aerosolized metaproterenol and intravenous methylprednisolone, and randomized to receive either aminophylline or placebo (65). There was no significant change in the peak expiratory flow rate after 120 min of treatment; however, the hospital admission rates in patients treated with aminophylline was threefold lower (21% vs. 6%; $p = 0.016$) than those treated with placebo. Although there is some conflicting data about the effect of aminophylline in acute asthma, the therapeutic effect is greatest when used in combination with inhaled β agonists in patients with FEV_1 less than 1 L (5).

V. TOXICITY

The incidence of theophylline side effects is difficult to assess but is estimated at an overall rate of 21% in patients taking theophylline (66). There is significant overlap of the therapeutic and toxic serum ranges for theophylline. As a result, symptoms of toxicity can be seen at levels within the conventional therapeutic window of 10–20 μg/mL. In 1995, the American Association of Poison Control Centers reported 2338 cases of theophylline toxicity, with 19 fatalities (67).

At therapeutic dosage, drug levels follow first-order kinetics in which a constant fraction of drug is eliminated per unit of time. In the high therapeutic and toxic ranges, mixed first- and zero-order kinetics can occur resulting in lengthened half-lives. Zero-order kinetics occurs when normal mechanisms of elimination are saturated and rather than eliminate a constant fraction of total drug, a constant amount of drug is excreted. This amount may be a progressively smaller fraction of the total drug, resulting in decreased elimination over time (11). Half-lives of up to 20 hr have been reported (12,15,68). It is important to recall those factors that may lead to alterations in the metabolism of theophylline and closely follow serum levels in their presence (see Table 1).

Symptoms of minor toxicity include nausea, vomiting, diarrhea, abdominal pain,

Table 1 Factors Altering Theophylline Clearance

Factors decreasing theophylline elimination by 20% or more	Factors increasing theophylline elimination by 20% or more
Environment	
Prolonged fever	Cigarette/marijuana smoking
Hepatitis/cholestasis	Adolescents with cystic fibrosis
Cirrhosis	Hyperthyroidism
Cardiac decompensation	Eating charcoal-broiled meats
Cor pulmonale	
Septic shock	
Viral infections	
Drugs	
Alopurinol (600 mg/d)	Carbamazepine
Cimetidine	Isoproterenol (IV)
Ciprofloxin	Isoniazid
Clarithromycin	Phenobarbital
Disulfiram	Phenytoin
Erythromycin	Rifampin
Estrogen/oral contraceptives	Sulfinpyrazone
Interferon	Terbutaline
Methotrexate	
Mexiletine	
Nortriptyline	
Propranolol	
Thiabendazole	
Ticlopidine	
Troleandomycin	
Verapamil	

headache, irritability, and insomnia. These are commonly seen by the time drug levels exceed 15–20 μg/mL, but may occur at levels as low as 5 μg/mL. When these symptoms are seen during initial therapy, they are usually transient and can be prevented with gradual increments to the desired dose (69).

Major toxicity includes such events as cardiac dysrhythmias, cardiovascular collapse, and seizures and have been reported at a variety of drug levels. Although there is a tendency toward more serious events/toxicity with increased drug levels, these events may occur at any measured level. Once seizures or cardiac events have taken place, they are often intractable and death may ensue. Importantly, these events may occur without any preceding minor toxicity symptoms, especially in patients with chronic intoxications. Severe cardiac dysrhythmias and seizures are more frequently seen, and at lower serum levels, in patients with chronic intoxication compared to acute ingestions. However, patients with acute ingestions are more apt to suffer severe hypotension, hypokalemia, hyperglycemia, and lactic acidosis presumably due to intracellular shifts. Patients over the age of 60 are at greater risk for major toxicity (11,12,15,66,68,69).

The exact mechanism of toxicity is unknown. Theophylline is known to inhibit phosphodiesterase and increase intracellular cAMP (11,12). It causes release of endogenous catecholamines at toxic levels and may stimulate β-adrenergic receptors (68,70).

Symptoms of minor toxicity may be seen at ''normal'' serum levels of 10–20 μg/

mL or less. Levels in the 20–40 μg/mL range or greater may be associated with symptoms of major toxicity. An acute oral ingestion of 50 mg/kg or more may potentially result in a level greater than 100 μg/mL and significant toxicity. Symptoms may be delayed 12 hr or more following ingestions of slow-release formulations. Some commercial assays may be falsely elevated in the event of acute caffeine toxicity, which may present with a similar clinical picture.

Initial management in suspected theophylline overdose should focus on preventing further administration or absorption of the drug. Gastric lavage should be performed in acute ingestions when the patient presents less than four hours after ingestion and has not been vomiting (68). There may be some benefit to lavage after 4 hr in ingestions involving slow release forms.

Administration of activated charcoal is of great benefit as it avidly binds to theophylline still in the gut. It has also been shown to decrease serum levels after parenteral administration of aminophylline; thus it not only decreases absorption but also increases clearance (68,69). Clearance is increased due to interruption of the enterohepatic cycle and passive trapping of theophylline in the gut. Initial doses should be 50–75 g in adults and repeated doses are recommended at approximately 10 g/hr, which can be given continuously or as single doses every 1–2 hr (71). A cathartic such as sorbitol should be added to prevent constipation and enhance elimination of the theophylline/charcoal complex (12). Nasogastric administration may be required with concomitant use of antiemetics or ranitidine. The patient's airway patency must be considered and the airway secured and protected during this procedure as indicated. Forced diuresis is not useful (68).

Serum theophylline levels should be closely followed, every 2–4 hr for 16–18 hr or until a nontoxic level is reached. This is especially important with intoxication of slow-release preparations as there may be ongoing absorption.

Hypotension, tachycardia, and ventricular dysrhythmias are predominantly the result of excessive β-adrenergic stimulation. These symptoms may be treated with low doses of propranolol (0.01–0.03 mg/kg IV) or esmolol (25–50 μg/kg/min IV). Beta blockers should be used cautiously in these patients and the risk of bronchospasm cannot be ignored. Ventricular dysrhythmias may be treated with lidocaine as necessary (66,68,70).

Hypokalemia is the result of intracellular movement of potassium and does not usually indicate significant total body depletion. This is found in nearly all patients with acute theophylline overdose but less than half of those with chronic toxicity (64). In most cases, this spontaneously resolves without aggressive management (68) and is not felt to be related to vomiting or diuresis (64).

Seizures are associated with severe theophylline toxicity and are generally focal with secondary generalization (68). They are often very difficult to control and may be refractory to common anticonvulsant therapy. Diazepam, phenytoin, or clonazepam should be given initially. If these agents are unsuccessful, general anesthesia with thiopental should be considered (11,12).

Extracorporeal hemoperfusion is the elimination technique of choice when needed for theophylline elimination. Clearances of 150–300 mL/min may be achieved; charcoal hemoperfusion is somewhat more effective than resin hemoperfusion. Hemodialysis is less effective but can achieve clearances of 100–120 mL/min (68). There is significant variability in the literature concerning the indications for hemoperfusion. Established major toxicity in the form of intractable seizures, persistent hypotension, or refractory dysrhythmias are considered criteria by most authors regardless of the serum level (68). Clinical circumstances known to decrease theophylline clearance such as age greater than 60, cardiac decompensation, and hepatic disease also warrant consideration of hemoperfusion. Theophylline levels greater than 60 μg/mL in chronic intoxications or greater than 100 μg/mL in acute ingestions are also criteria for hemoperfusion by most authors. Serum levels less than 30–40 μg/mL generally do not justify the use of hemoperfusion (66,68).

VI. DRUG INTERACTIONS

Some drugs interact with theophylline in ways that do not alter pharmacokinetics. Oral β-adrenergic antagonists potentiate adverse side effects because they are synergistic with theophylline (15,66,72). Ketamine may lower the seizure threshold and fluorinated volatile anesthetics such as halothane may cause ventricular dysrhythmias (73). Theophylline may antagonize the effects of adenosine, benzodiazepines, and nondepolarizing agents such as pancuronium (15).

VII. SUMMARY

Interpretation of the studies regarding aminophylline is complicated by the facts that most of them had small numbers of patients, treated patients in a manner that is not consistent with the current management of asthma, and only followed patients for short periods of time. Most of these studies did not use the frequent dosing of albuterol that is typical today, and some did not routinely administer corticosteroids. A review of the results of these studies demonstrates that many of them found a small advantage to combination treatment with aminophylline, although in any one study, these results did not reach statistical significance. Littenberg compiled 13 relevant studies evaluating the use of aminophylline in the treatment of acute asthma to perform a meta-analysis (74). Pooling all of the studies together, Littenberg found that there was a slight advantage to the addition of aminophylline to treatment with other sympathomimetic agents. They note that, given the size of the studies they were able to evaluate, they had only a 25% chance of detecting a 20% difference in treatment with aminophylline compared to control. Littenberg concluded that there were inadequate data to determine whether or not aminophylline should be added to treatment with other adrenergic agents.

Given the information available to date on the use of theophylline for both acute and chronic asthma, some suggestions can be made with the caveats that reasonable alternative strategies exist. Theophylline generally should not be considered as first-line therapy for acute asthma. Patients with mild to moderate asthma are best managed with inhaled β-agonists and inhaled corticosteroids acutely and with inhaled corticosteroids for more persistent symptoms. Theophylline may be considered for patients with moderate to moderately severe asthma when adequate control can not be achieved with inhaled β agonists and inhaled corticosteroids. Theophylline may also be considered for patients who are unable or unwilling to utilize inhaled β agonists or in children who can not tolerate oral albuterol syrup. In addition, theophylline may be useful for control of exercise-induced asthma or nocturnal asthma. The relative efficacy of oral theophylline as compared to long acting β agonists (such as salmeterol) in the treatment of nocturnal asthma has yet to be established. When used for nocturnal asthma, the pharmacokinetics of theophylline should be taken into account so that peak levels are achieved at the time of nocturnal symptoms. Theophylline should also be considered in patients with moderately severe to severe asthma in whom adequate control was not obtained with regular doses of inhaled β agonists, inhaled corticosteroids, and short courses of steroids. The use of theophylline may also allow a decrease in oral steroids in patients with moderately severe to severe asthma.

When used for chronic asthma, theophylline should be administered initially in low doses. A total initial adult starting dose of 400 mg per day in divided doses may minimize adverse effects. Theophylline doses may be increased based on serum levels (see Table 2). Patients should be cautioned not to self-adjust their theophylline. In addition, patients should be cautioned about the variety of factors that may affect the theophylline clearance including medications such as cimetidine or erythromycin, viral illness, smoking cessation, or the occurrence of congestive heart failure or liver disease.

The role of aminophylline in the treatment of acute asthma appears to be more limited. Standard therapy for acute asthma should initially be used for patients, consisting of frequent administration of nebulized albuterol and early administration of corticosteroids in patients who are unresponsive to initial treatment. Aminophylline may be considered for patients who are resistant to this therapy, although there are few data to suggest it will be effective in these circumstances. When administered, the dose of aminophylline should be based on a measured theophylline level. Using an empiric formula to gauge the

Table 2 Dosing of Intravenous Aminophylline

Dosing variable	Maximal dose (weight adjusted)	Comments
Intravenous dosing	Load: 5 mg/kg over 20–30 min followed by maintenance dose: • initial maintenance dose 0.4 mg/kg/hr in adult nonsmokers • 0.6 mg/kg/hr in smokers • 0.2 mg/kg/hr in CHF or liver disease • 0.8 mg/kg/hr in children 1–9 years old • 0.6 mg/kg/hr in children >9 years old	Measure serum level 4–6 hr after initiating treatment
Oral dosing		
Initial	10–12 mg/kg/d max. 300–400 mg/d	Adults and children >1 yr
First increase	13–16 mg/kg/d max. 450–600 mg/d	If tolerated, increase no sooner than 3 days later.
Second increase	16–22 mg/kg/d max. 600–800 mg/d	Measure serum level after 3 days at max. dose.

Serum concentration	Directions
<10 μg/mL	Increase 25%
10–20 μg/mL	Maintain dose *if tolerated*
20–25 μg/mL	Skip dose and decrease 10–25%
>25 μg/mL	Skip next two doses and decrease 50%

loading dose for aminophylline is likely to lead to errors in drug administration. Additional bronchodilation may occur by targeting a theophylline level in the high therapeutic range. This should be done cautiously, based on repeated theophylline levels and carries with it an increased risk of side effects. Aminophylline may be given by continuous infusion for patients requiring prolonged treatment for acute asthma. The dosing must take into account the patient's smoking status, ideal body weight, and complicating factors such as congestive heart failure or liver disease. Theophylline levels should be monitored. The switch from intravenous therapy to oral therapy should be made by discontinuing intravenous aminophylline at the time the first oral dose is given (see Table 2).

In spite of years of experience with aminophylline, its mechanism of action and role in the treatment of asthma continue to be debated. Ready availability of drug levels and a better understanding of pharmacokinetics afford safer means of dosing aminophylline. Although more potent and selective agents exist, aminophylline still has a role in the treatment of asthma.

REFERENCES

1. Javaheri S, Parker TJ, Wexler L, Liming JD, Lindower P, Roselle GA. Effect of theophylline on sleep disordered breathing in heart failure. N Engl J Med 1996; 335:562–567.
2. Hermann G, Aynesworth MB. Successful treatment of persistent extreme dyspnea''status asthmaticus''; use of theophylline ethylene diamine (aminophylline, USP) intravenously. J Lab Clin Med 1937; 23:135–148.
3. Brown EA. New type of medication to be used in bronchial asthma and other allergic conditions. N Engl J Med 1940; 223:843–846.
4. Fanta CH, Rossing TH, McFadden ER. Emergency room treatment of asthma; relationships among therapeutic combinations, severity of obstruction and time course of response. Am J Med 1982; 72:416–422.
5. Rossing TH, Fanta CH, Goldstein DH, Snapper JR, McFadden ER, and the Medical Hospital Staff of the Peter Bent Brigham Hospital. Emergency therapy of asthma: comparison of the acute effects of parenteral and inhaled sympathomimetics and infused aminophylline. Am Rev Respir Dis 1980; 122:365–371.
6. Josephson GW, MacKenzie EJ, Lietman PS, Gibson G. Emergency treatment of asthma: a comparison of two treatment regimes. JAMA 1979; 242(7):639–643.
7. Appel D, Shim C. Comparative effect of epinephrine and aminophylline in the treatment of asthma. Lung 1981; 159:243–254.
8. Siegel D, Sheppard D, Gleb A, Weinberg PF. Aminophylline increases the toxicity but not the efficacy of an inhaled beta-adrenergic agonist in the treatment of acute exacerbations of asthma. Am Rev Respir Dis 1985; 132:283–286.
9. Bresnick E, Woodard WK, Sageman CB. Fatal reactions to intravenous administration of aminophylline: report of three cases. JAMA 1948; 136:397–398.
10. Merrill GA. Aminophylline deaths. JAMA 1943; 123:1115.
11. Rall T. Drugs used in the treatment of asthma: the methylxanthines, cromolyn sodium and other agents, In: Goodman and Gilman, eds., Goodman and Gilman's the Pharmacological Basis of Therapeutics, New York: Pergamon Press, 1990, pp. 20–47, 618–630.
12. Meich R, Stein M. Respiratory pharmacology. Clin Chest Med 1986; 7(3):331–340.
13. Weinberger M. Therapeutic indications and rationale for theophylline in the management of asthma. Allergy Proc 1994; 15(6):275–282.
14. Shaw Phillips M. Criteria for the use of theophylline in inpatients and outpatients with pulmonary disease. Clin Pharmacol 1992; 11:1033–1038.

15. Weinberger M, Hendeles L. Theophylline in asthma. N Engl J Med 1996; 334(21):1380–1388.
16. Litovitz TL, Felberg L, White S, Klein-Schwartz W. Annual report of the American association of poison control centers toxic exposure surveillance system. Am J Emerg Med 1996; 14(5): 487–537.
17. Jenne J. Theophylline use in asthma. Clin Chest Med 1984; 5(4):645–658.
18. Taburet AM, Schmit B. Pharmacokinetic optimization of asthma treatment. Clin Pharmacokinet 1994; 27(5):396–418.
19. Jones J, McMullen MJ, Dougherty J, Cannon L. Repetitive doses of activated charcoal in the treatment of poisoning. Am J Emerg Med 1987; 5:305–311.
20. Asmus MJ, Weinberger MM, Milavetz G, et al. Pharmacokinetics and drug disposition. Apparent decrease in population clearance of theophylline: implications for dosage. Clin Pharmacol Ther 1997; 62:483–489.
21. Duncan PE, Griffin JP, Solomon SS. Bronchodilator drug efficacy via cyclic AMP. Thorax 1975; 30:192–196.
22. Butcher RW, Sutherland EW. Adenosine 3′-5′ phosphate in biological materials. J Biol Chem 1962; 1244–1250.
23. Polson JB, Krazanowski JJ, Goldman AL, et al. Inhibition of human pulmonary phosphodiesterase activity by therapeutic levels of theophylline. Clin Exp Pharmacol Physiol 1978; 5: 535–539.
24. Polson JB, Krazanowski JJ, Anderson WH, et al. Analysis of the relationship between pharmacological inhibition of cyclic nucleotide phosphodiesterase and relaxation of canine tracheal smooth muscle. Biochem Pharmacol 1979; 28:1391–1395.
25. Fredholm BB. Theophylline actions on adenosine receptors. Eur J Respir Dis 1980; 61(suppl 109):29–36.
26. Rossing TH. Methylxanthines in 1989. Ann Intern Med 1989; 110(7):502–504.
27. Scordamaglia A, Ciprandi G, Ruffoni S, et al. Theophylline and the immune response: in vitro and in vivo effects. Clin Immunol Immunopathol 1988; 48:238–246.
28. Kidney J, Dominguez M, Taylor PM, Rose M, Chung KF, Barnes PJ. Immunomodulation by theophylline in asthma: demonstration by withdrawal of therapy. Am J Respr Crit Care Med 1995; 151:1907–1914.
29. Magnussen H, Reuss G, Jorres R. Theophylline has a dose-related effect on the airway response to inhaled histamine and methacholine in asthmatics. Am Rev Respir Dis 1987; 136: 1163–1167
30. Sullivan P, Bekir S, Jaffar Z, Page C, Jeffery P, Costello J. Anti-inflammatory effects of low-dose oral theophylline in atopic asthma. Lancet 1994; 343:1006–1008.
31. Kraft M, Torvik JA, Trudeau JB, Wenzel SE, Martin R. Theophylline: potential anti-inflammatory effects in nocturnal asthma. J Allergy Clin Immunol 1996; 97(6):1242–1246.
32. Shohat B, Volovitz B, Varsano I. Induction of suppressor T-cells in asthmatic children by theophylline treatment. Clin Allergy 1983; 13:487–493.
33. Lahat N, Nir E, Horenstien L, Colin A. Effects of theophylline on the proportion and function of T-suppressor cells in asthmatic children. Allergy 1985; 40:453–457.
34. Ward AJ, McKenniff M, Evans JM, Page CP, Costello JF. Theophylline an immunomodulatory role in asthma? Am Rev Respir Dis 1993; 147:518–523.
35. Metenko PA, Ogilvie RE. Rational intravenous doses of theophylline. N Engl J Med 1973; 289:600–603.
36. Fairshter RD. How much theophylline is enough? Am J Med 1988; 85(suppl 1B):54–59.
37. Hendeles L, Jenkins J, Temple R. Revised FDA labeling guideline for theophylline oral dosage forms. Pharmacotherapy 1995; 15:409–427.
38. Aubier M, DeTroyer A, Sampson M, et al. Aminophylline improves diaphragmatic contractility. N Engl J Med 1981; 305:249–252.
39. Murciano D, Aubier M, Lecocguic Y, et al. Effects of theophylline on diaphragmatic strength

and fatigue in patients with chronic obstructive pulmonary disease. N Engl J Med 1984; 311: 349–353.
40. Matthay RA, Berger HJ, Loke J, et al. Effects of aminophylline upon right and left ventricular performance in chronic obstructive pulmonary disease: noninvasive assessment by radionuclide angiocardiography. Am J Med 1978; 65:903–910.
41. Segal MS, Levinson L, Bresnick E, et al. Evaluation of therapeutic substances employed for the relief of bronchospasm. J Clin Invest 1949; 28:1190–1195.
42. Jezek V, Ourednik A, Stepanek J, et al. the effect of aminophylline on the respiration and pulmonary circulation. Clin Sci 1970; 38:549–554.
43. Pollock J, Kiechel F, Cooper D, Weinberger M. Relationship of serum theophylline concentration to inhibition of exercise-induced bronchospasm and comparison with cromolyn. Pediatrics 1977; 60:840–844.
44. Anderson S, Seale JP, Ferris L, Furukawa C, Lindsay DA. An evaluation of pharmacotherapy for exercise-induced asthma. J Allergy Clin Immunol 1979; 64(pt2):612–614.
45. Fairshter RD, Bhola R, Thomas R, et al. Comparison of clinical effects and pharmacokinetics of one-daily Uniphyl and twice-daily Theo-Dur in asthmatic patients. Am J Med 1985; 79(suppl 6A):48–53.
46. Barnes PJ, Greening AAP, Neville L, Timmers J, Poole GW. Single dose slow-release aminophylline at night prevents nocturnal asthma. Lancet 1982; 1:299–301.
47. Neuenkirchen H, Wilkens JH, Oellerich M, Saybrecht GW. Nocturnal asthma: effect of a once per evening dose of sustained release theophylline. Eur J Respir Dis 1985; 66:196–204.
48. Weinberger MM, Bronsky EA. Evaluation of oral bronchodilator therapy in asthmatic children. J Pediatr 1974; 84:421–427.
49. Weinberger MM, Bronsky EA, Bensch GW, et al. Interaction of ephedrine and theophylline. Clin Pharmacol Ther 1975; 17:585–592.
50. Hambleton G, Weinberger MM, Taylor J, et al. Comparison of cromoglycate (cromolyn) and theophylline in controlling symptoms of chronic asthma: a collaborative study. Lancet 1977; 1:381–385.
51. Nassif EG, Weinberger MM, Thompson R, et al. The value of maintenance theophylline for steroid dependent asthma. N Engl J Med 1981; 304:71–75.
52. Barclay J, Whiting B, Addis GH. The influence of theophylline on maximal response to salbutamol in severe chronic obstructive pulmonary disease. Eur J Clin Pharmacol 1982; 22:389–393.
53. Barclay J, Whiting B, PA Meredith, et al. Theophylline-salbutamol interaction: bronchodilator response to salbutamol at maximally effective plasma theophylline concentrations. Br J Clin Pharmacol 1981; 11:203–208.
54. Svedmyr K. β_2-adrenoceptor stimulants and theophylline in asthma therapy. Eur J Respir Dis 1981; 116(suppl):1–48.
55. Rachelefsky GS, Katz RM, Mickey MR, et al. Metaproterenol and theophylline in asthmatic children. Ann Allergy 1980; 45:207–212.
56. Rossing TH, Fanta CH, McFadden ER. Med Staff of the Peter Bent Brigham Hospital. A controlled trial of the use of single versus combined-drug therapy in the treatment of acute episodes of asthma. Am Rev Respir Dis 1981; 123:190–194.
57. Carter E, Cruz M, Chesrown S, Shieh G, Reilly K, Hendeles L. Efficacy of intravenously administered theophylline in children hospitalized with severe asthma. J Pediatr 1993; 122: 470–476.
58. Pearson WE, Bierman CW, Stamm SJ, VanArsdel PP. Double-blind trial of aminophylline in status asthmaticus. Pediatrics 1971; 48:642–646.
59. DiGiulio GA, Kercsmar CM, Krug SE, Alpert SE, Marx CM. Hospital treatment of asthma: lack of benefit from theophylline given in addition to nebulized albuterol and intravenously administered corticosteroid. J Pediatr 1993; 122(3):464–469.
60. Strauss RE, Wertheim DL, Bonagura VR, Valacer DJ. Aminophylline therapy does not im-

prove outcome and increases adverse effects in children hospitalized with acute asthmatic exacerbations. Pediatrics 1994; 2:205–210.

61. Murphy DG, McDermott MF, Rydman RJ, Sloan EP, Zalenski RJ. Aminophylline in the treatment of acute asthma when β_2-adrenergics and steroids are provided. Arch Intern Med 1993; 153:1784–1788.
62. Rodrigo C, Rodrigo G. Treatment of acute asthma: lack of therapeutic benefit and increase of the toxicity from aminophylline given in addition to high doses of salbutamol delivered by metered-dose inhaler with a spacer. Chest 1994; 106(4):1071–1076.
63. Zainudin BM, Ismail O, Yusoff K. Effect of adding aminophylline infusion to nebulized salbutamol in severe acute asthma. Thorax 1994; 49:267–269.
64. Huang D, O'Brien RG, Harman E, Aull L, Reents S, Visser J, Shieh G, Hendeles L. Does aminophylline benefit adults admitted to the hospital for an acute exacerbation of asthma? Ann Intern Med 1993; 119(12):1155–1160.
65. Wrenn K, Slovis CM, Murphy F, Greenberg RS. Aminophylline therapy for acute bronchospastic disease in the emergency room. Ann Intern Med 1991; 115(4):241–247.
66. Shannon M. Predictors of major toxicity after theophylline overdose. Ann Intern Med 1993; 119:1161–1167.
67. Litovitz TL, Feldberg L, White S, Klein-Schwartz W. Annual report of the American association of poison control centers toxic exposure surveillance system. Am J Emerg Med 1996; 14(5):487–537.
68. Stegeman CA, Jordans JGM. Theophylline intoxication: clinical features, treatment, and outcome: a case report and a review of the literature. Neth J Med 1991; 39:115–125.
69. Nasser SS, Rees PJ. Theophylline: Current thoughts on the risks and benefits of its use in asthma. Drug Safety 1993; 8(1):12–18.
70. Hendeles L, Massanari M, Weinberger M. Update on the pharmacodynamics and pharmacokinetics of theophylline. Chest 1985; 88(2):S103–S111.
71. Jones J, McMullen MJ, Dougherty J, Cannon L. Repetitive doses of activated charcoal in the treatment of poisoning. Am J Emerg Med 1987; 5:305–311.
72. Milgrom H, Bender B. Current issues in the use of theophylline. Am Rev Respir Dis 1993; 147:S33–S39.
73. Hirshman CA, Kreiger W, Littlejohn G, Lee R, Julien R. Ketamine-aminophylline-induced decrease in seizure threshold. Anesthesiology 1982; 56:464–467.
74. Littenberg B. Aminophylline treatment in severe, acute asthma: A meta-analysis. JAMA 1988; 259:1678–1684.

22

Steroids

Robert Silverman
Albert Einstein College of Medicine, Bronx, and Long Island Jewish Medical Center, New Hyde Park, New York

I. INTRODUCTION

Asthma is a chronic illness characterized by inflammation of the lungs and airways. The inflammation can cause edema and production of mucus, which leads to airway narrowing and plugging. As the airway diameter becomes reduced, patients will have difficulty ventilating and develop increasing asthma symptoms. Steroids are highly effective pharmacological agents that were first used around 1950 for controlling the inflammation associated with asthma (see Chapter 1). Steroids have since become the mainstay of therapy. Potent inhaled agents are now the treatment of choice for controlling chronic asthma and systemic steroids are used to treat patients with worsening symptoms, acute episodes and asthma that cannot be controlled by other inhaled or oral agents. This chapter will address issues related to steroid use for acute or uncontrolled asthma that requires urgent evaluation.

II. MECHANISMS OF ACTION

The mechanisms of action of steroids in asthma, while not fully elucidated, are becoming better understood. Glucorticoids are potent anti-inflammatory agents whose beneficial effects do not appear linked to any single pathway (1). Steroids decrease activation and recruitment of inflammatory cells, as well as inhibit the release of inflammatory mediators. Inhibition of the inflammatory process appears to occur at a number of different cellular sites with overall beneficial effect due to modulation of new protein synthesis. This includes the decreased production of proinflammatory mediators as well as the increased production of proteins that help to control the inflammatory response (1). A number of cells that actively participate in the cycle of inflammation are also directly inhibited by

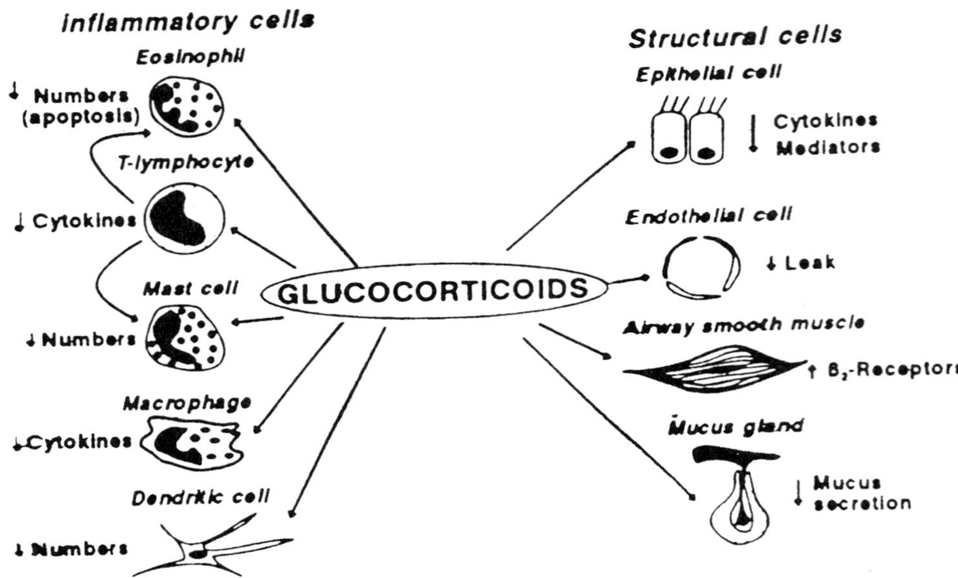

Figure 1 Effect of glucocorticoids on target cells. (From Ref. 1.)

the actions of glucorticoids (Figure 1). By controlling various aspects of the inflammatory process, steroids have proven to be a valuable tool for treating asthma.

Molecular actions of the glucocorticoids can be explained by modulation of protein synthesis at the site of the gene. Glucocorticoids bind to specific receptors on the cell membranes of airway epithelium or a variety of inflammatory cells. Activated glucorticoid receptors are transported into the cell cytoplasm and nucleus and may (1) upregulate transcription and therefore increase protein synthesis by linking to specific DNA receptors in the promoter region of the gene, (2) bind to a site that represses gene transcription and therefore directly suppress protein synthesis or, more likely, (3) interfere with the transcription factors AP-1 and NF-κB and thereby downregulate gene expression. AP-1 is a sequence specific transcriptional activator that promotes gene induction and is induced by a variety of stimuli, including cytokines (2). NF-κB is a particularly important transcriptional factor that is responsible for the activation of a wide variety of immunoregulatory genes, including IL-1β, TNF-α, IL-2, IL-6, IL-8, GM-CSF, IL-2 receptor, ICAM-1*, MCP-1†, RANTES†, and E-selectin* (3–5) (see Chapter 4). Glucocorticoids interfere with the transcriptional activity of both AP-1 and NF-κB, and this may explain most of the antiinflammatory effect.

Proteins synthesized in response to glucocorticoids include a variety of enzymes and regulators such as lipocortins, β_2-adrenergic receptors, and specific cytokines that regulate inflammation. Lipocortin-1 inhibits phospholipase A2, resulting in a decreased production of leukotrienes, prostaglandins and platelet-activating factor (1). Glucocorti-

* Molecules that cause the adherence of leukocytes.

† Chemokines that cause the chemotaxis of leukocytes.

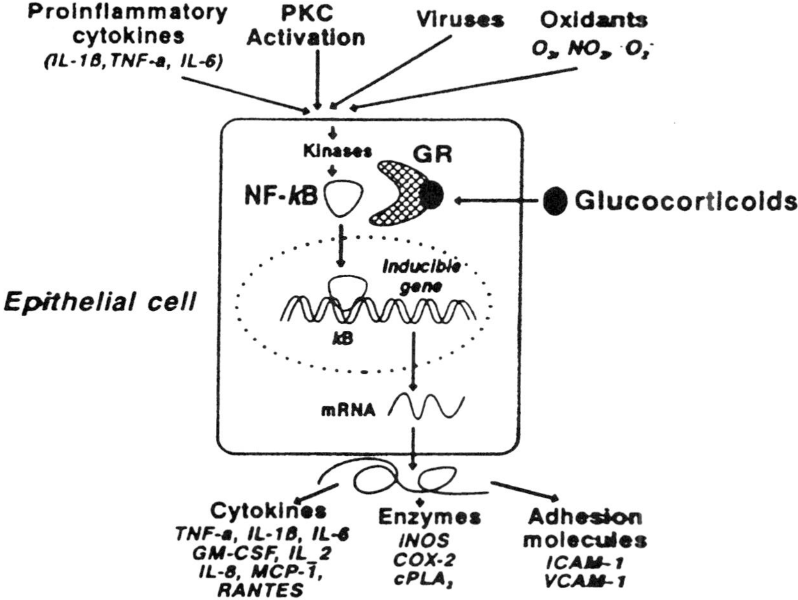

Figure 2 Various mediators or environmental triggers activate NF-κB, which results in the induction of multiple inflammatory genes. A "unifying" hypothesis places the role of glucorticoid as blocking the activation of NF-κB, leading to control of inflammation from the surface of the airway. (From Ref. 1.)

coids increase the rate of production of β_2-receptors (6). In laboratory animals, steroids prevent the downregulation seen with the prolonged use of β-adrenergic agents (7). Steroids can also cause induction of an IL-1 decoy receptor, which can neutralize the proinflammatory cytokine IL-1 (8).

The effects of glucorticoids are noted in a variety of cells that participate in the inflammatory process. Circulating eosinophils are reduced either as a result of diminished bone marrow production or the influence on cytokines that affect eosinophil survival time (9). Mast cells will be decreased in number as a result of steroid treatment, and the influx of eosinophils and T lymphocytes into the lung will be reduced.

A hypothesis that attempts to establish a link between NF-κB , various asthma triggers or inflammatory mediators and steroids has been proposed by Barnes (1) (Figure 2). Viral infections, atmospheric pollutants, superoxide anions and proinflammatory cytokines activate NF-κB found in airway epithelial cells which in turn stimulates a number of proinflammatory genes. Glucocorticoids, by interfering with the activity of NF-κB, block the synthesis of a number of inflammatory mediators. If this proves to be a key step, then the development of agents that specifically block NF-κB may help to control asthma.

III. PHARMACOLOGY

Preparations of glucorticoids differ in their anti-inflammatory properties, sodium retention, and biological half-life (10). (Table 1). Prednisone and prednisolone are the most com-

Table 1 Properties of Corticosteroid Preparations

Steroid	Anti-inflammatory relative potency	Plasma half-life (hr)	Biological half-life (hr)	Equivalent dose (mg)	Sodium-retaining potency
Short acting					
Hydrocortisone	1	2	12	20.0	2+
Cortisone	0.8	0.5	—[a]	25.0	2+
Intermediate acting					
Prednisone	3.5	1	—[a]	5.0	1+
Prednisolone	4	2–3.5	12–36	5.0	1+
Triamcinolone	5	2–3.5	12–24	4.0	0
Methylprednisolone	5	2–3.5	12–36	4.0	0
Prolonged acting					
Betamethasone	25–30	5	24–28	0.6–0.75	0
Dexamethasone					

[a] Prednisone and cortisone must be first converted to prednisolone and hydrocortisone before being active; the half-lives are then compared to the initial compound.

Source: Ref. 10.

monly prescribed oral agents and the tablet preparations are bioequivalent (15). In the emergency department (ED) there are sometimes reasons to choose one preparation over another. In patients prone to hypertension, hypokalemia, or congestive heart failure, methylprednisolone may be superior to prednisone due to the mineralicorticoid effects associated with prednisone. Prednisone must first be converted in the liver to the biologically active compound prednisolone although the presence of severe liver disease does not appear to significantly impair this conversion (11). The bioavailability after oral administration of prednisolone or prednisone ranges from 50 to 90% in a variety of populations with significant individual variability noted (11). The large interindividual variability may be related to differences in absorption, first-pass metabolism, or a combination of both effects (12). Substantial serum levels of prednisone are found one-half hour after oral ingestion with peak levels occurring approximately 1 hr after ingestion (13,14). When prednisone or prednisolone is given intravenously, the time to maximum serum concentration ranges from several minutes to half an hour (13,14). The maximum serum concentration is up to several times greater for the same amount of steroids given intravenously when compared to oral administration (14,15).

IV. ADRENAL AXIS

Suppression of the hypothalamic-pituitary-adrenal axis is a potential complication of sustained glucorticoid use. The adrenal cortex hypofunction results from loss of endogenous adrenocorticotropic hormone (ACTH) and is termed secondary adrenocortical insufficiency. Depending on the duration of exogenous corticosteroid administration, the adrenals may produce less cortisol but still enough to maintain homeostasis, even during times of stress. With prolonged suppression severe adrenal atrophy may result with the body unable to produce adequate amounts of cortisol even to meet the needs of acute medical problems. An adrenal crisis can occur and replacement with stress doses of glucorticoids and volume is needed to reverse severe systemic symptoms or shock.

Patients with chronic asthma who have not used systemic steroids have normal hypothalamic-pituitary-adrenal function (16). The endogenous production of glucorticoid is equivalent to approximately 7.5–10 mg of prednisolone daily and, if doses higher than this are administered, adrenal suppression may result. Adrenal function typically becomes suppressed days after the administration of corticosteroids. After short-term glucorticoid treatment (e.g., 3 weeks or less) full recovery of adrenal function occurs 5–10 days after steroids are stopped. This has been demonstrated in several studies, including healthy individuals and asthmatic children and adults. Among healthy adults given 50 mg daily of prednisolone for 5 days, adrenal suppression was noted 2 days after the steroids were stopped, and almost full recovery was noted 5 days after the steroids were stopped (17). Among asthmatic children given 2 mg/kg/day of prednisone for 5 days, blunting of peak corticosteroid responses occurred 3 days after completion of the steroid course (18). At 10 days after steroids were discontinued, adrenal function returned to normal. In another study patients with chronic airflow obstruction were given a 3-week course of prednisolone, 40 mg per day, and adrenal function fully recovered 5 days after stopping corticosteroids (19). In an attempt to determine if periodic bursts of steroids influenced adrenal function, children with chronic asthma who did not recently receive systemic steroids were studied. Those who received three or fewer bursts of steroids in the past 12 months had normal adrenal function. Among the children who received four or more bursts of steroids in the past year, there were some who had a subnormal adrenal stress test, although the number of patients in this latter group were too few to draw general conclusions (20).

Chronic steroid use may prolong recovery of the hypothalamic-pituitary-adrenal axis with an impaired response to adrenal stimulation as long as one or more years after steroids have been discontinued. In several asthmatic patients on 5–20 mg of daily prednisone for 2–17 years, evidence of adrenal suppression was found even 36 months after stopping therapy (21). In a group of patients with either adrenocortical tumors or ingesting exogenous corticosteroids for more than one year, adrenal function took up to 9 months to recover after the sources of the increased steroid were removed (22). Among children on large daily doses of steroids for 0.5–5 years, weaning of steroids over a 4- to 8-week period led to improved adrenal responses (23). Normal cortisol responses were seen 1–2 weeks after complete discontinuation of corticosteroid treatment. It is not clear if this more rapid restoration occurred because the adrenals of children have shorter recovery times than adults.

Although adrenal suppression is a concern, clinical signs of adrenal insufficiency in patients presenting with severe asthma is uncommon, and deaths in asthmatics due to adrenal suppression are considered rare. Still, patients who have been treated with long-term systemic steroids should be considered at risk for adrenal insufficiency and coverage for stress instituted even up to several years after glucorticoids are discontinued. Among patients given short bursts of steroids, replacement therapy should be considered if a significant stress occurs within 5–10 days of discontinuation.

V. GENERAL ACUTE CLINICAL EFFECTS OF STEROIDS

Steroids are effective in the treatment of chronic asthma, reducing inflammation, lessening symptoms, improving pulmonary function, and decreasing the need for ED visits or hospitalizations. Studies of the use of steroids in acutely ill ED patients, however, have provided conflicting results. Some trials have demonstrated benefit several hours after administration, prompting recommendations for ED asthmatics to receive steroids as soon as possible. Based on these studies, clinicians could expect to see improvement in pulmonary function while the patient is treated in the ED, thereby decreasing the need for hospitalization or even an intensive care unit (ICU) admission in more severely ill patients. Unfortunately not all studies have demonstrated a rapid (e.g., 6 hr or less) benefit from systemic steroids. Some studies even question the efficacy of steroids within 12 hr or more after administration. An overview of some of the published clinical trials can help to better understand the issues, and why the reported time to achieve a clinically meaningful improvement from steroids has varied.

VI. WHEN DO STEROIDS BEGIN TO WORK?

The question of when steroids begin to improve acute asthma remains largely unanswered. Three clinical trials in adults have not demonstrated any benefit occurring within approximately 6 hr of ED steroid administration (24–26) while two studies reported some benefit (27,28). In a study by McFadden et al., 38 patients were given placebo or intravenous hydrocortisone in doses ranging from 250 to 1000 mg, and there was no improvement in pulmonary function at 6 hr (24). Stein and colleagues gave 81 patients either placebo or

125 mg of intravenous methylprednisolone, and a disposition was made by 12 hr (25). No difference in admission rate was noted, although results may have been influenced by the relatively high baseline peak expiratory flow rate (PEFR) in the study population, as well as the administration of steroids to any patient who was not admitted by 6 hr. In a study by Rodrigo and Rodrigo, 98 patients with an $FEV_1 < 50\%$ predicted on ED arrival received either 500 mg of intravenous hydrocortisone or placebo (26). After up to 6 hr of treatment there was no difference in admission rate, pulmonary function or use of β agonists, suggesting that severity of pulmonary obstruction did not influence response to steroids (Figure 3).

Among the studies in adults demonstrating benefit, Littenberg and Gluck reported a reduction in hospital admissions of 44% in patients receiving 125 mg methylprednisilone as compared to 9% among patients receiving placebo (27). In this study there was no reported time limit to the ED stay, and although the final FEV_1 was greater in the steroid group, the differences did not reach statistical significance. In a trial by Schneider et al., 54 patients received either 30 mg/kg methylprednisolone or placebo as part of a standardized treatment protocol (28). Fewer patients receiving steroids required admission (19%) when compared to placebo (44%), although these differences did not reach statistical significance ($p = 0.08$)

ED studies evaluating the early efficacy of steroids in children with acute asthma have generally shown favorable results. In a pediatric trial of 140 patients, 3% of those receiving oral prednisone were admitted compared to 30% of children receiving placebo after several hours of treatment (29). In a post hoc analysis, the beneficial effect of steroids was noted several hours after dosing (Figure 4). The dose of prednisolone was 30 mg in children under 5 years, otherwise it was 60 mg. In another pediatric study of 75 ED patients the 4-hr admission rate in the placebo group was 49% versus 31% in the patients receiving 2 mg/kg of oral prednisone ($p = 0.10$) (30). When a subset of children with more severe

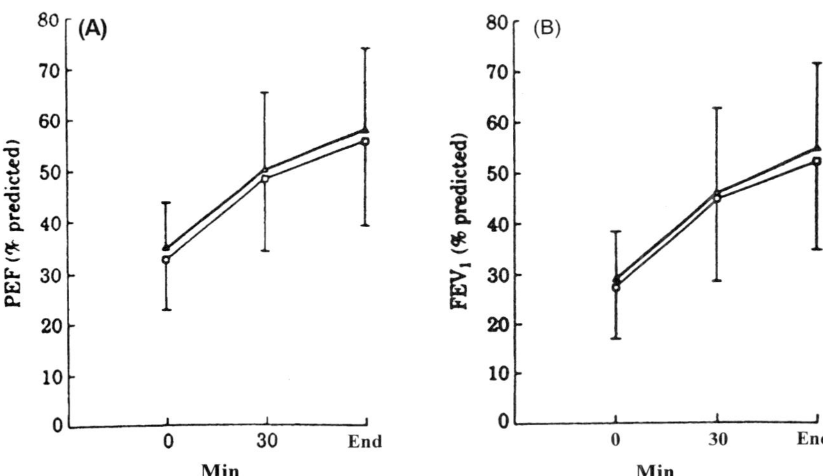

Figure 3 Pulmonary function after up to 6 hr of treatment with 125 mg methylprednisolone (△) or placebo (□). Mean values for peak expiratory flow rate (PEF) and forced expiratory volume in 1 sec (FEV_1) are expressed as percentage of predicted. (From Ref. 26, with permission of W.B. Saunders Co.)

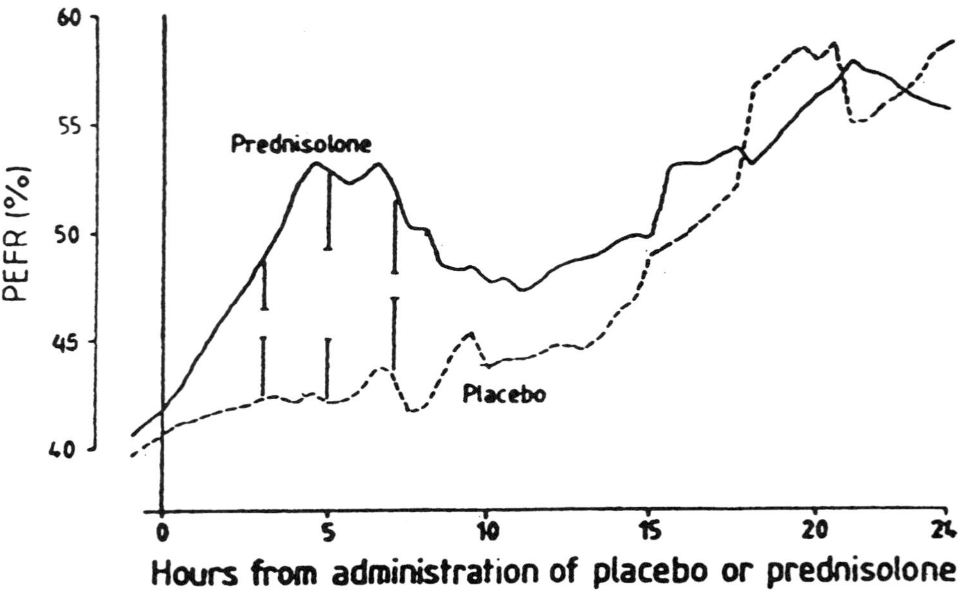

Figure 4 The mean onset and duration of effect of prednisolone in children receiving placebo or prednisolone. Patients were retrospectively paired to obtain these data, and pairs were excluded if patient was discharged or received further steroids. There were 29 pairs initially, 20 at 5 hr and 10 at 10 hr. SE is indicated at 3, 5, and 7 hr. (From Ref. 29.)

asthma was analyzed, prednisone appeared to significantly reduce the need for hospitalization. In another trial of infants and toddlers aged 6 to 60 months, treatment with 4 mg/kg of intramuscular methylprednisilone was associated with a significant reduction of admissions at 3 hr (31).

A number of studies evaluated the effects of steroids in acutely ill patients 12 hr or more after administration and benefits could not be consistently demonstrated. Four clinical trials noted improvement from steroids while two did not. Fanta and colleagues administered 2 mg/kg hydrocortisone or placebo to a total 20 adults and found statistically significant improvement in pulmonary function after 12 hours (32) (Figure 5). In an outpatient study of 16 children, greater improvement in pulmonary function as compared to placebo was noted at 12 hr, the first time point measured (33). In 49 children hospitalized for asthma, those receiving 1 mg/kg of methylprednisolone every 6 hr had improvement in a clinical index at 24 hr, but not 12 hr, after admission (34). The results of pulmonary function testing were, however, not significantly different at 24 hr after admission. Another study in children did not demonstrate any benefit from intravenous methylprednisolone after 48 hr of inpatient treatment (35). Evaluation of single-dose treatment in pediatric outpatient populations also had varying results. In a study of 86 outpatient children, a single dose of 2 mg/kg prednisone or placebo was given at home early during an asthma attack. The use of prednisone was actually associated with an increase in outpatient visits relative to placebo (36). In a second study of 72 children who presented to the clinic with mild to moderate asthma episodes, patients receiving prednisone had greater improvements in clinical criteria at 24 hr, which was the first time point measured (37).

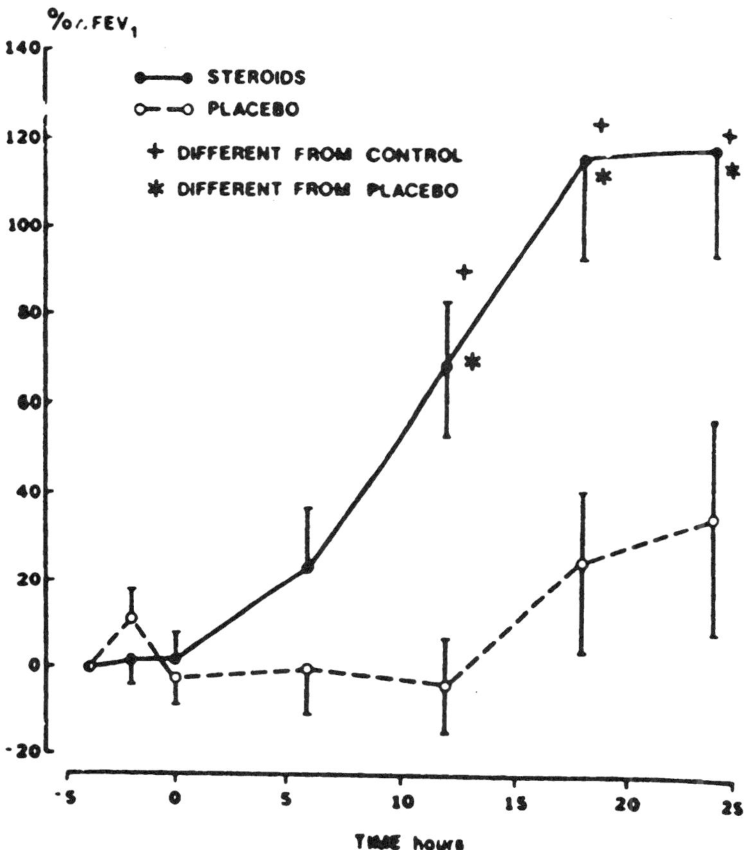

Figure 5 The effect of hydrocortisone 2 mg/kg bolus followed by 0.5 mg/kg/h for 24 hr on 20 adults hospitalized with acute asthma, as compared to placebo. Solid line indicates hydrocortisone; dashed line indicates placebo. The relative percentage of improvement from baseline forced expiratory volume in 1 sec (FEV_1) was recorded every 6 hr. Statistically significant differences were noted in this small group of patients at 12, 18, and 24 hr after the initial bolus. (From Ref. 32.)

A number of study design issues may contribute to the inconsistent findings among acute asthma trials, including sample size (relatively few patients were included in many studies, leading to chance observations), different treatment protocols (including dose, route of administration and types of steroids used), differences in patient assessment and study endpoints, as well as the wide spectrum of illness severity. Another important factor to consider is that any early beneficial effects may be masked by the more robust and immediate responses to β agonists. In observational studies where bronchodilators were not given, steroids improve pulmonary function in chronic asthma within 2 hr and in acute asthma within 6–8 hr (38,39). Even when bronchodilators are given, the maximal improvements from steroids are best measured over days and not hours (Figure 6).

Factors influencing the time to beneficial effects include the mechanisms of steroid action. Steroids cause synthesis of new proteins to be modulated, and this may require some time. Even if the production of proinflammatory mediators can be rapidly decreased

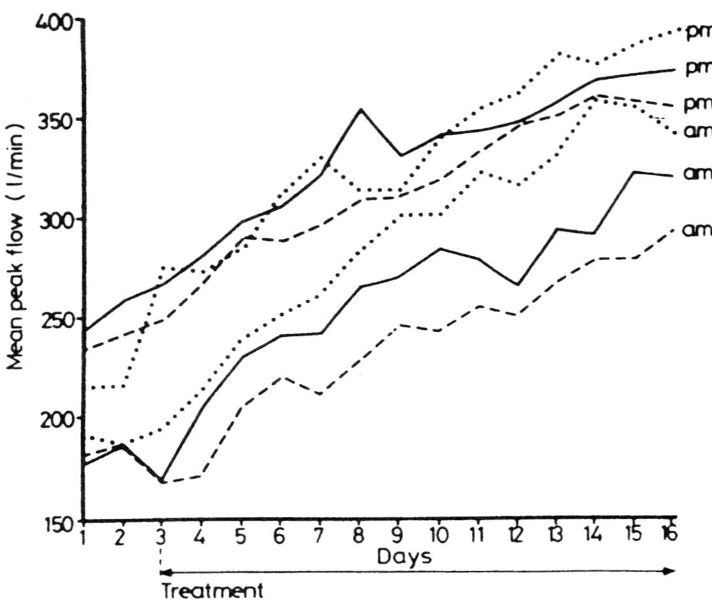

Figure 6 Peak flow measures (L/min) for morning (am) and evening (pm) evaluating 3 different doses of prednisolone treatment in 10 patients during three separate exacerbations. Low dose prednisolone (---) equals 0.2 mg/kg; medium dose (—) equals 0.4 mg/kg; high dose (····) equals 0.6 mg/kg. Treatment with steroids began at day 3. (From Ref. 50.)

by the administration of steroids, the airway swelling and mucous plugging would take some time to resolve, and this would vary from patient to patient. It is also possible that there are patients who are more steroid responsive and benefit early, but in studies of limited sample size it is difficult to identify them. Given all of these conditions it is not that surprising that results from clinical studies vary greatly, and, when evaluating the literature, it can be difficult to assess the acute benefits of steroid administration.

In summary, the time of onset for steroid action is not certain but may prove to be as variable as the patient population. The earlier steroids are given, the sooner they will have their effect; whether this is hours after administration for some patients or days later for others. It is important to remember that steroids are potent anti-inflammatory agents, and, although when they begin to work continues to be debated, there is no question they are important therapeutic agents and should be used routinely in patients with acute asthma.

VII. ORAL VS. INTRAVENOUS STEROIDS

There have not been any published studies that directly compare the efficacy of oral to intravenous steroids in the first few hours of ED asthma care. Ratto and colleagues did find that FEV_1 was similar in patients receiving oral or intravenous methylprednisolone at 6 hr after ED treatment and up until 72 hr or hospital discharge (40). Since absorption of the oral agent is fairly rapid, the standard ED dose is relatively large, and steroids likely require at least hours to cause any clinical benefit, there does not appear to be a need for most patients to receive steroids intravenously. It is possible, however, that some patients do not absorb oral agents effectively and the decreased bioavailability may not allow maximum benefit. As the optimal dose of steroids is not known and much serum higher levels are reached when the agents are given intravenously, some asthmatics may benefit more from intravenous (IV) steroids. Since studies have not addressed these issues, in situations where the clinician needs to be certain that maximal levels are reached as soon as possible, such as in the critically ill patient, intravenous rather than oral agents may be warranted.

VIII. INITIAL DOSE

The optimal initial dose of steroids administered to acutely ill patients has not been well studied. A typical oral dose in the United States would be 40–80 mg of prednisone and a typical IV dose would be 40–125 mg methylprednisolone. Giving higher systemic doses has not been shown to be useful, as Emerman and Cydulka demonstrated that 500 mg methylprednisolone was as effective as 100 mg methylprednisolone (41). Although higher doses in the ED are not more beneficial, it is still unclear what is the lowest appropriate dose, as dose-response curves for this population has not been established.

IX. WHO SHOULD RECEIVE STEROIDS IN THE ED?

Any patient with airway inflammation associated with an acute asthma episode should receive steroids in the ED. Of course, the clinician cannot accurately assess the degree of inflammation, and there is evidence that almost all cases of acute asthma are associated with some degree of acute inflammation. Because of this, many clinicians will give systemic steroids to every patient presenting to the ED with acute asthma. An argument can be made for withholding steroids in patients that present with acute onset of mild illness and that respond completely to one or two bronchodilator treatments. The rationale is that these patients do not have significant inflammation, although this has not been well studied. There should be no question about giving steroids early on to the vast majority of ED patients with asthma. This includes patients with significant risk factors, such as severe airway obstruction, inadequate response to initial β-agonist treatment, frequent ED visits or hospitalizations, past history of endotracheal intubation, and prolonged acute illness, and those asthmatics presently receiving outpatient steroids.

X. DISCHARGE ON STEROIDS

Although patients presenting to the ED with acute asthma may improve enough to be discharged, this does not mean they have recovered from the episode. Often symptoms will persists for days or weeks after ED discharge. Relapse, or the need for urgent asthma treatment or hospitalization after an acute episode, is fairly common. Relapse rates of 10% 7 days after ED discharge and up to 31% within the first 10 to 21 days after ED discharge have been reported (42–45). It should be noted that while relapse is common

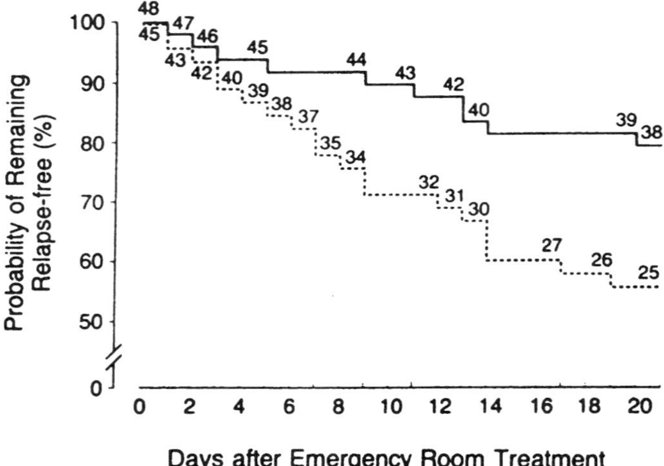

Figure 7 Kaplan-Meier Survival Curve showing the probability of remaining relapse-free after ED treatment for patients receiving prednisone (solid line) and those receiving placebo (dashed line). Values shown are numbers of subjects remaining relapse-free at the beginning of the days on which a relapse occurred. (From Ref. 48, © 1991 Massachusetts Medical Society.)

it is likely that there are many discharged patients whose condition has either not improved or even worsened but do not seek medical care. In a small series of patients followed for up to 2 months after ED discharge, half the patients had their highest FEV_1 recorded in the ED, and one-third of patients had an FEV_1 <50% predicted 1 month after leaving the ED (46) (see Chapter 31).

Up until the 1980s, steroid treatment for most patients presenting to the hospital with acute asthma was limited to inpatient therapy, and patients were often not sent home from the ED on steroids. Short courses of systemic steroids have since shown to decrease relapse rates in patients discharged from the ED. An 8-day tapering dose of prednisone lowered the incidence of relapse at 10 days from 24% in the placebo group to 6% in the treatment group (48) (Figure 7). In another study, an 8-day tapering course of methylprednisolone had 10-day relapse rates of 21% in the placebo group as compared to 6% in the methylprednisolone group (49). The subgroup of patients who have an immediate and almost complete recovery from one or two βagonist treatments in the ED would seem to be the group least likely to need a burst of steroids, but this has not been studied.

XI. DURATION OF STEROIDS TREATMENT ON ED DISCHARGE

Although oral steroids are routinely prescribed to patients discharged from the ED, the optimal dose or duration of therapy is not known. It takes approximately 8 days for patients with chronic asthma to achieve maximum benefit from oral steroid use (47). It is likely that patients with acute asthma, many who may have mucous plugging and worsening inflammation, would also need at least this long a course. The shortest course of ED discharge steroids tested in clinical trials of adults was 8 days (48,49). Chapman and colleagues discharged patients on an 8-day dose tapering from 40 to 0 mg of prednisone and Fiel and colleagues discharged patients on oral methylprednisolone, starting at 32 mg twice a day and decreasing to 0 mg over 8 days. Other data suggests that it takes 14 days of oral steroid treatment to reach a plateau in PEFR following an asthma exacerbation (50) (see Figure 6). In this small study dose response was also evaluated. Doses approximating 14, 28, or 42 mg daily of prednisolone were given, and patients receiving the higher doses had greater improvement in pulmonary function at the end of 2 weeks.

The clinician discharging the patient has several goals, including preventing relapse, optimizing therapy so the patient will have a more speedy recovery, and allowing the patient to reach a plateau of improvement. For some patients a very short course of steroids may be sufficient, and it is possible that there are patients who would do well without any steroids at all. For others, a more prolonged course of treatment may be needed to optimize therapy and prevent relapse. This may include patients who have prolonged symptoms, incomplete responses to β-agonists, frequent past ED visits or hospitalization for asthma, or a past history of severe attacks. Still, it is difficult if not impossible to predict the optimal regimen of outpatient steroids for any individual patient, and this can only be determined through follow-up evaluation. It would seem reasonable to discharge most patients on at least 7 days of systemic steroids and to urge a follow-up visit before the course is completed to determine whether steroids are required for a longer (or shorter) duration. It is possible that the addition of inhaled steroids would decrease the need for more prolonged courses of systemic agents, and several ongoing clinical trials are addressing this issue.

XII. OUTPATIENT TAPERING OF ORAL STEROIDS

The issue of whether steroids should be tapered after ED discharge has not been resolved. Tapering steroids is the practice of administering higher amounts initially and gradually decreasing the dose, either over days or weeks. The rationale for tapering, the practice of which began in the mid-1950s, was the concern that abrupt withdrawal of steroids may precipitate an asthma exacerbation or, even worse, an adrenal crisis. There is, however, no substantial evidence in the literature of either occurring when steroids are prescribed for short periods of time. Recovery in adrenal function is rapid even after a 3-week course of oral steroids is given (19).

Several studies have addressed the need for outpatient tapering although the selection of subjects was from an inpatient population. After hospitalization for acute asthma, a 7-day oral steroid taper was similar in efficacy to a 7-week taper (51). In this study patients received 8 days of high-dose inpatient steroid treatment before entering the randomized outpatient portion of the trial, and, therefore, even the "short" taper group had already received substantial amounts of steroids. Similarly, in two studies that found outpatient tapering unnecessary, substantial doses of inpatient steroids were given for 6–10 days, and patients discharged on placebo also received continued outpatient treatment with inhaled steroids (52,53).

The argument for not tapering is that patients will receive a larger dose of steroids for a longer period of time and that compliance to medication is potentially greater with simpler dosing schedules. Given the lack of published evidence in the ED population, the general question of whether of tapering is necessary remains unanswered.

XIII. THE IM ROUTE

Studies have suggested that the intramuscular (IM) injection of repository steroids is effective in improving asthma symptoms and preventing relapse after an acute asthma episode. In one trial, patients were discharged from the ED receiving either IM saline placebo or 240 mg methylprednisolone acetate suspension (54). Of the 56 patients who were contacted on 7-day follow-up, relapse occurred in 7% of patients who received IM steroids and in 31% of placebo recipients. A study involving 154 patients found 7-day relapse rates among patients receiving 40 mg triamcinolone diacetate IM similar to those receiving 5 days of oral prednisone (55). In an outpatient study of patients with severe chronic asthma, a total of 360 mg of triamcinolone given intramuscularly over 3 days was more effective than low dose daily prednisone given for 3 months in decreasing ED visits and hospitalizations (56).

A single IM injection of steroids is not dependent on patient compliance and may be a reasonable alternative to oral therapy for some patients, especially those with difficulty adhering to outpatient regimens. The clinician should be aware of the disadvantages to IM treatment, which include the inability to alter doses in the case of adverse reactions. Also, the long-term steroid induced side effects are not known when repeated injections of IM steroids are given. As with all steroid regimens, further study is needed to determine optimal dosing.

XIV. INHALED STEROIDS

Presently, oral steroids remain the treatment of choice for acute episodes of asthma although there is evidence that inhaled steroids may eventually have a role in the management of acute asthma and actually work faster than systemic steroids. Rodrigo and Rodrigo found that patients with acute moderate to severe asthma had significant benefits from very large doses of the potent inhaled steroid flunisolide, and this effect was seen 2 hr after administration (57). If further study confirms this observation, then it raises the possibility that other mechanisms than those previously described are responsible for the acute beneficial effect of inhaled corticosteroids.

For patients with chronic asthma, inhaled steroids have been shown to improve pulmonary function and decrease the need for hospitalization, urgent asthma visits, and rescue with oral steroids. The use of inhaled steroids can also reduce the need for prolonged systemic use. Based on their benefits in chronic asthma, consensus guidelines recommend that inhaled steroids be prescribed to patients discharged from the ED (58,59). This brings up other issues, including inadequate outpatient treatment of patients presenting to the ED. Only 30–40% of asthmatics presenting to the ED with asthma have been taking inhaled steroids as part of a long-term management strategy, and far more should have been using these agents (60,61). This is further complicated by the observation that many patients consider the ED their source of primary asthma care and may not seek further follow-up care after discharge (60,61) (see Chapter 37). To avoid the dilemma of providing chronic care to patients—a situation that the ED is not set up to handle—while assuring proper short and long-term treatment, the discharging physician should either provide inhaled corticosteroids with arrangements for follow-up care or recommend prompt outpatient follow-up care so that inhaled corticosteroids can be started before the course of oral steroids are completed.

XV. STEROID RESISTANCE

Although most patients with symptoms of asthma will respond to treatment with steroids, there are a small number of patients who have been characterized as ''steroid resistant.'' Assuming the label is correctly applied, these patients may improve only when given very large doses of steroids, and some may prove unresponsive at any dose. In the ED, the lack of response to steroids may simply represent the known delayed onset of the drug and not ''steroid resistance.'' If a patient known to have steroid resistance becomes acutely ill, the management will be more complicated. The patient may need very high doses of steroids, as well as aggressive management with bronchodilators, and is more likely to require hospitalization. Long-term management may involve trials of other anti-inflammatory agents and maximization of bronchodilator treatment to reduce the dose of daily steroid intake. Steroid resistant asthma may also indicate that the diagnosis of asthma is not correct and other diagnoses should be considered, such as vocal cord dysfunction (see Chapter 13).

XVI. COMPLICATIONS

Treatment with steroids results in a leukocytosis that is first noted a few hours after administration and reaches maximal intensity within 2 weeks of continued treatment (62–64). Steroids cause a granulocytosis by decreasing the egress of cells from the blood granulocyte pool, as well as increasing the influx of cells from the bone marrow (62). A shift to the left or appearance of toxic granulocytes is more likely to be seen in infection rather than steroid-induced leukocytosis (64).

An acute necrotizing myopathy has been described in severely ill asthmatics that required mechanical ventilation and received corticosteroids (65–67). Clinical findings range from mild diffuse weakness to complete paralysis. Cranial nerves are sometimes involved and recovery could take up to 6 months (68). The use of corticosteroids combined with a neuromuscular blocking agent is far more likely to be associated with this syndrome than patients who received steroids alone. In one study diffuse weakness occurred in 20 of 69 patients who received both agents (71). Neuromuscular blocking agents suspected of causing a myopathy include vecuronium, as well as pancuronium, atracurium, and doxacurium (65,69–71). Aminoglycosides also potentiate neuromuscular blockade and may contribute to the weakness (72). It has been suggested that ventilated patients with acute severe asthma who require neuromuscular blocking agents should be given intermittent boluses rather than constant infusions, be weaned, if possible, from the ventilator within 48 hours, and be given the lowest therapeutic doses of steroids possible (69). For prolonged muscle relaxation, alternative methods including propofol or a combined benzodiazepine-narcotic or propofol-narcotic infusion have been suggested (71).

Steroids are soluble in cell membranes and readily cross the blood brain barrier (73). A variety of psychiatric symptoms have been reported, ranging from alterations of mood to frank psychotic states. Among patients given 75–125 mg of IV methylprednisolone daily for 8 days, 18/50 (36%) fulfilled Diagnostic and Statistical Manual of Mental

Disorders (DSM) III criteria for organic mood disorders (74). Most of the affective disorders occurred within the first three days with 13/18 patients exhibiting mild manic symptoms and 5/18 symptoms of mild to moderate depression. A number of other studies also found that corticosteroids cause a variety of mood disorders 3–5 days after starting, including euphoria, sadness, restlessness, and anxiety (75–77). For most of these studies, the first observational point was 3 days after initiation of steroids, and the onset of symptoms was not timed before that. In one study where mood was assessed 24 hr after 4 mg of dexamethasone was administered to healthy volunteers, subjects felt more ''activated'' and less fatigued (78).

There appears to be a dose-response relationship for prednisone and acute psychiatric reactions. Among hospitalized patients, 1.3% experienced acute psychiatric reactions after receiving $\leq$ 40 mg daily prednisone, 4.6% of patients after receiving 41 to 80 mg prednisone, and 18% of patients who received >80 mg prednisone daily had acute psychiatric side effects (79). There have been also reports of acute psychotic behavior after steroid administration. These severe reactions occur infrequently, 2% of patients in one study and less than 1% in another, and are more likely to occur within the first 5 days of treatment (77,79).

Patients with chronic obstructive pulmonary disease (COPD) who received 30 mg of prednisone daily for 14 days had generalized improvement in mood states within 3 days that was not associated with improvement in FEV_1 (80). It would be of interest in patients with acute asthma to determine if these mood-altering effects occur concomitantly with objective measures of asthma improvement. In an ED study of acutely ill asthmatics, admission rates and subjective symptoms significantly improved after IV steroids, but the improvement in FEV_1 did not reach significance (29). Whether the mood altering effect of steroids may have in part influenced the admission rates for this and other studies warrants further investigation.

A number of other steroid-induced side effects have been noted. Although corticosteroids are often used to treat allergic reactions, allergies to the steroids have been reported (81,82). Short courses of steroids of less than 5–7 days duration appear to pose little risk for infection, while patients treated for more than 3–4 weeks may be at higher risk (83,84). After treatment with prednisone or methylprednisolone followed by prednisone, stomach upset (45% of patients), facial flush (17%), sleep disturbance (49%), or weight gain (mean 1 to 1.5% increase from baseline) is noted 4–15 days after initiation of treatment (77). The causal relationship between steroid use and the development of peptic ulcer or GI hemorrhage continues to be debated, although, if a relationship exists, the risk is probably small (85–89).

REFERENCES

1. Barnes PJ. Mechanisms of action of glucocorticoids in asthma. Am J Respir Crit Care Med 1996; 154:S21–S27.
2. Angel P, Karin M. The role of Jun, Fos and the AP-1 complex in cell proliferation and transformation. Biochem Biophys Acta 1991; 1072:129–157.
3. Siebenlist U, Franzoso G, Brown K. Structure, regulation and function of NF-κB. Ann Rev Cell Biol 1994; 10:405–455.
4. Grilli M, Chiu JJ, Lenardo MJ. NF-κB and Rel: Participants in a multiform transcriptional regulatory system. Int Rev Cytol 1993; 143:1–62.

5. Didonato JA, Saatcioglu F, Karin M. Molecular mechanisms of immunosuppression and anti-inflammatory activities by glucocorticoids. Am J Respir Crit Care Med 1996; 154:s11–15.
6. Mak JC, Nishikawa M, Barnes PJ. Glucocorticoids increase beta-2 adrenergic receptor transcription in human lung. Am J Physiol 1995; 268:L41–L46.
7. Mak JC, Nishikawa M, Shirasaki H, Miyayasu K, Barnes PJ. Protective effects of a glucocorticoid on down regulation of pulmonary β2-adrenergic receptors *in vivo*. J Clin Invest 1995; 96:99–106.
8. Re F, Muzio M, De Rossi M, Polentarutti N, Giri JG, Mantovani A, Colotta F. The type II ''receptor'' as a decoy target for interleukin 1 in polymorphonuclear leukocytes: characterization of induction by dexamethasone and ligand binding properties of the released decoy receptor. J Exp Med 1994; 179:739–743
9. Wallen N, Kita H, Weiler D, Gleich GJ. Glucocorticoids inhibit cytokine-mediated eosinophil survival. J Immunol 1991; 147:3490–3495.
10. Chung KF, Wiggins J, Collins J. Corticosteroids, In: Weiss EB and Stein M, eds., Bronchial Asthma: Mechanisms and Therapeutics, 3rd Ed., Boston: Little Brown and Co., 1993.
11. Frey BM, Frey FJ. Clinical pharmacokinetics of prednisone and prednisolone. Clin Pharmacokinet 1990; 19:126–146.
12. Pickup ME. Clinical pharmacokinetics of prednisone and prednisolone. Clin Pharmacokinet 1979; 4:111–128.
13. DiSanto AR, DeSante KA. Bioavailability and pharmacokinetics of prednisone in humans. J Pharm Sci 1975; 64:109–112.
14. Bergrem H, Grottum P, Rugstad HE. Pharmacokinetics and protein binding of prednisolone after oral and intravenous administration. Eur J Clin Pharmacol 1983; 24:415–419.
15. Ferry JJ, Horvath AM, Bekersky I, Heath EC, Ryan CF, Colburn WA. Relative and absolute bioavailability of prednisone and prednisolone after separate oral and intravenous doses. J Clin Pharmacol 1988; 28:81–87.
16. Morrish DW, Sproule BJ, Aaron TH, Outhet D, Crockford PM. Hypothalamic-pituitary-adrenal function in extrinsic asthma. Chest 1979; 75:161–166.
17. Streck WF, Lockwood DH. Pituitary adrenal recovery following short-term suppression with corticosteroids. Am J Med 1979; 66:910–914.
18. Zora JA, Zimmerman D, Carey TL, O'Connell EJ, Yunginger JW. Hypothalamic-pituitary-adrenal axis suppression after short-term, high dose glucocorticoid therapy in children with asthma. J Allergy Clin Immunol 1986; 77:9–13.
19. Webb J, Clark TJ. Recovery of plasma corticotropin and cortisol levels after a three-week course of prednisolone. Thorax 1981; 36:22–24.
20. Dolan LM, Kesarwala HH, Holroyde JC, Fischer TJ. Short-term, high-dose, systemic steroids in children with asthma: The effects on the hypothalamic-pituitary-adrenal axis. J Allergy Clin Immunol 1987; 80:81–87.
21. Harrison BDW, Rees LH, Cayton RM, Nabarro JDN. Recovery of hypothalamo-pituitary-adrenal function in asthmatics whose oral steroids have been stopped or reduced. Clin Endocrinol 1982; 17:109–118.
22. Graber AL, Ney RL, Nicholson WE, Island DP, Liddle GW. Natural history of pituitary-adrenal recovery following long-term suppression with corticosteroids. J Clin Endocrinol 1965; 25:11–16.
23. Morris HG, Jorgensen JR. Recovery of endogenous pituitary-adrenal function in corticosteroid-treated children. J Pediatrics 1971; 79:480–488.
24. McFadden ER, Jr., Kiser R, deGroot WJ, Holmes B, Kiker R, Viser G. A controlled study of the effects of single doses of hydrocortisone on the resolution of acute attacks of asthma. Am J Med 1976; 60:52–59.
25. Stein L, Cole R. Early administration of corticosteroids in emergency room treatment of acute asthma. Ann Intern Med 1990; 112:822–827.

26. Rodrigo C, Rodrigo G. Early administration of hydrocortisone in the emergency room treatment of acute asthma: a controlled clinical trial. Respir Med 1994; 88:755–761.
27. Littenberg B, Gluck EH. A controlled trial of methylprednisolone in the emergency treatment of acute asthma. N Engl J Med 1986; 314:150–152.
28. Schneider SM, Pipher A, Britton HL, Borok Z, Harcup CH. High dose methylprednisolone as initial therapy in patients with acute bronchospasm. J Asthma 1988, 25:189–193.
29. Storr J, Barrell E, Barry W, Lenney W, Hatcher G. Effect of a single dose of prednisolone in acute childhood asthma. Lancet 1987; 1:879–882.
30. Scarfone RJ, Fuchs SM, Nager AL, Shane SA. Controlled trial of oral prednisone in the emergency department treatment of children with acute asthma. Pediatrics 1993; 92:513–518.
31. Tal A, Levy N, Bearman JE. Methylprednisolone therapy for acute asthma in infants and toddlers: A controlled clinical trial. Pediatrics 1990; 86:350–356.
32. Fanta CH, Rossing TH, McFadden ER. Glucocorticoids in acute asthma: A critical controlled trial. Am J Med 1983; 74:845–851.
33. Loren ML, Chai H, Leung P, Rohr C, Brenner AM. Corticosteroids in the treatment of acute exacerbations of asthma. Ann Allergy 1980; 45:67–71.
34. Younger RE, Gerber PS, Herrod HG, Cohen RM, Crawford LV. Intravenous methylprednisolone efficacy in status asthmaticus of childhood. Pediatrics 1987; 80:225–230.
35. Morell F, Orriols R, de Gracia J, Curull V, Pujol A. Controlled trial of intravenous corticosteroids in severe acute asthma. Thorax 1992; 47:588–591.
36. Grant CC, Duggan AK, DeAngelis C. Independent parental administration of prednisone in acute asthma: A double-blind placebo-controlled, crossover study. Pediatrics 1995; 96:224–229.
37. Horowitz I, Zafrir O, Gilboa S, Berger I, Wolach B. Acute asthma. Single dose oral steroids in paediatric community clinics. Eur J Pediatr 1994; 153:526–530.
38. Ellul-Micallef R. The acute effects of corticosteroids in bronchial asthma. Eur J Respir Dis 1982; 122(suppl):118–125.
39. Collins JV, Clark TJ, Brown D, Townsend J. The use of corticosteroids in the treatment of acute asthma. Q J Med 1975; 44:259–273.
40. Ratto D, Alfaro C, Sipsey J, Glovsky MM, Sharma OP. Are intravenous corticosteroids required in status asthmaticus? JAMA 1988; 260:527–529.
41. Emerman CL, Cydulka RK. A randomized comparison of 100-mg vs 500-mg dose of methylprednisolone in the treatment of acute asthma. Chest 1995; 107:1559–1563.
42. Emerman C, Cydulka R, Gibbs MA, et al. Prospective, multicenter study of relapse following treatment for acute asthma among adults presenting to the emergency department. Acad Emerg Med 1998; 5(abstr):375.
43. Rodrigo G, Rodrigo C. A new index for early prediction of hospitalization in patients with acute asthma. Am J Emerg Med 1997; 15:8–13.
44. Ducharme FM, Kramer MS. Relapse following emergency treatment for acute asthma: Can it be predicted or prevented? J Clin Epidemiol. 1993; 46:1395–1402.
45. Emerman CL, Cydulka RK. Factors associated with relapse after emergency department treatment for acute asthma. Ann Emerg Med 1995; 26:6–11.
46. Silverman R, Kumlin M, Yoon D, Larsson L, Dahlen SE. LTE4 excretion during an acute asthma episode. Acad Emerg Med 1997; 4(abstr):482.
47. Webb J, Clark TJ, Chilvers C. Time course of response to prednisolone in chronic airflow obstruction. Thorax 1981; 36:18–21.
48. Chapman KR, Verbeek PR, White JG, Rebuck AS. Effect of short course of prednisone in the prevention of early relapse after the emergency room treatment of acute asthma. N Engl J Med 1991; 324:788–794.
49. Fiel SB, Swartz MA, Glanz K, Francis ME. Efficacy of short-term corticosteroid therapy in outpatient treatment of acute bronchial asthma. Am J Med 1983; 75:259–262.
50. Webb, JR. Dose response of patients to oral corticosteroid treatment during exacerbations of asthma. Br Med J Clin Res Ed 1986; 292:1045–1047.

51. Lederle FA, Pluhar RE, Joseph AM, Niewoehner DE. Tapering of corticosteroid therapy following exacerbations of asthma. Arch Intern Med 1987; 147:2201–2203.
52. O'Driscoll BR, Kalra S, Wilson M, Pickering CA, Carroll KB, Woodcock AA. Double-blind trial of steroid tapering in acute asthma. Lancet 1993; 341:324–327.
53. Hatton MQ, Vathenen AS, Allen MJ, Davies S, Cooke NJ. A comparison of 'abruptly stopping' with 'tailing off' oral corticosteroids in acute asthma. Respir Med 1995; 89:101–104.
54. McNamara RM, Rubin JM. Intramuscular methylprednisolone acetate for the prevention of relapse in acute asthma. Ann Emerg Med 1993; 22:1829–1835.
55. Schuckman H, DeJulius DP, Blanda M, Gerson LW, DeJulius AJ, Rajaratnam M. Comparison of intramuscular triamcinolone and oral prednisone in the outpatient treatment of acute asthma: A randomized controlled trial. Ann Emerg Med 1998; 31:333–338.
56. Ogirala RG, Aldrich TK, Prezant DJ, Sinnett MJ, Enden JB, Williams MH, Jr. High-dose intramuscular triamcinolone in severe, chronic, life-threatening asthma. New Engl J Med 1991; 324:585–589.
57. Rodrigo R, Rodrigo C. Inhaled flunisolide for acute severe asthma. Am J Respir Care Med 1998; 157:698–703.
58. Beveridge RC, Grunfeld AF, Hodder RV, Verbeek PR. Guidelines for the emergency management of asthma in adults. Can Med Assoc J 1996; 155:25–37.
59. Guidelines for the diagnosis and management of asthma. Expert panel report 2. NIH publication No. 97-4051, National Heart, Lung and Blood Institute, July 1997.
60. Silverman R, Chiang W, Osborn H, Gallagher EJ. Survey of patient home treatment for asthma exacerbations. Am J Respir Crit Care Med 1996;A860 (abstr).
61. Camargo CA. First multicenter asthma research collaboration. Acad Emerg Med 1997; 4:470 (abstr).
62. Bishop CR, Athens JW, Boggs DR, Warner HR, Cartwright GE, Wintrobe MM. A non-steady state kinetic evaluation of the mechanism of cortisone-induced granulocytosis. J Clin Invest 1968; 47:249–260.
63. Cream JJ. Prednisolone induced granulocytosis. Br J Haematol 1968; 15:259–267.
64. Schoenfeld Y, Gurewich Y, Gallant LA, Pinkhas J. Prednisone-induced leukocytosis: Influence of dosage, method and duration of administration on the degree of leukocytosis. Am J Med 1981; 71:773–778.
65. Douglass J, Tuxen D, Horne M, et al. Myopathy in severe asthma. Am Rev Respir Dis 1992; 146:517–519.
66. Dekhuijzen PNR, Decramer M. Steroid-induced myopathy and its significance to respiratory disease: A known disease rediscovered. Eur Respir J 1992; 5:997–1003.
67. Shee CD. Risk factors for hydrocortisone myopathy in acute severe asthma. Respir Med 1990; 84:229–233.
68. Op de Coul AA, Verheul GA, Leyten AC, Schellens RL, Teepen JL. Critical illness polyneuropathy after artificial respiration. Clin Neurol Neurosurg 1991; 93:27–33.
69. Nates JL, Cooper DJ, Day B, Tuxen DV. Acute weakness syndromes in critically ill patients—A reappraisal. Anaesth Intensive Care 1997; 25:502–513.
70. Marik PE. Doxacurium-corticosteroid acute myopathy: Another piece to the puzzle. Crit Care Med 1996; 24:1266–1267.
71. Leatherman JW, Fluegel WL, David WS, Davies SF, Iber C. Muscle weakness in mechanically ventilated patients with severe asthma. Am J Respir Crit Care Med 1996; 153:1686–1690.
72. Coakley J. Prolonged paralysis in critically ill patients. Intensive Care Med 1995; 21:387.
73. Barnes DM. Science 1986; 232:1344–1345.
74. Naber D, Sand P, Heigl B. Psychopathological and neuropsychological effects of 8 days corticosteroid treatment. A prospective study. Psychoneuroendocrinology 1996; 21:25–31.
75. Wolkowitz OM, Rubinow D, Doran AR, et al. Prednisone effects on neurochemistry and behavior: Preliminary findings. Arch Gen Psychiatry 1990; 47:963–968.

76. Cameron OG, Addy RO, Malitz D. Effects of ACTH and prednisone on mood: Incidence and time of onset. Int J Psychiatr Med 1985–86; 15:213–223.
77. Chrousos GA, Kattah JC, Beck RW, Cleary PA. Side effects of glucocorticoid treatment: Experience of the Optic Neuritis Treatment Trial. JAMA 1993; 269:2110–2112.
78. Plihal W, Krug R, Pietrowsky R, Fehm HL, Born, J. Corticosteroid receptor mediated effects on mood in humans. Psychoneuroendocrinology 1996; 21:515–523.
79. Boston Collaborative Drug Surveillance Program. Acute adverse reactions to prednisone in relation to dosage. Clin Pharmacol Ther 1972; 13:694–698.
80. Swinburn CR, Wakefield JM, Newman SP, Jones PW. Evidence of prednisilone induced mood change (''steroid euphoria'') in patients with chronic obstructive airways disease. Br J Clin Pharmacol 1988; 26:709–713.
81. Preuss L. Allergic reactions to systemic glucocorticoids: Intolerance to hydrocortisone. Ann Allergy 1985; 55:772–775.
82. Kounis NG. Untoward reactions to corticosteroids: Intolerance to hydrocortisone. Ann Allergy 1976; 36:203–206.
83. Aucott JN. Corticosteroids and infection. Endocrinol Metabol Clin North Am 1994; 23:655–671.
84. Wiest PM, Flanigan T, Salata RA, Shlaes DM, Katzman M, Lederman, MM. Serious infectious complications of corticosteroid therapy for COPD. Chest 1989; 95:1180–1184.
85. Spiro HM. Is the steroid ulcer a myth? N Engl J Med 1983; 309:45–47.
86. Messer J, Reitman D, Sacks HS, Smith H, Jr, Chalmers TC. Association of adrencorticosteroid therapy and peptic-ulcer disease. N Engl J Med 1983; 309:21–24.
87. Piper JM, Ray WA, Daugherty JR, Griffin MR. Corticosteroid use and peptic ulcer disease: Role of nonsteroidal anti-inflammatory drugs. Ann Intern Med 1991; 114:735–740.
88. Guslandi M, Tittobello A. Steroid ulcers: A myth revisited. Br Med J 1992; 304:655–656.
89. Conn HO, Poynard T. Corticosteroids and peptic ulcer: Meta-analysis of adverse events during steroid therapy. J Intern Med 1994; 236:619–632.

23

Anticholinergics and Asthma

Jill P. Karpel
Albert Einstein College of Medicine and Montefiore Medical Center, Bronx, New York

Richard M. Nowak
Henry Ford Health Systems, Detroit, Michigan

I. INTRODUCTION

Since the time of the ancient Greeks, patients with ''wheezing'' disorders have been treated with the inhalation of various anticholinergic alkaloids. Patients were literally advised to inhale smoke from the leaves of plants containing atropine or similar alkaloids (1) (see Chapter 1). Although popular for centuries, this form of therapy was largely abandoned with the advent of other classes of bronchodilators, such as β-agonists and methylxanthines. As these latter medications had more clearly defined therapeutic windows, and therefore fewer adverse effects, atropine and its derivatives were forgotten until the 1970s. At that time, there was a new understanding of the important role that the parasympathetic system played in maintaining airway tone. Additionally, synthetic quartenary anticholinergic compounds were developed, which were not systemically absorbed and therefore did not result in serious adverse effects.

As a result, academic interest in redefining the role of anticholinergic medications in treating obstructive airways disease emerged. The use of anticholinergic medication for patients with asthma and chronic obstructive pulmonary disease (COPD) has been extensively studied in many clinical trials. Although there is consensus that anticholinergics are first line medications for patients with COPD, either in the emergency department (ED) or for chronic therapy (2–7), their use in asthma has remained controversial (8).

In the following discussion, we will review the current literature concerning the use of anticholinergics for asthma.

A. Physiology

Asthma is currently thought to be primarily an inflammatory disease that secondarily involves airway bronchoconstriction, edema, and mucus production. However, airway tone, which is increased in asthma, is predominantly under the control of the parasympathetic (vagal) nerves, which cause contraction of smooth muscle when acetylcholine is released from motor nerve terminals (9). Thus, stimulation of the muscarinic receptors by acetylcholine results in bronchconstriction and increased mucus production, the clinical hallmarks of asthma.

Atropine and its related compounds effectively block acetylcholine at the receptor level. However, anticholinergics do not block the effect of other inflammatory mediators, such as histamine and the leukotrienes, and consequently do not have anti-inflammatory properties. Furthermore, to the extent that noncholinergic mechanisms are responsible for bronchoconstriction and mucus production, β-agonists may be more effective therapy for asthma. However, some degree of cholinergic bronchoconstriction is responsible for airway narrowing in acute asthma, and therefore anticholinergics could be effective in preventing or reversing this component. Therefore, clinical investigations into the precise role of anticholinergic therapy in treating asthma has been a subject of much interest.

B. Muscarinic Receptors

Although as many as five distinct muscarinic receptors have been identified, it is currently believed that only three are involved in maintaining airway tone (10) (Figure 1).

The M_1 receptor is found in autonomic ganglia and has high affinity for the muscarinic antagonist, piperazine (11). M_1 receptors may be found in human cholinergic nerves in airways, but their role in maintaining airway tone is not yet defined, and the current available anticholinergics, such as ipratropium bromide, have little blocking effect on this receptor.

The M_2 receptors are present in the gut, and are located prejunctionally on the postganglionic parasympathetic nerves. M_2 receptors are also found in human airway smooth muscle. They can inhibit acetylcholine release and it has been postulated that this may be due to a functional defect in these M_2 receptors that would result in reflex cholinergic bronchoconstriction. Currently available anticholinergics are nonselective. Therefore, it

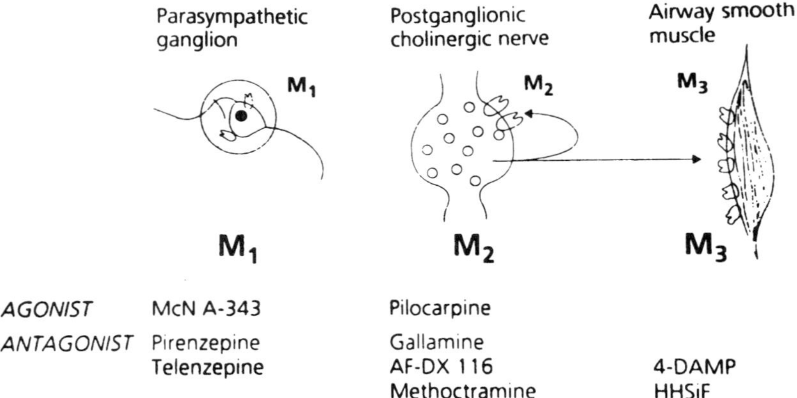

	M_1	M_2	M_3
AGONIST	McN A-343	Pilocarpine	
ANTAGONIST	Pirenzepine Telenzepine	Gallamine AF-DX 116 Methoctramine	4-DAMP HHSiF

Figure 1 Three subtypes of muscarinic receptor can be distinguished pharmacologically: M_1, M_2, and M_3. 4-DAMP = 4-diphenyl-acetoxy-N-methyl-piperidine methiodide. HHSiF = hexahydrosiladifenidol. (Adapted from Ref. 55.)

is possible that more acetylcholine could be released during cholinergic nerve stimulation (prejuctionally) and this might not be sufficient to overcome postjunctional blockade (M_3 receptor), resulting in less bronchodilatation (or possibly paradoxical bronchoconstriction) (10,11). A more selective anticholinergic drug that is specific for the M_3 receptor would theoretically avoid this problem.

The M_3 receptors are found in the walls of both large and small bronchial smooth muscles of airways and submucosal glands (10,11) and are postjunctional. The development of new drugs that would be selective for the M_3 receptor would be clinically important because they would be more potent and not result in paradoxical bronchoconstriction and other adverse effects that have occurred with nonselective blockade of M_2 and M_1 receptors. One such drug, tiotropium bromide, is currently under investigation. In the future, more M_3 selective drugs may provide more effective treatment of obstructive airways disease.

II. PHARMACOLOGY

The anticholinergic drugs are antagonists of acetylcholine and other muscarinic agonists. They block the muscarinic receptors mentioned above, and by altering cholinergic tone can result in bronchodilatation and decreased mucus production.

Atropine, the prototypic agent, is a tertiary ammonium compound. It is available in several forms, the most common being 1% atropine sulfate. It is extracted from the nightshade plant.

When given systemically, atropine's usefulness as a bronchodilator is limited due to its well-known adverse effects including dry mouth, blurred vision, tachycardia, flushed skin, urinary retention, confusion, and delirium. In an attempt to limit these unpleasant and potentially serious adverse effects, several investigators nebulized atropine solution and delivered it locally to the airways. When inhaling atropine sulfate bronchodilating effects may be seen within 15 min and persist up to 4–6 hr. The adverse effects encountered will depend on the route of administration and dose. Most have reported that 1 mg of atropine sulfate is well tolerated when nebulized (12). In a study by Karpel and colleagues (13), nebulized atropine sulfate (3.2 mg nebulized twice at 30-min intervals; total 6.4 mg) was administered to patients with acute asthma exacerbations in the ED. No serious adverse effects were noted, but the majority of the patients complained of dry mouth, blurred vision and/or headache (13). Furthermore, atropine is only available as a solution and requires a nebulizer to deliver the medication as there is no metered dose inhaler (MDI) available.

To summarize, the major disadvantages of atropine sulfate are that: (1) it is rapidly absorbed from the bronchial tree when inhaled and so has the potential to cause significant systemic toxicity, (2) it is only available as a nebulizer solution, and (3) it is less potent than the synthetic anticholinergic compounds that have been developed or are under development. As such, atropine sulfate solution should no longer be used to treat obstructive airways disease.

The synthetic anticholinergics that are currently available include ipratropium bromide, oxitropium bromide, atropine methonitrate, and glycopyrolate. Tiotropium bromide is a newer, longer-acting, more selective anticholinergic that is currently under investigation. Additionally, Combivent, which is a combination of ipratropium bromide and, the β-agonist, albuterol, has recently been approved by the Food and Drug Administration

Table 1 Anticholinergics

Drug	Form	Dose	Duration (hr)
Atropine sulfate	NS[a]	0.025 mg/kg	6–8
Ipratropium bromide	NS	500 μg	4–6
	MDI[b]	36–120 μg	4–6
Combivent (ipratropium bromide and albuterol)	MDI NS (not available in U.S.)	36 μg of ipratropium bromide and 90 μg albuterol sulfate	4–6
Atropine methonitrate	NS	1.5 mg	6–10
Glycopyrronium bromide	NS	0.21–1.0 mg	6–12
Oxitropium bromide	MDI	0.0–0.5 mg	8–10

[a] Available as wet nebulizer solution.
[b] Available as metered-dose inhaler.

(FDA) for the treatment of COPD. Only ipratropium is available as both an MDI and nebulizer solution. In the United States, the only FDA approved anticholinergic for the treatment of obstructive airways disease is ipratropium bromide. The dosages, duration of action, and formulations of these anticholinergics are noted in Table 1.

Ipratropium bromide is the drug that has been the most widely studied for treatment of obstructive airways disease. When using the nebulizer solution, 500 μg (only 10–30% of which is actually delivered to the patient) appears to provide maximum bronchodilatation (Figure 2) while 2–4 puffs (36–72 μg) are recommended by most investigators when the drug is administered via MDI (14). We have given three puffs via an MDI and spacer to patients with COPD in the ED and found excellent results (5,6). The duration of action is approximately 6 hr. The time to peak bronchodilatation may be up to 90 min in patients

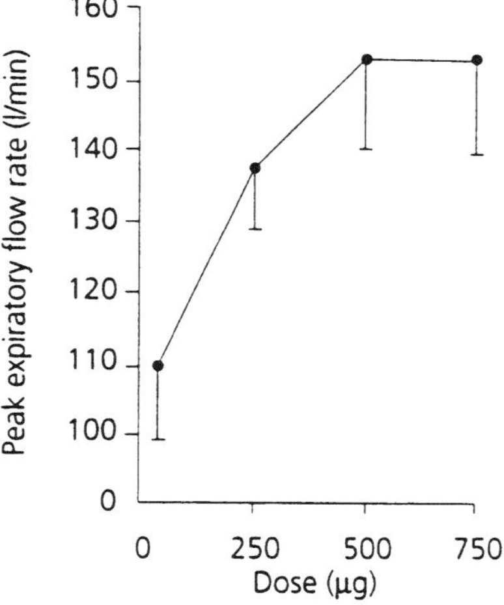

Figure 2 Dose-response curve for nebulized ipratropium bromide in acute asthma. Values are mean ± SEM. (Adapted from Ref. 4.)

with severe COPD, but effects as early as 15–30 min have been reported for patients with asthma (5,6,11).

Adverse effects associated with the inhalation of ipratropium are clinically insignificant and rarely necessitate discontinuing the medication. However, when administering ipratropium with the MDI, patients should be warned not to spray into the eye, and, when using nebulizer solution, the face mask should fit tightly. This is to avoid the potential risk of precipitating glaucoma. Additionally, physicians should be aware of the extremely rare occurrence of paradoxical bronchoconstriction, which can worsen cough and symptoms. As with any treatment, the medication should be discontinued if patients appear to worsen following treatment.

Although the continuous use of β-agonists may result in tachyphylaxis, with a diminished bronchodilator response, ipratropium bromide has not been reported to induce tolerance at the receptor level. In long-term studies (90 days), the bronchodilator response appears to be well preserved for patients with COPD (4,15).

In the upper respiratory tract, ipratropium can cause drying of the mucosa, with some nasal discomfort. Rarely, does this result in discontinuation of the medication. Although atropine itself can slow mucociliary clearance and depress ciliary beat frequency, ipratropium bromide does not alter lower airway mucus secretion, velocity, or viscosity (16). Importantly, it does not result in mucous plugging, which could potentially cause exacerbations of obstructive airways disease.

Although it has been postulated that anticholinergic bronchodilators would predominantly have their major effect on large airways while β-agonists would affect small, peripheral airways, studies have not substantiated this finding when pulmonary function data is analyzed (FEV_1 compared to midflow rates) for patients with either acute exacerbations of COPD or asthma or when clinically stable (5,6,17).

In conclusion, the inhaled synthetic anticholinergic compounds have predominantly local effects on the airways, with virtually no systemic adverse effects. They have a wide therapeutic margin, are extremely well tolerated, and are safe.

III. CLINICAL EXPERIENCE

Three types of clinical studies have been conducted with anticholinergic medications and asthma patients. These include provocative challenge studies, pulmonary function laboratory studies with stable patients, and ED or hospital studies conducted during acute exacerbations of asthma.

A. Provocative Challenge Studies

Anticholinergics are obviously very effective in blocking the deterioration in pulmonary function that would be induced by all types of cholinergic agents. In contrast, their effectiveness in blocking the bronchoconstrictor response to histamine, exercise, and various allergens has varied as addressed by different investigators (18). Of clinical interest, anticholinergics can be useful in reversing bronchospasm induced by beta-blockade (18).

B. Stable Patients with Asthma

The majority of these studies were performed by having patients withhold their routine bronchodilator medications and then inhaling anticholinergic drugs, β-agonists, or some combination of the two in the pulmonary function laboratory.

Early studies by Altouynan and Snow and coworkers compared isoproterenol and atropine and reported them to be equally effective bronchodilators, but atropine had a later peak onset and longer duration of action (19,20). Further studies comparing ipratropium bromide with isoproterenol reported equal bronchodilatation, but longer duration of action with ipratropium (21–23). One problem with some of these early studies, such as Altouynan, was that they did not differentiate between patients with COPD and asthma. As such, some of their findings may not be comparable to later studies, which clearly separate these different groups of patients.

When comparing anticholinergics to more selective β-agonists in stable patients, two studies reported equivalent bronchodilatation of ipratropium and salbutamol (24,25). In contrast, several other studies found ipratropium to be a less effective bronchodilator than the selective β-agonists, but with a longer duration of action (21–23).

The additive and/or synergistic effects of anticholinergics administered concurrently or sequentially with β-agonists has also been investigated (19–23,25,26). The majority of these have demonstrated either improvement in pulmonary function or greater duration of action when combination therapy was used (19–23,25,26). Theoretically, the β-agonist provides rapid relief of airway obstruction while the anticholinergic increases the magnitude and/or duration of the bronchodilator response.

Areas of continuing controversy include whether or not older patients with more fixed airway obstruction respond better to anticholingerics, whether atopic individuals respond differently, and whether the degree of airway obstruction correlates with anticholinergic responsiveness (19,26,27).

Consensus among investigators has been that anticholinergics are not as effective bronchodilators for chronic asthma as β-agonists and should not be used alone to treat chronic asthma. Specific recommendations concerning chronic asthma therapy and anticholinergic drugs are the following: anti-inflammatory medications, usually inhaled corticosteroids, are first line medications, while β-agonists are to be used on an as needed basis (28). In a stepwise fashion, if symptoms are not controlled, pulmonary function remains abnormal, or the patient is requiring systemic corticosteroids, then a trial of anticholinergic medication could be initiated as a third step or as a fourth step following other drugs, such a long-acting β-agonist, theophylline, or cromolyn sodium. We recommend following pulmonary function [home peak expiratory flow rates (PEFRs) and spirometry] along with the patient's asthma symptoms to document the efficacy of the anticholinergic. If there is no improvement, the anticholinergic should be discontinued, as it adds additional complexity and expense to the patient's asthma regimen.

C. Acute Exacerbations

Although increased vagal tone plays an important role in acute exacerbations of asthma, and theoretically anticholinergic medications should be quite effective in treating the associated bronchospasm, the results of numerous clinical studies have yielded conflicting results.

Initially, investigators compared anticholinergic medications directly to β-agonists for the acute treatment of asthma, and the majority found the β-agonist to be superior (8,13,14,17,29–33). In an ED study by Karpel et al., high-dose atropine sulfate (6.4 mg) was not as effective a bronchodilator as metaproterenol sulfate (30 mg) when administered

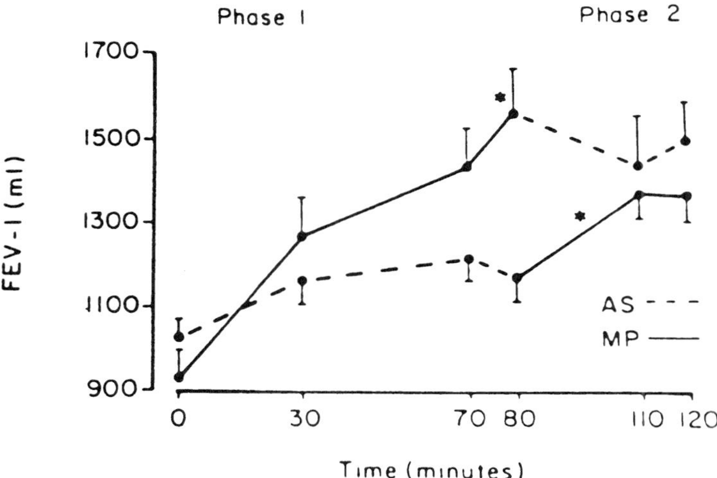

Figure 3 Changes in FEV_1 (mean ± SEM) versus time from baseline after initial treatment with nebulized AS (6.4 mg) or nebulized MP (30 mg) for phase 1 and after crossover (phase 2) with AS (3.2 mg) or MP (15 mg). Asterisks indicate significant differences between the groups ($p < 0.05$). (Adapted from Ref. 13.)

by wet nebulizer solution (Figure 3) to patients with moderate to severe airway obstruction (13). In fact, 40% of the patients did not respond to atropine, whereas all responded and improved their flow rates after inhaling metaproterenol (13). Furthermore, we did not demonstrate any synergy after the sequential administration of the two drugs.

In six additional studies comparing a β-agonist to ipratropium bromide alone, all but one found that the β-agonist produced superior bronchodilatation to ipratropium (14,17,29–32). Additionally, ipratropium had a slower onset of action. The one study that differed found that 0.5 mg of ipratropium resulted in equivalent bronchodilatation to 10 mg salbutamol (14).

In a meta-analysis by Ward (Figure 4) analyzing the same six studies, he concluded that the β-agonist produced significantly more bronchodilatation than ipratropium alone. The effect size was 0.28 with 95% confidence interval (CI) of +0.28 to +0.54 (8).

Although anticholinergics may result in bronchodilatation in some patients with acute asthma, they should not be used alone. They are clearly not superior bronchodilators to traditional β-agonists.

Given these findings, investigators questioned whether there might be synergistic actions when concurrently administering an anticholinergic with a β-agonist to patients experiencing acute exacerbations of asthma. This led to nine initial clinical trials comparing ipratropium bromide and a β-agonist to β-agonist alone (14,17,29–35).

Two separate meta-analyses analyzed these clinical trials and both found a small advantage to combination therapy (8,33). Higggins and coworkers reported the results of their own clinical trial, which found no difference in response to either nebulized salbutamol alone or salbutamol and ipratropium (33). However, they also defined acceptable clinical responses and found that more patients responded to combination therapy than to

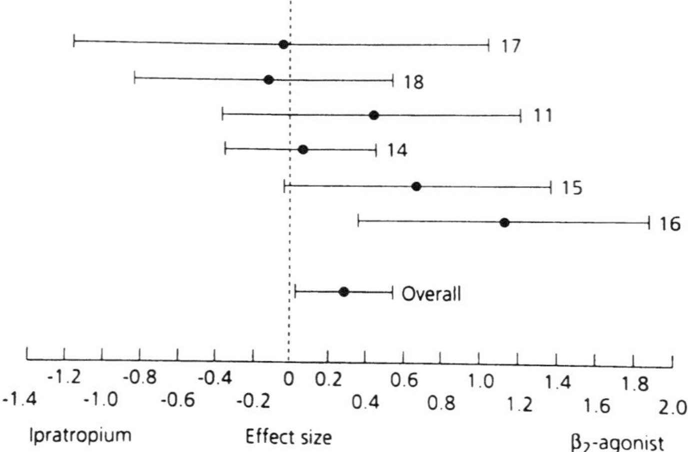

Figure 4 Diagram showing the effect size and its 95% confidence interval for studies comparing ipratropium with a β_2-agonist in acute severe asthma. The pooled result is also shown. Reference numbers are given on the right. (Adapted from Ref. 8.)

salbutamol alone. When they performed a meta-analysis that included their study and several others, they reported a 12.5% improvement in pulmonary function for combination therapy versus β-agonist alone (33).

Ward performed a later meta-analysis (Figure 5) and again reported a statistically significant, but clinically small, advantage for combination therapy when treating acute exacerbations of asthma (8). He suggested that combination therapy with ipratropium and

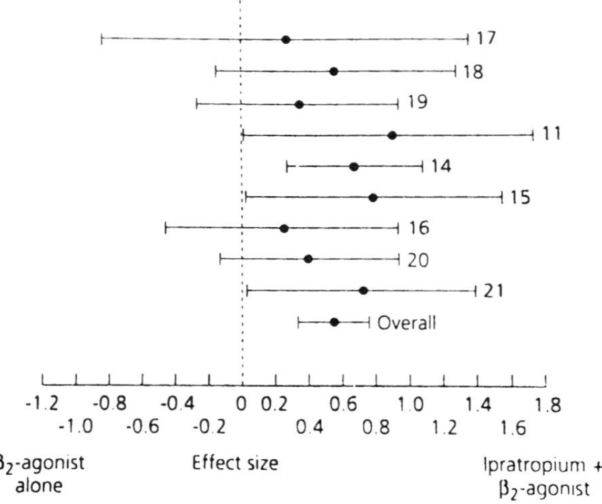

Figure 5 Diagram showing the effect size and its 95% confidence interval for studies comparing ipratropium and a β_2-agonist alone. The pooled result is also shown. Reference numbers are given on the right. (Adapted from Ref. 8.)

β-agonist conferred an additional 0.55 standard deviation units (PEFR or FEV_1) compared to β-agonist alone (8). This represented an additional mean increase in PEFR of approximately 44 L/min during the various ED studies for a duration of up to 4 hr.

Two studies also have demonstrated that for patients with severe airways obstruction as defined by $FEV_1 < 1.0$ L or PEFR < 140 L/min, combination therapy with ipratropium and salbutamol or fenoterol resulted in greater improvement than the β-agonist administered alone (14,34). The mean increase in FEV_1 was 55.6% for combination therapy vs. 38.9% with fenoterol alone (14). Both of these studies involved small numbers of patients.

The study by Ward et al. that demonstrated an advantage for combination therapy (salbutamol 10 mg and ipratropium 0.5 mg) also showed that patients experienced less adverse effects (specifically tachycardia and tremor) compared to high-dose salbutamol alone (20 mg) (14).

In both COPD and asthma, the inhalation of an anticholinergic drug has not been associated with oxygen desaturation as has been demonstrated for β-agonists (5). The explanation(s) and the clinical significance of this finding remains unexplained.

As the results of these meta-analyses showed only small, but statistically significant benefits for combination therapy compared to β-agonist alone, there still remained an important issue as to whether combination therapy is truly advantageous or of real clinical benefit. To address this issue, three recent clinical trials have been performed comparing ipratropium bromide and albuterol (Combivent) to albuterol alone (36–38).

The first of these to be published was performed in three university-affiliated hospitals, including our own (36): 380 patients presenting to the ED with acute exacerbations of asthma were randomized to receive either 3 mL of nebulized 0.02% ipratropium bromide (2.5 mL) and 0.5% albuterol (0.5 mL) or 0.5% albuterol (0.5 mL) and 2.5 mL of normal saline. Patients received initial treatment at entry into the study and at 45 min following the first treatment. The two groups of patients began the study with similar pulmonary function (initial FEV_1 was approximately 1.22 and 1.25 L, respectively), asthma medications, and other demographics. There was no significant difference in improvement in FEV_1 at the end of the 90-min study between the groups treated with combination therapy versus albuterol alone (Figure 6).

Additionally, when data were analyzed by subdividing both treatment groups into those patients with FEV_1 greater than 1.0 L and 1.0 L or less, no advantage for combination therapy could be demonstrated even among the most obstructed patients. This was in contrast to the two studies mentioned above (37,38).

A positive finding was that at 45 min, the proportion of responders, as defined as those patients with a 15% improvement in FEV_1 above initial baseline, was significantly greater for the group receiving combination therapy compared to albuterol alone (85% vs. 78%, respectively). At 90 min, this difference was no longer significant. There was also no significant difference in the number of patients requiring additional therapy in the ED or hospitalization. Thus, in this population of inner city asthmatics, no additive benefit could be demonstrated for combination therapy.

Two other publications have also investigated this issue. While the Canadian Combivent Study confirmed our findings, the New Zealand Combivent Study favored combination therapy with albuterol and ipratropium (37,38). The study design of the latter two studies differed from ours, as all the patients received hydrocortisone during the study, and only one treatment with albuterol or albuterol and ipratropium was administered during the study.

In an effort to reconcile the differences in these data, a pooled analysis of all 1064

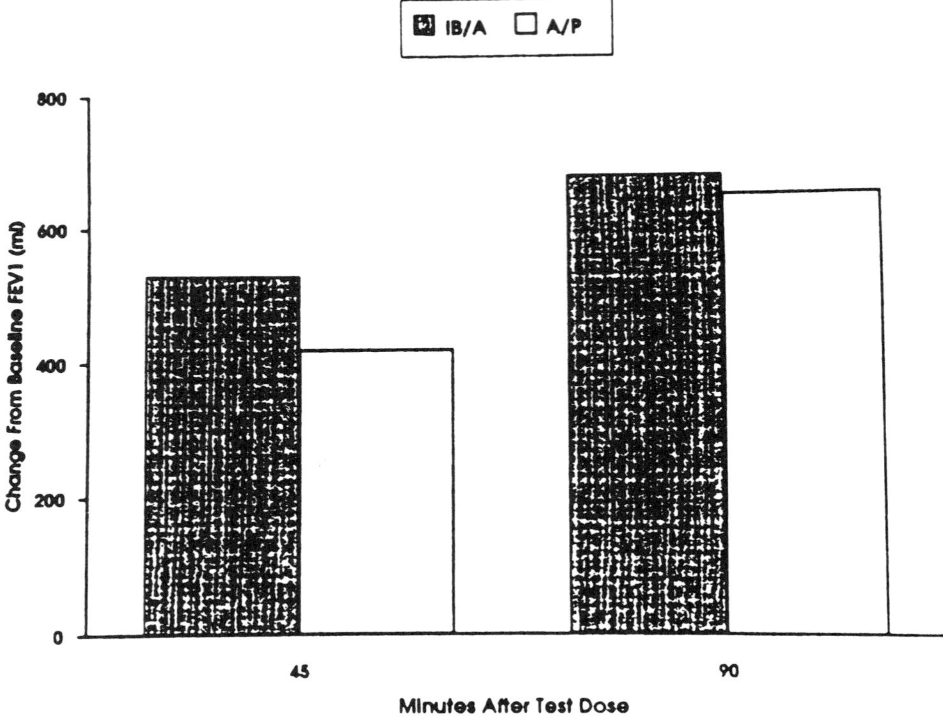

Figure 6 The median change from baseline FEV_1 at 45 min following the first dose and 45 min following the second dose of nebulized ipratropium and albuterol (IB/A) or albuterol and saline solution (A/P). (Adapted from Ref. 36.)

patients with acute asthma enrolled in these three trials is being conducted. The data suggest a trend for improved pulmonary function (47 mL mean improvement in FEV_1 from initial baseline, 95% confidence interval = −28,122) with the combination of ipratropium bromide and albuterol compared to albuterol alone (39). The difference in the proportion of patients having at least a 20% improvement in FEV_1 was 7.4% ($p = 0.02$) in favor of combination therapy. Patients receiving combination therapy also had 17% lower risk of relapse with hospitalizaton 24 hr after treatment (relative risk = 0.83, 95% confidence interval = 0.63, 1.1). Interestingly, a subgroup of patients with recent history of upper respiratory infection appeared to have an even greater improvement in FEV_1 with combination therapy (130 mL; $p = 0.02$) (39).

In conclusion, when treating adult patients with acute exacerbations of asthma in the ED, combination bronchodilator therapy with a β-agonist and ipratropium bromide may confer a small improvement in pulmonary function and other secondary outcomes compared to monotherapy with a β-agonist alone. In this age of cost-effective care, the cost of combination therapy should be factored into the decision to treat patients with acute asthma with combination therapy. Pulmonary function should be monitored in the ED, and if the patient is not responding to combination therapy, then β-agonist treatment alone might be continued. Additionally, systemic corticosteroids should be started early for any patients responding poorly to either β-agonists or combination therapy. Previous studies have targeted this group of nonresponders as those asthmatics most likely to require systemic steroids, more frequent β-agonist treatments, and hospitalization (40–42).

Finally, the National Asthma Education and Prevention Program (NAEPP) Expert Panel Report II (1997) has stated that ipratropium bromide may provide some additive benefit to inhaled β-agonists in severe asthma exacerbations and may be considered an alternative bronchodilator for patients who do not tolerate inhaled β-agonists. These recommendations for the use of inhaled anticholinergic medication as "quick relief" bronchodilators is new compared to the original 1991 guidelines.

IV. PEDIATRIC ASTHMA AND ANTICHOLINERGICS

As with the adult population, ipratropium bromide has been found to be quite safe for pediatric patients. However, several investigators have demonstrated the optimal dose to be 250 μg of ipratropium bromide (43–45). Ipratropium can be administered either as a nebulized solution or with an MDI attached to a holding chamber or spacer device. For infants, the holding chamber can be fitted with a face mask for ease of administration.

The majority of studies in children have compared combination therapy with ipratropium bromide and a β-agonist to β-agonists alone. Beck and coworkers studied 25 children age 6 or older with initial FEV_1 less than 50% predicted and demonstrated that adding ipratropium bromide 60 min after initial treatment with salbutamol resulted in additional improvement compared to those children given placebo and additional salbutamol (45).

In a similar population of asthmatic children presenting to the ED with FEV_1 less than 50% predicted, Reisman and coworkers compared treatment with the combination of salbutamol and ipratropium and salbutamol alone administered at entry, 40, and 80 min. They found superior bronchodilation with combination therapy compared to salbutamol alone (46).

In a more recent ED study by Schuh and coworkers, 120 children ages 5–17 years old with $FEV_1 < 50\%$ predicted normal were treated with either three doses of nebulized ipratropium (250 μ/dose within 60 min), one dose of ipratropium at 60 min or placebo. All of the patients received three doses of nebulized albuterol (0.15 mg/kg per dose) within 60 min (47). The study demonstrated that repeated doses of ipratropium added to albuterol resulted in significantly greater bronchodilation than did albuterol alone (48). This was amplified further in patients with $FEV_1 < 30\%$ predicted normal. Additionally, for those patients with $FEV_1 < 30\%$ predicted normal, the number of patients hospitalized was reduced in the high-dose ipratropium and albuterol group compared to albuterol alone (48). The authors concluded that the combination of high-dose albuterol and repeated doses of ipratropium bromide for pediatric patients with acute severe was superior to treatment with albuterol alone. No significant adverse effects were associated with the ipratropium therapy.

Of note, two dissenting studies found no benefit from combination therapy (48,49). The study designs of these investigations have been questioned, and the majority of opinion supports the use of combination therapy for pediatric patients with acute asthma. One could postulate that pediatric patients have significantly more cholinergic tone during acute attacks of asthma than do adult asthmatics. This might possibly explain the different response to anticholinergic medications between these two groups of patients with acute asthma.

V. CHRONIC PEDIATRIC ASTHMA

As with adult asthmatics, studies with asthmatic children have yielded conflicting results concerning the role of anticholinergics in chronic therapy. Although some studies have not documented any benefit to adding ipratropium to regimens of inhaled corticosteroids, β-agonists, and theophyllines, one study did suggest a longer duration of bronchodilator effect (50–53). The recommendations from a consensus committee concerning anticholinergic therapy and chronic pediatric asthma were that ipratropium bromide could be added as a third-line medication when additional bronchodilatation was required or when maximum bronchodilatation could not be achieved with β-agonists without adverse effects (54).

VI. CONCLUSIONS

Although anticholinergic medications are the oldest form of pharmacological therapy for treating obstructive airways disease, its role in asthma therapy remains controversial. Practical suggestions concerning the use of this class of medications are as follows. First, nebulized atropine sulfate should no longer be used as the anticholinergic of first choice, as it is easily absorbed from the bronchial tree and has the potential for greater systemic toxicity. It is also less potent than the newer, synthetic compounds. Ipratropium bromide, which is available either as an MDI or nebulizer solution, is the only anticholinergic currently approved by the FDA for the treatment of obstructive airways disease and is therefore the drug of choice in the United States. In other countries, oxitropium bromide is commonly used.

When treating adult patients with acute asthma, anticholinergics should not be used alone, as β-agonists have clearly been proven to be the superior bronchodilator. Should a patient be unable to tolerate β-agonists due to adverse effects, then a trial of anticholinergic therapy should be considered with pulmonary function monitoring to demonstrate significant bronchodilator response.

For adult patients with acute asthma, combination therapy with ipratropium bromide and albuterol produces a small trend towards superior improvements in pulmonary function and other important secondary outcomes compared to β-agonists alone (39). As there are no significant adverse effects associated with combination therapy, patients presenting to the ED with acute asthma may safely be treated with combination therapy. The true clinical benefit of combination therapy remains to be defined.

In contrast to adults, pediatric patients appear to obtain significant benefit from combination therapy, as reflected in improved flow rates and reduced hospitalizations.

Future directions in anticholinergic therapy include the development of newer, more potent drugs, which may prove to be more effective bronchodilators. As clinical investigation continues to refine the role of these medications for asthma therapy, recommendations concerning the acute (and chronic) management of asthma may change. At present, we can fairly state that anticholinergics are efficacious and safe adjuncts to asthma therapy for both adult and pediatric patients.

REFERENCES

1. Herxheimer H. Atropine cigarettes in asthma and emphysema. Br J Med 1959; 2:167–171.
2. Gross N. Ipratropium bromide. N Engl J Med 1988; 319:486–494.
3. Braun SR, McKenzie WN, Copeland C, Knight L, et al. Comparison of the effect of ipratropium bromide and albuterol in the treatment of chronic obstructive airways disease. Arch Intern Med 1989; 149:544–547.
4. Tashkin DP, Ashutosh K, Britt EJ, Cugell DW, et al. Comparison of the anticholinergic bronchodilator ipratropium bromide with metaproterenol in chronic obstructive pulmonary disease. A 90-day multi-center trial. Am J Med 1986; 81(suppl 5A):81–89.
5. Karpel JP, Pesin J, Greenberg D, Gentry E. A comparison of the effects of ipratropium bromide and metaproterenol sulfate in acute exacerbations of COPD. Chest 1990; 98:835–839.
6. Karpel JP. Bronchodilator responses to the effects of ipratropium bromide and beta-adrenergics in acute and stable COPD. Chest 1991, 99:871–876.
7. Combivent Inhalational Aerosol Study Group. In chronic obstructive pulmonary disease, a combination of ipratropium and albuterol is more effective than either agent alone: an 85-day multi center trial. Chest 1994; 105:1411–1419.
8. Ward MJ. The role of anticholinergic drugs in acute asthma. In: Gross N, ed. Anticholinergic therapy in obstructive airways disease. London, UK: Franklin Scientific Publications, 1993; 155–162.
9. Bleeker ER. Cholinergic and neurogenic mechanisms in obstructive airways disease. Am J Med 1986; 81(suppl 5A):93–99.
10. Hulme EC, Birdsall NJM, Buckley NJ. Muscarinic receptor subtypes. Ann Rev Pharmacol 1990; 30:633–673.
11. Minette PA, Barnes PJ. Muscarinic receptor subtypes in the lung. Am Rev Respir Dis 1990; 141(suppl):S165.
12. Fairshter RD, Habib MP, Wilson AF. Inhaled atropine sulfate in acute asthma. Respiration 1981; 42:263–272.
13. Karpel JP, Appel D, Breidbart D, Fusco MJ. A comparison of atropine sulfate and metaproterenol sulfate in the emergency treatment of asthma. Am Rev Respir Dis 1986; 133:727–729.
14. Ward MJ, Fenton PH, Smith WHR, Davies D. Ipratropium bromide in acute asthma. Brit Med J 1981; 282:598–600.
15. Rennard S, Serby CW, Ghafouri M, Johnson PA, Freidman M. Extended therapy with ipratropium bromide is associated with improved lung function in patients with COPD. Chest 1996; 110:62–70.
16. Foster WM, Bergifsky EH. Airway mucus membrane: effect of beta-adrenergic and anticholinergic stimulation. Am J Med 1986; 81(suppl 5A):28–35.
17. Rebuck AS, Chapman KR, Abboud R, et al. Nebulized anticholinergic and sympathomimetic treatment of asthma and chronic obstructive airway disease in the emergency room. Am J Med 1987; 82:59–64.
18. Gross NJ, Skorodin MS. Anticholinergic, muscarinic bronchodilators. Am Rev Respir Dis 1984; 29:856–870.
19. Altouynan REC. Variation of drug action on airway obstruction in man. Thorax 1964; 19: 406–415.
20. Snow RW, Miller WC, Blair HT, Rice DL. Inhaled atropine in asthma. Ann Allergy 1979; 42:286–289.

21. Ruffin RE, Mc Intyre E, Crockett AJ, Zielonka K, et al. Combination bronchodilator therapy in asthma. J Allergy Clin Immunol 1982: 69:60–62.
22. Bruderman I, Cohen-Aronovskin R, Smorzik J. A comparative study of various combinations of ipratropium bromide and metaproterenol in allergic asthmatic patients. Chest 1883; 83: 208–210.
23. Elkwood RK, Abboud RT. The short-term bronchodilator effects of fenoterol and ipratropium in asthma. J Allergy Clin Immunol 1982: 69:467–473.
24. Firstater E, Mizrachi E, Topilsky M. The effect of vagolytic drugs on airway obstruction in patients with bronchial asthma. Ann Allergy 1981; 46:332–335.
25. Pierce RJ, Allen CJ, Cambell AH. A comparative study of atropine methonitrate, salbutamol and their combination in airways obstruction. Thorax 1979; 34:45–50.
26. Petrie GR, Palmer KNV. A comparison of aerosol ipratropium bromide and salbutamol in chronic bronchitis and asthma. Br Med J 1975; 1:430–432.
27. Ullah MI, Newman GB, Saunders KB. Influence of age on response to ipratropium and salbutamol in asthma. Thorax 1981; 36:523–529.
28. U.S. Department of Health and Human Services. Guidelines for the diagnosis and management of asthma: expert panel report. Bethesda, MD: Department of Health and Human Services, 1991, NIH Publication No. 91-3042A.
29. Bryant DH. Nebulizer ipratropium bromide in the treatment of acute asthma. Chest 1985; 88; 24–29.
30. Watson WTA, Becker AB, Simons FER. Comparison of ipratropium solution, fenoterol solution, and their combination administered by nebulizer and face mask to children with acute asthma. J Allergy Clin Immunol 1988; 82:1012–1018.
31. Leahy B, Gomm SA, Allen SA. Comparison of nebulized salbutamol with nebulised ipratropium in acute asthma. Br J Dis Chest 1983; 77:159–163.
32. Summers Q, Tarala RA. Nebulized ipratropium in the treatment of acute asthma. Chest 1990; 97:425–427.
33. Higgins RM, Stradling JR, Lane DJ. Should ipratropium bromide be added to beta-agonist in the treatment of acute, severe asthma? Chest 1988; 94:718–722.
34. O'Driscoll BR, Taylor RJ, Horsley MG, Chambers DK, Bernstein A. Nebulised salbutamol with and without ipratropium bromide in acute airflow obstruction. Lancet 1989; 1:1418–1420.
35. Rosler J, Reynaert MS. A comparison of fenoterol and fenoterol ipratropium nebulisation treatment in acute asthma. Act Therapeutica 1987; 13:571–576.
36. Karpel JP, Schacter EN, Fanta C, Levey D, Spiro P, Aldrich TK, Menjjoge SS, Witek T. A comparison of ipratropium and albuterol vs albuterol alone for the treatment of acute asthma. Chest 1996; 110:611–616.
37. FitzGerald JM, Grunfeld A, Pare PD, et al. The clinical efficacy of combination nebulized anticholinergic and adrenergic bronchodilators vs nebulized adrenergic bronchodilator alone in acute asthma. Canadian Combivent Study Group. Chest 1997; 111:311–315.
38. Garnett JE, Town I. For the New Zealand Combivent Study Group. Nebulised salbutamol with and without ipratropium bromide in acute asthma. Am Rev Respir Dis 1995; 151(abstr): A270.
39. Lanes SF, Garrett JE, Wentworth CA, Fitzgerald JM, Karpel JP. The effect of adding ipratropium bromide to salbutamol in the treatment of acute asthma: A pooled analysis of three trials. Chest 1998; 114:365–372.
40. Appel DA, Karpel JP, Sherman M. Epinephrine improves flow rates in patients with asthma who do not respond to inhaled metaproterenol sulfate. J Allergy Clin Immunol 1989; 84:90–98.
41. Stein L, Cole R. Early administration of corticosteroids in the emergency treatment of acute asthma. Ann Intern Med 1990; 112:822–827.
42. Karpel JP, Aldrich TK, Prezant DJ, Guguchev K, Gaitan-Salas A, Pathiparti R. Emergency

treatment of acute asthma with albuterol metered-dose-inhaler plus holding chamber: How often should treatments be administered? Chest 1996; 110:39S.
43. Lenney W, Evans NMP. Nebulised and salbutamol and ipratropium bromide in asthmatic children. Br J Dis Chest 1986; 80:59–65.
44. Friberg S, Graff-Lonnevig V. Ipratropium (Atrovent) in childhood asthma: a cumulative dose-response study. Ann of Allergy 1989; 62:131–134.
45. Beck R, Robertson C, Galdes-Sevaldt M, Levinson H. Combined salbutamol and ipratropium by inhalation in the treatment of severe acute asthma. J Pediatr 1985; 107:605–608.
46. Reisman J, Galdes-Sevaldt M, Kazim F, Canny G, Levison H. Frequent administration by inhalation of salbutamol and ipratropium bromide in the initial management of severe acute asthma in children. J Allergy Clin Immunol 1988; 81:16–20.
47. Schuh S, Parkin P, Rajan A, Canny G, Healy R, Rieder M, et al. High-versus low dose frequently administered nebulized albuterol in children with severe acute asthma. Pediatrics 1989; 83:513–518.
48. Storr J, Lenney W. Nebulized ipratropium and salbutamol in asthma. Arch Dis Child 1986; 61:602–603.
49. Boner AL, De Stephano G, Niero F, Vallone G, Gaburro D. Salbutamol and ipratropium bromide solution in the treatment of bronchospasm in children. Ann Allergy 1987; 58:54–58.
50. Mann NP, Hiller EJ. Ipratropium bromide in children with asthma. Thorax 1982: 37:72–74.
51. Sly PD, Landau LI, Olinsky A. Failure of ipratropium bromide to modify diurnal variation of asthma in asthmatic children. Thorax 1987: 42:357–360.
52. Freeman J, Landau LI. The effects of ipratropium bromide and fenoterol nebulizer solutions in children with asthma. Clin Pediatr 1989: 28:556–560.
53. Vichynond P, Slade WA, Sur S, Hill MR, Seefiss SJ, Nelson HS. Efficay of atropine methinitrate alone and in combination with albuterol in children with asthma. Chest 1990; 98:637–642.
54. Levinson H, ed. Treatment of pediatric asthma: A Canadian Consensus. Toronto: Medicine Publishing Foundation Symposium Series, 29, September 1990.
55. Barnes PJ. Theoretical aspects of anticholinergic treatment. In: Gross N, ed., Anticholinergic Therapy in Obstructive Airways Disease, Franklin Scientific Publishing, 1993.

24

Magnesium

Robert Silverman
Albert Einstein College of Medicine, Bronx, and Long Island Jewish Medical Center, New Hyde Park, New York

I. INTRODUCTION

The increasing morbidity associated with asthma has focused attention on methods to improve treatment of the acutely ill emergency department (ED) patient. Hospitalization of patients with asthma is common with approximately 20% of adults presenting to the ED with acute episodes requiring admission (see Chapter 5). In addition asthmatics with especially severe airway compromise may require intensive care unit (ICU) admission or endotracheal intubation. The present mainstay of treatment in the ED consists of β-agonists and systemic steroids, although steroids may take a number of hours or longer to improve pulmonary function. The clinician is constantly searching for additional treatments that will improve the patient's condition, prevent hospitalization, or further clinical deterioration. Magnesium is an agent that has clinical promise as an adjunct to standard care in the acutely ill patient.

II. PHARMACOLOGY

A. Background

Magnesium, the second most common cation found in intracellular fluid and the fourth most common cation in the human body, has many important metabolic roles in humans (1). The majority of the estimated 21–28 g (approximately 2000 mEq) total body magnesium is found in the bones and muscle, with an estimated 1% found in the extracellular space (1,2). Serum magnesium is 32% protein bound, 13% complexed to anions, and 55% found in the free ionized or diffusible form (3). Magnesium is absorbed primarily in the small intestine, and gastrointestinal absorption is in part dependent on the amount of magnesium in the diet as well as total body stores. Magnesium excretion is primarily regulated by the kidney. The kidney retains magnesium in the presence of deficiency by increasing tubular reabsorption. High serum levels of magnesium are difficult to sustain in the presence of normal renal function, since renal excretion increases in proportion to the amount filtered through the kidney (1).

Intracellular magnesium is a crucial cofactor in many cellular enzymatic reactions including those involving the production and utilization of ATP. Biological processes as diverse as glycolysis, deoxyribonucleic acid (DNA) transcription, and protein synthesis require magnesium. In addition to acting as a enzymatic cofactor for energy producing reactions, magnesium influences nerve conduction, maintains the integrity of cell membranes, and helps to operate cellular transport channels.

B. Proposed Mechanisms of Action in Asthma

The clinical manifestations of asthma are the results of inflammatory mediators acting on cells in the airway, neural transmission, and smooth muscle constriction (see Chapters 3 and 4). A variety of experimental evidence offers explanation for the potential benefits of magnesium in the treatment of asthma. Magnesium causes relaxation of bronchial smooth muscle in vitro (4). Magnesium has been found to decrease the amount of neurotransmitter released at motor nerve terminals, diminish the depolarizing action of acetylcholine at the neuromuscular end plate, and depress excitability of smooth muscle membranes (5). There is evidence that prostaglandin mediated smooth muscle contraction is magnesium dependent (6). In neutrophils taken from patients with asthma, magnesium decreases superoxide radical production, suggesting a possible anti-inflammatory effect (7). Magnesium is necessary for the binding of the β-agonist/receptor complex with GS protein, a step that leads to activation of adenyl cyclase and smooth muscle relaxation (8,9). Increasing concentrations of magnesium in vitro has also been found to overcome β-adrenergic desensitization of lymphocytes, suggesting a complimentary role of β-agonists and magnesium (10). This may have clinical importance given the decrease in serum magnesium noted after treatment with β-agonists (11), as well as the common finding of magnesium deficiency in patients with asthma (35).

Any consideration of the role of magnesium in pulmonary health or illness must also consider the important role of calcium (12,13). Calcium is a cation essential for smooth muscle contraction by binding to calmodulin and activating myosin light chain kinase. Reactions involving inflammatory pathways, mast cell release of histamine, nerve impulse initiation, and conduction of vagal fibers are also calcium dependent (13). Magnesium plays an important role in the regulation of calcium. At the cellular level, magnesium may act as a calcium antagonist by influencing the movement of calcium across the cell membrane. Magnesium limits calcium bioavailability by causing a redistribution of calcium within the sarcolemma (14,15). In smooth muscle, magnesium may also compete with calcium for nonspecific binding sites and therefore limit maximal tension (16).

III. CLINICAL EXPERIENCE IN ASTHMA

In 1912, Trendelenberg noted that magnesium caused relaxation of isolated cow bronchial smooth muscle. It was not until 1936 that magnesium was first reported as a potential treatment for asthma (17). A patient hospitalized with severe acute illness was not responding to the commonly used therapies of the time, including belladonna and epinephrine. After the patient's condition further worsened and shaking of the extremities started, magnesium sulfate was given as a treatment for presumed seizures. Shortly after magnesium was injected, the patient's respiratory condition markedly improved. In 1940, Haury also reported two hospitalized patients whose asthma was worsening despite epinephrine therapy (18). After a dose of intravenous (IV) and intramuscular (IM) magnesium sulfate, the respiratory symptoms ''immediately'' improved.

For many years there was little further mention of magnesium in the literature, possibly as a result of the widespread use of bronchodilators, such as adrenergic agents and aminophylline. The next reports of magnesium as a treatment for asthma came in 1987 when Okayama and colleagues found intravenous magnesium to transiently improve pulmonary function in 10 asthmatics presenting to an outpatient clinic with moderate obstruction (19). Rolla in 1988 noted a transient bronchodilating effect of $MgSO_4$ in a crossover study of 10 outpatients with asthma (20). Noppen and colleagues in 1989 found 3 grams of $MgSO_4$ produced bronchodilatation in hospitalized patients with asthma and the effects were additive to β-agonist treatment (21). A number of case reports subsequently reported magnesium prevented intubation in severely ill ED patients (22,23).

The first placebo controlled trial of patients with acute bronchospasm was performed in 1989, when Skobeloff and colleagues studied 38 ED patients with moderate to severe asthma (24). After a treatment period that included β-agonists and steroids, patients were given 1.2 gm $MgSO_4$ or placebo and observed for 45 min. Patients receiving magnesium had significant improvements of peak flow and had a reduction in admission rates. Green and Rothrock conducted a larger trial in which 120 ED patients with airway obstruction, ranging from mild to severe, were given 2 g $MgSO_4$ or placebo as part of a treatment protocol (25). In this single-blinded study, no improvements in pulmonary function or admission rates were seen in the magnesium group. Tiffany and colleagues randomized 48 ED patients into one of three treatment groups that included either placebo, 2 g magnesium, or 2 g $MgSO_4$ with a 4 hr infusion and found that magnesium was not beneficial (26). Of interest, there was a trend toward improved pulmonary function in patients with lower initial FEV_1 (personal communication, Brian Tiffany, 1998).

In 1994, Bloch and colleagues studied 145 acutely ill ED asthmatics with an FEV_1 $< 75\%$ of predicted both before and after a single β-agonist treatment was administered (27). Two grams $MgSO_4$ were given as part of a 4-hr standardized treatment protocol. Overall, magnesium did not change FEV_1 or admission rates (Figure 1). When the 35 patients with severe asthma, defined as an initial $FEV_1 < 25\%$ predicted, were analyzed separately, this group had significant improvement in pulmonary function as well as decreased admissions (Figure 1). These results suggested that magnesium was effective only in patients with acute severe asthma and helped to explain some of the conflicting data found previously.

A study to validate the observations that patients with severe pulmonary obstruction respond to magnesium was recently completed (28). In a multicenter clinical trial, 245 patients with acute severe asthma, defined as an $FEV_1 < 30\%$ predicted on ED arrival, were given 2 g $MgSO_4$ or placebo as part of a standardized assessment and treatment protocol. In this 4-hr protocol, which included early administration of IV steroids and frequent administration of nebulized β-agonists, improvements in FEV_1 were noted at all time points following the infusion of magnesium. At 4 hr, patients who received magnesium had an FEV_1 of 49% predicted versus 43% in those receiving placebo ($p = 0.017$).

When the data were further stratified, the greatest improvements in pulmonary function were found in the patients with an initial $FEV_1 < 25\%$ predicted, similar to the

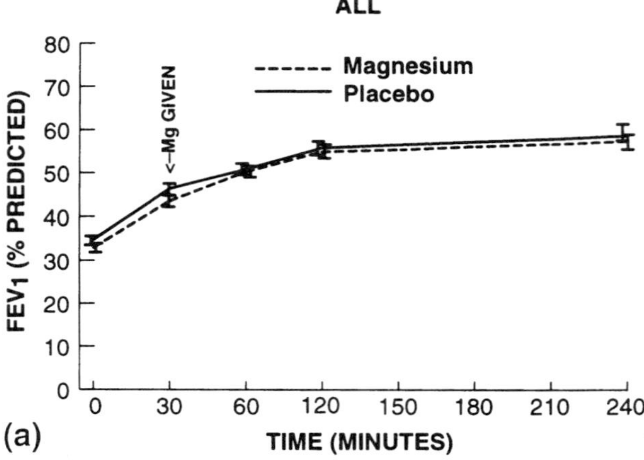

Figure 1 FEV_1, percent predicted as a function of time, where time 0 is ED arrival and magnesium or placebo is given at 30 min. Albuterol is given at 0, 30, 60, 120, and 180 min. Steroids were also administered (27). (a) All patients; (b) severe = patients with FEV_1 less than 25% of predicted at time 0; and (c) moderate = patients with FEV_1 25–75% of predicted at time 0. Results are expressed as mean ± SEM. (From Ref. 27.)

study by Bloch et al. Among the 90 patients with an initial FEV_1 between 25 and 30% predicted, very little improvement in pulmonary function was noted. Only patients with an $FEV_1 < 25\%$ predicted had significant improvements in FEV_1, and further analysis revealed that the lower the baseline FEV_1 the greater the improvement in pulmonary function. This further confirmed the hypothesis that patients with the most compromised pulmonary function were more likely to respond to magnesium.

Several observations can be made from the literature. Magnesium is a bronchodilator as demonstrated by the immediate improvement in pulmonary function when used as the sole agent. However, when used as part of a treatment protocol in patients with acute episodes, clinical benefit is demonstrated only in patients with severe illness as defined by pulmonary function testing. Two grams of magnesium sulfate does not appear to improve pulmonary function when given with β-agonists in patients with mild to moderate asthma episodes.

Among severely ill patients there is an overall improvement in pulmonary function, which is greater in patients with the lowest FEV_1. Even among the more severely ill, some will respond better than others, and some patients do not respond at all to magnesium. This individual variability in response to magnesium may be related to the mechanisms of action of magnesium or the fact that significant airway swelling and mucous plugging limits the rapidity of improvement.

Based on the current literature, magnesium should not be viewed as a "magic bullet" but as an agent that has potential benefit to some patients with severe acute asthma.

IV. INHALED MAGNESIUM

The use of nebulized $MgSO_4$ as a therapy has been studied. Pretreatment with $MgSO_4$-attenuated histamine or methacholine-induced bronchospasm in stable asthmatics (29–

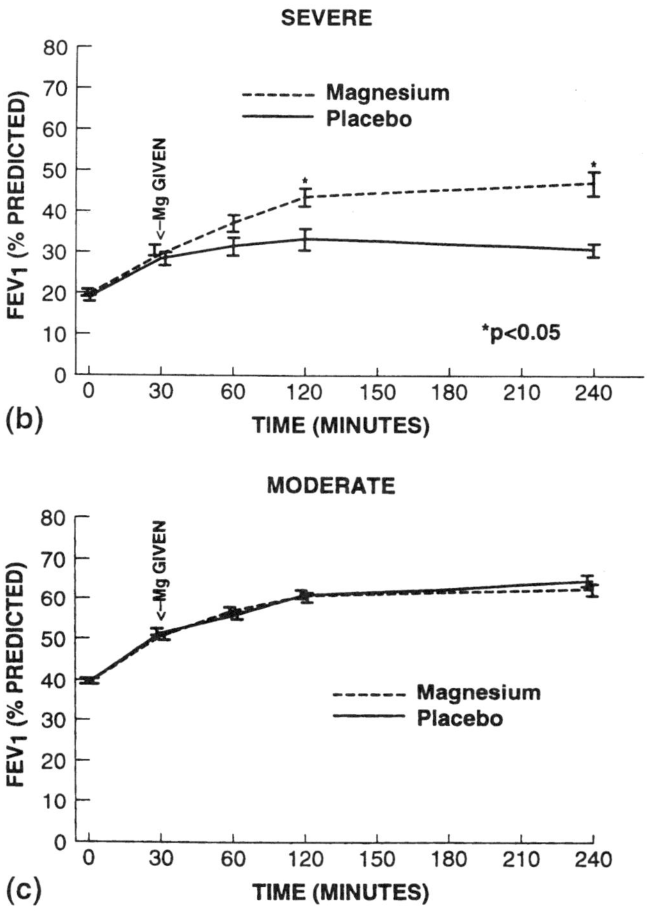

31). Another study, however, found doses of 3 mL $MgSO_4$ (268 mmol/L) had a minimal effect on reversing methacholine induced bronchospasm. Yet another study of stable asthmatics found that inhaled doses ranging from 90 to 360 mg $MgSO_4$ did not cause bronchodilation (32,33). It is not clear why magnesium was not uniformly effective in preventing bronchospasm given the clinical evidence that magnesium is a bronchodilator when given intravenously. As there have not been adequate clinical trials in acutely ill patients, $MgSO_4$ cannot presently be recommended for inhaled use.

V. USE FOR COPD

In a placebo-controlled study of patients with chronic obstructive pulmonary disease (COPD), 1.2 g $MgSO_4$ was found to improve pulmonary function during acute exacerbations when the initial peak expiratory flow rate (PEFR) was less than 250 L/min (34). The magnesium infusion was not given at the same time as the albuterol treatment in this study, and therefore it is not known whether patients would have had the same benefit from magnesium had they received simultaneous treatment with β-agonists.

VI. SERUM LEVELS

It is not known whether the benefits of magnesium are due to replacement of deficient stores, a direct pharmacological effect, or both. In the study that evaluated magnesium efficacy in patients with severe asthma, serum levels did not predict response to treatment (28). However, it should be pointed out that determining magnesium deficiency is difficult, since serum levels may not reflect intracellular or total body stores, and a patient with a normal serum level may actually be magnesium deficient (1). One study that measured intracellular magnesium levels found that patients with asthma are more likely to be magnesium deficient (35). Another investigation that measured total body stores of magnesium in stable asthmatics, using intravenous magnesium infusions, found that magnesium deficiency was common in mild asthmatics, although the prevalence did not differ from the healthy controls (36).

VII. WHO SHOULD RECEIVE MAGNESIUM?

Patients with acute severe airway obstruction, specifically when $FEV_1 < 25\%$ predicted on ED arrival, should receive magnesium. It is possible that other indices of disease severity, including poor response to multiple β-agonist treatments, may also predict response to magnesium, but this has not been well studied. Since the patients clinical appearance may not be indicative of the degree of airway obstruction, the peak flow or FEV_1 should be measured on arrival to the ED, and magnesium administered to those with severe obstruction (see Chapter 14). If peak flow or FEV_1 cannot be obtained, and clinical signs of severe obstruction are present, then the patient should also be considered for magnesium. Without performing objective measures of air movement and only relying on clinical assessment, some patients with severe obstruction will not receive magnesium when they may possibly benefit. Likewise, many other patients with less severe airway obstruction but who appear to be uncomfortable will receive magnesium and probably have no clinical improvement.

VIII. HOW SHOULD IT BE GIVEN AND AT WHAT DOSE?

The only clinical trials that demonstrate efficacy used doses of 1.2 or 2.0 g magnesium sulfate, with the greatest number of patients having been enrolled in protocols that used 2.0 g. The rates of infusion studied varied from 10 to 20 min and the $MgSO_4$ was administered in 50–100 cc of NS or D5W. A dose-response curve in the acutely ill population has not been performed, and the optimal dose is not known. It is also unknown whether repeat doses or constant infusions are beneficial in selected populations. The recommendations are to administer 2 g of $MgSO_4$ in 50–100 mL D5W or NS over 10 min.

IX. SIDE EFFECTS OF MAGNESIUM

The downside of administering magnesium is usually limited to the time, additional costs, and discomfort to the patient of intravenous cannula placement. Relatively minor side effects of magnesium infusions are common and include flushing, lethargy, nausea, and burning at the site of IV infusion. There are two cases in the literature of patients who developed urticaria during the infusion of magnesium (37). The rash resolved soon after the magnesium was discontinued. It is not clear whether it was the magnesium compound that caused these reactions or a carrier used in the preparation of the solution. Serious side effects in the healthy population are rare when 2 g magnesium are administered over 5–10 min or longer and have not been reported in any of the clinical trials.

Hypermagnesemia may cause serious neuromuscular, central nervous system, and cardiac complications. Normal serum levels are between 1.5 and 2.5 mEq/L. At serum levels of 7–10 mEq/L, deep tendon reflexes are lost, hypotension may occur, and lethargy or stupor can be noted. With serum levels of 12–15 mEq/L or higher, respiratory paralysis and malignant arrhthymias can appear, and death has been reported at levels of 15–25 mEq/L (1,38). High doses of magnesium when given rapidly are more likely to cause respiratory failure or cardiac arrest than an overdose involving a slow infusion.

There have been anecdotal reports of patients with extremely severe asthma quickly improving when rapid "boluses" of magnesium sulfate are given (39). Caution when infusing magnesium too rapidly is warranted, as it has been the experience of the writer that some patients will develop a transient sensation of extreme fatigue or faintness when even 2 g of magnesium are given over 2–3 min. These symptoms will rapidly resolve, although in a severe asthmatic it can sometimes be difficult to distinguish them from impending respiratory failure. Another note of caution is warranted for patients with renal failure and pre-existing hypermagnesemia, as parenterally administered magnesium is excreted almost exclusively by the kidneys.

X. UNANSWERED QUESTIONS

A number of important questions regarding the use of magnesium remain unanswered. These include the optimal dose, speed of administration, use as a continuous infusion, or the benefits of treatment with repeated doses. To date there have not been any dose-response studies performed in patients with acute illness. Patients with more moderate illness did not benefit from 2 g of magnesium, and perhaps a different dose would provide benefit. Reasons why magnesium appears to be most beneficial in patients with more severe illness need to be understood. Importantly the variables that will allow the clinician to determine which patients truly benefit from magnesium needs to be further investigated. A greater understanding of the therapeutic actions of magnesium will help to identify patients most likely to benefit.

There have not been any studies evaluating the role of magnesium in preventing endotracheal intubation or decreasing the time on a respirator. The use of magnesium in hospitalized patients to improve pulmonary function and decrease length of stay should be considered. Studies evaluating the potential use as an inhalant in the severely ill patient also need to be done, although determining the appropriate doses to test also poses a difficult challenge.

XI. SUMMARY

Magnesium sulfate appears to benefit asthmatic patients with acute, severe airway compromise. The lower the FEV_1, the greater the improvement. Magnesium has not been shown to improve pulmonary function in patients with more moderate disease when used as an adjunct to standard therapy of β-agonists and steroids. It is possible that magnesium will show benefit when other markers are used, such as lack of response to aggressive bronchodilator therapy, but this has not been well studied. Given the low risks associated with intravenous magnesium therapy and the potential benefit in the sickest population, its use should be strongly considered in patients with acute severe asthma.

REFERENCES

1. Reinhart RA. Magnesium metabolism. A review with special reference to the relationship between intracellular content and serum levels. Arch Intern Med 1988; 148:2415–2420.
2. Widdowson EM, McCance RA, Spray CM, et al. Chemical composition of the human body. Clin Sci 1951; 10:113–125.
3. Walser M. Magnesium metabolism. Ergeb Physiol 1967; 59:185–296.
4. Spivey WH, Skobeloff EM, Levin RM. Effect of magnesium chloride on rabbit bronchial smooth muscle. Ann Emerg Med 1990; 19:1107–1112.
5. del Castillo J, Engbaek L. The nature of the neuromuscular block produced by magnesium. J Physiol 1954; 124:370–384.
6. Altura BM, Altura BT, Waldemar Y. Prostaglandin-induced relaxations and contractions of arterial smooth muscle: effects of magnesium ions. Artery 1976; 2:326–336.
7. Cairns CB, Kraft M. Magnesium attenuates the neutrophil respiratory burst in adult asthmatic patients. Acad Emerg Med 1996; 3:1093–1097.
8. Ransnas LA, Jasper JR, Leiber D, Insel PA. Beta-adrenergic-receptor-mediated dissociation and membrane release of the Gs protein in S49 lymphoma-cell membrane: Dependence on Mg^{2+} and GTP. Biochem J 1992; 283:519–524.
9. Brandt DR, Ross EM. Catecholamine-stimulated GTPase cycle. Multiple sites of regulation by beta-adrenergic receptor and Mg^{2+} studied in reconstituted receptor-Gs vesicles. J Biol Chem 1986; 261:1656–1664.
10. Feldman RD. Beta-adrenergic desensitization reduces the sensitivity of adenylate cyclase for magnesium in permeabilized lymphocytes. Molecular Pharmacology 1989; 35:304–310.
11. Bodenhamer J, Bergstrom R, Brown D, Gabow P, Marx JA, Lowenstein SR. Frequently nebulized beta-agonists for asthma: effects on serum electrolytes. Ann Emerg Med 1992; 21:1337–1342.
12. Iseri LT, French JH. Magnesium: Natures physiologic calcium blocker. Am Heart J 1984; 108: 188–193.
13. Mathew R, Altura BM. Magnesium and the lungs. Magnesium 1988; 7:173–187.
14. Dunnett J, Nayler WG. Calcium efflux from sarcoplasmic reticulum: effects of calcium and magnesium. J Mol Cell Cardiol 1978; 10:487–498.
15. Stephenson EW, Podelsky RJ. Regulation by magnesium of intracellular calcium movement in skinned muscle fibers. J Gen Physiol 1977; 69:1–16.
16. Potter D, Robertson SP, Johnson JD. Magnesium and regulation of muscle contraction. Fed Proc 1981; 40:2653–2656.
17. Roselló HJ, Plá JC. Sulfato de magnesio en la crisis de asma. Prensa Méd Argent 1936; 23: 1677–1680.

18. Haury VG. Blood serum magnesium in bronchial asthma and its treatment by administration of magnesium sulfate. J Lab Clin Med 1940; 26:340–344.
19. Okayama H, Aikawa T, Okayama M, Sasaki H, Mue S, Takishima T. Bronchodilating effects of intravenous magnesium sulfate in bronchial asthma. JAMA 1987; 257:1076–1078.
20. Rolla G, Bucca C, Caria E, et al. Acute effect of intravenous magnesium sulfate on airway obstruction of asthmatic patients. Ann Allergy 1988; 61:388–391.
21. Noppen M, Vanmaele L, Impens N, Schandevyl W. Bronchodilating effect of intravenous magnesium sulfate in acute severe bronchial asthma. Chest 1990; 97:373–376.
22. Kuitert LM, Kletchko SL. Intravenous magnesium sulfate in acute, life-threatening asthma. Ann Emerg Med 1991; 20:1243–1245.
23. McNamara RM, Spivey WH, Skobeloff E, Jacubowitz S. Intravenous magnesium sulfate in the management of acute respiratory failure complicating asthma. Ann Emerg Med 1989; 18: 197–199.
24. Skobeloff EM, Spivey WH, McNamara RM, Greenspon L. Intravenous magnesium sulfate for the treatment of acute asthma in the emergency department. JAMA 1989; 262:1210–1213.
25. Green SM, Rothrock SG. Intravenous magnesium for acute asthma: failure to decrease emergency treatment duration or need for hospitalization. Ann Emerg Med 1992; 21:260–265.
26. Tiffany BR, Berk WA, Todd IK, White SR. Magnesium bolus or infusion fails to improve expiratory flow in acute asthma exacerbations. Chest 1993; 104:831–834.
27. Bloch H, Silverman R, Mancherje N, Grant S, Jagminas L, Scharf SM. Intravenous magnesium sulfate as an adjunct in the treatment of acute asthma. Chest 1995; 107:1576–1581.
28. Silverman R, Osborne H, Runge J, et al. Magnesium Sulfate as an adjunct to standard therapy in severe asthma. Acad Emerg Med 1996; 3(abstr):467.
29. Rolla G, Bucca C, Bugiani M, et al. Reduction of histamine induced bronchoconstriction by magnesium in asthmatic subjects. Allergy 1987; 42:186–188.
30. Rolla G, Bucca C, Arossa W, et al. Magnesium attenuates methacholine induced bronchoconstriction in asthmatics. Magnesium 1987; 6:201–204.
31. Rolla G, Bucca C, Caria E. Dose-related effect of inhaled magnesium sulfate on histamine challenge in asthmatics. Drugs Exp Clin Res 1988; 14:609–612.
32. Chande VT, Skoner DP. A trial of nebulized magnesium sulfate to reverse bronchospasm in asthmatic patients. Ann Emerg Med 1992; 21:1111–1115.
33. Hill J, Britton J. Dose-response relationship and time-course of the effect of inhaled magnesium sulfate on airflow in normal and asthmatic subjects. Br J Clin Pharmacol 1995; 40:539–544.
34. Skorodin, MS, Tenholder MF, Yetter B, et al. Magnesium sulfate in exacerbations of chronic obstructive pulmonary disease. Arch Intern Med 1995; 155:496–500.
35. de Valk HW, Kok PTM, Struyvenberg A, et al. Extracellular and intracellular magnesium concentrations in asthmatic patients. Eur Respir J 1993; 6:1122–1125.
36. Silverman RA, Skobeloff E, Altura BT, et al. Detection of magnesium deficiency in asthmatics using an intravenous magnesium loading test. Chest 1994; 106:110S.
37. Thorp JM, Katz VL, Campbell D, Lefalo RC. Hypersensitivity to magnesium sulfate. Am J Obstet Gynecol 1989; 161:889–890.
38. Magnesium, Drug Facts and Comparisons, 1998 Edition, Facts and Comparisons, St. Louis, MO: Wolters and Kluwer, 1998, 152–153.
39. Schiermeyer RP, Finkelstein JA. Rapid infusion of magnesium sulfate obviates need for intubation in status asthmaticus. Am J Emerg Med 1994; 12:164–166.

25

Medical Management of Severe Acute Asthma

Edward A. Panacek
University of California, Davis, Sacramento, California

Charles V. Pollack Jr.
Maricopa Medical Center, Phoenix, Arizona

Acute severe asthma (ASA) is characterized by severe bronchospasm refractory to the usual outpatient treatment. "Status asthmaticus" is generally used in reference to those episodes in which the degree of airflow obstruction is severe and not relieved by aggressive therapy within 30–60 min (1). The discussion of the standard therapy of acute asthma occurs in Chapters 18 and 19. This chapter concerns treatment of ASA and "refractory status asthmaticus," a term generally reserved for those cases in which the patient's condition further deteriorates despite aggressive pharmacological interventions. Approximately 5–10% of the general asthmatic population will experience an episode of status asthmaticus at some point (2). Of those who require intubation and admission to an intensive care unit (ICU), the mortality rates can approach 10–20% (3). Increases in the general prevalence of asthma have been recognized with a corresponding increase in cases of ASA, refractory asthma, and asthma deaths (4). Most asthma deaths are due to underrecognition and poor patient education, but some are also due to undertreatment in the acute setting (5).

The natural history of ASA symptoms varies from hours to weeks. Generally there are two types of ASA; type I, or slow-onset asthma; and type II, or sudden-onset asthma. Sudden narrowing of the airways with mucus plugging appears to be a feature of the type II group (6). The more common presentation is type I, i.e., a gradual deterioration superimposed on a background of relatively chronic and poorly controlled asthma. Though less common, type II is the relatively more dangerous group.

This chapter will review the evaluation of a patient with ASA and discuss the management strategies for adults with ASA up to the point of intubation. Two points deserve early and repeated emphasis. First, initiating therapy should not wait until the evaluation is completed. Patient assessment and initial interventions should occur concurrently. Second, these patients can be extremely ill and can suddenly deteriorate. The management strategy should start with standard therapies initiated in all patients with ASA. Those who do not

Table 1 The Therapy of Acute Severe Asthma

I. Routine Care
Inhaled β_2-agonists at continuous or high doses
e.g., albuterol (5–15 mg/hr)
Early steroid administration (PO, IM, or IV)
e.g., prednisone ($\geq$60 mg, or equivalent)
Inhaled anticholinergics
e.g., ipratroprium (0.5–1.0 mg)
II. Second-Line Therapies
Magnesium
Aminophylline
Systemic catecholamines
III. Third-Line Therapies
Heliox
Ketamine
CPAP/BLPAP

quickly respond to those therapies or who deteriorate should have second-line therapies added. However, some patients simply will not respond to the first-line or second-line interventions. In such cases, there should be a fallback plan to try to prevent the need for intubation, or even patient death. Which of the ''third-line options'' preferred as the fallback plan will depend on individual physician experience, combined with the constraints existent within an individual institution. Discussion of management strategies in this chapter are organized along these lines (Table 1).

I. PATIENT ASSESSMENT

There is usually little doubt about the clinical diagnosis of acute severe asthma. These patients generally carry an established diagnosis of asthma and have already tried their regular treatment before presenting to the emergency department (ED) or other acute care setting. The patient is usually sitting upright, profusely diaphoretic, with obvious and marked respiratory distress, and able to speak only a few words at a time or not at all. The respiratory rate can be variable but most patients are hyperventilating in proportion to the severity of the attack. Hypoventilation is a poor sign and worrisome for imminent respiratory arrest (5,6).

The initial examination generally shows hyperinflation of the lungs, accessory muscle use in both inspiration and expiration, and widespread wheezes. A relatively ''silent chest'' is another worrisome sign, because it represents the patient's inability to generate enough airflow to produce wheezing. Tachycardia, hypertension, and various levels of pulsus paradoxus are also relatively common.

Objective measures of asthma severity, such as forced expiratory volume in 1 sec (FEV_1) and peak expiratory flow rate (PEFR), are usually reduced to less than a quarter of the expected values or less than 120 L/min for the PEFR in an adult. Severely distressed patients (those who can barely speak) do not need to undergo these tests; their flow rates are assumed to be very low and in the ''severe'' range.

Arterial blood gases (ABGs) are also rarely necessary, as the severity of these patients is clinically evident. If checked, they may initially show respiratory alkalosis with a low $Paco_2$, but the Pco_2 will rise as the severity of the asthma increases. Trends in the $Paco_2$ may be more important than a single isolated level that does not always correlate well with severity of the asthma itself (7). However, a ''normal'' $Paco_2$ is not normal in a patient in the midst of a severe attack. It represents CO_2 retention and correlates with a worse prognosis and possible need for intubation.

Initiation of therapy should not await completion of history or physical exam, but rather should be concurrent. Important points in history include previous hospitalizations, particularly ICU admissions, and history of medications recently used, started, or discontinued (e.g. steroid use). History of prior intubations also can correlate with predicted severity (8).

Further diagnostic investigations in patients with ASA generally include a chest X-ray to exclude other causes for their dyspnea including pulmonary barotrauma or pneumonia. However these are best done as a portable exam or deferred until the most acute phase of bronchospasm has resolved. Basic serum chemistries are appropriate in patients in which admission is anticipated, but commonly only reveal hypokalemia, secondary to the β-agonist use. A 12-lead electrocardiograph (EKG) may occasionally reveal other causes for the patients symptoms, but generally just shows sinus tachycardia and sometimes right heart strain. Patient assessment is described in further detail in Chapter 13.

II. PATIENT MANAGEMENT

Because of their severity, patients with ASA should be on continuous EKG monitors and pulse oximetry and receive frequent estimations of their respiratory rate, blood pressure, and mental status. They should all immediately receive supplemental oxygen.

Part of the initial management of patients with acute severe asthma involves reassurance. These patients can become very anxious, and confidence in their treating physician is important. An experienced, organized, prepared medical team should ideally direct the care and evaluate the effects of treatment in such patients. There should be a systematic plan of treatment that begins with routine care involving the use of agents that have clearly established efficacy in the treatment of ASA. Many patients will respond to these first-line agents. However, many others will not respond and will require the rapid application of more aggressive (second-line) measures. Such therapies are those that have generally shown benefit in the care of such patients, although their efficacy is not as firmly established. When both routine (first-line) and second-line therapies are unsuccessful and the patient's condition continues to deteriorate, third-line options should be considered in an effort to prevent intubation. Each of these options (and others listed as ''special or unconventional therapies'') can also be applied after intubation when there are ongoing problems with adequate ventilation. Plans for these contingency options are best considered and organized in advance. The smooth coordination of the necessary resources at the time of an absolute emergency can be difficult, and sometimes impossible.

III. ROUTINE CARE

The following are first-line therapies that should be used immediately in all patients presenting with ASA. They have a proven efficacy when used appropriately. They are similar to the medications used in patients presenting with less severe asthma symptoms; the difference is the aggressiveness with which they are used.

A. β_2-Agonists

It has been suggested that β_2-adrenergic agonist use in chronic asthma may be detrimental (9). However, this association appears to be weak, if at all, and does not apply to the treatment of acute asthma. There is no question that inhaled β_2-agonists remain the primary mainstay of immediate treatment of acute severe asthma (10). Despite agreement on the importance of inhaled β_2-agonists in this setting, there is not clear consensus on the route of administration or the optimal dose. Importantly, recent β_2 agonist administration by the patient should not affect the dose or frequency of further drug administered in the ED or other acute care setting. Even when their home inhalers are not providing benefit, most patients with acute severe asthma respond to increasing doses of β_2-adrenergic agents at the hospital. This may be due to the unpredictability of home nebulization systems or the patient use of empty or near empty metered dose inhaler (MDI) canisters. However, more commonly it is related to reduced sensitivity of β_2-receptors in severe asthma, and probable downregulation of those receptors. There is some evidence that steroids can upregulate those same receptors. Continuous nebulization of the β_2-agonist dose is as effective as intermittent doses in both the ordinary dose range as well as at higher doses (11,12). The newer β_2-agonists are surprisingly safe drugs, even when used in high doses. No maximum dose limit for inhaled albuterol has been established. The side effects of β_2-agonists are similar regardless of route and appear to plateau despite increasing doses. These common side effects include tachycardia, nausea, vomiting, and tremor. They are discussed in further detail in Chapter 19.

Continuous nebulized albuterol has shown advantages over intermittent administration in those patients who have an FEV_1 less than 50% (12) or adults with a PEFR less than 200 (13). Some investigators have reported that MDIs are more efficient than nebulizers in the treatment of acute asthma (14). However, proper use of the MDI in the acute setting requires patient concentration and cooperation, which is not always possible in individuals with ASA. Proper use of the MDI in the acute setting requires the continuous bedside presence of a nurse or respiratory therapist. Even with that assistance, some patients are so severe they simply cannot use an MDI, even with a holding chamber. Therefore, for the most severe patients continuous nebulization is preferable.

There are a number of different inhaled β-adrenergic agonists. They vary slightly in terms of their pharmacokinetics, but also in terms of their relative β_2 selectivity. This selectivity may be important in terms of minimizing cardiovascular and central nervous system (CNS) side affects. Albuterol and salbutamol appear to be more β_2 selective than earlier agents such as terbutaline and metaproterenol and are commonly preferred. Albuterol is generally given as a dose of 2.5–5 mg nebulized every 20 min as needed. Continuous albuterol treatments have been shown to be safe and well tolerated. The most common dosages are 5–15 mg over 60 min, diluted in up to 70 mL of saline (13,15). Of note, intermittent positive pressure ventilation (IPPB) administration of β-agonists has not been shown to be advantageous over simple nebulization (16). However, particularly in children, there is experience with giving albuterol in dosages much higher than the Food and Drug Administration (FDA) approved dose range, without problematic toxicity (17). Again, it should be emphasized that there is no known maximum acceptable dose for the use of agents such as albuterol. Patients with severe acute asthma exacerbations should receive aggressive intermittent or continuous albuterol at a dose of at least 7.5 mg/hr until improved.

B. Corticosteroids

These medications are discussed in greater length in Chapter 22. It is worth noting here that although bronchodilators are directed at the symptoms of acute asthma, corticosteroids primarily treat the cause. Inflammation is central to the pathogenesis of asthma and corticosteroids are the most effective treatment (18). Several studies have demonstrated the effectiveness of steroids in acute severe asthma (19–21). Though occasional studies have suggested slightly earlier effects (22), generally the response to steroid administration occurs 6–12 hr after a dose (23). Because of this delay, steroids should be given as early as possible in the course of treatment of ASA. The route by which the steroids are given is not important, but it must be reliable. If there is any question regarding the effectiveness of oral administration, they should be given intramuscularly or intravenously. In those patients who already have an IV, the preference is intravenous administration.

There is no evidence that higher doses (greater than 80 mg of prednisone every 6 hr) are more effective than moderate doses (23). In addition, the higher doses can be associated with an increased incidence of side effects. The use of inhaled steroids for acute exacerbations is an intriguing area of investigation but is not yet proven in the treatment of acute severe asthma. It is best avoided outside of an investigational protocol, due to risks of inducing paroxysms of coughing and acutely worsening bronchospasm.

C. Anticholinergic Agents

Anticholinergic agents block muscarinic receptors, inhibit vagal tone, and thereby promote bronchodilation. This is discussed in greater detail in Chapter 23. The effect of these drugs in acute asthma treatment is not as clearly established as for β_2-agonists or steroids. However, the majority of studies have shown that ipratroprium, and perhaps other anticholinergic agents, has a small additive benefit, especially in children (24–26) (see Chapter 27). As a result, they warrant use in the routine care of acute severe asthma.

Three anticholinergic agents have been used in asthma: atropine, glycopyrrolate, and ipratropium bromide. Ipratropium has shown the most consistent benefits in asthma. It has very little systemic absorption and is often considered to be the ''topical anticholinergic.'' Anticholinergic agents generally have a slower onset than β-agonists but a more prolonged effect (24,27). With ipratropium, bronchodilation begins in approximately 20 min and maximal effect is seen in 60–120 min. The cholinergic receptors are primarily located in the larger and more proximal airways, while the β_2 receptors are generally found more distal in the smaller airways. Therefore, the effects of anticholinergics would logically be supplemental to the β-agonists. Anticholinergic agents have shown greater benefit in the management of chronic obstructive pulmonary disease (COPD) than in asthma. The distinction between acute exacerbations of asthma and COPD, however, is not always clear, particularly in older patients or smokers. As such, anticholnergics warrant use in the routine care of patients with ASA. Additionally, it has been shown that ipratropium can safely be mixed with albuterol (data on file, Boehringer Ingelheim, Ridgefield, CT) so their administration need not delay or interfere with the administration of inhaled β_2-agonists.

IV. SECOND-LINE THERAPIES

When a patient with ASA deteriorates or fails to quickly improve in response to routine measures, a more aggressive therapeutic approach is necessary. This involves the addition of one or more second-line therapies, which are summarized in Table 1. These are therapies which are not as consistently efficacious for the treatment of ASA as the routine care measures, but have generally shown benefits that exceed their toxicity or side effects.

A. Magnesium

Trials with magnesium sulfate ($MgSO_4$) have been inconsistent. Some have shown improvement in flow rates in asthma after β-agonist treatments have failed (28). However, generally it has not shown benefit in patients with mild, moderate, or moderately severe asthma (29,30). The greatest benefit appears to be in those patients with the most severe symptoms, e.g., with an $FEV_1 \leq 25\%$ of predicted (31). It is established that magnesium relaxes smooth muscle and dilates bronchial rings, perhaps in addition to other effects. However, its effects as a smooth muscle relaxant are relatively short lived (perhaps only 30 min) and best seen at relatively higher dosages (at least 2–5 g) than was used in many of the comparative trials. Though the true benefits of magnesium have not been clearly defined, it has been established as a relatively safe adjunct to first-line therapies in the treatment of asthma. The effect of magnesium on bronchodilation is likely modest, temporary, variable, and most commonly seen only with severe exacerbations. This is discussed in much greater detail in Chapter 24.

B. Aminophylline

Once a part of the standard treatment of all patients with recurrent asthma symptoms, the value of aminophylline in ASA has been questioned. Its exact mechanism of action is an area of some debate. At therapeutic concentrations, the inhibition of phosphodiesterase is minimal and it is a relatively weak bronchodilator (32,33). It has a low therapeutic index and a high incidence of side effects, including serious cardiac dysrhythmias and seizures. It has been suggested that the addition of aminophylline to high dose β-agonist therapy is more likely to increase side effects than to achieve bronchodilation. However, this was most evident in patients already on theophylline (34). The risk–benefit ratio may be different for those not already on the medication. Whether the other actions of aminophylline, including enhanced diaphragmatic contractility, pulmonary and systemic vasodilation, cardiac stimulation and diuresis, have any clinical relevance in ASA treatment remains speculative. Nonetheless, if the patient is not responding to standard care measures, aminophylline may be used. Its efficacy may be more likely in older patients with underlying congestive heart failure or whose asthma has elements of COPD (35). In these patients, the nonbronchodilator effects of the drug may be the source of benefit, e.g., via enhanced diuresis. The loading dose is 5–6 mg/kg if the patient is not already taking theophylline. Otherwise obtain a ''stat'' theophylline level and administer 1 mg/kg to raise the serum level by 2 μg/ml. The maintenance dose varies between 0.2 and 0.8 mg/kg/hr. There are wide variations in the elimination of aminophylline in individual patients, so serum concentrations should be checked regularly, and dosing adjusted. Toxicity and efficacy are related more closely to the serum concentrations (goal 10–15 mg/dL) than to the administered dose.

C. Systemic Catecholamines

It is theorized that, in some patients, air flow is so compromised that inhaled bronchodilators cannot reach the most important areas, but perhaps systemic catecholamines could reach those receptors. Multiple studies have demonstrated the advantages of inhaled over systemic β-agonists individually (36,37). However, the value of systemic catecholamines added to optimal inhaled treatment is less clear (38). In the United States, administration of systemic catecholamines to patients with ASA generally means the subcutaneous use of epinephrine (0.3–0.5 mg, 1:1000 solution) every 20 min, up to 3 doses, or terbutaline (0.25–0.5 mg). Epinephrine has a wide range of β_1, β_2, and also α-stimulatory effects. Cydulka et al. showed that the use of subcutaneous epinephrine was safe, even in older adults (up to the age of 96) and without adverse effects (39). However, there remain concerns regarding increased myocardial ischemia when used in patients with underlying coronary disease. As such, its use has generally been superseded by the more specific β_2-agonist agent, terbutaline. However, epinephrine may increase airway diameter not only through β_2-agonist activity, but through other mechanisms, including possible alpha mediated vasoconstriction of vessels in the bronchial mucosa. This is controversial (see Chapter 20).

The intravenous use of epinephrine in treating severe life-threatening asthma is much more common in Australia and in Europe. There, it is administered as intermittent boluses (2–10 mL of 1:10,000 concentration solution over 5 min) or more often as an infusion (1–20 μg/min) if there is felt to be benefit after the initial bolus dose (40).

Most of the clinical experience with intravenous β-agonist agents comes from the pediatric population, where the majority of studies support efficacy in that age group. Early reports of the use of intravenous (IV) isoproterenol indicated that children normally requiring intubation showed improvement with the infusion and avoided intubation. There were no reported drug-related deaths. However, others have reported evidence of myocardial injury and elevation in cardiac enzymes after the use of intravenous isoproterenol for the treatment of ASA, and have strongly cautioned against its use, even in children (41). In addition, a death in an adult asthmatic has been directly been attributed to the use of IV isoproterenol (42).

The more β_2-selective agent salbutamol is available in an intravenous form in Europe. Comparative trials there have again demonstrated efficacy in the pediatric population with ASA (43). Specifically, investigators reported that salbutamol produced less effect on heart rate, more lasting bronchodilation, and sustained reduction in carbon dioxide levels. They used a loading dose of 1 μg/kg over 10 min, followed by a 0.2 μg/kg/min infusion. They also did not see the same tachyphylaxis reported with the intravenous use of isoproterenol. The British Thoracic Society recommends the use of intravenous β_2-selective agonists in adults with refractory asthma (e.g., IV salbutamol 200 μg or terbutaline 250 μg over 10 min, then infusion of 3–12 μg/min) (44).

V. THIRD-LINE THERAPIES

When ASA patients continue to deteriorate or simply fail to respond to both first-line and second-line therapies, third-line or ''fall-back'' therapies should be implemented. These are therapeutic options that are either investigational in nature or involve complicated logistics, making them more difficult to administer in the emergency department setting. The ''investigational'' agents in this category have either theoretical or anecdotal support for their use. In general, these should be considered alternative therapies used in a last effort to prevent intubation. Instituting these measures is most effective when they are thought about and planned in advance. Mobilizing the necessary resources in an absolute emergency is not always possible.

A. Heliox

The clinical use of helium mixtures was described as early as 1935 (45). Subsequently, numerous reports have indicated that the inclusion of helium, a low-density gas, as part of inhaled gas mixtures lowers airway resistance and decreases respiratory work (46–48). Inhalation of helium-oxygen mixtures has resulted in temporary improvement in patients with airway obstruction due to a number of obstructive lesions, including asthma, COPD, bronchiectasis, and even pulmonary fibrosis. In asthma treatment, studies performed in patients after intubation have consistently shown improvements in peak airway pressures and effective ventilation (45,47). More recently there have been reports of the benefits of Heliox used in nonintubated patients with ASA. These have been relatively small reports and generally focused in the pediatric population. Kudukis et al. showed significant improvements in pulsus paradoxus, dyspnea scores, peak flow rates, and need for intubation in 18 patients with ASA, aged 16 months to 16 years (48). However, Carter et al. had less success with the use of a 30/70 Heliox mixture in children 5–18 years of age with acute severe asthma requiring hospitalization (49). All patients received standardized therapy and the Heliox mixture, or air, for 15 min in random order. He found no significant differences in most parameters, except for the FEF 25–75, and those differences were relatively small.

There have been a few reports of an impressive response to Heliox therapy in adults, both intubated and nonintubated. Austan reported the case of a 28 year old woman in extremis who refused oral tracheal intubation and was placed on Heliox by nonrebreathing mask. Within 2 hr of treatment the patient's condition improved and Heliox was discontinued without further incident (50). Kass reported a case series of 12 adults who all presented to the ED with acute respiratory acidosis. Five patients received Heliox through the ventilator and seven via face mask. Eight of the 12 responded to therapy. They tended to be patients who had a shorter duration of their ASA symptoms and a lower baseline pH on ABG. Three of the four nonresponders reported prolonged duration of symptoms ($\geq$ 96 hr). Responders showed improvement within 1 hour (51). Some investigators have used the Heliox mixture as the carrier for the nebulized bronchodilator treatments. More commonly, it was simply applied during, or in between bronchodilator treatments. Such use is not so much a ''treatment'' of asthma as a means to ''buy time'' while medications can exert their effects. The helium percentage in these mixtures varies from 50%–80%, though the most common combination is a 30% oxygen, 70% helium mixture. As the oxygen concentration rises, it is expected that the helium effectiveness declines. This is a therapy very much in need of large prospective randomized clinical trials. However, the existing literature to date demonstrates absolutely no adverse effects from the use of Heliox and supports its empiric use as a second-line therapy. It also has a role in the intubated patient who is extremely difficult to ventilate. It is commonly available in most hospitals and the cost is only modestly higher than a tank of oxygen. The current infrequent use of Heliox appears to be largely due to lack of physician familiarity.

B. Ketamine

Ketamine is a parenteral dissociative anesthetic that was structurally derived from phencyclidine in 1963. It has been reported, in anecdotal cases, to prevent the need for intubation and mechanical ventilation (52,53). Ketamine has multiple effects and all of its activities in asthma may not be fully understood. Its mechanism as a bronchodilator is generally thought to be mediated through two effects; potentiation of catecholamines (which then are bronchodilators), as well as a more direct effect on bronchial smooth muscle (54). However, ketamine also increases cerebral blood flow and intracranial pressure and is a myocardial depressant, which could cause problems in some patients with ASA. In addition, its use in adults has been modulated by its potential to increase airway secretions and cause emergence reactions (54). Benzodiazepines are useful in preventing the emergence problems (55). Because of its effect on increasing bronchial secretions, ketamine is best administered in combination with an anticholinergic agent, preferably given systemically. Most of the reports supporting the use of ketamine are case series in intubated patients (56–58). One prospective, randomized, comparative study in nonintubated adults with ASA showed improved symptom scores, but not improvement in other objective measures, with use of IV ketamine (59). They used a dose of 0.1–0.2 mg/kg bolus, then an infusion of 0.5 mg/kg/hr, for 3 hr. In intubated patients, the doses of ketamine most commonly used are 0.5–1.5 mg/kg as an initial bolus. This bolus can either be repeated in 20 min or followed by a 1–5 mg/kg/hr infusion. The upper limit on hourly infusion rates is less clear.

C. Pressure Support and Noninvasive Ventilation

In the patients with inadequate ventilation but intact airway, noninvasive ventilation may avoid endotracheal intubation. Clearly when endotracheal intubation is indicated (see Chapter 26), such as patients with apnea, airway patency difficulty, or altered mental status, it should not be delayed. Endotracheal intubation of the patient with acute asthma, however, is fraught with risk both in the ED as well as in the ICU. In the ED complications of a difficult intubation, hypotension, paralysis, or barotrauma may be immediately life-threatening. Once the patient is intubated in the ED, the length of hospitalization and cost of care is increased, as well as the risks of nosocomial infection, barotrauma, hypotension, endotracheal tube plugging, kinking, or respirator malfunction in the intensive care unit. In addition noninvasive ventilation has been considered a good method for administering inhalant medications in asthmatics in general, since the devices may reduce respiratory muscle fatigue.

Earliest efforts to employ pressure support for the treatment of bronchospasm utilized intermittent positive pressure breathing via face mask or mouthpiece. With IPPB, a pressure-cycled ventilator would deliver positive pressure flow, triggered by patient inspiratory efforts. It was usually given to deliver bronchodilator treatments, arguing that the aerosol particles were driven deeper into the distal airways by the IPPB pressure (60,61). It was also argued that IPPB decreased the work of breathing (62) and reduced the volume and tenacity of airway secretions in acute asthma (63). However, there were occasional reports of IPPB treatment causing decreased cardiac output and barotrauma (63,64). In

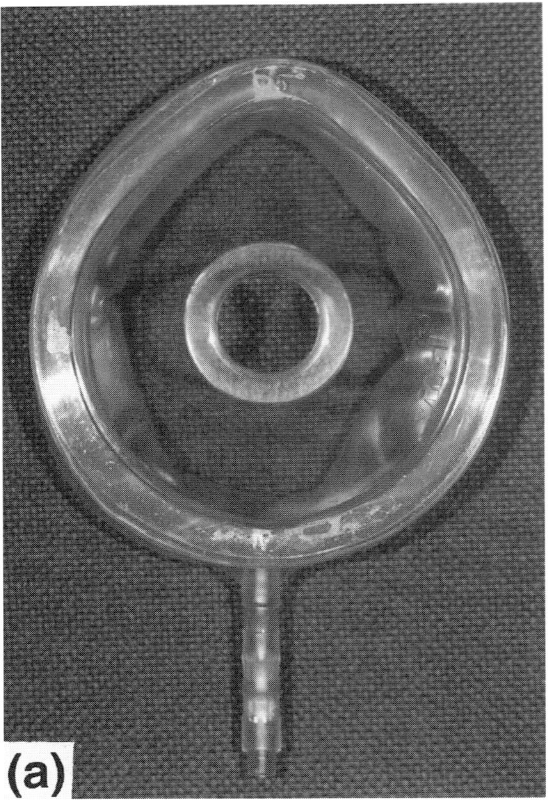

Figure 1 (a) Continuous high-flow full-face nasal CPAP mask. (b) Full-face CPAP with option to provide volume-cycled pressure support. (Photographer Francis Dayrit, M.D.)

addition, the cost of establishing and maintaining an IPPB therapy program was felt to be quite expensive (63). More importantly, there was lack of proven efficacy for IPPB and evidence that it did not actually result in deeper deposition of the aerosolized particles (65,66). It also seemed counterintuitive to use positive pressure breathing to treat a problem already characterized by hyperinflation, air trapping, and a propensity toward barotrauma.

The use of continuous positive airway pressure (CPAP) in asthma has also been reported. CPAP provides a constant ''background'' positive pressure beyond which the pressure in the patient's upper airway is not allowed to drop. Theoretically, CPAP improves oxygenation by increasing the functional residual capacity (FRC) and lung compliance (67). CPAP can be applied noninvasively via nasal or facial masks (Figures 1a and b). Similar to IPPB, concerns have been raised that CPAP could decrease venous return and thereby decrease cardiac output (67). In addition, it is possible that CPAP could induce or exaggerate dynamic hyperinflation of the lungs. However, it has also been suggested that CPAP could supply some of the inflating pressure needed during inspiration, potentially ''off-loading'' the inspiratory muscles and reducing fatigue (68). Studies of adults

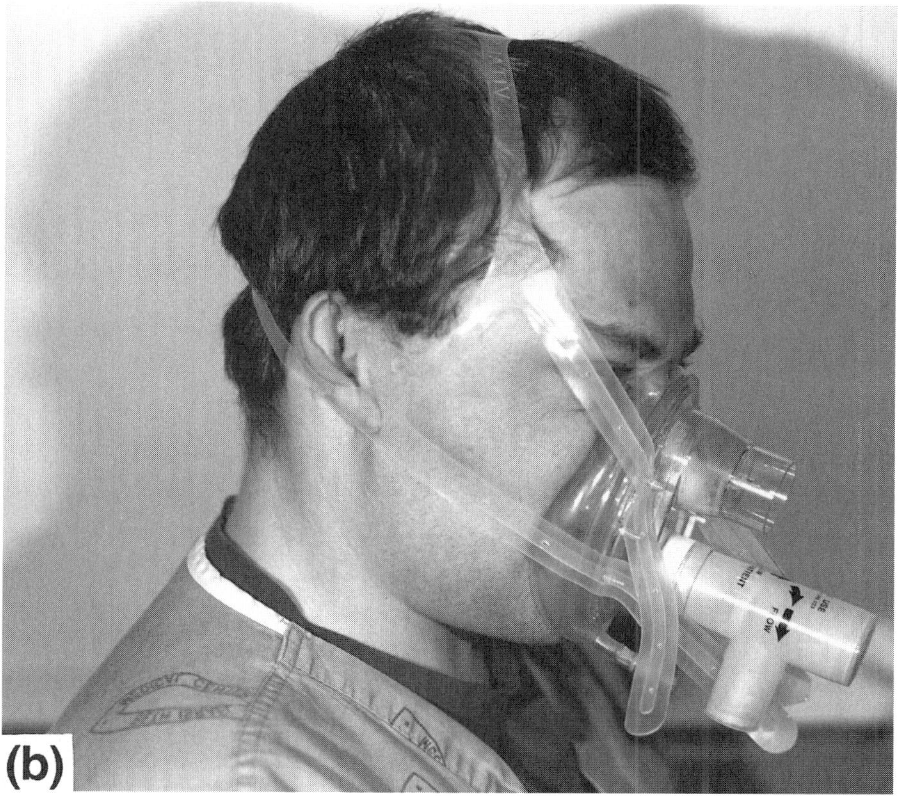

with acute severe asthma requiring hospitalization noted a maximal breathing comfort at a CPAP of 5.3 ± 2.8 cmH_2O, but nonwheezing control subjects were most comfortable at a CPAP of 1.6 ± 2.5 (69). Evaluation of a simple positive expiratory pressure device, which provided no inspiratory flow pressure, however, showed no benefit in asthma (70). This again suggested that CPAP assisted inspiratory muscles and lessened fatigue in asthma. Additionally, it was postulated that any additional inspiratory benefits of higher levels of CPAP might be offset by reduced peak expiratory flow rates. CPAP may also have beneficial effects separate from mechanical airway pressure itself. A study of 16 asthmatic patients with methacholine-induced acute bronchospasm showed that nasal CPAP at 8 cmH_2O reduced bronchial reactivity and bronchial sensitivity and improved the bronchodilatory effects of β_2-agonist therapy (71).

In summary there is clinical evidence that suggests that noninvasive CPAP may be beneficial in acute asthma exacerbation. Levels of CPAP below 10 cmH_2O appear to improve inspiratory muscle efficiency and reduce bronchial sensitivity and subjective dyspnea sensation. There has been no large randomized trial that has measured each of these outcomes in patients with acute asthma. Until this is accomplished, CPAP support should be utilized with caution, and only as an adjunct to other aggressive therapies. Further investigation is needed.

A recently developed similar modality is that of bilevel positive airway pressure (BLPAP), which is similar to a combination of IPPB and positive end expiratory pressure

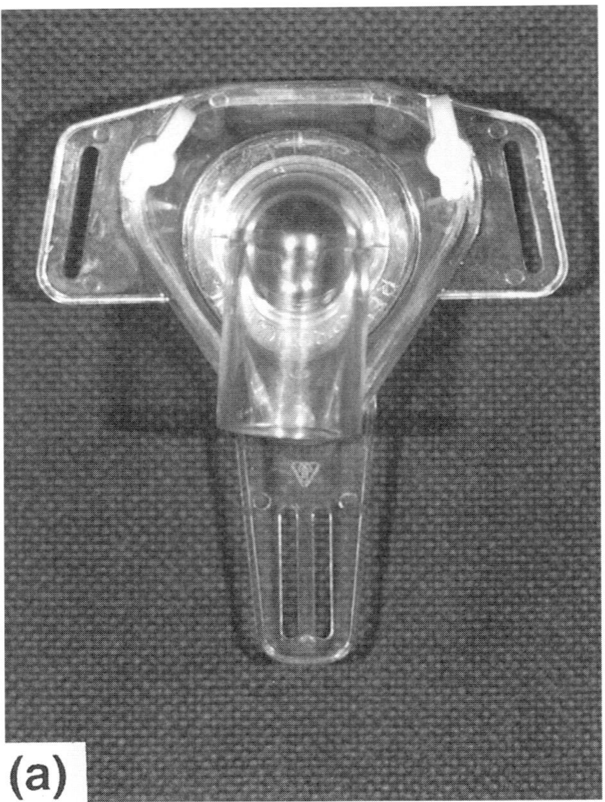

Figure 2 (a) Nasal BLPAP mask. (b) Nasal BLPAP applied to subject. (Photographer Francis Dayrit, M.D.)

(PEEP). It provides higher airway pressures during inspiration than during expiration, but always applies some positive pressure. In addition, the higher positive inspiratory support is generally applied for a longer duration than was true with IPPB. Its use may avoid endotracheal intubation and help reduce respiratory muscle fatigue in the acute asthmatic. One study investigated the use of BLPAP for delivery of inhaled β_2-adrenergic agents versus conventional aerosol therapy. In the study, the BLPAP circuit was set at an inspiratory pressure of 10 cmH_2O and an expiratory airway pressure of 5 cmH_2O, thereby providing a pressure support of 5 cmH_2O. These settings are equivalent to standard ventilator setting of 10 cmH_2O for inspiratory pressure and 5 cmH_2O for PEEP. Subsequent increases in absolute PEFR were greater in the BLPAP group, and this effect was clinically significant (72). This same group also reported on a small set of patients in status asthmaticus who were successfully supported noninvasively with BLPAP, rather than receiving intubation (73). With CPAP and BLPAP facial-skin necrosis with prolonged use was considered a problem. But with soft cushions and stoma paste, this has no longer been a problem. BLPAP can be given nasally adding to patient comfort and ease of access for airway secretions (Figures 2a and b). Also BLPAP is highly leak tolerant and therefore can be used in less-cooperative patients with good results and for longer periods of time without

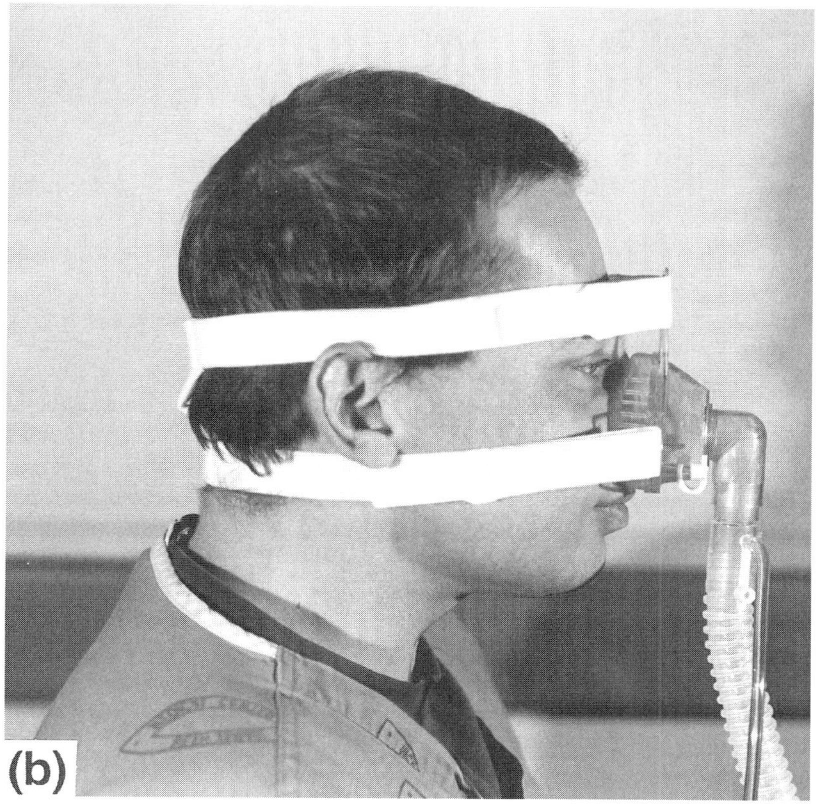

a significant risk of facial skin necrosis. Typically therapy is initiated with inspiratory positive airway pressure (IPAP) of 8–10 and expiratory positive airway pressure (EPAP) of 3–5 cmH_2O, respectively, resulting in a pressure support of 5 cmH_2O. Changes to IPAP and EPAP should be made concomitantly. Asthmatics need higher inspiratory pressure and in one study the final IPAP and EPAP for acute asthmatics was 16 and 5 cmH_2O, respectively (73). Though intriguing, more experience with this modality must be accrued before it can be recommended for ED asthma management.

VI. SPECIAL OR UNCONVENTIONAL THERAPIES

Table 2 lists other potential therapies that could be employed in patients with acute severe asthma not responding adequately to the more conventional therapies. These options may have an application in certain patients, or at individual institutions. Generally these are only a consideration after the patient has been intubated. In the future some of these options may have a more established role in the therapy of ASA, but they require further study. Ideally, most of these should not be employed outside the setting of an investigational protocol. However, it may be helpful for the emergency physician to be familiar with these options for use in particularly desperate situations.

Table 2 The Therapy of Acute Severe Asthma: Special or Unconventional Therapies

1. Inhaled anesthetics
2. Glucagon
3. Bronchoscopy
4. Leukotriene inhibitors
5. Nebulized lidocaine
6. Nitroglycerin
7. Nebulized clonidine
8. Nebulized calcium channel blockers
9. External chest compression
10. Extra corporeal membrane oxygenation
11. Induced hypothermia

A. Inhaled Anesthetic Agents

Volatile inhaled anesthetic agents work by relaxing bronchial smooth muscle directly as well as modulating histamine-induced bronchospasm. Unlike ketamine, they do not increase respiratory secretions, induce laryngeal irritation, or increase intracranial pressure. However, they can cause myocardial depression and induce cardiac dysrhythmias, particularly in the settings of acidosis and hypoxia which are common in ASA (74). Inhaled anesthetic agents have been used as a ''last resort'' treatment for severe asthma for over 100 years (see Chapter 1). Several studies have demonstrated their successful use in ASA, though essentially all the experience has been in intubated patients (75–77). The greatest volume of reported experience has been with inhaled halothane at a 1–2% concentration. However, cases have also been reported of status asthmaticus unresponsive to halothane at 2%, but responding dramatically to diethyl ether inhalation (78). Enflurane is less potent than halothane. Isoflurane and desflurane cause greater airway irritation and should be avoided. Sevoflurane is a newer agent that may be as effective as halothane with fewer cardiac side effects (79). The general efficacy of inhaled anesthetic agents is fairly well established and accepted. However, their use in nonintubated patients is essentially limited to induction in preparation for intubation. More importantly, inhalational anesthesia generally cannot be administered in the emergency department and requires specialized equipment found only in the operating room. Mobilizing those resources can be time consuming. As such, the emergency physician should plan on implementing third-line or other therapies even while attempting to mobilize the resources for inhaled anesthetics.

B. Glucagon

Though the data supporting its use in ASA are extremely limited, most emergency physicians are already familiar with using glucagon for other disorders. As such, it warrants mention as a potential agent in the treatment of acute refractory severe asthma. In a study reported in 1990, 1 mg of intravenous glucagon was shown to reverse acute severe bronchospasm in 8/14 (57%) of patients treated (80). This was accompanied with an increase within 10 min in the measured mean PEFR of over 100 L/min; there were no reported complications. It is deserving of further study.

C. Bronchoscopy

In many patients with ASA, a major cause of airway obstruction is mucus plugging. For this reason, therapeutic bronchoscopy with lavage has been used as an additional supportive measure in patients on mechanical ventilation (81). However, no controlled studies exist demonstrating clear benefit. It is not done routinely in ASA because worsening bronchospasm, i.e., refractory to conventional therapy, is a recognized complication. The procedure involves use of a fiberoptic bronchoscope with a large suction channel and the patient must be heavily sedated prior to the procedure. Airways that are heavily coated or blocked with thick secretions then undergo repeated saline lavage. In some cases, acetylcysteine is cautiously added to the lavage as a dilute (less than 1%) solution. Though this drug can also induce bronchospasm in asthmatics, it is felt to be beneficial in dissolving specific mucus plugs when used in this manner in selected cases (82). There are other potential complications from this procedure, and it should only be performed by practitioners skilled in the technique.

D. Anecdotal or Theoretical Therapies

There are some alternative therapies that have a theoretical basis, or that have been reported as anecdotally useful when all other conventional therapies have failed. Most of these would truly be considered ''last-ditch'' efforts or areas for development of an investigational protocol.

Lidocaine is well known as a local anesthetic. It is known to effectively blunt cough reflexes in the airway prior to tracheal intubation, and most commonly prior to fiberoptic bronchoscopy. In a study of fluids obtained by bronchoalveolar lavage from symptomatic patients with asthma, a potent inhibitor of eosinophils was noted and subsequently identified as the lidocaine used for topical anesthesia (83). Subsequent studies showed that lidocaine appeared to inhibit cytokine-induced eosinophil survival and in many ways mimicked the effects of glucocorticoid administration (84). Hunt and colleagues prospectively studied the effects of nebulized lidocaine (40–160 mg) four times daily in 20 patients with severe chronic asthma requiring high dose corticosteroids (85). These patients did not have acute exacerbations of their asthma. Three patients had no response, four achieved significant reduction in their corticosteroid requirement, and 13 were impressively able to discontinue all use of corticosteroid despite prolonged corticosteroid dependence (mean 6.6 years). There have been numerous anecdotal reports of the effectiveness of nebulized lidocaine in treating refractory, severe coughing disorders of multiple etiologies (86). There is also a case report of preventing the need for intubation in a 40 year old man who presented to an ED with ASA. The patient had severe, intractable coughing that became worse with albuterol treatment. The patient then became lethargic, cyanotic, and hypoxic and attempts at nasotracheal intubation were initiated. However, prior to passing the tube through the cords, 50 mg of lidocaine was injected into the patient's larynx. Within seconds, the coughing abruptly stopped, oxygen saturation improved and intubation was no longer necessary (87). There is also evidence that intravenous lidocaine has effects as a suppressant of coughing during tracheal intubation in some patients (88). There are no reports of complications and further investigation is warranted.

Nitroglycerin has been shown to produce bronchodilation in acute asthma (89). Prostacyclin production in endothelial cells and stimulation of adenyl cyclase have been proposed as possible mechanisms for the bronchodilation (90). Induced hypotension may be a prohibitive side effect (91).

Calcium channel blockers prevent the entry of calcium into the smooth muscle cells via voltage-dependent channels, thereby relaxing smooth muscle, and may therefore be of benefit in asthma (92). Nifedipine and verapamil are the agents that have been most widely reported, but there have been no formal comparisons between agents. Nifedipine does not modify the basal bronchial tone in patients with asthma but does prevent exercise-induced asthma (93). Verapamil, when used via inhalation in high doses (10–20 mg), can dilate the bronchi of both asthmatics and normal subjects (94). One limitation in the use of calcium channel blockers in acute asthma is the appearance of side effects, including hypotension.

Clonidine, an agonist of central and peripheral α_2-adrenergic receptors has shown promise as an aerosol adjunct in the early treatment of status asthmaticus (95). In asthmatic subjects, inhaled clonidine (75 μg via DeVilbiss #40 nebulizer) improved the basal respiratory function and reduced the inflammatory reactions induced by allergens in subjects with extrinsic asthma (96). Like calcium channel blockers, the hypotensive effect of this medication limits its use.

The leukotrienes, especially LTC_4, LTD_4, and LTE_4, have been strongly implicated in the pathophysiology of asthma and have been demonstrated to have multiple harmful effects, including the promotion of bronchoconstriction, mucous secretion, and airway mucosal edema (97). Agents that provide leukotriene-receptor blockade have been shown to improve both bronchospasm and subsequent inflammatory responses (98,99). Two of these agents have been extensively studied in clinical trials and have recently been approved for the chronic treatment of asthma. Zileuton, which inhibits the 5-lipoxygenase pathway, was shown to substantially improve the FEV_1 and decrease the need for β-agonist treatments in adults with mild to moderate asthma (100). Zafirlukast, a leukotriene receptor antagonist, was also shown to improve asthma symptom scores and pulmonary flow functions and decrease the need for β-agonist therapy in patients with mild to moderate asthma (101). In addition, adult and pediatric subjects presenting to the ED with acute asthma exacerbations have been shown to have elevated urinary levels of LTE_4 compared to normals (102,103). This suggests that leukotriene-antagonizing drugs may play an important role in the treatment of acute asthma exacerbations in some subjects. There are currently active trials involving both zileuton and zafirlukast, examining their roles in ED treatment of ASA. In addition, such agents may play a particularly important role in the treatment of patients with aspirin-sensitive asthma (104).

One report described the use of induced hypothermia to manage a particularly severe patient with ASA (105). The intention was to lower the metabolic rate substantially, resulting in decreased carbon dioxide production. This permitted adequate ventilation using smaller tidal volumes with resultant lower airway pressures. The patient survived. Another report described a case of status asthmaticus with severely elevated airway pressures and severe respiratory acidosis that was successfully treated with extracorporeal membrane oxygenation (ECMO). The patient was already refractory to sodium bicarbonate administration. The intention was to provide relatively short-term support to the patient until airway inflammation would respond to corticosteroids, and other therapies. This patient also survived (106).

In particularly severe cases of ASA, one of the problems with pulmonary mechanics is an inability to achieve adequate expiration. Manual compression of the chest and rib cage during expiration has been occasionally reported as a useful and potentially life-saving technique (107,108). In theory, manual expiratory compression of the rib cage could reduce the marked hyperinflation that exists in these patients, by increasing expiratory air flow. However, there have been only anecdotal or brief reports and no clear evidence that the technique is beneficial. There is also no clear evidence that expiratory air flow is actually increased through this maneuver. In theory, external thoracic pressure could actually worsen the patient's condition by further increasing intrathoracic pressure and causing hemodynamic impairment. The published reports describe manual expiratory rib cage compression in spontaneously breathing patients with severe acute asthma. They describe increased expiratory gas volume and suggest improved aerosol delivery. One laboratory investigation suggests that expiratory abdominal compression may be as effective and preferable due to improved cardiac effects (109).

E. Therapies to Use Cautiously and Not at All

In addition to therapies that are advocated in the treatment of ASA, there are also some therapies to be avoided. Historically, it was recommended that all patients with ASA receive aggressive IV fluids. It was thought that IV fluid administration would thin bronchial secretions and assist with their clearance. This effect of fluids on bronchial secretions is now known not to be true (110). Additionally, a subset of asthmatic patients are poorly tolerant of the additional IV fluids and can theoretically develop pulmonary edema through a combination of negative intrapleural pressures, hydrostatic forces, and hypo-osmolarity (111). In children, approximately 5% dehydration is common producing an appropriate secretion of antidiuretic hormone (112–114). Children who were dyspneic for more than 24 hr had more evidence of dehydration (113). Rehydration did not affect the rate of recovery from acute asthma, however. In children, the fluid infusions should be at 50 mL/kg/24 hr (114). At least in adults, IV fluids should only be provided at maintenance rates in patients with ASA, unless there is compelling evidence that they are dehydrated or develop hypotension. Dehydration theoretically could produce decreased perfusion, and asthma is characterized in part by areas of the lung that are ventilated but not perfused, which constitutes part of the dead space of the lung. Intravenous fluid infusion of only 250–500 mL has reduced the dead space by approximately 5% in mechanically ventilated severe asthmatics. Therefore, judicious treatment of dehydration even in adult severe asthmatics may be beneficial (115).

The use of mucolytic agents has presently no place in the acute treatment of severe asthma. These agents, such as n-acetylcysteine, can actually be irritating to the airways and cause increasing bronchoconstriction, as well as inducing nausea and vomiting (116). Similar precautions apply to the acute use of cromolyn. Some medications, such as morphine, promote histamine release and, in theory, may worsen asthma.

Sedatives also have no place in the ED treatment of patients with ASA, up to the point of intubation. Despite appearances of patient anxiety and the presence of tremors, sedatives have no benefit in acute severe asthma. Instead, they are more likely to cause respiratory depression and increase the frequency of intubation. At least one sedative agent, midazolam, has actually been shown to increase total pulmonary resistance, providing further evidence that sedative drugs are contraindicated in this setting (117).

F. Disposition

Most patients presenting to the emergency department with ASA will require subsequent admission to the hospital (see Chapter 31). A minority will demonstrate substantial improvement both subjectively as well as by objective measures after receiving routine care measures in the emergency department. Patients having flow rates in the "mild" range and remaining stable during a period of observation after completion of all bronchodilator treatments, can be discharged if they have a reliable home situation, including the ability to fill prescriptions and a means of return transport. Patients showing mild to moderate improvement to routine care therapies in the emergency department will generally require admission to an unmonitored hospital floor bed. However, those patients that persist with severe symptoms despite routine care therapies, or who require second- or third-line therapies, are safest admitted to a monitored bed. It must be a setting where the patients respiratory status can be monitored closely and frequent bronchodilator therapy reliably provided. The majority of patients, even in the most severe group, will show improvement over a 24 hr period. For those emergency departments with the option, admission to an ED observation unit may be just as effective for patients not deteriorating or approaching intubation.

Patients whose symptoms remain very severe or deteriorate, are best cared for in an ICU. These patients can require sudden intubation. They must be in a setting where respiratory monitoring is routine and the necessary resources for intubation immediately available. Failure to provide rapid intubation, when needed, is an identified cause of preventable mortality in ASA patients.

REFERENCES

1. Busey J, Fenger E, Hepper J, et al. Management of status asthmaticus. Am Rev Respir Dis 1968; 97:735–736.
2. Bone R, Calverley P, Chapman K, et al. The international clinical respiratory group: Special report. Chest 1992; 101:1420–1424.
3. Marquette C, Saulnier F, Leroy O, et al. Long-term prognosis of near-fatal asthma. Am Rev Respir Dis 1992; 146:76–81.
4. Burney PGJ. Asthma mortality: England and Wales. J Allergy Clin Immunol 1987; 80(pt2): 379–382.
5. Benatar S. Fatal asthma. N Engl J Med 1986; 314:423–428.
6. Strunk R, Mrazek D, Wolfson F, et al. Physiologic and psychological characteristics associated with deaths due to asthma in childhood. JAMA 1985; 254:1193–1198.
7. Mountain R, Heffner J, Brackett N, et al. Acid-base disturbances in acute asthma. Chest 1990; 98:651–655.
8. Rea HH, Scragg R, Jackson R, et al. A case control study of deaths from asthma. Thorax 1986; 41:833–839.
9. Mullen M, Mullen B, Carey M. The association between beta-agonist use and death from asthma: A meta-analytic integration of case-control studies. JAMA 1993; 270:1842–1845.
10. Ziment I. Beta-adrenergic agonist toxicity: Less of a problem, more of a perception. Chest 1993; 103:591–597.
11. Colacone A, Afilalo M, Wokove N, et al. The comparison of albuterol administered by metered dose inhaler and holding chamber or wet nebulizer in acute asthma. Chest 1993; 104: 835–841.
12. Lin R, Sauter D, Newman I, et al. Continuous versus intermittent albuterol nebulization in the treatment of acute asthma. Ann Emerg Med 1993; 22:1847–1853.
13. Rudnitsky G, Eberlein R, Schoffstall J, et al. comparison of intermittent and continuously nebulized albuterol for treatment of asthma in an urban emergency department. Ann Emerg Med 1993; 22:1842–1846.
14. Newhouse MT, Fuller HD. Rose is a rose is a rose? Aerosol therapy in ventilated patients:

Nebulizers versus metered dose inhalers-a continuing controversy. Am Rev Respir Dis 1993; 148:1444–1446.
15. Olshaker J, Jerrard D, Barish RA, et al. The efficacy and safety of a continuous albuterol protocol for the treatment of acute adult asthma attacks. Am J Emerg Med 1993; 11:131–133.
16. Intermittent Positive Pressure Breathing Trial Group. Intermittent positive pressure breathing therapy of chronic obstructive pulmonary disease: A clinical trial. Ann Intern Med 1983; 99:612–620.
17. Penna AC, Dawson KP, Manglick P, et al. Systemic absorption of salbutamol following nebulizer delivery in acute asthma. Acta Paediatr 1993, 82:963–966.
18. Morris HG. An update on treatment of asthma with inhaled steroids, Allergy Proc 1987; 8: 85–94.
19. Haskell R, Wong B, Hansen J. A double-blind, randomized clinical trial of methylprednisolone in status asthmaticus. Arch Intern Med 1983; 143:1324–1327.
20. Littenberg B, Gluck E. A controlled trial of methylprednisolone in the emergency treatment of acute asthma. N Engl J Med 1986; 314:1324–1327.
21. McNamara R, Rubin P. Intramuscular methylprednisolone acetate for the prevention of relapse in acute asthma. Ann Emerg Med 1993; 22:1829–1835.
22. Storr J, Barell E, Barry W, et al. Effect of a single oral dose of prednisone in acute childhood asthma. Lancet 1987; 1:879–882.
23. McFadden ER. Use of steroids in asthma. Am Rev Respir Dis 1993; 147:1306–1310.
24. Rebuck A, Chapman K, Abboud R, et al. Nebulized anticholinergic and sympathomimetic treatment of asthma and chronic obstructive airway disease in the emergency room. Am J Med 1987; 82:59–64.
25. Ward M, MacFarlane J, Davies D. A place for ipratropium bromide in the treatment of severe acute asthma. Br J Dis Chest 1985; 79:374–378.
26. Patrick D, Dales R, Stark R, et al. Severe exacerbations of COPD and asthma: Incremental benefit of adding ipratropium to usual therapy. Chest 1990; 98:295–297.
27. Oates J, Wood A. Ipratropium bromide. N Engl J Med 1988; 319:486–493.
28. Skobeloff E, Spivey W, McNamara R, et al. Intravenous magnesium sulfate for the treatment of asthma in the emergency department. JAMA 1989; 262:1210–1213.
29. Tiffany B, Berk W, Todd K, et al. Magnesium bolus or infusion fails to improve spirometric performance in acute asthma exacerbations [abstract]. Ann Emerg Med 1992; 21:646.
30. Green S, Rothrock S. Intravenous magnesium for acute asthma: Failure to decrease emergency treatment duration or need for hospitalization. Ann Emerg Med 1992; 21:260–265.
31. Bloch H, Silverman R, Mancheije N, et al. Intravenous magnesium sulfate as an adjunct in the treatment of acute asthma. Chest 1995; 107:1576–1581.
32. Milgrom H, Bender B. Current issues in the use of theophylline. Am Rev Respir Dis 1993; 147(suppl):S33–S39.
33. Barnes PJ. Endogenous catecholamines and asthma, J Allergy Clin Immunol 1986; 7:791–795.
34. Murphy D, McDermott M, Rydman R, et al. Aminophylline in the treatment of acute asthma when beta$_2$-adrenergics and steroids are provided. Arch Intern Med 1993; 153:1784–1788.
35. Wrenn K, Slovis C, Murphy F, et al. Aminophylline therapy for acute bronchospastic disease in the emergency room. Ann Intern Med 1991; 115:241–247.
36. Swedish Society of Chest Medicine. High dose inhaled versus intravenous salbutamol combined with theophylline in severe acute asthma. Eur Respir J 1990; 3:163–170.
37. Salmeron S, Brochard L, Mal H, et al. Nebulised versus intravenous albuterol in hypercapnic acute asthma. Am J Respir Crit Care Med 1994; 149:1466–1470.
38. Appel D, Karpel JP, Sherman M. Epinephrine improves expiratory flow rates in patients with asthma who do not respond to inhaled metaproterenol sulfate. J Allergy Clin Immunol 1989; 84:90–98.

39. Cydulka R, Davison R, Grammer I, et al. The use of epinephrine in the treatment of older adult asthmatics. Ann Emerg Med 1988; 17:322–326.
40. Bishop GF, Hillman KM. Acute severe asthma. Int Care World 1993; 10:166–171.
41. Matson JR, Loughlin GM, Strunk RC. Myocardial ischemia, complicating the use of isoproterenol in asthmatic children. J Pediatr 1978; 92:776–778.
42. Kurland G, Williams J, Lewiston N. Fatal myocardial toxicity during continuous infusion intravenous isoproterenol during therapy of asthma. J Allergy Clin Immunol 1979; 63:107–111.
43. Bohn D, Kalloghlian A, Jenkins J, et al. Intravenous salbutamol in the treatment of status asthmaticus in children. Crit Care Med 1984; 12:892–895.
44. British Thoracic Society. Guidelines for management of asthma in adults. II. Acute severe asthma. Br Med J 1990; 301:797–800.
45. Barach AL. The use of helium in the treatment of asthma and obstructive lesions in the larynx and trachea. Ann Intern Med 1935; 9:739–765.
46. McGee D, Wald DA, Hinchliffe S. Helium-oxygen therapy in the emergency department. J Emerg Med 1997; 15(3):291–296.
47. Gluck EH, Onorato DJ, Castriotta R. Helium-oxygen mixtures in intubated patients with status asthmaticus and respiratory acidosis. Chest 1990; 98:693–698.
48. Kudukis TM, Manthous CA, Schmidt GA, et al. Inhaled helium-oxygen revisited: effect of inhaled helium-oxygen during the treatment of status asthmaticus in children. J Pediatr 1997; 130(2):217–224.
49. Carter ER, Webb CR, Moffitt DR. Evaluation of heliox in children hospitalized with acute severe asthma. A randomized crossover trial. Chest 1996; 109(5):1256–1261.
50. Austan F. Heliox inhalation in status asthmaticus and respiratory acidemia: a brief report. Heart Lung 1996; 25(2):155–157.
51. Kass JE, Castriotta RJ. Heliox therapy in acute severe asthma. Chest 1995; 107(3):757–760.
52. Fisher M. Ketamine for status asthmaticus. Anesthesia 1977; 32:771–772.
53. Betts E, Parkin C. Use of ketamine in an asthmatic child. Anesth Analg 1971; 50:420–421.
54. Sarma V. Ketamine and asthma. Acta Scand 1992; 36:1507–1510.
55. Green S, Johnson N. Ketamine sedation for pediatric procedures. 2. Review and implications. Ann Emerg Med 1990; 19:1033–1046.
56. L'Homedieu C, Arens J. The use of ketamine for the emergency intubation of patients with status asthmaticus. Ann Emerg Med 1987; 16:568–571.
57. Rock M, De La Rocha R, L'Hommedieu C, et al. Use of ketamine in asthmatic children to treat respiratory failure refractory to conventional therapy. Crit Care Med 1986; 14:514–516.
58. Hemmingsen C, Kielsen P, Ordorico J. Ketamine in the treatment of bronchospasm during mechanical ventilation. Am J Emerg Med 1994; 12:417–420.
59. Howton JC, Rose J, Duffy S, et al. Randomized, double-blind, placebo-controlled trial of intravenous ketamine in acute asthma. Ann Emerg Med 1996; 27:170–175.
60. Choo-Kang YFJ, Grant IWB. Comparison of two methods of administering bronchodilator aerosol to asthmatic patients. Br Med J 1975; 2:119–120.
61. Cayton RM, Webber B, Paterson JW, Clark TJH. A comparison of salbutamol given by pressure-packed aerosol or nebulization via IPPB in acute asthma. Br J Dis Chest 1978; 72: 222–224.
62. Ayers SM, Kozam RL, Lukas DS. The effects of intermittent positive pressure breathing on intrathoracic pressure, pulmonary mechanics, and the work of breathing. Am Rev Respir Dis 1963; 87:370–379.
63. Gonzalez ER, Burke TG. Review of the status of intermittent positive pressure breathing therapy. Drug Intell Clin Pharm 1984; 18:974–976.

64. Murray JF. Review of the state of the art in intermittent positive pressure breathing therapy. Am Rev Resp Dis 1974; 110(suppl):193–199.
65. Dolovich MB, Dermott K, Wolff RK, et al. Pulmonary aerosol deposition in chronic bronchitis: Intermittent positive pressure breathing versus quiet breathing. Am Rev Respir Dis 1977; 397–402.
66. Fergusson RJ, Carmichael J, Rafferty P, et al. Nebulized salbutamol in life-threatening asthma: Is IPPB necessary? Br J Dis Chest 1983; 77:255–261.
67. Duncan AW, Oh TE, Hillman DR. PEEP and CPAP. Anaesth Intens Care 1986; 14:236–250.
68. Martin JG, Shore S, Engel LA. Effect of continuous positive airway pressure on respiratory mechanics and pattern of breathing in induced asthma. Am Rev Respir Dis 1982; 126:812–817.
69. Shivaram U, Donath J, Khan FA, Juliano J. Effects of continuous positive airway pressure in acute asthma. Respiration 1987; 52:157–162.
70. Christensen EF, Nørregaard O, Jensen LW, Dahl R. Inhaled $Beta_2$ agonist and positive expiratory pressure in bronchial asthma. Chest 1993; 104:1108–1113.
71. Lin H-C, Wang C-H, Yang C-T, et al. Effect of nasal continuous positive airway pressure on methacholine-induced bronchospasm. Respir Med 1995; 89:121–128.
72. Pollack CV, Fleisch KB, Dowsey K. Treatment of acute bronchospasm with Beta adrenergic agonist aerosols delivered by a nasal bilevel positive airway pressure circuit. Ann Emerg Med 1995; 26:552–557.
73. Pollack CV, Torres MT, Alexander L. Feasibility study of the use of bilevel positive airway pressure for respiratory support in the emergency department. Ann Emerg Med 1996; 27: 189–192.
74. Roizen M, Stevens W. Multiform ventricular tachycardia due to the interaction of aminophyline and halothane. Anesth Analg 1978; 57:738–741.
75. Saulnier FF, Durocher AV, Deturck RA, et al. Respiratory and hemodynamic effects of halothane in status asthmaticus. Intensive Care Med 1990; 16:104–107.
76. Bierman M, Brown M, Muren O, et al. Prolonged isoflurane anesthesia in status asthmaticus. Crit Care Med 1986; 14:832–833.
77. Echeverria M, Gelb AW, Wexler Hr, et al. Enflurane and halothane in status asthmaticus. Chest 1986; 89:152–154.
78. Robertson C, Steedman D, Sinclair C, et al. Use of ether in life-threatening acute severe asthma. Lancet 1985; 1:187–188.
79. Mitchell RG, Nichol N, Goldie AS, et al. Inhalational anaesthesia in emergency medicine using a new volatile—sevoflurane. J Accid Emerg Med 1997; 14:328–330.
80. Wilson JE, Nelson RN. Glucagon as a therapeutic agent in the treatment of asthma. J Emerg Med 1990; 8:127–130.
81. Smith DL, Deshazo RD. Bronchoalveolar lavage in asthma. Am Rev Respir Dis 1993; 148: 523–526.
82. Millman M, Millman FM, Goldstein IM, et al. Use of acetylcysteine in bronchial asthma-another look. Ann Allergy 1985; 54:294–296.
83. Ohashi Y, Motojima S, Fukuda T, et al. Airway hyperresponsiveness, increased intracellular spaces of bronchial epithelium, and increased infiltration of eosinophils and lymphocytes in bronchial mucosa in asthma. Am Rev Respir Dis 1992; 145:1469–1476.
84. Wallen N, Kita H, Weiler D, et al. Glucocorticoids inhibit cytokine-mediated eosinophil survival. J Immunol 1991; 147:3490–3495.
85. Hunt LW, Swedlund HA, Bleich GJ. Effective nebulized lidocaine on severe glucocorticoid-dependent asthma. Mayo Clin Proc 1996; 71:361–368.
86. Trochenberg S. Nebulized lidocaine and the treatment of refractory cough. Chest 1994; 105: 1592–1594.

87. Rabold M, Tintinalli J. Tracheal lidocaine stops airway hyper responsiveness (letter). Ann Emerg Med 1995; 25:432.
88. Yukioka H, Hayashi M, Terai T, et al. Intravenous lidocaine as a suppressant of coughing during tracheal intubation in elderly patients. Anesth Analg 1993; 77:309–312.
89. Kennedy T, Summer WR, Sylvester J, et al. Airway response to sublingual nitroglycerin in acute asthma. JAMA 1981; 246:145–147.
90. Goldstein JA. Nitroglycerin therapy of asthma. Chest 1984; 3:449–450.
91. Levin RI, Jaffe EA, Weksler BB, et al. Nitroglycerin stimulates synthesis of prostacyclin by cultured human endothelial cells. J Clin Invest 1981; 67:762–679.
92. Russi EW, Ahmed T. Calcium and calcium antagonist in airway disease. A review. Chest 1984; 86:475–482.
93. Cuss FM, Barnes PJ. The effect of inhaled nifedipine on bronchial reactivity to histamine in man. J Allergy Clin Immunol 1985; 76:718–723.
94. Popa VT, Somani P, Simon V. The effect of inhaled verapamil on resting bronchial tone and airway contractions induced by histamine and acetylcholine in normal and asthmatic subjects. Am Rev Respir Dis 1984; 130:1006–1013.
95. Lindgren BR, Ekstrom T, Andersson RG. The effect of inhaled clonidine in patients with asthma. Am Rev Respir Dis 1986; 134:266–269.
96. Lindgren BR, Brundin A, Andersson RG. Inhibitory effects of clonidine on the allergen-induced wheal-and-flare reactions in patients with extrinsic asthma. J Allergy Clin Immunol 1987; 79:941–946.
97. Griffin M, Weiss W, Leitch A, et al. Effects of leukotriene D on the airways in asthma. N Engl J Med 1983; 308:436–439.
98. Barnes N, Piper P, Costello J. Comparative effects of inhaled leukotriene C_4, leukotriene D_4, and histamine in normal human subjects. Thorax 1984; 39:500–504.
99. Jones T, Zamboni R, Belley M. Pharmacology of L-660,711 (MF-571): a novel potent and selective leukotriene D_4 receptor antagonist. Can J Physiol Pharmacol 1988; 67:17–28.
100. Israel E, Reuben P, Kemp JP, et al. The effect of inhibition of five-lypoxygenase by Zileuton in mild-to-moderate asthma. Ann Intern Med 1993; 119:1059–1066.
101. O'Byrne PM, Israel E, Drazen JM. Antileukotrienes in the treatment of asthma. Ann Intern Med 1997; 127:472–480.
102. Sampson AP, Green CP, Spencer DA, et al. Leukotrienes in the blood and urine in children with acute asthma. An NY Acad Sci 1991; 629:437–439.
103. Drazen JM, O'Brien J, Sparrow D, et al. Recovery of leukotriene E_4 from the urine of subjects with airway obstruction. Am Rev Resp Dis 1992; 146:104–108.
104. Israel E, Fischer AR, Rosenberg MA, et al. The pivotal role of five-lipoxygenase products and the reaction of aspirin-sensitive asthmatics to aspirin. Am Rev Respir Dis 1993; 148: 1447–1451.
105. Browning D, Goodrum DT. Treatment of acute severe asthma assisted by hypothermia. Anaesthesia 1992; 47:223–225.
106. Shapiro MB, Kleaveland AC, Bartlett RH. Extracorporeal life support for status asthmaticus. Chest 1993; 103:1651–1655.
107. Watts JM. Thoracic compression for asthma. Chest 1984; 86:505.
108. Fisher MM, Bowey CJ, Ladd-Hudson K. External chest compression in acute asthma: a preliminary study. Crit Care Med 1989; 17:686–687.
109. Van Der Touw T, Tully A, Amis TC, et al. Cardio-respiratory consequences of expiratory chest wall compression during mechanical ventilation and severe hyperinflation. Crit Care Med 1993; 21:1908–1914.
110. Marchette LC, Marchette BE, Abraham WM et al. The effect of systemic hydration on normal and impaired mucociliary function. Pediatr Pulmonol 1985; 1:107–111.
111. Stalcup SA, Mellins RB. Mechanical forces producing pulmonary edema in acute asthma. N Engl J Med 1977; 297:592–596.

112. Straub PW, Buhlman AA, Rossier PW. Hypovolaemia in status asthmaticus. Lancet 1969; 2:923–926.
113. Iikura Y, Odajima Y, Akazawa A, et al. Antidiuretic hormone in acute asthma in children: effects of medication on serum levels and clinical course. Allergy Proc 1989; 10:197–201.
114. Potter PC, Klein M, Weinberg EG. Hydration in severe acute asthma. Arch Dis Child 1991; 66:216–219.
115. Manthous CA, Goulding P. The effect of volume infusion on dead space in mechanically ventilated patients with severe acute asthma. Chest 1997; 112:843–846.
116. Bernstein IL, Ausdenmoore RW. Iatrogenic bronchospasm occurring during clinical trials of a new mucolytic agent, acetylcysteine. Am Rev Respir Dis 1964; 46:469–473.
117. Molliex S, Dureuil B, Montravers P, et al. Effects of midazolam on respiratory muscles in humans. Anesth Analg 1993; 77:592–597.

26

Intubation of the Asthma Patient

Martin S. Kohn
The Brooklyn Hospital Center, member of New York–Presbyterian Hospitals, Weill Medical College of Cornell University, Brooklyn, and New York University School of Medicine, New York, New York

In most cases of life-threatening respiratory distress, endotracheal intubation is a rapid and appropriate way of avoiding catastrophe with relatively little adverse consequence. In the case of the asthmatic patient, however, endotracheal intubation creates its own set of difficult problems. The decision to intubate the asthmatic patient in the emergency department (ED) requires a refined judgment of risks and benefits that is, essentially, unique. Controversy exists with respect to the decision to intubate, the method of intubation, and postintubation management.

Fortunately, the vast majority of asthmatic patients can be managed without endotracheal intubation. Aggressive therapy will reverse even very severe bronchospasm in most patients. Numerous series indicate that only small percentages of asthmatic patients need to be intubated. Braman and Kaemmerlen reported that of 2094 patients admitted for asthma over a 10-yr period (1978–1987), 80 were admitted to the intensive care unit (ICU), and only 24 required mechanical ventilation (1). Mountain and Sahn, in reviewing patients that presented with hypercapnia, noted that only 5 of 61 required intubation (2). Clearly, the intubation of an asthmatic patient is, and should be, a rare event.

The purpose of this discussion is to review airway management principles in asthma, specifically with respect to indications for endotracheal intubation, potential adverse consequences of intubation, the intubation process itself, and the immediate postintubation period. Generally the indications for intubation of the asthmatic patient fall into four categories, which are listed Table 1. The first two categories are obvious and demand no clinical judgment. The latter two categories are the ones that are the challenge.

In the past, it was argued that the development of respiratory acidosis, or a rising $Paco_2$, was an indication for intubation. As was the case with many "standards," when the axiom was actually studied, it did not hold up. Most asthmatics with respiratory acidosis can be managed without intubation (3). Even a very high $Paco_2$, in and of itself, may not require intubation, as long as the patient has a normal mental status and is responsive

Table 1 Categories for Intubation Indications

1. Cardiac arrest
2. Respiratory arrest or profound bradypnea
3. Physical exhaustion
4. Altered mental status

to therapy. Progressively increasing $Paco_2$, unresponsive to therapy, and usually associated with a changing mental status, is an indication for intubation.

Numerous efforts have been made to codify the criteria for intubation, resulting in lengthy arrays of indications. The sets compiled by various authors usually have several indications in common, and then several unique ones. The lengthy lists of criteria seem to be an effort to quantitate the general categories 3 and 4 from Table 1. Examples typical of the list of indications are present in Table 2 and Table 3.

As can be seen, some of the criteria, such as "persistent lactic acidosis," by virtue of both time frame and practicality, are not applicable to the ED. Inherent in the nature of EDs is the tenet that an asthma patient's tenure will be relatively brief. A patient will arrive, and either improve and be discharged within a few hours, or not improve and be admitted to the hospital within about 4–6 hr. The style of previous decades, when an asthma patient might frequently spend 12 or 24 hours under the care of the emergency physician, is much less common.

For most patients with bronchospasm in the ED, blood gases are not necessary. If a patient is sick enough to merit a blood gas, the question of intubation has probably been considered. In such a patient, the observation of the patient's clinical condition is more valuable than laboratory testing (6). In the more recent literature, the role of clinical assessment and observation of the patient's course, as indicators for intubation, rather than specific criteria, have begun to dominate (7,8). Although blood gases continue to have a role, such as in a patient who is overtly hypoxic ($po_2 < 60$ mmHg) despite maximum oxygen delivery, clinical observation will likely be the determinant in intubating the asthma patient. With the hypercarbic patient, intubation is appropriate only if the patient does not respond to maximal pharmacological therapy, as most patients will reverse a respiratory acidosis within 2–4 hr (2).

All the indicators in Table 4 are inherently subjective, and although different authors

Table 2 Indications for Mechanical Ventilation (1990)

Respiratory rates climbing > 40
Inability to speak
Pulsus paradoxus climbing or falling in the exhausted patient
Patient subjective sense of exhaustion
Altered sensorium
Barotrauma complicating status asthmaticus
Unresolving lactic acidosis
Diaphoresis in the recumbent position
Silent chest despite respiratory effort
Elevation of pco_2 with progressive dyspnea

Source: Ref. 4, Table 4.

Table 3 Indications for Intubation and Mechanical Ventilation (1984)

Clinical findings[a]
Diminished level of consciousness
Diminished response to pain
Progressive exhaustion
Absent breath sounds and wheezing
Fixed chest
Pulsus paradoxus
Arterial blood gas levels
pH less than 7.2
Carbon dioxide pressure
Increasing by more than 5 mm Hg/hr
Greater than 55 to 70 mm Hg
Oxygen pressure less than 60 mm Hg
Evidence on chest X-ray films
Pneumothorax
Pneumomediastinum
Results of spirometric tests
Forced expiratory volume in 1 second less than 500 ml or vital capacity less than 1000 ml and failing to improve with bronchodilators.

[a] Combined with decreasing arterial blood gas levels.
Source: Ref. 5, Table 1.

may propose threshold values for some of the laboratory-based criteria, there is little, if any, support in the literature for any firm cutoff value. The clinical criteria need to be invoked with care. For example, under appropriate circumstances an asthmatic patient who was comfortable in the recumbent position could indicate that symptoms are minimal. Most patients in acute respiratory distress will want to sit up. Recumbency, with diaphoresis or other signs of discomfort, may represent progressive exhaustion, because the patient is too tired to sit up (9). Other manifestations of physical exhaustion, could include decreasing respiratory effort, head nod, or the patient's complaint of feeling tired. Altered mental status may manifest as confusion, inability to follow instructions or respond to questions, agitation, or combativeness. Such changes could result from a combination of hypoxia, acidosis or fatigue. What is clear, no matter how difficult or ambiguous the criteria might be, is that once a patient demonstrates the need for intubation delay is dangerous. Since so few asthmatic patients ever need to be intubated, few emergency

Table 4 Consensus Indicators for Intubation

Clinical
Cardiac arrest
Respiratory arrest
Altered mental status
Progressive exhaustion (3)
Silent chest (3)
Laboratory
Severe hypoxia with maximal oxygen delivery
Failure to reverse severe respiratory acidosis despite intensive therapy

physicians will have a substantial experience with the situation, which makes decision making more difficult. Some authors have grouped critically ill asthmatic patients (those who were candidates for intubation) into categories that may give some guidance in the clinical decision-making area.

It has been observed that the asthmatic who gets into serious trouble shows one of three temporal patterns (10–12). First, there is the group that comes to the ED with a sudden and extremely severe bout of bronchospasm. The second is a group that shows gradual, persistent deterioration. The third is a group that presents to the ED with relatively severe, and perhaps labile bronchospasm, that may respond minimally to therapy and then experiences an abrupt deterioration. Such a classification meets most of our intuitive feelings about the presentation of acute asthmatic patients.

In the first group, the time between onset of symptoms and intubation was reported as averaging three hours (10). Breath sounds were either absent or markedly diminished, and mental status was altered. Fortunately, this group of patients also responded well to intubation, and corrected more quickly than patients in the other two groups. The other two groups were characterized by patients who had previous history of similar severe episodes of asthma with similar patterns of deterioration. The experience in such groups of patients emphasizes the value of clinical history. If a patient describes previous episodes of deterioration, either abrupt or progressive, the patient could be in group at high risk for needing airway management.

There has been some effort to identify risk factors associated with the increased likelihood of a patient needing intubation. Although it is possible to identify factors that are associated with intubation, they seem to be similar to the factors that are generally associated with more severe asthma (3,13–17). Factors that contribute to increased risk of intubation include, not surprisingly, history of prior intubation, admission to the hospital for asthma, prior ED visit for asthma, respiratory infection, steroid dependence, and smoking. In younger patients, second-hand smoke seems be a precipitant (13). In addition, the existence of psychosocial problems or family dysfunction represent substantial risks (15). Curiously, LeSon's work seems to indicate that the likelihood of intubation is lower in the winter, when acute asthma is often more prevalent, than it is in the summer (13–16). Using his data in adults (age greater than 20, N = 375), for example, a statistical calculation shows the likelihood of intubation in the summer is greater than in the winter with a significance of $p < .004$ (16). The number of intubations was larger in the summer both in absolute terms and as a fraction of total patients. One possible explanation is that patients that have asthma symptoms in the summer have more severe disease than other patients, who usually improve during the summer. Although risk factors may provide some insight into the nature of severe asthma, the factors are a population statistic. Individual patients with none of the risk factors may still require intubation. Thus, close clinical observation of patients who either arrive in the ED in a serious state, or deteriorate in the ED, is still the most reliable method (3,6,7).

Once the decision to intubate has been made, controversy surrounds the method to achieve intubation. The literature reveals strong, but contradictory, preferences. The choices appear to be:

1. Nasotracheal intubation
2. Awake orotracheal intubation
3. Orotracheal intubation with sedation
4. Orotracheal intubation with sedation and neuromuscular blockade

The authorities who prefer nasotracheal intubation cite the minimal need for sedation, rapidity of preparation, greater postintubation comfort for the awake patient and the maintenance of semiupright posture, maintenance of spontaneous respiration, and decreased likelihood of aspiration as compelling advantages (3,8). However, they generally advocate orotracheal intubation in the most critical situations. Contraindications to nasotracheal intubation are nasal polyps, which may occur in up to one-third of asthma patients (18), coagulation disorder or thrombocytopenia or abnormal nasal anatomy. In addition to topical anesthetics and vasoconstrictors in the nose, topical hypopharyngeal anesthesia is necessary to minimize reactive bronchospasm.

The advocates of orotracheal intubation prefer the advantages of a larger sized endotracheal tube, direct visualization, and the relative ease of obtaining pharyngeal anesthesia (4,5,19). They also express concern about the complications of nasotracheal intubation, including profuse epistaxis and purulent sinusitis. There have not been any direct comparisons between the two techniques in the asthmatic patient, and given the infrequency with which asthma patients must be intubated, it is unlikely that there will be such a study.

The issue of sedation and/or neuromuscular blockade is similarly marked by strong advocates of opposing positions. Bellomo prefers "awake" intubation, i.e., without sedation, either orally or nasally, with only local anesthesia (11). An underlying concept for advocates for intubation without sedation is the concern about rendering a patient apneic. If the patient can then not be intubated, you are left with supporting ventilation by bag-valve-mask in an apneic patient with severe bronchospasm, which is a difficult task.

On the other hand, once you have decided that the patient needs intubation, sedation often allows for a more rapid, less traumatic control of the airway. If sedation is advisable, an intravenous benzodiazepine (midazolam or diazepam), ketamine (often in concert with a benzodiazepine, to minimize the disassociative reaction that may follow use of ketamine), is commonly recommended (4,5,11,19,20). Midazolam has the advantage of being shorter acting than diazepam, which gives some measure of protection if the intubation is difficult. The recommended doses for midazolam vary, with some authors recommending repeated 1 to 2 mg boluses, and others advocating initial doses of up to 5 mg. Initial doses for diazepam are generally 5–10 mg, with increments of 2.5 to 10 mg as needed. On occasion large doses may be necessary (4–6,21).

Ketamine is valuable in the critically ill asthma patient because it is known to reduce bronchospasm both directly, by a possible effect on bronchial smooth muscle, and indirectly, by increasing levels of catecholamines (20). Ketamine has been reported to relieve bronchospasm in mechanically ventilated patients when the patients were not responding to other therapy (20,22). Since ketamine may induce bronchorrhea in children, premedication with atropine (0.01 mg/kg, with a minimum of 0.1 mg) is used.

Walls is a strong advocate of rapid sequence intubation, using succinylcholine [1.5 mg/kg intravenous (IV) push], followed immediately by ketamine (1.0–1.5 mg/kg IV) to obtain optimal intubation conditions (23). The use of lidocaine (1.0 mg/kg IV immediately before giving succinylcholine) may help reduce airway reactivity and can be supplemented with topical anesthesia. Alternatively, lidocaine may be administered via the endotracheal tube. He further argues that, since most intubated asthmatic patients will be sedated and likely paralyzed, there is no contraindication to sedation and paralysis for the intubation process.

The authorities who recommend neuromuscular blockade sometimes prefer a nondepolarizing blocker (such as vecuronium) to a depolarizing blocker (succinylcholine) because of a concern that succinylcholine causes more histamine release, with the potential for worsening bronchospasm (5). Despite the widely expressed concerned about histamine release precipitated by succinylcholine, there is no recent report of any adverse consequence from the use of succinylcholine in an acute asthmatic patient. Succinylcholine also may cause an increase in vagal tone, particularly in children. Therefore, in young patients prophylactic treatment with atropine (0.1 mg/kg, with a minimum of 0.1 mg) is frequently given.

Assessment of the risk of succinylcholine as a precipitant of bronchospasm is difficult because every aspect of airway intervention can irritate the airway. The tube itself, or airway manipulation, may be irritants that trigger bronchospasm (3–5,24). Wheezing has been associated with sedative-hypnotic agents and, in the operative environment, with inhalation anesthetics (24,25). Studies comparing the response of both asthmatic and non-asthmatic patients to anesthesia induction determined that bronchospasm can occur in both groups of patients (24,25). Thus, it has to be assumed that although the use of neuromuscular blockers may carry a risk of increased bronchospasm, that risk is small, and needs to be balanced against the need for rapid, atraumatic airway control.

The risk-benefit decision could be made easier by the use of an additional medication that could reduce or eliminate the risk of worsening bronchospasm. Pizov et al. reported on wheezing in asthmatic and nonasthmatic patients given succinylcholine and one of three sedatives prior to intubation for surgery (25). Fifteen of 59 asthma patients developed wheezing during induction, while six of 96 nonasthmatics wheezed. The patients had been given either a barbiturate or propofol as sedative. None of the 48 patients receiving propofol (2.5 mg/kg), either asthmatic [16] or nonasthmatic [32], developed wheezing, whereas 15 of 43 patients receiving a barbiturate developed wheezing, suggesting possible value for propofol as the sedative agent for asthmatics. In all cases, the wheezing was mild, and even those patients treated with β-adrenergic inhalants resolved with 5 min. In a group of 41 asthmatic patients undergoing bronchoscopy, 21 sedated with propofol and 20 sedated with midazolam, none developed bronchospasm or hypotension, and the incidence of desaturation was similar with the two drugs. Propofol was found to be a safe and effective sedative agent for bronchoscopy in asthma (26). Propofol was given at 60 to 80 mg per min, up to 2 mg per kg, while midazolam was given in an initial dose of 2 mg over 30 sec. Thus, ketamine and propofol may well be favored sedative agents for airway management in the acutely asthmatic patient (6,25,26).

The rapid onset and short duration of action of succinylcholine (paralysis generally achieved within 60 sec, resolution usually about 10 min) are compelling advantages, leading to its use in many centers (11,22,23). Even some of those who are concerned about the issue of histamine will use succinylcholine in the most critical situations (19).

For vecuronium, when it is used to prepare the patient for intubation, the dose is 0.15 mg/kg IV. It may take up to 3 min to get adequate paralysis, and the paralysis will last up to 30 min. If large-dose vecuronium is used (0.3 mg/kg), paralysis occurs in about 90 sec, but may last 2 hr or more, which could be problematic if the intubation is difficult.

The controversy over intubation, and the optimal method for intubation, will undoubtedly continue. Review of the literature suggests that the complications resulting from the use of neuromuscular blockade are few and rarely serious. The advantages of sedation and controlled respiration are substantial, especially considering that many patients are sedated and paralyzed postintubation. In the author's experience, the use of neuromuscular blockade in the critically ill asthmatic patient is valuable and appropriate, subject to the usual caveats inherent in the use of neuromusclar blockers in any patient. For example, if the patients airway anatomy suggests a very difficult intubation (e.g., inability to widely open the mouth, large overbite, etc.), then the relative contraindication to pharmacologically induced apnea exists irrespective of bronchospasm. The concern about worsening bronchospasm applies to all patients, both with and without known asthma. The incidence of bronchospasm appears to be limited by the use of ketamine, and now, propofol.

Postintubation sedation is frequently provided by a benzodiazepine, and pancuronium is commonly advocated for paralysis. Pancuronium is a nondepolarizing blocker (with less likelihood of histamine release). Given at a dose of 0.05–0.10 mg/kg, the paralytic effect will last 1–2 hr.

Because of the prolonged expiratory phase in severe asthmatics, and the concern about overpressure injury, mechanical ventilation must be managed carefully. If a patient abruptly deteriorates during mechanical ventilation, pneumothorax, hypovolemia, and dynamic hyperinflation must be considered. Dynamic hyperinflation is the name given to the phenomenon of progressively increasing pulmonary inflation and intrathoracic pressure as the result of air trapping in an asthmatic patient receiving mechanical ventilation. It is typically the result of insufficient exhalation time (3,27–29). It is important to control tidal volume and time for exhalation, and the ventilator parameters listed below will allow dynamic hyperinflation to be limited. As a result of the high pressures sometimes used to achieve ventilation, pneumothorax—which can evolve to a tension pneumothorax—is a constant risk. Immediate intervention to identify and deflate the pneumothorax is essential. Since many critically asthmatics will have been ill for hours, if not days, with concomitant decrease of fluid intake, hypovolemia is likely. In the face of increased intrathoracic pressure from mechanical ventilation, decreased venous return and reduced cardiac output is always a risk. If hypotension occurs shortly after the initiation of mechanical ventilation, the rapid infusion a bolus of crystalloid (500 cc) may be helpful. Some authorities recommend briefly disconnecting the patient from the ventilator, to see if cardiac output improves when intrathoracic pressure is reduced. If blood pressure rises during the test, then volume resuscitation is appropriate. Since most such patients will be at least marginally volume depleted anyway, preemptive hydration without the stress of separating the patient from the ventilator seems justified. If the patient does not respond to fluid, look again for pneumothorax.

Low respiratory rates (8–12/min), modest tidal volumes (5–8 cc/kg), with high flow rates with decelerating wave forms (60–70 L/m) to provide adequate exhalation time, would be a reasonable initial effort. Peak inflation pressure initially should be limited to 50 cmH_2O, to reduce the chances of pulmonary barotrauma (4,8,19,29,30). If ventilation is not adequate and auto-PEEP is greater than 15 mmHg, then high flow rates (60 L/min) with a square wave pattern should be instituted. Peak inflation pressures may be allowed to rise quite substantially in this circumstance (see Chapter 30).

Since intubating the patient does not resolve the bronchospasm, continued pharmacological therapy is required. Inhaled bronchodilators can be given to the intubated patients by several methods. Nebulized albuterol (0.5 mL of 0.5% solution, diluted in 3 mL saline) is effective (31). The successful use of direct endotracheal administration of albuterol has been reported, with an initial dose of 0.5 mL albuterol diluted with 2.5 mL of saline placed in the endotracheal tube and diffused with five forceful insufflations (32). A second dose of 1.0 mL diluted in 3.0 mL of saline was given. A metered dose inhaler can also be used. One description requires three puffs from the inhaler, 1 min apart. Each puff is distributed by slow manual lung inflation with increased volume maintained for several seconds (31).

The resistance to air flow that is inherent in severe asthma has prompted some to consider the use of helium-oxygen mixtures for ventilation (33,34). Since helium is less dense than nitrogen, it will flow past obstruction more readily then a nitrogen-oxygen mixture. The reports claim improvement attributable to the use of helium, but the small numbers of patients and the absence of controls leave the role of helium-oxygen option intriguing but ill-defined. A more extensive discussion of helium-oxygen therapy appears in Chapter 25.

Endotracheal intubation for the asthmatic patient clearly can be life-saving. The fundamental issues—when to intubate and how to intubate—remain controversial and will probably remain so. The final decision will be one of clinical judgment, based on the individual's skills and interpretation of the literature.

REFERENCES

1. Braman S, Kaemmerlen J. Intensive care of status asthmaticus—A 10-year experience. JAMA 1990; 264:366–368.
2. Mountain RD, Sahn SA. Clinical features and outcome in patients with acute asthma presenting with hypercapnia. Am Rev Respir Dis 1988; 138:535–539.
3. Leatherman J. Life-threatening asthma. Clin Chest Med 1994; 15:453–479.
4. Hall JB, Wood LDH. Management of the critically ill asthmatic patient. Med Clin N Am 1990; 74:779–796.
5. Dales RE, Munt PW. Use of mechanical ventilation in adults with severe asthma. Can Med Assoc J. 1994; 130:391–395.
6. Corbridge TC, Hall JB. The assessment and management of adults with status asthmaticus. Am J Respir Crit Care Med 1995; 151:1296–1316.
7. Zimmerman JL, Dellinger RP, Shah AN, et al. Endotracheal intubation and mechanical ventilation in severe asthma. Crit Care Med 1993; 21:1727–1730.
8. Duncan SR, Raffin TA. Status asthmaticus: ventilatory management. Current Respiratory Care, BC Decker, 1988.
9. Brenner BE, Abraham E, Simon RR. Position and diaphoresis in acute asthma. Am J Med 1983; 74:1005–1009.
10. Wasserfallen JB, Schaller MD, Feihl F, et al. Sudden asphyxic asthma: a distinct entity? Am Rev Respir Dis 1980; 142:108–111.
11. Bellomo R, McLaughlin P, Tai E, et al. Asthma requiring mechanical ventilation a low morbidity approach. Chest 1994; 105:891–896.
12. Kallenbach JM, Frankel AH, Lapinsky SE, et al. Determinants of near fatality in acute severe asthma. Am J Med 1993; 95:265–272.
13. LeSon S, Gershwin ME. Risk factors for asthmatic patients requiring intubation. i. observations in children. J Asthma 1995; 32:285–294.
14. LeSon S, Gershwin ME. Risk factors for asthmatic patients requiring intubation. ii. observations in teenagers. J Asthma 1995; 32:379–389.
15. LeSon S, Gershwin ME. Risk factors for asthmatic patients requiring intubation. iii. observations in young adults. J Asthma 1995; 33:27–35.
16. LeSon S, Gershwin ME. Risk factors for intubation of adult asthmatic patients. J Asthma 1995; 32(2);97–104.
17. Pacht ER, Lingo S, St. John RC. Clinical features, management and outcome of patients with severe asthma admitted to the intensive care unit. J Asthma 1995; 32:373–377.
18. Brenner BE. Bronchial asthma in adults: presentation to the emergency department—part II. Am J Emerg Med 1983; 3:306–333.
19. Mansel JK, et al. Mechanical ventilation in patients with acute severe asthma. Am J Med 1990; 89:42–48.

20. L'Hommedieu CS, Arens JJ. The use of ketamine for the emergency intubation of patients with status asthmaticus. Ann Emerg Med 1987; 16:568–571.
21. Einarsson O, Rochester CL, Rosenbaum S. Airway management in respiratory emergencies. Clin Chest Med 1994; 15;13–34.
22. Rock MJ, Reyes de la Rocha S, L'Hommedieu CS, et al. Use of ketamine in asthmatic children to treat respiratory failure refractory to conventional therapy. Crit Care Med 1986; 14:514–516.
23. Walls RM. Advanced airway management. ACEP Scientific Assembly, 1995.
24. Olsson GL. Bronchospasm during anaesthesia. A computer-aided incidence study of 136929 patients. Act Anaesthiol Scand 1987; 31:244–252.
25. Pizov R, Brown RH, Weiss YS, et al. Wheezing during induction of general anesthesia in patients with and without asthma—a randomized, blinded trial. Anesthesiology 1995; 82: 1111–1116.
26. Clarkson K, Power CK, O'Connell F, et al. A comparative evaluation of propofol and midazolam as sedative agents in fiberoptic bronchoscopy. Chest 1993; 104:1029–1031.
27. Tuxen DV, Lane S. The effects of ventilatory pattern on hyperinflation, airway pressures, and circulation in mechanical ventilation of patients with severe air-flow obstruction. Am Rev Respir Dis 1987; 136:872–879.
28. Williams TJ, Tuxen DV, Scheinkestel CD, et al. Risk factors for morbidity in mechanically ventilated patients with acute severe asthma. Am Rev Respir Dis. 1992; 146:607–615.
29. Tuxen DV. Detrimental effects of positive end-expiratory pressure during controlled mechanical ventilation of patients with severe airflow obstruction. Am Rev Respir Dis 1989; 140: 5–9.
30. Tuxen DV, Williams TJ, Scheinkestel CD, et al. Use of a measurement of pulmonary hyperinflation to control the level of mechanical ventilation in patients with acute severe asthma. Am Rev Respir Dis 1992; 146:1136–1142.
31. Gay PC, Patel HG, Nelson SB, et al. Metered dose inhalers for bronchodilator delivery in intubated, mechanically ventilated patients. Chest 1991; 99:66–71.
32. Verbeek PR, Gareau AB, Rubes CJ. Treat of asthma-related respiratory arrest with endotracheal albuterol. Ann Emerg Med 1988; 17:358–360.
33. Gluck EH, Onorato DJ, Castriotta R. Helium-oxygen mixtures in intubated patients with status asthmaticus and respiratory acidosis. Chest 1990; 98:693–698.
34. Kass JE, Castriotta RJ. Heliox therapy in acute severe asthma. Chest 1995; 107:757–760.

27

Management of Acute Asthma in Children

Richard J. Scarfone
MCP-Hahnemann School of Medicine and St. Christopher's Hospital for Children, Philadelphia, Pennsylvania

Susan Fuchs
Northwestern University Medical School, Chicago, Illinois

Asthma is one of the most common diseases for which children seek care in the emergency department (ED). The management of acute asthma is ever-evolving as research advances allow clinicians to fine tune treatment strategies. This chapter will serve to discuss options in the emergency treatment of acute asthma in children with an emphasis on newer approaches such as metered dose inhalers (MDIs) with holding chambers, nebulized dexamethasone, ipratropium bromide, continuously nebulized albuterol, and magnesium sulfate.

I. PATIENT ASSESSMENT

Patient assessment should begin with a brief and focused history. The clinician should ascertain the duration of symptoms and their severity compared to previous exacerbations. Also, inquiries about recent medication use should be made. A more comprehensive history should be delayed until after treatment has been initiated. Points of the past medical history that are particularly important include prior ED visits and hospitalizations for asthma, previous admissions to an intensive care unit (ICU) or need for intubation, and other medical conditions, especially pulmonary or cardiac.

Decisions about therapeutic options should be made on the basis of the severity of the asthma exacerbation. Several asthma scoring systems exist to aid the practitioner in assessing degree of illness including the complete respiratory assessment score developed by the National Institutes of Health (NIH), as well as scores developed by Woods-Downes and Becker (1–3). None of these scores is universally accepted and each has drawbacks. For example, the complete respiratory assessment score includes variables such as pulsus paradoxus and peak expiratory flow (PEF), which may be difficult to measure in young children and which have not been systematically studied (1); while the Becker score has only been validated in those under age 6 (3).

An alternative to using a formal scoring system in assessing degree of illness is to evaluate the child for specific signs and symptoms indicative of respiratory distress. The exam should begin with an assessment of mental status and recording of vital signs. In addition, the phase(s) of respiration during which wheezing is heard should be noted as well as the use of accessory muscles, inspiratory-to-expiratory ratio, and the oxygen saturation in room air. The sum total of this information will allow the clinician to determine the severity of the exacerbation, provide a starting point from which management can begin, and help insure that appropriately aggressive therapy is administered to the most severely ill patients. Of course, during the ED stay, the degree of illness may change, so frequent examinations to assess response to therapy are critically important.

II. MILD EXACERBATION

Presenting signs and symptoms of mild bronchospasm in children may be subtle and can include decreased activity, poor feeding, or persistent coughing. Undoubtedly, many children with a mild exacerbation of asthma do not seek medical care because the problem is not recognized by caretakers or appropriate therapy is initiated at home. A mild exacerbation is characterized by alertness, slight tachypnea, expiratory wheezing only, minimal accessory muscle use, an inspiratory-to-expiratory ratio of 1:1, or an oxygen saturation of 97% or greater in room air.

The initial therapy for a mild exacerbation is a short-acting β_2-agonist, usually albuterol. The NIH Expert Panel has stated that ''the repetitive or continuous administration of inhaled short-acting beta$_2$-agonists is the most effective means of reversing airflow obstruction'' (4). Albuterol is a selective β_2-agonist that provides clinically significant improvement in pulmonary function in less than 5 min and has become the drug of choice for the initial treatment of acute asthma.

Considerations in the use of albuterol include the delivery system, optimal dose, and frequency of administration. Traditionally albuterol has been delivered by hand-held jet nebulizers. These have a reservoir for the drug, an ''in-port'' for flow of air or oxygen, and an ''out-port'' through which aerosolized drug is inhaled. Schuh has found that a nebulized dose of 0.15 mg/kg (max 5 mg) is more effective and as safe as lower doses (5,6). Several studies have shown that the volume of drug aerosolized increases with increasing diluent volumes and nebulizer flow rate (7–11). In general, a total solution volume (drug plus diluent) of 3–4 mL driven at a flow rate of 6–8 L/min seems to optimize drug delivery (12). In addition, it is preferable to employ a mouthpiece rather than a face mask for children who are old enough to use the mouthpiece. This helps avoid nasal deposition of the drug and creates a more closed system, thus decreasing the amount of drug lost to the environment (13).

Several studies from the adult literature have demonstrated the effectiveness of delivering albuterol by MDIs with a holding chamber or spacer (14–23). There is a growing experience in children as well (24–28). Kerem et al. found no difference in objective and subjective outcomes among mild to moderately ill children treated with albuterol either by nebulization or via MDI with a spacer (24). In that study, the dose ratio for albuterol by MDI-spacer versus nebulizer was 1:5. Advantages to MDI-spacer include lower costs and decreased administration time.

It is imperative to utilize a holding chamber/spacer since children have difficulty coordinating the delivery of mist from the MDI with the inhalation phase of respiration.

In addition, for children who are too young to hold the holding chamber in their mouths, a face mask should be employed to achieve a seal over the mouth and nose. The medication is delivered into the chamber and several breaths are taken by the child. Precise coordination between the administration of drug into the chamber and the phase of respiration is not needed and the chamber decreases the deposition of large aerosol particles in the upper airway. The optimal dose to administer via MDI has not been precisely defined, but the NIH Expert Panel recommends 4–8 puffs per dose every 20 min, 90 μg per puff (4).

Whether the delivery system is a hand-held jet nebulizer or a MDI with holding chamber, albuterol should be administered every 20 min (4). After each treatment, the patient should be reassessed, and a decision should be made regarding the need for additional treatments. The child should be observed for 30–40 min after the most recent albuterol treatment before disposition decisions are made to assure that wheezing and respiratory symptoms do not recur. If after 1–3 treatments there has been a good response, as evidenced by a decreased respiratory rate, no retractions, no dyspnea, and alertness with good color, then the episode can be considered mild and arrangements can be made to send the child home. The ability of the child to perform a peak expiratory flow rate (PEFR) value >80% of predicted or personal baseline value would confirm therapeutic success.

After discharge from the ED, patients should continue to receive albuterol every 3–4 hr for 3–5 days and resume taking their other asthma medications. The initiation of oral corticosteroids at home should be considered for patients who had been already receiving daily β_2-agonists on arrival to the ED, have frequent relapses or hospitalizations (29), or have been on corticosteroids in the past after asthma exacerbations. A usual course is 2 mg/kg/day for 5 days, with no need to taper the dose since there will not be significant adrenal suppression (30). Contact with the primary care physician should be encouraged not only if symptoms recur but for decisions regarding the need for long-term medication.

III. MODERATE EXACERBATION

Children who are experiencing a moderate asthma exacerbation usually have several of the following clinical characteristics. Typically, they are somewhat breathless and tachypneic, with inspiratory and expiratory wheezing, moderate suprasternal and intercostal retractions, an inspiratory-to-expiratory ratio of 1:2 or an oxygen saturation of 92–97% in room air. Oxygen should be administered to maintain a saturation above 92%.

The general management scheme for these patients is outlined in Figure 1. As with the child having a mild exacerbation, a more moderately ill patient should receive albuterol either by nebulization or via MDI with a holding chamber. The NIH Expert Panel Report recommends that corticosteroids be given to any asthmatic child who does not improve after one hour of β_2-agonist therapy (4). However, for moderately ill children we favor administering corticosteroids immediately following the initial albuterol treatment. Clinical benefits from steroids are delayed (31–34) and all moderately ill children will require steroids whether or not they require hospitalization. Therefore, it seems more prudent to administer steroids soon after ED arrival in an attempt to hasten clinical improvement and perhaps prevent the need for hospitalization (31–35).

We favor treating moderately ill asthmatic children who do not require intravenous access for some other reason with 2 mg/kg of oral prednisone (max 60 mg). The NIH Expert Panel has advised that oral prednisone is preferred because it is less invasive with effects equivalent to parenterally administered corticosteroids (4). We have shown that

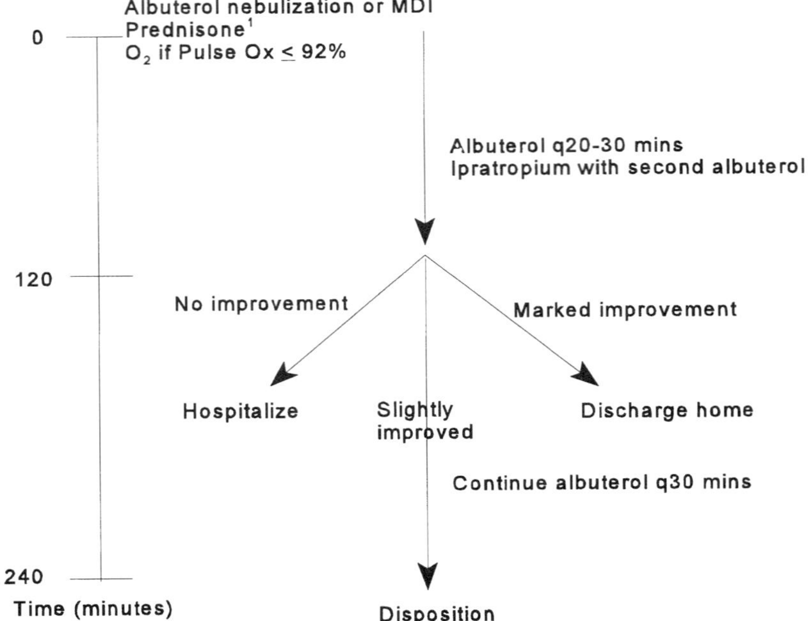

Figure 1 General management scheme for patients with moderate exacerbations.

oral prednisone reduces the need for hospitalization among a subset of moderately to severely ill children treated aggressively with β_2-agonists (those with an initial pulmonary index >10); this benefit was achieved within four hours of the administration of prednisone (Table 1). Oral prednisone is rapidly and completely absorbed, and advantages include the potential for prehospital administration and decreased frequency of minor complications associated with parenteral therapy. Most importantly, routine use of prednisone for all moderately ill children in the ED will avoid delays in corticosteroid delivery pending the insertion of an intravenous line. It follows then that oral administration would result in an increased utilization of corticosteroids among children in the ED.

For patients who have been vomiting at home prior to the ED visit or who vomit

Table 1 Hospitalization Rates

	Predisone[a]	Placebo[a]	*P* value
All patients	11/36 (31)	19/39 (49)	.10
Patients with initial PI > 10	7/22 (32)	13/18 (72)	<.05

[a] Values expressed as number hospitalized/total (%).
PI = pulmonary index.
Source: Ref. 31.

the oral prednisone within 15 minutes of its administration, options include single doses of either 4 mg/kg of intramuscular methylprednisolone (32) or 1.5 mg/kg of nebulized dexamethasone (35). We found that a subset of moderately ill children who received dexamethasone sodium phosphate solution delivered by nebulization were able to be discharged home from the ED sooner than those receiving prednisone (Figure 2).

Albuterol treatments should be continued every 20–30 min with clinical reassessment preceding each nebulization. For the second nebulized treatment, we favor adding 250–500 μg of ipratropium bromide to the albuterol. Alternatively, ipratropium may be administered via MDI with spacer immediately after the second albuterol is given by MDI. Ipratropium has local anticholinergic effects with little systemic absorption. Bronchodilation is achieved within 20 min and peaks at 60–120 min (36). Several studies in children have found that its use in combination with albuterol results in a degree of bronchodilation above that achieved with albuterol alone (37–40). In the largest of these studies, the addition of repeated doses of 250 μg of nebulized ipratropium to frequent high-dose albuterol among moderately ill asthmatic children resulted in significant objective benefits (37). However, children in this study were not treated concurrently with corticosteroids. In a more recent study, two 500 μg doses of ipratropium along with frequent nebulized albuterol and oral corticosteroids was compared to albuterol and steroids alone for moderately ill asthmatic children. The ipratropium group experienced a significant improvement in pulmonary function at 120 min (40).

As yet, the optimal dose and frequency of ipratropium treatments are not well established. As more experience with the use of ipratropium accumulates, its niche in the treatment of acute asthma will become clearer. The available data seem to support its use for moderately to severely ill patients either as a single dose or given repeatedly with each albuterol treatment.

Once therapy has been initiated for moderately ill children, decisions about laboratory studies can be made. The presence of fever, respiratory rate above 60, an asymmetric pulmonary examination persisting after therapy, or a concern about foreign body aspiration or pneumothorax would all be reasonable indications for a chest radiograph to be obtained (41).

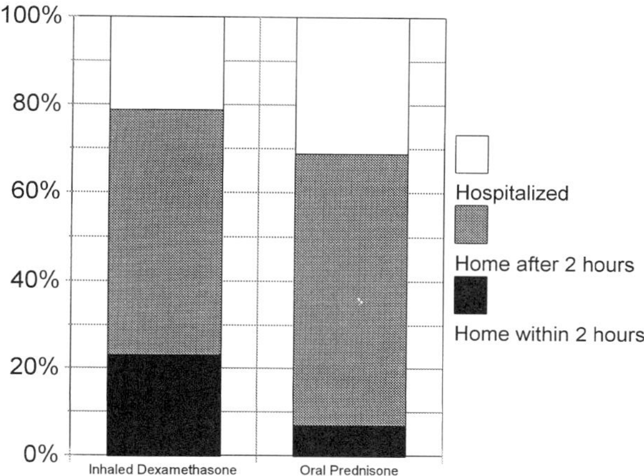

Figure 2 Patient outcomes among moderately ill children. (From Ref. 35.)

If this is the first episode of wheezing in an infant, a chest radiograph may be obtained to look for other etiologies of wheezing such as congestive heart failure, pneumonia, congenital airway or lung abnormalities, foreign body aspiration, cystic fibrosis, or tumor. Routine acquisition of chest radiographs for older children who are wheezing for the first time is not recommended (41).

Other studies, such as complete blood count or serum electrolytes rarely provide useful information in managing the asthmatic child. For patients receiving theophylline prior to presentation, a measurement of serum theophylline concentration is warranted.

Much has been written about the role of aminophylline in the ED treatment of acute asthma. A meta-analysis of 13 trials found no difference between the aminophylline-treated and control groups (42). While the data do not allow one to conclude that a child who is unresponsive to conventional therapy will not benefit from aminophylline, the preponderance of evidence suggests that aggressive use of inhaled β_2-agonists and corticosteroids obviates the need for aminophylline (43). As stated by the NIH Expert Panel, "There is no evidence that theophylline adds to the bronchodilation achieved with beta$_2$-agonists in the first 4 hours in the ED" (4). Given this, as well as the narrow therapeutic window of aminophylline, it is not recommended as a routine component of therapy for those presenting with a moderate exacerbation.

The clinician should use the patient's clinical response to decide the duration of ED therapy as well as the disposition. Those who show prompt improvement early in their ED management may be discharged home. However, it is wise to delay a disposition decision until 30–40 min after the most recent albuterol treatment so that a clinical relapse may be noted. Albuterol should be prescribed for all such patients, as described earlier. In addition, 5 days of oral prednisone is recommended for all children who present with a moderate exacerbation, even if they were readily responsive to albuterol in the ED or had not been receiving albuterol prior to their ED visit.

On the other hand, 90–120 min after arrival in the ED, most children should have received 3–4 albuterol treatments, corticosteroids, and ipratropium. When subjective and objective measures reveal that the degree of respiratory distress is unchanged at this point, then hospitalization is warranted. One should have a lower threshold for admitting those children who have had numerous previous admissions, severe prior exacerbations, inexperienced caretakers at home, or difficulty returning in case of relapse (see Chapters 32 and 35).

Perhaps the group of patients for which clinicians can have the greatest impact is that subset of moderately ill children who experience some degree of clinical improvement at this stage, but are not quite well enough to be sent home. We tend to continue to treat such children with albuterol every 30 min for a total of 3–4 hr. We found that among prednisone-

Table 2 Outcome for Patients with a Preliminary Disposition (PD) of "Admit"

	PD of "admit"	Final disposition for those with PD of "admit"
Prednisone[a]	20/36 (56)	9/20 (45)
Placebo[a]	18/39 (46)	15/18 (83)
P value	.42	<.05

[a] Values expressed as number (%).
Source: Ref. 31.

treated children who would have been hospitalized after 2 hr of ED therapy, less than half were actually hospitalized when aggressive β_2-agonist therapy was continued for an additional 2 hr (Table 2). Presumably, the onset of the effects of prednisone allowed these children to avoid hospitalization. Thus, if staffing and space allows, moderately ill children showing slow and steady improvement should continue to be treated for up to four hours.

IV. SEVERE EXACERBATION

A severe exacerbation is characterized by breathlessness, agitation or lethargy, extreme tachypnea, loud wheezing audible without a stethoscope, significant use of accessory muscles with suprasternal and intercostal retractions, a markedly prolonged expiratory phase or an oxygen saturation <92% in room air. Some children with a severe exacerbation may have a slowed respiratory rate because of a prolonged expiratory phase, and wheezing may not be audible if aeration is markedly decreased.

The general management scheme for these patients is outlined in Figure 3. Continuous monitoring of heart and respiratory rates, pulse oximetry, and blood pressure should be performed. Supplying oxygen and promptly administering a β_2-agonist are the initial steps to take in the treatment of severely ill children. To achieve an oxygen saturation of 92% or greater, it may be necessary to employ a nonrebreathing face mask. Ipratropium bromide should be administered soon after the initial albuterol treatment with consideration given for repeat doses.

For children with poor inspiratory flow or who are extremely agitated and uncooperative, inhaled albuterol will not be effectively delivered to the small airways; thus, subcutane-

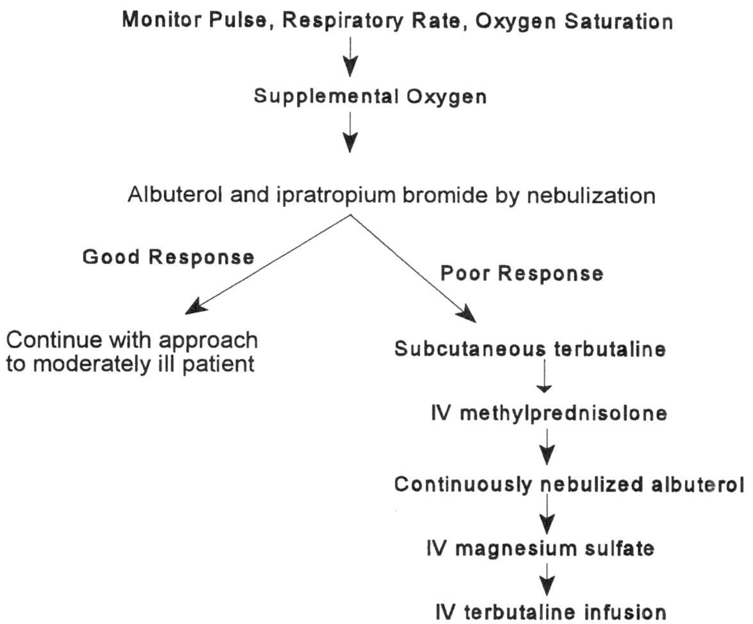

Figure 3 General management scheme for patients with severe exacerbations.

ous epinephrine or terbutaline may be used in this setting. Terbutaline is a selective β_2-agonist and an appropriate dose is 0.01 mL/kg with a maximum of 0.5 mL in adolescents.

An intravenous line should be established as soon as possible and 2 mg/kg methylprednisolone administered. An arterial blood gas will be helpful to evaluate arterial carbon dioxide tension in a patient suspected to be hypoventilating.

Based on the response to these initial therapeutic interventions, the emergency physician must decide on the degree of escalation of care. Children who demonstrate considerable improvement may be managed as moderately ill children, as discussed previously. For those who are poorly responsive, therapeutic options include albuterol delivered by continuous nebulization, the intravenous administration of magnesium sulfate, and sympathomimetics administered by continuous intravenous infusion.

Studies in adults evaluating the efficacy of continuously nebulized albuterol versus intermittently nebulized albuterol in the ED have shown that the continuous route was as safe and as effective as the intermittent route with fewer side effects (44–46). Two of the studies demonstrated that continuously nebulized albuterol was more beneficial than intermittently nebulized albuterol in those patients with more severe distress (44,45). However, in each of these studies there has been a wide variability in the doses used for continuous nebulization as well as the frequency with which intermittently nebulized albuterol was delivered.

Continuously nebulized albuterol has been used in the pediatric intensive care setting for children with impending respiratory failure for several years. One of the initial studies in the ICU setting demonstrated that patients receiving continuously nebulized albuterol improved more rapidly, had shorter hospital stays, and required less respiratory therapy time at the bedside then those children receiving intermittently nebulized albuterol (47). Another study found that continuously nebulized albuterol reduced the need for mechanical ventilation and the use of intravenous β-agonist infusions (48). Regarding side effects, creatinine phosphokinase (CPK) levels were monitored in two pediatric ICU-based studies, and were elevated in three of 17 and three of 19 patients. Although a total of three patients had elevated CPK-MB fractions, no patients had electrocardiogram (ECG) evidence of ischemia or dysrhythmias during treatment including those with isoenzyme elevations (47,49,50). Although there is a theoretical concern for hypokalemia after long-term use of continuous nebulization, this was not demonstrated in the Papo study.

A recent study assessed the use of continuously nebulized albuterol to treat children in the ED with moderate to severe asthma. Compared were 0.3 mg/kg/hr of albuterol versus 0.15 mg/kg/dose delivered every 30 min. Although there were no differences in admission rates or side effects, there was a greater reduction in asthma score and in respiratory therapy time for those patients receiving continuously nebulized albuterol (45). In addition, similar to the studies in adults, among a subpopulation with more severe disease, there was a trend toward a reduced admission rate among those receiving continuously nebulized albuterol.

Potential advantages of using continuously nebulized albuterol include greater bronchodilation occurring with smaller, more frequently nebulized doses of β_2-agonists, better drug distribution, a wide therapeutic index compared to the intravenous route, diminished respiratory therapy time, and cost savings (45,51). Potential disadvantages of its use include young children not being able to tolerate wearing a face mask for a prolonged period of time and physicians failing to assess children who are receiving ongoing therapy (45).

For severely ill asthmatic children who have a suboptimal response to initial therapeutic options, we advocate the use of continuously nebulized albuterol at a dose of 0.5

mg/kg/hr (max 15 mg). These patients require frequent assessments to ensure that there is not a deterioration in their respiratory status while they are receiving this therapy. There are several methods of delivery, but a simple and readily available one uses a HEART (high-output extended aerosol respiratory therapy) nebulizer (B&B Medical Technologies, Inc., Orangevale, CA), which has a large reservoir and can hold several hours of medication (44,45,51). Another delivery method is a small-particle aerosol generator (Spag unit, ICN Pharmaceuticals, Costa Mesa, CA), often used for the administration of antiviral aerosol medication (51). While patients are receiving continuously nebulized albuterol, they should continue to be monitored closely for dysrhythmias or blood pressure changes.

Currently, there are few large clinical trials assessing the use of magnesium sulfate in children. In one double-blinded and placebo-controlled trial, moderately to severely ill asthmatic children treated with intravenous magnesium sulfate demonstrated significant improvements in pulmonary function studies and rate of discharge from the ED compared to the placebo group (52). Studies performed in adults have had conflicting results, most likely due to wide variability in both degree of illness of patients and magnesium dosing. Okayama et al. and Rolla et al. each demonstrated modest improvements in pulmonary function studies among adult asthmatics treated with intravenously administered magnesium sulfate (53,54). Skobeloff et al. found that among adult asthmatics refractory to initial beta-agonist therapy, there was a demonstrable improvement in peak expiratory flow rates as well as hospitalization rates among those treated with magnesium sulfate (55). On the other hand, a larger study failed to identify a magnesium benefit among adults with status asthmaticus (56).

When magnesium sulfate is reserved for use in only the most severely ill patients, perhaps mild degrees of bronchodilation brought about by the drug are not discernible. In addition, since very ill asthmatics are treated concurrently with many forms of aggressive therapy, it may not be possible to distinguish which component of the patient's therapy is leading to a clinical benefit.

Magnesium sulfate has been shown to be safe. The side effects are mild and, if they occur, are more pronounced immediately during the infusion (57). This includes transient sensation of facial warmth, flushing, nausea and vomiting, dry mouth, and malaise (57). Early signs of more significant magnesium toxicity such as hypotension do not appear until serum levels of greater than 8 mg/dL are achieved. Yet, at doses of 50–75 mg/kg, levels of 2–4 mg/dL are usually achieved (57). We are currently studying the use of 75 mg/kg (max 2.5 g) of intravenous (IV) magnesium sulfate administered over 20 min for severely ill children. We continuously monitor heart rate and blood pressure and none of the 30 subjects enrolled to date have had significant adverse effects.

At this time magnesium sulfate cannot be recommended as a routine therapy for all asthmatics. However, given that there are data demonstrating its efficacy in children and adults treated with aggressive β_2-agonist therapy and given its wide therapeutic window, the risk-benefit ratio favors its use for severely ill children with status asthmaticus who are not responding to more conventional therapy.

A small subset of children treated with continuously administered albuterol and a bolus of magnesium sulfate will continue with significant respiratory distress and may require intravenous sympathomimetics to stave off the need for mechanical ventilation. Studies comparing nebulized and intravenously administered sympathomimetics have had conflicting results. Some have demonstrated the nebulized route to be either greater (58,59) or equal (60–62) in efficacy to the parenteral route, while others have had more success with intravenous administration (63). It is difficult to draw conclusions from these studies because of variability in particular agents compared, degree of illness of patients, and dosages selected.

Bohn found that in 11 of 16 children admitted to an ICU with severe asthma, the use of intravenous salbutamol averted the need for mechanical ventilation (64). This therapy reduced the group's mean $Paco_2$ from 60 to 50 after 1 hr and to 42 after 2.5 hr.

To date, there are limited data comparing continuously nebulized albuterol alone versus albuterol and intravenous sympathomimetics. Based on the existing literature, because of the concern for toxicities, there is no justification for initiating therapy with intravenous sympathomimetics, even for severely ill children. However, for those who are poorly responsive to the aggressive treatment outlined previously, the risk–benefit ratio shifts toward the use of intravenous therapy. For these children with tight bronchoconstriction, theoretically, the drug will be delivered by the systemic circulation to distal airway sites.

Isoproterenol had been the drug of choice in the past. However, its use was associated with frequent and severe complications such as dysrhythmias, hypertension, and myocardial ischemia. The selective β_2-agonist terbutaline should be used in this setting. A recommended dose is 10 μg/kg over 30 min followed by an infusion of 0.1 μg/kg/min (65). The dose can be increased in 15 to 20 min intervals by increments of 0.3–0.5 μg/kg/min to a maximum of 4.0 μg/kg/min. This dose is largely empiric however since there are few dose-response studies correlating bronchodilating effects with plasma levels in children (66). In one such study, 4.5 μg/kg/hr was found to be the optimal dose producing maximal bronchodilation. However, just 10 children were studied and the plasma level correlating with maximal bronchodilation varied widely among subjects. Therapeutic doses will result in side effects such as tachycardia, increased systolic and decreased diastolic blood pressures, flushing, headaches, and tremors. Patients should be monitored for dysrhythmias, hypokalemia, hyperglycemia, and hypophosphatemia. Children with a severe asthma exacerbation should, of course, be admitted to the intensive care unit.

Asthma is a potentially serious disorder seen commonly in the pediatric ED. The clinician is called upon to rapidly assess a child's degree of illness and institute appropriate therapy. This chapter has provided an overview of assessment and management recommendations with an emphasis on some of the newer treatment options available. It is only through more effective preventative measures and timely and appropriate institution of treatment that we can hope to reverse the current trends in morbidity and mortality.

REFERENCES

1. Global Strategy for Asthma Management and Prevention, National Heart, Lung, and Blood Institute of the National Institutes of Health, Publication Number 95-3659, Jan. 1995.
2. Wood DW, Downes JJ, Lecks HI. A clinical scoring system for the diagnosis of respiratory failure. Am J Dis Child 1972; 123:227–228.
3. Becker AB, Nelson NA, Simons FE. The pulmonary index: assessment of a clinical score for asthma. Am J Dis Child 1984; 138:574–576.
4. National Asthma Education Program, Expert Panel Report. Guidelines for the diagnosis and management of asthma. Bethesda, MD: National Heart, Lung, and Blood Institute of the National Institutes of Health, 1991, Publication No. 91-3042.
5. Schuh S, Parkin P, Rajan A, et al. High versus low dose, frequently administered nebulized albuterol in children with severe, acute asthma. Pediatrics 1989; 83:513–518.

6. Schuh S, Reider MJ, Canny G, et al. Nebulized albuterol in acute childhood asthma: Comparison of two doses. Pediatrics 1990; 86(4):509–513.
7. Clay MM, Pavia D, Newman SP, et al. Assessment of jet nebulizers for lung aerosol therapy. Lancet 1983; 2:592–594.
8. Hess D, Horney D, Snyder T. Medication-delivery performance of eight small-volume, hand-held nebulizers: effects of diluent volume, gas, flow rate, and nebulizer model. Respir Care 1989; 34:717–723.
9. Wood JA, Wilson RS, Bray C. Changes in salbutamol concentration in the reservoir solution of a jet nebulizer. Br J Dis Chest 1986; 80:164–169.
10. Clay MM, Pavia D, Newman SP, Clarke SW. Factors influencing the size distribution of aerosols from jet nebulisers. Thorax 1983; 38:755–759.
11. Douglas JG, Leslie MJ, Brompton GK, Grant IW. Is the flow rate used to drive a jet nebulizer clinical important? (letter). Br Med J Clin Res 1985; 290:29.
12. Kacmarek RM, Hess D. The interface between patient and aerosol generator. Respir Care 1991; 36(9):952–976.
13. American Association for Respiratory Care, Aerosol Consensus Statement—1991. Respir Care 1991; 36(9):916–921.
14. Turner JR, Corkery KJ, Eckman D, et al. Equivalence of continuous flow nebulizer and metered-dose inhaler with reservoir bag for treatment of acute airflow obstruction. Chest 1988; 93:476–481.
15. Salzman GA, Steele MT, Pribble JP, RM, et al. Aerosolized metaproterenol in the treatment of asthmatics with severe airflow obstruction: comparison of two delivery methods. Chest 1989; 95:1017–1020.
16. Mestitz H, Copland JM, McDonald C. Comparison of outpatient nebulized vs. metered-dose inhaler terbutaline in chronic airflow obstruction. Chest 1989; 96:1237–1240.
17. Pendergast J, Hopkins J, Timms B, Asperen PP. Comparative efficacy of terbutaline administered by Nebuhaler and by nebulizer in young children with asthma. Med J Aust 1989; 151: 406–408.
18. Summer W, Elston R, Tharpe L, et al. Aerosol bronchodilator delivery methods: relative impact on pulmonary function and cost of respiratory care. Arch Intern Med 1989; 149:618–623.
19. Shim CS, Williams MH. Effect of bronchodilator therapy in administration by canister versus jet nebulizer. J Allergy Clin Immunol 1984; 73:387–390.
20. Jasper AC, Mohsenifar Z, Kahan S, et al. Cost-benefit comparison of aerosol bronchodilator delivery methods in hospitalized patients. Chest 1987; 91:614–618.
21. Benton G, Thomas RC, Nickerson BG, et al. Experience with a metered-dose inhaler with a spacer in the pediatric emergency department. Am J Dis Child 1989; 143:678–681.
22. Bowton DL, Goldsmith WM, Haponik EF. Substitution of metered-dose inhalers for hand-held nebulizers: success and cost savings in a large, acute care hospital. Chest 1992; 101:305–308.
23. Idris AH, McDermott MF, Raucci JC, et al. Emergency department treatment of severe asthma: metered dose inhaler is equivalent in effectiveness to nebulizer. Chest 1993; 103:665–672.
24. Kerem E, Levison H, Schuh S, et al. Efficacy of albuterol administered by nebulizer versus spacer device in children with acute asthma. J Pediatr 1993; 123(2):313–317.
25. Colacone A, Afilalo M, Wolkove N, Kreisman H. A comparison of albuterol administered by metered dose inhaler (and holding chamber) or wet nebulizer in acute asthma. Chest 1993; 104(3):835–841.
26. Batra V, Sethi GR, Sachdev HP. Comparative efficacy of jet nebulizer and metered dose inhaler with spacer device in the treatment of acute asthma. Indian Pediatr 1997; 34:497–503.
27. Chou KJ, Cunningham SJ, Crain EF. Metered dose inhalers with spacers vs. nebulizers for pediatric asthma. Arch Pediatr Adolesc Med 1995; 149:201–205.

28. Kerem E, Levison H, Schuh S, et al. Efficacy of albuterol administered by nebulizer versus spacer device in children with acute asthma. J Pediatr 1993; 123:313–317.
29. Brunette MG, Lands L, Thibodeau LP. Childhood asthma: prevention of attacks with short-term corticosteroid treatment of upper respiratory tract infection. Pediatrics 1988; 81:624–629.
30. Zora JA. The use of corticosteroids in childhood asthma. J Asthma 1989; 26(3):159–165.
31. Scarfone RJ, Fuchs S, Nagers AL, Shane SA. Controlled trial of oral prednisone in the emergency department treatment of children with acute asthma. Pediatrics 1993; 92:513–518.
32. Tal A, Levy N, Bearman JE. Methylprednisolone therapy for acute asthma in infants and toddlers: a controlled clinical trial. Pediatrics 1990; 86:350–356.
33. Littenberg B, Gluck EH. A controlled trial of methylprednisolone in the emergency treatment of acute asthma. N Engl J Med 1986; 314:150–152.
34. Storr J, Barrell E, Barry W, et al. Effect of a single oral dose of prednisolone in acute childhood asthma. Lancet 1987; 1:879–882.
35. Scarfone RJ, Loiselle JM, Wiley JF, et al. Nebulized dexamethasone versus oral prednisone in the emergency treatment of asthmatic children. Ann Emerg Med 1995; 26(4):480–486.
36. Gross NJ. Ipratropium bromide. N Engl J Med 1988; 319:486–494.
37. Schuh S, Johnson DW, Callahan S, et al. Efficacy of frequent nebulized ipratropium bromide added to frequent high-dose albuterol therapy in severe childhood asthma. J Pediatr 1995; 126(4):639–645.
38. Reisman J, Galdes-Sebalt M, Kazim F, et al. Frequent administration by inhalation of salbutamol and ipratropium bromide in the initial management of severe acute asthma in children. J Allergy Clin Immunol 1988; 81(1):16–20.
39. Beck R, Robertson C, Galdés-Sebaldt M, Levison H. Combined salbutamol and ipratropium bromide by inhalation in the treatment of severe acute asthma. J Pediatr 1985; 107(4):605–608.
40. Qureshi F, Zaritsky A, Lakkis H. Efficacy of nebulized ipratropium in severe asthmatic children. Ann Emerg Med 1997; 29(2):205–211.
41. Gershel JC, Goldman HS, Stein RE, et al. The usefulness of chest radiographs in first asthma attacks. N Engl J Med 1983; 309(6):336–339.
42. Littenberg B. Aminophylline treatment in severe, acute asthma. JAMA 1988; 259(11):1678–1684.
43. Weinberger M. Theophylline: When should it be used? J Pediatr 1993; 122:403–405.
44. Rudnitsky GS, Eberline RS, Schoffstall JM, et al. Comparison of intermittent and continuously nebulized albuterol for treatment of asthma in an urban emergency department. Ann Emerg Med 1993; 22:1842–1846.
45. Khine H, Fuchs SM, Saville AL. Continuous vs. intermittent nebulized albuterol for emergency department management of asthma. Acad Emerg Med 1996; 3:1019–1024.
46. Colacone A, Wolkove N, Stern E, et al. Continuous nebulization of albuterol (salbutamol) in acute asthma. Chest 1990; 97:693–697.
47. Papo MC, Frank J, Thompson AE. A prospective, randomized study of continuous versus intermittent nebulized albuterol for severe status asthmaticus in children. Crit Care Med 1993; 21:1479–1486.
48. Craig VL, Bigos D, Briglia F, et al. Continuous albuterol therapy in children with status asthmaticus (abstract). Crit Care Med 1994; 22:A182.
49. Craig VL, Bigos D, Brilli RJ. Efficacy and safety of continuous albuterol nebulization in children with severe status asthmaticus. Pediatr Emerg Care 1996; 12:1–5.
50. Katz RW, Kelly HW, Crowley MR, et al. Safety of continuous nebulized albuterol for bronchospasm in infants and children. Pediatrics 1993; 92:666–669.
51. Portnoy J, Nadel G, Amado M, et al. Continuous nebulization for status asthmaticus. Ann Allergy 1992; 69:71–79.
52. Ciarallo L, Sauer AH, Shannon MW. Intravenous magnesium therapy for moderate to severe

pediatric asthma: results of a randomized, placebo-controlled trial. J Pediatr 1996; 129(6): 809–814.
53. Okayama H, Aikawa T, Okayama M, et al. Bronchodilating effect of intravenous magnesium sulfate in bronchial asthma. JAMA 1987; 257:1076–1078.
54. Rolla G, Bucca C, Bugiani M, et al. Reduction of histamine-induced bronchoconstriction by magnesium in asthmatic subjects. Allergy 1987; 42:186–188.
55. Skobeloff EM, Spivey WH, McNamara RM, Greenspon L. Intravenous magnesium sulfate for the treatment of acute asthma in the emergency department. JAMA 1989; 262;1210–1213.
56. Green SM, Rothrock SG. Intravenous magnesium for acute asthma: failure to decrease emergency treatment duration or need for hospitalization. Ann Emerg Med 1992; 21:260–265.
57. Monem GF, Kissoon N, DeNicola L. Use of magnesium sulfate in asthma in childhood. Pediatric Ann 1996; 25(3):139–144.
58. Salmeron S, Brochard L, Mal H, et al. Nebulized versus intravenous albuterol in hypercapnic acute asthma. Am J Respir Crit Care Med 1994; 149:1466–1470.
59. Swedish Society of Chest Medicine, High-dose inhaled versus intravenous salbutamol combined with theophylline in severe acute asthma. Eur Respir J 1990; 3:163–170.
60. Lawford P, Jones BJM, Milledge JS. Comparison of intravenous and nebulized salbutamol in initial treatment of severe asthma. Br Med J 1978; 1:84.
61. Bloomfield P, Carmichael J, Petrie GR, et al. Comparison of salbutamol given intravenously and by intermittent positive-pressure breathing in life-threatening asthma. Br Med J 1979; 1: 848–850.
62. Williams SJ, Winner SJ, Clark TJH. Comparison of inhaled and intravenous terbutaline in acute severe asthma. Thorax 1981; 36:629–632.
63. Cheong B, Reynolds SR, Rajan G, Ward MJ. Intravenous agonist in severe acute asthma. Br Med J 1988; 297:448–450.
64. Bohn D, Kalloghlian AV, Jenkins J, et al. Intravenous salbutamol in the treatment of status asthmaticus in children. Crit Care Med 1984; 12(10):892–896.
65. DeNicola LK, Monem GF, Gayle MO, Kissoon N. Treatment of critical status asthmaticus in children. Pediatr Clin N Am 1994; 41(6):1293–1324.
66. Fuglsang G, Pedersen S, Borgenström L. Dose-response relationships of intravenously administered terbutaline in children with asthma. J Pediatr 1989; 114(2):315–320.

28

Acute Asthma in Pregnancy

Richard Sinert, Karen L. Stavile, and Jin H. Han
State University of New York Health Science Center at Brooklyn Kings County Hospital Center, Brooklyn, New York

I. INTRODUCTION

The pregnant patient with an exacerbation of asthma presents many challenges to the emergency physician. Alterations in respiratory physiology during pregnancy and the additional concerns for preventing fetal hypoxia requires increased vigilance. The risks of asthma therapy to the developing fetus must be balanced with the risks of maternal and fetal hypoxia. Patient education and appropriate outpatient follow-up aimed at preventing recurrent attacks takes on an added importance in this patient population.

Asthma occurs in 1–4% of all pregnancies, representing one of the most common serious medical complications of pregnancy (1,2). Many large studies during pregnancy have established that mild (2–4) and even well-controlled steroid dependent asthma (5,6) have little untoward effects on either the mother or fetus. Yet, status asthmaticus, which occurs in 0.05–0.2% of all pregnancies, is associated with significantly higher frequencies of maternal death, fetal loss, prematurity, and intrauterine growth retardation (1,7–9).

II. RESPIRATORY PHYSIOLOGY WITH PREGNANCY

Progesterone elevation during pregnancy results in maternal hyperventilation (10). By term there is a 40% increase in minute ventilation, from 6.6 L preterm to 9.2 L by 39 weeks (11). Respiratory rate remains unchanged (10) but tidal volume increases from 0.4 L in the nonpregnant state to 0.6 L at term (10). Decreases in total lung volume (4–6%), residual volume and functional residual capacity (15–25%) cannot be completely accounted for by the mechanical effects from a gravid uterus (12).

Airway mechanics, FEV_1, and closing volumes remain unchanged during pregnancy (13). Predicted peak expiratory flow rates in pregnancy remain in normal ranges between

380 and 550 L/min (14). Pulmonary diffusion capacity increases during pregnancy, which is not explained by alterations in hemoglobin concentration, alveolar volume, or estrogen concentration (15).

Arterial blood gas (ABG) measurements are consistent with a compensated chronic respiratory alkalosis reflecting maternal hyperventilation. Normal blood gases during pregnancy reveal a normal range pH (7.40–7.45) a decreased pco_2 (28–30) and a higher po_2 (100–106) (16–18).

These changes in respiratory physiology have important implications in the emergent treatment of the pregnant asthmatic. Maternal hyperventilation is often interpreted by the patient as shortness of breath, leading to the condition known ''dyspnea of pregnancy,'' which has been reported by up to 76% of nonasthmatic pregnant patients (19). The differentiation of an early acute exacerbation of asthma versus ''dyspnea of pregnancy'' may present a clinical challenge to the emergency department (ED) physician.

Bronchospasm is accompanied by an increase in minute ventilation in order to maintain an adequate oxygen exchange. A pregnant patient with baseline chronic hyperventilation may have less of a respiratory muscle reserve during an asthmatic attack. Since maternal pco_2 is normally less than 30 mmHg, physicians must readjust their normal ranges so that a pco_2 of 40 mmHg represents severe hypoventilation in these patients. In the example below, I have attempted to give a typical scenario of ABGs during an asthma attack in a pregnant patient. Early in the course of an acute asthma attack acute respiratory alkalosis adds to pregnant patient's chronic respiratory alkalosis. If alveolar hypoventilation occurs, the typical rapid fall in arterial pH and rise of pco_2 may not be seen and respiratory failure must be diagnosed on the basis of this very normal appearing ABG. Clinical correlation with the knowledge of changes in respiratory physiology will aid the ED physician in correctly identifying respiratory failure in the pregnant patient (Figure 1).

Although airway resistance and mechanics are unchanged during pregnancy, alterations in body position has been shown to have significant respiratory effects in the full-term pregnant patient. FEV_1 was found to be significantly lower in the supine compared to sitting position (20). The alveolar-arterial oxygen gradient also increased by changing position from the sitting to supine (21). The ED physician is recommended to always maintain the pregnant asthmatic in a sitting and never a supine position.

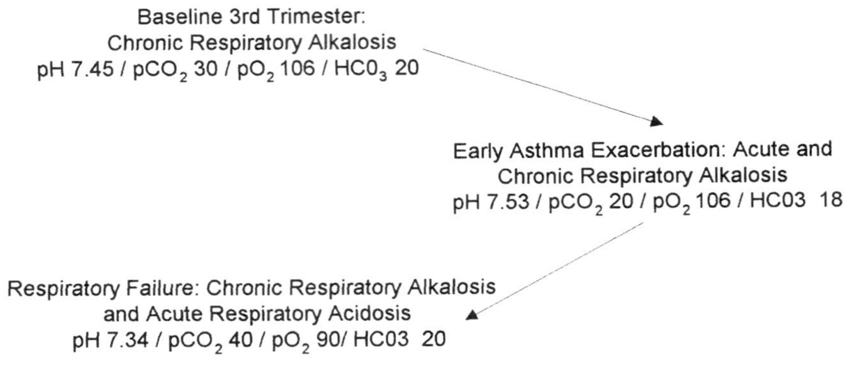

Figure 1 ABGs in pregnant asthmatics.

III. MATERNAL FETAL OXYGEN EXCHANGE

The urteroplacental circulation is a countercurrent exchange system resulting in significant arteriovenous oxygen shunting (22). The fetus thrives in a continual state of hypoxia, with an umbilical artery po_2 (11 mmHg) and vein po_2 (32 mmHg) while the woman breathes room air (23). This low fetal arterial po_2 combined with the rightward shift of the fetal hemoglobin-oxygen dissociation curve leaves the fetus with only a 2-min oxygen reserve (24). Compensations to prevent fetal hypoxia include: (1) fetal shunts (i.e., ductus arteriosus, venosus, and foramen ovale), which direct the majority of blood flow to vital organs; (2) fetal oxygen-hemoglobin dissociation favors more oxygen uptake and release in the normally acidic fetal environment; and (3) the ability to increase blood flow rates from fetus to placenta (25).

A high degree of correlation exists between maternal and fetal po_2 (23). This leaves the fetus extremely vulnerable to hypoxia during an asthma attack, and has led to the recommendation for monitoring maternal oxygen saturation in these patients. Since increasing maternal Po_2 has been shown to increase fetal po_2 (23), supplemental oxygen should be given to all pregnant patients with an asthma exacerbation.

Fetal hypoxia can also occur independently of maternal hypoxia as result of only an exacerbation of maternal hyperventilation (23,26–28). This hypoxia has been ascribed to the decreasing pco_2 by itself (23). An increasing pH can decrease uterine blood flow, and increase maternal hemoglobin affinity for oxygen compared to the fetus, leading to fetal hypoxia (26–28).

These increased risks to fetal hypoxia have led to the recommendation for fetal heart rate monitoring in the ED in severe asthma attacks (29). Fetal heart rate decelerations or absent variability would then provide for an early warning of fetal hypoxia and point to a more aggressive approach to maternal oxygenation.

IV. HOW PREGNANCY AFFECTS ASTHMA

Physiological changes during pregnancy may have significant effects on the course of asthma. These effects can be divided into factors that have the potential to improve or exacerbate asthma during pregnancy.

A. Factors That May Improve Asthma During Pregnancy

During pregnancy an increase in β-agonist reactivity has been ascribed to increased levels of estrogen and progesterone (30). Plasma free-cortisol levels are increased in pregnancy, secondary to a combination of decreased clearance by estrogen (31) and displacement of cortisol from transcortin by progesterone (32). Serum histamine levels decrease during pregnancy as a result of its increased enzymatic breakdown (33). Increases in cyclic adenosine monophosphate (cAMP) during pregnancy have also been reported (34).

Decreases in cell-mediated immunity with pregnancy occur as evidenced by a reduction in maternal lymphocyte response to phytohemagglutinin (35). Immunoglobulin E (IgE) levels have been shown to decrease during pregnancy (3). The failure to decrease IgE levels during pregnancy has been shown to be associated with a higher frequency of asthma exacerbations (3). The prostaglandins, PGE (36) and PGI_2 (37), which decrease bronchospasm, are also increased with pregnancy (38).

B. Factors That May Exacerbate Asthma During Pregnancy

As with the other prostaglandins, PGF_2 also increases with pregnancy (38). Unlike PGE and PGI_2, PGF_2 has been linked to bronchconstriction (39).

Gastrointestinal reflux, a common complication of pregnancy, is highly correlated with asthma exacerbations (40). A prospective study that decreased reflux in asthmatics reported significant decreases in FEV_1 and Asthma Severity Scores (41).

Sinusitis, another condition associated with asthma exacerbations (42), occurs more frequently during pregnancy. Sinusitis was estimated in one study to occur in 1.5% of all pregnancies, a six-fold increase in incidence as compared to the general population (43).

A number of medications occasionally used during pregnancy have been reported to cause bronchospasm. Ergonovine, used to stimulate uterine contraction to reduce postpartum or postabortion bleeding, has been reported to cause bronchconstriction in asthmatics (44). Prostaglandins used in second-term abortions and to induce labor in incomplete abortions have also been known to exacerbate asthma (45). It is recommended that Ergonovine and prostaglandins should be avoided if possible in all patients with a history of asthma.

C. Clinical Studies of the Effects of Pregnancy on Asthma

The final analysis of the effects of pregnancy on the course of asthma must rely on clinical observations. Many large studies of asthma during pregnancy have confirmed the general rule that one-third of patients remain unchanged, one third deteriorate, and one third improve (3,46). Yet other studies have reported large variations in asthma improvement from 18% to 69%, and deterioration in 6% to 42% during pregnancy (47,48).

These variations in outcomes of asthma during pregnancy can be explained by variations in study populations, in the choice of measures of asthma severity, and in study design. Demographic variations are very significant because of the reported higher asthma severity in the adolescent (49) and African-American populations (50).

A common theme in many studies is that women with more severe asthma prior to their pregnancies tend to have an increased frequency of attacks during their pregnancies (3,46,48). Changes in asthma severity with pregnancy are also consistent in individual women during successive pregnancies (46).

The timing of asthma improvement and deterioration during the course of the pregnancy has also been studied. As a general rule, asthma improves during the second half of the pregnancy (3,46). In patients who suffered a deterioration of their asthma, weeks 24–36 were the most common time for asthma exacerbation (46). During weeks 37–40, improvement is asthma symptoms occurs across all groups of patients (46). Asthma exacerbations are rarely reported during labor and delivery (46).

V. HOW ASTHMA AFFECTS PREGNANCY

Several historical studies reporting on the effects of asthma in pregnancy conducted prior to the 1980s showed an increased incidence of low birthweight and increased frequency of perinatal mortality (7,9). Adverse maternal outcomes included hyperemesis, hemorrhage, preeclampsia, chronic hypertension, complicated labor, hypoxia, hypocapnia, and alkalosis (4,9). The poor maternal and fetal outcomes frequently cited in these studies was probably the result of lack of steroid treatment for asthma.

Published data from the Collaborative Perinatal Project by Gordon et al. in 1970 reviewed outcomes in a cohort of 277 pregnant asthmatics compared to 30,861 controls (7). A significant increase in perinatal mortality (5.9% vs. 3.2%) was found among pregnant asthmatics, but no difference in prematurity rates or low birthweights was found. There were six maternal deaths, five attributed to asthma. Gordon concluded that severe asthma was a high risk for both mother and fetus.

In 1972, a retrospective study of pregnancy outcomes in 381 asthmatics compared to 112,530 patients without disease found an increased incidence of prematurity, low birthweights, and neonatal mortality (9). There also was noted an increased incidence of hyperemesis, hemorrhage, and preeclampsia in the asthmatic patients. Malformation, stillbirths, and perinatal mortality were not increased in their study.

In more recent studies, with continued advances in asthma therapy, control of disease, and good prenatal care, complications from asthma appear to have become less problematic than previously reported. Asthmatic women treated aggressively during pregnancy have shown improved maternal and fetal outcomes. There is compelling evidence to support the fact that prevention of repeated asthma exacerbations and status asthmaticus during pregnancy promotes favorable maternal-fetal outcomes (51,52).

In a prospective study by Fitzsimmons et al. in 1986, a statistically increased incidence of low birthweight and small-for-gestational-age births were found among eight infants born to women who experienced status asthmaticus during pregnancy compared with 41 infants born to women who did not experience status asthmaticus (51). There were no malformations, neonatal deaths, or maternal deaths. Thus the prevention of status asthmaticus resulted in a more favorable outcome for the fetus.

A prospective study by Stenius-Aarniala et al. in 1988 found no difference in gestational age, birthweight, or perinatal mortality among 181 pregnant asthmatics during 198 pregnancies compared to 198 controls (47). Elective cesarean sections were increased particularly in the most severely affected asthmatic women. Emergency cesarean sections were performed with equal frequency in asthmatic and control patients. Severe asthma and/or systemic corticosteroid treatment appeared to increase the incidence of mild preeclampsia in the mother and hypoglycemia in the infant. The authors concluded that close monitoring of asthma during pregnancy and labor is warranted and should prevent the most serious maternal and fetal complications.

In a recently concluded prospective case-controlled study of 486 asthmatic women and 486 controls followed over the course of 12 years by Schatz et al. found chronic hypertension to be significantly more common among asthmatics than controls (53). There were no statistical differences in the incidence of perinatal mortality, low-birthweight infants, intrauterine growth retardation, congenital malformations, or maternal preeclampsia. Cases and controls were matched for such variables as age, smoking status, parity, and year of delivery. Schatz et al. concluded that "the overall prognosis for women with well managed asthma during pregnancy is comparable to that found for the nonasthmatic population."

Serious complications due to uncontrolled asthma in pregnancy have reportedly been associated with numerous adverse outcomes to both the infant and mother. With the current armamentarium of asthma medications available, most pregnant asthmatics can be managed with minimal complications. Close monitoring and aggressive treatment of the more severe cases in collaboration with careful obstetrical management should preclude many of the adverse outcomes typically associated with pregnant asthmatics in the majority of cases.

VI. MANAGEMENT OF ASTHMA IN PREGNANCY

A. General Principles

Clark (54) has summarized a set of general principles for the treatment of the pregnant asthmatic from The National Institutes of Health (NIH) Working Group on Asthma: (1) monitoring of maternal lung function and fetal well being; (2) avoidance of environmental triggers; (3) pharmacological treatment; and (4) patient education (14).

B. Pharmacological Management

The generally accepted philosophy of avoiding unnecessary medications during the first trimester of pregnancy also applies to the asthmatic. Avoiding environmental triggers as in all asthmatics is the first line therapy in preventing exacerbations. Once an asthma attack occurs the emergency physician should not be hesitant to use pharmacological interventions as the benefits clearly outweigh the potential risks. A recent NIH study on asthma during pregnancy found that physicians and mothers often have unwarranted fears of these drugs' teratogenicity resulting in under treatment and noncompliance (14).

The pharmacological management of asthma in pregnancy is almost identical to that in nonpregnant patients. The Use-in-Pregnancy Ratings of the Food and Drug Administration (FDA) (see Table 1) classifies drugs according fetal risk based on animal and human data. The FDA considers no antiasthma drugs absolutely safe during pregnancy and includes none in Category A. Most asthma drugs are classified as Category B or C. Drugs in Category B can be used with less fear, since these agents do not have evidence of risk

Table 1 Federal Drug Administration Use-in-Pregnancy Ratings

Category	Interpretation
A	Controlled studies show no risk. Adequate, well-controlled studies in pregnant women have failed to demonstrate risk to the fetus.
B	No evidence of risk in humans. Either animal findings show risk, but human findings do not; or if no adequate human studies have been done, animal findings are negative.
C	Risk cannot be ruled out. Human studies are lacking, and animal studies are either positive for fetal risk or lacking as well. However, potential benefits may justify the potential risk.
D	Positive evidence of risk. Investigational or postmarketing data show risk to the fetus. Nevertheless, potential benefits may outweigh the potential risk.
X	Contraindicated in pregnancy. Studies in animals or human, or investigational or postmarketing reports have shown fetal risk that clearly outweighs any possible benefit to the patient.

in humans. Category C drugs have been shown to have teratogenic effects only in animals at supratherapeutic dosages (55) and thus may not be relevant to humans. The final decision to administer Category C drugs should be based on published clinical experiences. Category D drugs have evidence of risk to both animals and humans. No asthma medication in Category D is so exceptionally effective so as to be currently recommended for pregnant patients. Category X drugs show definite risk but little benefit and have no rational use in pregnancy.

VII. OVERVIEW OF ASTHMA MEDICATIONS IN PREGNANCY

A. β-Agonists

As in the nonpregnant patients, the use of β-agonists are first line therapy for acute asthma exacerbations in pregnant patients. β-agonists, especially terbutaline, have been extensively studied clinically in pregnant patients as tocolytic agents. This long-term experience with terbutaline has earned β-agonists an FDA Category B rating for safety in pregnancy. The tocolytic as compared to the bronchodilator dose of β-agonists is much higher and should assure an extra margin of safety for the asthmatic mother and her fetus. It should be remembered, however, that tocolytics are prescribed exclusively in the third trimester and extrapolating their high degree of safety to other intervals of gestation may be an overstatement.

β-agonists may be administered in oral, parenteral, and inhaled formulations. The use of parental administration have been advocated by some physicians for severe attacks, because, theoretically, severe obstruction may prevent some of the drug from entering smaller airways (56). However, studies have not shown subcutaneous administration to be anymore beneficial than inhalation (57,58). Inhaled bronchodilators have been found to be safe in pregnancy (59). The inhaled route is recommended over parental administration because of a more rapid onset of action, higher peak effects, lower plasma levels, with less side effects (60). For the lactating mother, although it is unknown if inhaled β-agonists are found in breast milk, oral and parenteral administration result in detectable levels (61).

The majority of clinical reports of complications with β-agonists have occurred at tocolytic not asthma dosages. Subcutaneous and intravenous administration of β-agonists for tocolysis has been linked to noncardiogenic pulmonary edema (62–65), hypokalemia (66,67), and neonatal hypoglycemia (68). When used to treat asthma, β-agonists have been associated with hypotension (69) and cerebral ischemia (70).

Epinephrine, because of its α-agonist properties, deserves special note. Epinephrine given parenterally has been reported to cause marked decreases in urteroplacental blood flow after low doses of epinephrine in cows, rabbits, and monkeys (71–73). Although this vasoconstrictive effect of epinephrine has not been reproduced in humans further studies seem warranted (74). In rodents, epinephrine has been linked to intrauterine growth retardation (75), fetal survival (76), emotional lability, and learning deficits (77,78). In humans maternal epinephrine has been associated with a statistically higher incidence of congenital defects (79).

B. Corticosteroids

As in nonpregnant asthmatics, the importance and effectiveness of corticosteroids in pregnancy is well established. Corticosteroids reduces the risk of acute asthma attacks during pregnancy (80) and when given at discharge reduces serious exacerbations (81).

The FDA has given steroids a Category C rating. Though, animal studies have shown teratogenic risks such as cleft-palate formation in rabbits, there is little evidence to support teratogenicity in humans (82). Recent studies have shown the safety of corticosteroids in pregnancy and congenital malformations were similar to the general population when asthmatic symptoms were well controlled (51,47). In fact, chronic maternal pulmonary function and not corticosteroid usage were found to determine infant birthweight (83).

For the lactating mother oral and parenteral administration of corticosteroids results in transfer of steroids into breast milk, inhaled formulations have yet to be well studied (84).

Chronic corticosteroid administration may lead to hypothalamic-pituitary-adrenal suppression in both the mother and fetus. This becomes clinically significant only during periods of stress, such as during labor and delivery. Mothers receiving long-term corticosteroids should be given a stress dose of steroids (100 mg hydrocortisone intravenously) during labor. The neonate should then be observed very carefully for signs and symptoms of hypoadrenalism.

C. Methylxanthines

The methylxanthines (aminophylline and theophylline) have be given an FDA Category C rating. Although some animal studies with methylxanthines have demonstrated congenital defects (85,86) recent studies have shown no significant increase in risk (87–89). However, it has been recommended reducing theophylline dosage in the first trimester during fetal organogenesis (47).

Efficacy remains the same during pregnancy, however plasma levels may change during gestation. There appears to be a marked decrease in theophylline clearance (90) in the third trimester secondary to decrease in protein-binding to albumin (91,92). If theophylline is to be given during pregnancy, plasma levels must be carefully monitored.

Theophylline is found in breast milk and may cause may cause irritability or other signs of toxicity in the infant (93). Because there is a potential for serious adverse reactions, caution must be taken when nursing.

D. Anticholinergic Agents

Ipratropium bromide is rated by the FDA in Category B. Though well-controlled, human studies have not been done, there have been no reported teratogenic effects in animals (94). Safety in lactating mothers has not been reported; we recommend caution in use in these patients.

E. Cromolyn Sodium

There is no evidence of teratogenic effects in both humans and animals, and thus has been given a Category B rating. It is not known whether or not cromolyn sodium enters the breast milk. It should be used with caution.

VIII. SUMMARY

Changes in respiratory physiology with pregnancy complicate the diagnosis and clinical evaluation of asthma. Pregnancy requires ED physicians to concern themselves with both the maternal and fetal consequences of an asthma exacerbation. Fetal hypoxia can be caused by decreases in maternal Po_2 or Pco_2 alone. Poorly controlled asthma is associated with higher incidences of preeclampsia and maternal and fetal death. After the introduction of steroid therapy for asthma, aggressively treated pregnant asthmatics should now expect a complication rate no different from the nonasthmatic population. Risks of fetal hypoxia from undertreated asthma should always be balanced with the knowledge that no asthma medication is completely safe in pregnancy. Patient education and close follow-up are the cornerstone of effective therapy for the pregnant asthmatic.

IX. CONCLUSION

Although the pregnant asthmatic patient presents challenges to the ED physician, knowledge of respiratory physiological changes with pregnancy and the safety of asthma therapies provide for successful treatment of these complex patients.

REFERENCES

1. Hernandez E, Angell CS, Johnson JW. Asthma in pregnancy: current concepts. Obstet Gynecol 1980; 55(6):739–743.
2. Weinstein AM, et al. Asthma and pregnancy. JAMA 1979; 241(11):1161–1165.
3. Gluck JC, Gluck P. The effects of pregnancy on asthma: A prospective study. Ann Allergy 1976; 37(3):164–168.
4. Schatz M, et al. The safety of inhaled beta-agonist bronchodilators during pregnancy. J Allergy Clin Immunol 1988; 82(4):686–695.
5. Schatz M, et al. Corticosteroid therapy for the pregnant asthmatic patient. JAMA 1975; 233(7): 804–807.
6. Greenberger PA, Patterson R. Beclomethasone diproprionate for severe asthma during pregnancy. Ann Intern Med 1983; 98(4):478–480.
7. Gordon M, et al. Fetal morbidity following potentially anoxigenic obstetric conditions. VII. Bronchial asthma. Am J Obstet Gynecol 1970; 106(3):421–429.
8. Greenberger PA, Patterson R. The outcome of pregnancy complicated by severe asthma. Allergy Proc 1988; 9(5):539–543.
9. Bahna SL, Bjerkedal T. The course and outcome of pregnancy in women with bronchial asthma. Acta Allergol 1972; 27(5):397–406.
10. Cagal DW, Frank NR, Gaensler EA, et al. Pulmonary function in pregnancy. I. Serial observations in normal women. Am Rev Tuberc 1953; 67;568–597.
11. Rees GB, et al. A longitudinal study of respiratory changes in normal human pregnancy with cross-sectional data on subjects with pregnancy-induced hypertension. Am J Obstet Gynecol 1990; 162(3):826–830.
12. Alaily AB, Carrol KB. Pulmonary ventilation in pregnancy. Br J Obstet Gynaecol 1978; 85(7): 518–524.
13. Baldwin GR, et al. New lung functions and pregnancy. Am J Obstet Gynecol 1977; 127(3): 235–239.
14. National Asthma Education Program Working Group on Asthma and Pregnancy. National

Management of Asthma During Pregnancy. Bethesda, MD, NIH Publication No. 93-3279A, 1992.
15. Milne JA, et al. The effect of human pregnancy on the pulmonary transfer factor for carbon monoxide as measured by the single-breath method. Clin Sci Mol Med 1977; 53(3):271–276.
16. Fadel HE, et al. Normal pregnancy: a model of sustained respiratory alkalosis. J Perinat Med 1979; 7(4):195–201.
17. Liberatore SM, et al. Respiratory function during pregnancy. Respiration 1984; 46(2):145–150.
18. Templeton A, Kelman GR. Maternal blood-gases, PA_{O_2}—Pa_{O_2}, hysiological shunt and VD/VT in normal pregnancy. Br J Anaesth 1976; 48(10):1001–1004.
19. Milne JA, Howie AD, Pack AI. Dyspnoea during normal pregnancy. Br J Obstet Gynaecol 1978; 85(4):260–263.
20. Norregaard O, et al. Lung function and postural changes during pregnancy. Respir Med 1989; 83(6):467–470.
21. Awe RJ, et al. Arterial oxygenation and alveolar-arterial gradients in term pregnancy. Obstet Gynecol 1979; 53(2):182–186.
22. Meschia G. Physiology of transplacental diffusion. Obstet Gynecol Annu 1976; 5:21–38.
23. Wulf KH, Kunzel W, Lehmann V. Clinical aspects of placental gas exchange. In, Long LD, Bartesl H, eds., Respiratory Gas Exchange and Blood Flow in the Placenta. Bethesda, MD: National Institutes of Health, Public Health Service, U.S. Department of Health, Education and Welfare, 505–521, DHEW Publication no. (NIH)73-361, 1972.
24. Longo LD, Hill EP, Power GG. Factors affecting placental oxygen transfer In: Long LD, Bartesl H, eds., Respiratory Gas Exchange and Blood Flow in the Placenta. Bethesda, MD: National Institutes of Health, Public Health Service, U.S. Department of Health, Education and Welfare, 345–391, DHEW Publication No. (NIH)73-361, 1972.
25. Weinstein AM, et al. Asthma and pregnancy. JAMA 1979; 241(11):1161–1165.
26. Moya F, Morishima HO, et al. Influence of maternal hyperventilation on newborn infants. Am J Obstet Gynecol 1965; 91:76.
27. Motoyama EK, Acheson F, Rivard G, Cook CD. Adverse effect on maternal hyperventilation on the fetus. Lancet 1966; I:286.
28. Levinson G, et al. Effects of maternal hyperventilation on uterine blood flow and fetal oxygenation and acid-base status. Anesthesiology 1974; 40(4):340–347.
29. Chazotte C. Asthma in pregnancy: a review. J Assoc Acad Minor Phys 1994; 5(3):107–110.
30. Foster PS, Goldie RG, Paterson JW. Effect of steroids on beta-adrenoceptor-mediated relaxation of pig bronchus. Br J Pharmacol 1983; 78(2):441–445.
31. Nolten WE, et al. Diurnal patterns and regulation of cortisol secretion in pregnancy. J Clin Endocrinol Metab 1980; 51(3):466–472.
32. Burke CW, Roulet F. Increased exposure of tissues to cortisol in late pregnancy. Br Med J 1970; 1(697):657–659.
33. Resnik R, Levine RJ. Plasma diamine oxidase activity in pregnancy: a reappraisal. Am J Obstet Gynecol 1969; 104(7):1061–1066.
34. Taylor AL, et al. Factors influencing the urinary excretion of 3′,5′-adenosine monophosphate in humans. J Clin Endocrinol Metab 1970; 30(3):316–324.
35. Purtilo DT, Hallgren HM, Yunis EJ. Depressed maternal lymphocyte response to phytohemagglutinin in human pregnancy. Lancet 1972; 1(754):769–771.
36. Melillo E, et al. Effect of inhaled PGE2 on exercise-induced bronchconstriction in asthmatic subjects. Am J Respir Crit Care Med 1994; 149(5):1138–1141.
37. Bianco S, et al. Effects of prostacyclin on aspecifically and specifically induced bronchconstriction in asthmatic patients. Eur J Respir Dis Suppl 1980; 106:81–87.
38. Whalen JB, et al. Plasma prostaglandins in pregnancy. Obstet Gynecol 1978; 51(1):52–55.
39. O'Sullivan S, Dahlen B, et al. Increased urinary excretion of the prostaglandin D2 metabolite 9

alpha, 11 beta-prostaglandin F2 after aspirin challenge supports mast cell activation in aspirin-induced airway obstruction. J Allergy Clin Immunol 1996; 98(2):421–432.
40. Richter JE. Gastroesophageal reflux disease: An overlooked cause of asthma. Cleve Clin J Med 1995; 62(3):146–147.
41. Harding SM, et al. Asthma and gastroesophageal reflux: acid suppressive therapy improves asthma outcome. Am J Med 1996; 100(4):395–405.
42. Fuller CG, et al. Sinusitis in status asthmaticus. Clin Pediatr (Phila) 1994; 33(12)712–719.
43. Sorri M, Hartikainen-Sorri AL, Karja J. Rhinitis during pregnancy. Rhinology 1980; 18(2): 83–86.
44. Louie S, et al. Effects of ergometrine on airway smooth muscle contractile responses. Clin Allergy 1985; 15(2):173–178.
45. Partridge BL, Key T, Reisner LS. Life-threatening effects of intravascular absorption of PGF2 alpha during therapeutic termination of pregnancy. Anesth Analg 1988; 67(11):1111–1113.
46. Schatz M, et al. The course of asthma during pregnancy, post partum, and with successive pregnancies: a prospective analysis. J Allergy Clin Immunol 1988; 81(3):509–517.
47. Stenius-Aarniala B, Piirila P, Teramo K. Asthma and pregnancy: a prospective study of 198 pregnancies. Thorax 1988; 43(1):12–18.
48. White RJ, et al. A prospective study of asthma during pregnancy and the puerperium. Respir Med 1989; 83(2):103–106.
49. Apter AJ, Greenberger PA, Patterson R. Outcomes of pregnancy in adolescents with severe asthma. Arch Intern Med 1989; 149(11):2571–2575.
50. Sherman CB, et al. Airway responsiveness in young black and white women. Am Rev Respir Dis 1993; 148(1):98–102.
51. Fitzsimons R, Greenberger PA, Patterson R. Outcome of pregnancy in women requiring corticosteroids for severe asthma. J Allergy Clin Immunol 1986; 78(2):349–353.
52. Greenberger PA, Patterson R. The management of asthma during pregnancy and lactation. Clin Rev Allergy 1987; 5:317–324.
53. Schatz M, Zeiger RS, Hoffman CP, et al. Perinatal outcomes in the pregnancies of asthmatic women: a prospective controlled analysis. Am J Respir Crit Care Med 1995; 151:1170.
54. Clark SL. Asthma in pregnancy. National Asthma Education Program Working Group on Asthma and Pregnancy. National Institutes of Health, National Heart, Lung and Blood Institute [see comments]. Obstet Gynecol 1993; 82(6):1036–1040.
55. Burdon JG, Goss G. Asthma in Pregnancy (editorial). Aust NZ J Med 1993; 24(1):3–4.
56. Larson S, Svedmyr N. Bronchodilating effect and side effects of $beta_2$-adrenoceptor stimulants by different modes of administration (tablets, metered aerosol, and combinations thereof). Am Rev Respir Dis 1977; 116:861–869.
57. Zehner WJ Jr, Scott JM, Iannolo PM, Ungaro A, Terndrup TE. Terbutaline versus albuterol for out-of-hospital respiratory distress: randomized, double-blind trial. Acad Emerg Med 1995; 2:686–691.
58. Youngchaiyud P, Charoenratanakul S. Terbutaline pressurized aerosol inhaled via a Nebuhaler—An effective alternative to subcutaneous adrenaline for treatment of acute severe asthma. Eur J Respir Dis 1987; 70:284–292.
59. Schatz M. The safety of inhaled B-agonists during pregnancy. J Allergy Clin Immunol 1988; 82:686–695.
60. Chapman KR, Smith DL, Rebuck AS, Leenen FH. Hemodynamic effects of an inhaled beta-2 agonist. Clin Pharmacol Ther 1984; 35:762–767.
61. Lindberg C, Boreus LO, de Chateau P, Lindstrom B, Lonnerholm G, Nyberg L. Transfer of terbutaline into breast milk. Eur J Respir Dis (suppl) 1984; 134:87–91.
62. Mabie WC, Pernoll ML, Witty JB, Biswas MK. Pulmonary edema induced by betamimetic drugs. South Med J 1983; 76(11):1354–1360.
63. Benedetti TJ, Hargrove JC, Rosene KA. Maternal pulmonary edema during premature labor inhibition. Obstet Gynecol 1982; 59(6 suppl):33S–37S.

64. Guernsey BG, Villarreal Y, Snyder MD, Gabert HA. Pulmonary edema associated with the use of betamimetic agents in preterm labor. Am J Hosp Pharm 1981; 38(12):1942–1948.
65. Katz M, Robertson PA, Creasy RK. Cardiovascular complications associated with terbutaline treatment for preterm labor. Am J Obstet Gynecol 1981; 139(5):605–608.
66. Cotton DB, Strassner HT, Lipson LG, Goldstein DA. The effects of terbutaline on acid base, serum electrolytes, and glucose homeostasis during the management of preterm labor. Am J Obstet Gynecol 1981; 141(6):617–624.
67. Hurlbert BJ, Edelman JD, David K. Serum potassium levels during and after terbutaline. Anesthesia & Analgesia. 1981; 60(10):723–725.
68. Epstein MF, Nicholls E, Stubblefield PG. Neonatal hypoglycemia after beta-sympathomimetic tocolytic therapy. J Pediatr 1979; 94(3):449–453.
69. Margulies JL, Kallus L. Terbutaline-induced hypotension in a pregnant asthmatic patient. Am J Emerg Med 1986; 4(3):218–221.
70. Rosene KA, Featherstone HJ, Benedetti TJ. Cerebral ischemia associated with parenteral terbutaline use in pregnant migraine patients. Am J Obstet Gynecol 1982; 143(4):405–407.
71. Barron MD, Killam AP, Aexchai G. Response of ovine uterine blood flow to epinephrine and norepienephrine. Proc Soc Exp Biol Med 1974; 145:996–1003.
72. Carter AM, Olin T. Effects of adrenergic stimulation and blockade in the uteroplanceal circulation and uterine activity in the rabbit. Reprod Fertil 1972; 29:251–260.
73. Misenhimer HR, Marguiles SI, Pange IM, et al. Effects of vasoconstrictive drugs on the placental cirulation of the Rhesus monkey. A preliminary report. Invest Radiol 1971; 7:496–499.
74. Albright GA, Iuoppila R, Hollmen AL, et al. Epinephrine does not alter human intervillous blood flow during epidural anestheia. Anethesiology 1981; 54:131–135.
75. Weit K. Effects on the weights of fetuses and fetal lymphoid organs of adrenaline given to rabbits at a critical period of pregnancy: Observations on spontaneous and induced runting. Anat Rec 1965; 153:373–375.
76. Aluetta FL. Effect of epinephrine on implantatontion and fetal survival in the rabbit. J Reprod Fertl 1971; 27:281–285.
77. Crist T, Hulka IF. Influence of maternal epinephrine on behavior of off-spring. Am J Obstet Gynecol 1964; 58:309–311.
78. Young RD. Effect of parenteral maternal injection of epinephrine on post-natal offspring behavior. J Comp Physiol Pshchol 1963; 56:292–293.
79. Heinomen OP, Slone D, Shapiro S. Birth defects and drugs in pregnancy. Littleton, MA: Publishing Sciences Group, 345–348, 1977.
80. Stenius-Aarniala B, Hedman J, Teramo KA. Acute asthma during pregnancy. Thorax 1996; 51:411–414.
81. Wendel PJ, Ramin SM, Barnett-Hamm C, Rowe TF, Cunningham FG. Asthma treatment in pregnancy: A randomized controlled study. Am J Obstet Gynecol 1996; 175(1):150–154.
82. Fainstat T. Cortisone-induced congenital cleft palate in rabbits. Endocrinology 1954; 55:502–508.
83. Schatz M, Zeiger RS, Hoffman CP. Intrauterine growth is related to gestational pulmonary function in pregnant asthmatic women. Chest 1990; 98:389–392.
84. Pearlman WH. Glucocorticoids in milk: a review. Endocrinol Exp 1983; 17(3–4):165–74.
85. Gilbert EF, Bruyere HJ, Ishikawa S, et al. The effect of methylxanthine on catecholamine-stimulated and normal chick embryos. Teratology 1977; 16:47–52.
86. Ishikawa S, Gilbert EF, Bruyere HJ, et al. Aortic Aneurysms associated with cardiac defects in theophylline stimulated chick embryos. Teratology 1978; 18:23–30.
87. Stenius-Aarniala B, Riikonen S, Teramo K. Slow-release Theophylline in Pregnant Asthmatics. Chest 1995; 107(3):642–647.
88. Neff RK, Levitan A. Maternal theophylline consumption and the risk of stillbirth. Chest 1990; 97:1266–1267.

89. Labovitz G, Spector S. Placental theophylline transfer in pregnant asthmatics. JAMA 1982; 247:786–788.
90. Carter BL, Driscoll CE, Smith GD. Theophylline clearance during pregnancy. Obstet Gynecol 1986; 68(4):555–559.
91. Connelly TJ, Ruo TI, Frederiksen MC, et al. Characterization of the theophylline binding to serum proteins in pregnant and nonpregant women. Clin Pharamcol Ther 1990; 47:68–72.
92. Gardner MJ, et al. Longitudinal effects of pregnancy on the pharmacokinetics of theophylline. Eur J Clin Pharmacol 1987; 32(3):289–295.
93. Berlin CM Jr. Excretion of methylxanthines in human milk. Semin Perinatol 1981; 5(4):389–394.
94. Massey KL, Gotz VP. Ipratropium Bromide. Drug Intell Clincal Pharm 1985; 19:5–12.

29

Out-of-Hospital Asthma Care

Samuel J. Stratton
Los Angeles County EMS Agency, Los Angeles, and Harbor–UCLA Medical Center, Torrance, California

I. INTRODUCTION

Actions taken in the out-of-hospital (field) setting help determine the success in ongoing acute asthma management. Objectives for management of asthma in the field are efficient assessment, patient stabilization, initiation of efforts to interrupt bronchospasm, and safe, rapid transport to emergency center care. Excessive assessment time, use of unproven treatments, and high risk–low benefit maneuvers are to be avoided in the uncontrolled out-of-hospital environment. With these principles as a basis, rational approaches to the out-of-hospital management of acute asthma are discussed in this chapter.

Out-of-hospital data on the management of acute asthma is minimal. Therefore, this chapter relies on emergency department (ED) and other studies as well as out-of-hospital data resources. Because there are so few published studies focused on such a common disease, the out-of-hospital management of acute asthma is an area that presents ample opportunity for future research.

II. OUT-OF-HOSPITAL ASSESSMENT

Emergency personnel responding to a victim with acute asthma can add unique information to the patient assessment (Table 1). A quick survey of the scene can provide caregivers with information that otherwise may not be available. Reporting smoke, fumes, dust, or air pollution at the scene can be helpful for those receiving the patient from the field. Patient medication bottles should be gathered and brought to the ED. A quick overall assessment of patient psychological factors may prove helpful for those treating the patient's acute attack. Finally, an assessment of the patient's living or working conditions

Table 1 Out-of-Hospital Acute Asthma Scene Evaluation

Environment
Dust or pollutants noted
Fumes (paint, gasoline, solvents, etc.)
Tobacco smoke or fireplace-heater smoke
Pets and/or plants noted
Housecleaning in progress
Condition of carpet, furniture, and window coverings
Social
Emotional stress level
Evidence of alcohol and/or drug use
Evidence of tobacco use by patient

The out-of-hospital scene evaluation can provide information that cannot be obtained elsewhere. Documentation of possible precipitants of the acute asthma attack help primary care providers develop treatment plans for the prevention of future asthma attacks.

can be extremely helpful for identifying possible causes of exacerbation of a patient's asthma.

At the scene, a directed asthma history should be obtained and documented. The field history should be focused to determine the length of time for the present attack, any atypical aspects of the attack, precipitating factors, and current therapy including doses and frequency of use of medications. Previous hospitalizations and intubations as a result of asthma and recent use of steroids are also important facts to obtain in the field history. In addition, history of medical problems other than asthma (particularly cardiac) and known allergies and past drug reactions should be obtained.

Tachypnea and appreciation of wheezing on lung auscultation are the primary signs for field recognition of acute asthma. In addition to the primary signs, the secondary signs of accessory muscle use, breathlessness causing inability to speak, diaphoresis, posturing to augment breathing, tachycardia, and palpable pulsus paradoxus are important for the field recognition of acute asthma. The prolongation of the expiratory phase of breathing is also valuable for field recognition of acute asthma. Fever, cough, vomiting, and other signs of illness complicating asthma should also be noted. Documenting and reporting the initial signs of severe asthma are important because the signs may abate as treatment of bronchospasm is started in the field.

Severe bronchospasm with minimal breath sounds and loss of the primary sign of wheezing presents a difficult field assessment situation. History of asthma is often most helpful in decreasing confusion in this situation. Hyperinflation and recognition of the secondary signs of bronchospasm also allow for rapid out-of-hospital identification of acute asthma presenting with minimal breath sounds.

It is essential that those managing acute asthma in the out-of-hospital environment be familiar with the physical signs of respiratory failure. A shallow, labored breathing pattern, central cyanosis, bradypnea, staring facies, diaphoresis, a recumbent position because of exhaustion from the work of breathing, and poor perfusion secondary to hyperinflation causing decreased right heart filling are important field signs of impending respiratory arrest. It has been this author's field observation that uncontrolled head bobbing or relaxation of the neck allowing the head to lean forward while a patient is being moved on a stretcher or during ambulance transport signals exhaustion and impending respiratory arrest. Mental status changes—either as agitation, confusion, or somnolence—also should rapidly be recognized as important signs of hypoxia and impending respiratory arrest.

Pulse oximetry may add to the field assessment of the acute asthmatic. A 1989 survey of United States revealed that pulse oximetry was used in 6% of out-of-hospital systems (1). Despite risks of inaccuracy because of motion artifact and ambient light interference, pulse oximetry has been shown to be reliable for determination of hypoxia in the out-of-hospital setting (2–4). Reliability of pulse oximetry has also been shown when used in helicopter transports (5). A prospective study comparing ED admission oximetry with field assessment found that in 27 of 30 patients, hypoxia identified by pulse oximetry was not recognized by field physical assessment (6). Treating hypoxia is important, but it is of note that in-hospital pediatric studies show oximetry to be limited to identification of hypoxia and not necessarily indicative of the severity of an acute asthma attack (7–10). There are limitations to the accuracy of pulse oximetry from poor extremity perfusion, such as vasoconstriction secondary to cold ambient temperatures, and obstruction to the monitoring light beam, such as fingernail polish. Anemia has also been associated with erroneous pulse oximetry readings (11). (see Chapter 16). With recognition of its limitations, pulse oximetry can detect hypoxia in the field. Hypoxia identifies patients with severe asthma and risk of death and it is recommended that pulse oximetry be used in out-of-hospital asthma monitoring.

Measurement of peak expiratory flow rate (PEFR) is not widely used in out-of-hospital emergency medical service systems. PEFR measurements have been used without difficulty in field studies of asthma (12). In research of acute asthma, researchers should consider making initial pulmonary function measurements in the out-of-hospital setting because therapy begins in the field. Inexpensive, disposable PEFR meters are available and medical directors of out-of-hospital systems should consider using these devices to add to the field assessment information used for management of acute asthma patients.

III. OUT-OF-HOSPITAL TREATMENT

This section focuses on out-of-hospital treatment of acute asthma and its integration into the overall care of the patient. Discussion is directed toward the unique aspects of the field environment with recognition that more detailed treatment information is addressed in other chapters of this text. The primary goal in the out-of-hospital treatment of acute asthma is reversal of bronchospasm to provide normalization of pulmonary gas exchange. Bronchodilator therapy is therefore the primary field approach to management of acute asthma. Oxygen administration is also a standard field procedure. Anti-inflammatory therapy, such as oral or intravenous corticosteroids, are not known to be of immediate benefit in the field setting. With prolonged field times, as in the rural out-of-hospital setting, corticosteroids are sometimes included in treatment protocols so that there is not delay in initiation of anti-inflammatory therapy (13).

β_2-agonists are the agents of choice for the initial management of acute asthma and studies have shown that inhaled β_2-agonists are safe and effective in the out-of-hospital setting (14–17). β_2-agonists are the preferred initial bronchodilator because of fewer side effects when compared to other bronchodilators and a short onset of action within 5 min (18). The inhaled route is preferred because it has a more rapid onset of action when compared to oral administration and is as effective as the subcutaneous route (17,19–22). β_2-agonists are relatively safe when administered by inhalation, but out-of-hospital providers should be aware of the complications of the use of these drugs, which include cardiovascular stimulation, anxiety, and skeletal muscle tremor (19). There has not been a maximum dose established for β_2-agonists when used in the treatment of acute asthma, and they can be administered continuously by inhalation with discontinuation if adverse effects develop (23–28). Cardiac monitoring for dysrhythmias is important when aggressive continuous β_2-agonist therapy is used in the field for the management of acute asthma patients with known or potential cardiac disease. Studies, though, have not associated inhaled β_2-agonists use in acute asthma with increased ventricular ectopy (29,30).

The method of delivery of inhaled bronchodilators is of interest in out-of-hospital care. The field environment is a unique setting that requires safe, compact, and portable methods of delivery for treatments. With this in mind, there is question of whether a metered dose inhaler (MDI) or nebulizer is best for use in the field. Numerous studies have shown that bronchodilator delivery by metered dose inhaler with a spacer device is as effective as delivery by continuous nebulizer (31–42). With both techniques of aerosol delivery being equal, most out-of-hospital systems are left to choose the most cost effective and practical method. Interestingly, the literature bias is for MDIs with spacers, but in the out-of-hospital setting the nebulizer is commonly used. This is explained by the comparative low cost and compactness of the disposable plastic nebulizer. Disadvantages of the nebulizer include the need for concomitant oxygen delivery to drive the nebulizer because most out-of-hospital transport units do not carry compressed air. This concomitant supplemental oxygen delivery with nebulized therapy can result in potential respiratory depression for those with acute asthma complicated by chronic lung disease or carbon dioxide retention. Nebulizers also disperse aerosol into the closed environment of an ambulance and expose others to the drug. Metered dose inhalers, even with spacer chambers, are sometimes difficult for young and old patients to use. MDIs may have unpredictable aerosol delivery patterns at the extremes of temperatures that are encountered in the out-of-hospital environment and rarely have also been associated with paradoxical bronchospasm related to chlorofluorocarbons used to propel the drug from the canister (43,44).

Subcutaneous injection of epinephrine, terbutaline, or other adrenergic agents is used in many out-of-hospital systems as secondary therapy when aerosol therapy has failed to provide relief of acute asthma. Studies have shown that subcutaneous epinephrine or terbutaline are effective bronchodilators in acute asthma (17,45,46). It is also reported that subcutaneous injection of epinephrine improves expiratory flow rates for those patients who fail to respond to inhaled β-agonists (47). Although there is concern for causing serious cardiac side effects when using subcutaneous adrenergics for patients more than 40 years old, it has been reported that with caution these agents can be used in older patients (48). (see Chapter 20).

Oxygen is considered a mainstay in the field treatment of acute asthma and generally recommended in all but mild cases. When pulse oximetry is available, oxygen is recommended if the saturation is below 95%. Hypoxia is difficult to assess in the field and correlates poorly with severity of airflow obstruction (49). High flow (40% FiO_2 or greater) oxygen is usually used to supplement room air for acute asthma. Supplemental oxygen should be used with caution for those acute asthmatics who also have chronic lung disease. Whether using high- or low-flow oxygen for the management of acute asthma complicated by chronic lung disease, field personnel must be alert to the potential for oxygen to suppress respiratory drive.

There is little literature regarding the use of anticholinergics in the out-of-hospital setting. Ipratropium, available in MDIs, has minimal systemic absorption and proven bronchodilator effect (19). But studies of the benefit of adding anticholinergics to β-agonist in the ED setting have yielded conflicting results (50,51). Anticholinergics act on the parasympathetic system to provide secondary bronchodilation and clinical trials have shown inhaled anticholinergics to be inferior to a β_2-agonist in treating status asthmaticus (52). Therefore, anticholinergics have a secondary role to β_2-agonists if they are to be considered for use in the out-of-hospital setting.

Before the introduction of inhaled β_2-agonists, aminophylline was used extensively in the out-of-hospital setting. Concomitant with the introduction of β-agonists, the field use of aminophylline has become controversial due to the low therapeutic index for theophyllines. Although somewhat effective bronchodilators, several studies have questioned the benefit of theophyllines in the emergency setting (53–56). A primary concern is the risk of serious side effects and toxicity with the use of aminophylline in the relatively uncontrolled out-of-hospital environment. Aminophylline has a narrow therapeutic–toxic range and has multiple potential undesirable effects, including cardiac dysrhythmias and seizures (57–60). In addition, there is increased risk for complications when aminophylline is administered to patients already receiving maintenance theophylline preparations (59,61). This can complicate management of patients in the out-of-hospital setting who are taking unknown medications. With β_2-agonists available as effective out-of-hospital bronchodilators, the use of aminophylline in the field setting is questionable.

Systemic steroids are used in some out-of-hospital systems for the treatment of acute asthma (13). Steroids are currently the most effective method of reducing inflammation of the bronchi and are mainstays of treatment of acute asthma. A problem with the out-of-hospital use of steroids is that the anti-inflammatory effect takes hours, not minutes (52). Although steroids are safe and effective in the treatment of the acute asthmatic, it is unlikely that they have an immediate effect in the field setting. In situations of prolonged field treatment and transport times, such as occurs in rural out-of-hospital systems, the administration of oral or intravenous corticosteroids may be advantageous for overall patient management (see Chapter 22).

Magnesium sulfate produces bronchodilation and has been suggested by some to be effective in the management of acute asthma (62–64). Initial enthusiasm for magnesium in the treatment of acute asthma has decreased with further study (65,66). Intravenous magnesium sulfate has been shown to decrease hospital admission rate in patients with severe acute asthma but has not been shown to cause significant improvement in patients with moderate acute asthma (67). Side effects of magnesium include nausea, vomiting, and hypotension. Because of questionable efficacy when used in the routine treatment of acute asthma, the use of magnesium in the out-of-hospital management of acute asthma is unproven except in severe cases (see Chapter 24).

Past acute asthma management has encouraged early hydration based on the theory that increased respiratory rate and physical stress causes a relative state of dehydration resulting in thickened bronchial secretions that are difficult for a patient to clear. This theory is unsupported for adults or children who have usual access to oral fluids. In the out-of-hospital setting, fluid therapy is best based on the presence of circumstances and physical signs of dehydration and not on unproven theory of alteration in bronchial secretion viscosity (see Chapter 25).

IV. PEDIATRIC CONSIDERATIONS

The out-of-hospital management of acute asthma in children is similar to that already discussed in this chapter. Objective and subjective assessment parameters for children are subtle, making field assessment difficult in comparison to that of the adult. In general, field assessment of the asthmatic child is based on respiratory rate, degree of work in breathing, accessory muscle use, overall activity level, response to environment, pulse rate, palpable pulsus paradoxus, and assessment of breath sounds.

Respiratory rates in children can be difficult to assess because of age-related variation in normal breathing rates. Commonly in the out-of-hospital setting, a respiratory rate of greater than 35–40 per minute for a child over 1 year old is considered abnormal. Ideally, a reference chart of normal respiratory rates should be available in the field. A slow or irregular respiratory rate is a very serious sign of respiratory failure in the acutely ill child or infant. In addition to respiratory rate as an indication of breathlessness, the level of respiratory distress for a child who is able to verbalize can be assessed by determining if the child can speak in sentences or count to 10 without pausing to breathe.

Accessory muscle use in breathing correlates well with respiratory distress in childhood asthma (68). Because accessory muscle use is a reliable sign and quickly noted, it is a valuable assessment tool in the out-of-hospital setting. Palpable pulsus paradoxus is less valuable for field asthma assessment of children as compared to adults because the underlying respiratory and heart rate for children is often very rapid (see Chapter 13).

A decreased response to stimulation by parents and the environment is useful in determining level of fatigue. Decreased environmental response can also be an indication of hypoxia or poor cerebral perfusion. Fatigue, hypoxia, or poor cerebral perfusion causing abnormal environmental and parent response is a serious out-of-hospital sign that requires prompt stabilization and transport to an emergency center. Pulse oximetry on ambient air may help define hypoxia as a problem in the setting of decreased environmental response, but should not be relied upon to rule out respiratory fatigue and circulatory failure (7).

Wheezing indicates partial obstruction of small airways, but is of low sensitivity for the degree of obstruction (68). Auscultation of the child in the out-of-hospital setting is made more difficult than usual because of ambient noise. In severe airway obstruction, minimal airflow may result in absence of breath sounds. Because of these challenges, auscultation is often suboptimal and accurate field assessment of acute asthma in the child is based on a combination of assessment parameters.

Asthma, frequently related to respiratory syncytial virus, occurs in infants, and field assessment in this age group is particularly difficult. In addition to the parameters that are sought in assessing the older child, an infant may have poor feeding or suckling, weak cry, or interrupted sleeping patterns as manifestations of acute asthma. Out-of-hospital auscultation for lung sounds is particularly difficult in infants. Respiratory rates above 60 per minute should be considered abnormal in the field evaluation of the child from 1–12 months of age. Out-of-hospital management of infants with possible acute asthma should be conservative because of several anatomic and physiological differences that place them at risk for respiratory failure. These differences include increased peripheral airway resistance, spiral smooth muscle that extends into the peripheral airways, and decreased elastic recoil pressure within the airways and chest (69,70).

The basic out-of-hospital management of pediatric acute asthma is outlined in Table 2. As discussed in the general management of asthma earlier in this chapter, field pharmacological management of acute pediatric asthma is primarily inhaled β_2-agonists (25,28,71–73). Supplemental oxygen is also considered standard in moderate to severe asthma or for presence of signs of hypoxia. It is important to use a properly fitting mask when administering aerosols or oxygen to a child. If a child is in severe distress or has decreased mental status and is unable to adequately inhale β_2-agonists, it is recommended

Table 2 Out-of-Hospital Management of Pediatric Acute Asthma

Assess severity of attack
Airway patent?
Alert, aware of environment? Normal response to parents?
Rapid respiratory rate (use age-based reference chart)
Breathing slow or irregular?
Using accessory muscles?
Able to speak in sentences or count to 10 without breathlessness?
Tachycardia, palpable pulsus paradoxus?
Breath sounds = wheezing, decreased, absent?
Pulse oximetry $<$ 95%? Central cyanosis?
Bronchodilator therapy and oxygenation
Continuous β_2-agonist via nebulizer or inhaler with spacer
Supplemental oxygen (40% $F\text{IO}_2$)
Subcutaneous adrenergic if unable to inhale β_2-agonists (may repeat to total of 3 doses given every 20 min)
Considerations
Consider corticosteroids in prolonged field transports ($>$ 1 hr)
Also assess infants for decreased feeding or suckling, weak cry, or restlessness
Assess for evidence of other complicating illness (fever, vomiting)

that subcutaneous adrenergic be administered immediately (18). Anticholinergics add incremental bronchodilator effect when used in combination with β_2-agonists but should be considered as second line therapy to the β_2-agonists in the initial field management of pediatric acute asthma (74–76). A number of studies have shown that theophyllines are of little benefit and of high risk for adverse side effects in the initial phases of treatment of childhood acute asthma (77–79). Corticosteroids, as previously discussed, have a delayed onset of action and it is doubtful that they have an effect in other than circumstances of prolonged field transport times. Hydration of children with severe asthma to decrease viscosity of bronchial secretions and treat assumed dehydration from the stress of asthma has not been shown to be necessary (80).

V. SPECIAL CONSIDERATIONS

It is reported that fewer than 2% of ED visits for asthma result in admission to medical ICUs and even fewer require endotracheal intubation (52). Although rare, out-of-hospital intubation is sometimes required to stabilize the acute asthma patient. The indications for intubation of the acute asthmatic are acute respiratory failure or arrest and not different from other ventilatory emergencies, but there are some important aspects of mechanical ventilation of the asthmatic that must be considered.

For a complete discussion of endotracheal intubation of the acute asthmatic, refer to Chapter 26 on endotracheal intubation. Out-of-hospital intubation of the asthmatic is frequently difficult because the patient is usually semiconscious with increased jaw and facial muscle tone. Endotracheal tube placement in acute asthma may stimulate the airway and increase bronchospasm that can make ventilation more difficult (52). After intubation, the asthmatic airway poses further challenges. Overinflation of alveolar units can lead to local rupture, alveolar tissue damage, and—in extreme situations—to pneumothorax and

Table 3 General Out-of-Hospital Management of Acute Asthma

Assess severity of attack
- Airway patent?
- Increased respiratory rate, using accessory muscles?
- Central cyanosis, abnormal skin perfusion?
- Awake, alert?
- Diaphoretic, able to speak in sentences?
- Tachycardia, palpable pulsus paradoxus?
- Breathsounds = wheezing, decreased, absent?
- Pulse oximetry $< 95\%$?

Bronchodilator therapy and oxygenation
- Continuous β_2-agonist via nebulizer or inhaler
- Supplemental oxygen (caution in COPD) if:
  1. Pulse oximetry 95% saturation or below
  2. Moderate or severe attack
- Subcutaneous adrenergic if no response to inhaled β_2-agonist, may repeat to total of 3 doses given every 20 min

Considerations
- Consider corticosteroids in prolonged field transports (>1 hr)
- Constantly assess for need to assist ventilation or intubate
- Cardiac monitor if risk of cardiac disease

Summary of the basic out-of-hospital assessment and treatment of the acute asthmatic. Physical assessment is focused to determine the stability of the patient and need for field intervention. Field treatment is based on bronchodilator therapy with inhaled β_2-agonists, the preferred initial intervention.

pneumomediastinum (52). Air trapping from flow limiting segments of airways can lead to hyperinflation of the thorax and decreased ventilation. Because of air trapping, it is important for the out-of-hospital caregiver to provide an increased expiratory time as compared to inspiratory time to allow for adequate exhalation through partially obstructed airways. Considering the potential complications, intubation of the acute asthmatic in the out-of-hospital setting is dangerous and should only be considered in the most extreme of circumstances (see Chapter 30).

Theoretically, epinephrine, terbutaline, or other β_2-agonists can be administered endobronchially by instillation of the drug into an endotracheal tube when a severe asthmatic has been intubated. This technique for administering adrenergics has been adopted by some out-of-hospital systems (13). Further research is needed to establish the efficacy of this practice.

Air transport of the acute asthmatic introduces the risk of barotrauma. Theoretically, with rapid atmospheric pressure changes, hyperinflation can become extreme and lead to increased risk for pneumothorax and pneumomediastinum. Severe hyperinflation of the lungs can also lead to decreased right heart filling with resulting loss of cardiac output. There are few published data available regarding aerotransport of acute asthma victims. Because of potential complications, acute asthmatics being transported by rotary or fixed wing aircraft must be monitored closely by personnel trained in advanced life support and air transport procedures.

Helium-oxygen therapy has been suggested by some as potentially useful in the management of the out-of-hospital severe acute asthmatic. Preliminary studies have shown helium-oxygen to be possibly effective for short-term management to avoid intubation of the acute asthmatic (81,82). Although costly with limited indications, helium-oxygen may have application in the out-of-hospital setting and further study of this therapy is warranted.

VI. SUMMARY

The out-of-hospital management of acute asthma is based on rapid, efficient assessment of the patient and scene; ventilatory stabilization; initiation of treatment to interrupt bronchospasm; and safe transport to definitive medical care. Therapy (Table 3) is primarily adrenergic agents, usually β_2-agonists delivered by inhalation. The out-of-hospital caregiver must always be aware of the potential for rapid deterioration of the acute asthmatic and be prepared to act to stabilize the patient. Out-of-hospital situations that can lead to changes in atmospheric pressure are high risk and require particularly close monitoring.

REFERENCES

1. Lavery RF, Doran J, Tortella BJ, Cody RP. A survey of advanced life support practices in the United States. Prehospital and Disaster Medicine 1992; 7:144–150.
2. Silverston P. Pulse oximetry at the roadside: A study of pulse oximetry in immediate care. Br Med J 1989; 298:711–713.
3. Aughey K, Hess D, Eitel D, Bleecher K, Cooley M, Ogden C, Sabulsky N. An evaluation of pulse oximetry in prehospital care. Ann Emerg Med 1991; 20:887–891.
4. Cydulka RK, Shade B, Emerman CL, Gersham H, Kubincanek J. Prehospital pulse oximetry: useful or misused. Ann Emerg Med 1992; 21:675–679.
5. Valko PC, Campbell JP, McCarty DL, Martin D, Turnbull J. Prehospital use of pulse oximetry in rotary-wing aircraft. Prehospital and Disaster Medicine 1991; 6:421–428.
6. Brown LH, Manring EA, Kornegay HB, Prasad NH. Can prehospital personnel detect hypoxemia without the aid of pulse oximeters? Am J Emerg Med 1996; 14:43–44.
7. Gussack GS, Tacchi EJ. Pulse oximetry in the management of pediatric airway disorders. South Med J 1987; 80:1381–1384.
8. Geelhoed GC, Landau LI, LeSouef PN. Predictive value of oxygen saturation in emergency evaluation of asthmatic children. Br Med J 1988; 297:395–396.
9. Yamamoto LG, Wiebe RA, Anaya C, Chang RKS, Chang MA, Terada AM, Bray ML, Ching CY, Kim MY, Shinsato ET, Shomura LL. Pulse oximetry and peak flow as indicators of wheezing severity in children and improvement following bronchodilator treatments. Am J Emerg Med 1992; 10:519–524.
10. Mayefsky JH, El-Shinaway Y. The usefulness of pulse oximetry in evaluating acutely ill asthmatics. Ped Emerg Care 1992; 8:262–264.
11. Jubran A, Tobin MJ. Noninvasive respiratory monitoring. In: J.E. Parrillo and R.C. Bone, eds., Critical Care Medicine St. Louis, MO: Mosby, 1995, p. 159.
12. Rottman SJ, Robinson NE, Birnbaum ML. Comparison of inhaled metaproterenol via metered-dose inhaler and hand-held nebulizer in prehospital treatment of bronchospasm. Prehospital Disaster Medicine 1996; 11:280–284.
13. Westfal REJ. Paramedic Protocols, New York: McGraw-Hill, 1997, pp. 62–63.
14. Iscovich AL. Pre-hospital use of hand-held aerosol nebulizer. Ann Emerg Med 1985; 14:512.
15. Emerman C, Schade B, Kubincanek J. A controlled trial of nebulized isoetharine in the prehospital treatment of acute asthma. Am J Emerg Med 1990; 8:512–514.

16. Eitel DR, Meador SA, Drawbaugh R, Hess D, Sabulsky NK, Bernini R. Prehospital administration of inhaled metaproterenol. Ann Emerg Med 1990; 19:1412–1417.
17. Quadrel M, Lavery RF, Jaker M, Atkin S, Tortella BJ, Cody RP. Prospective, randomized trial of epinephrine, metaproterenol, and both in the prehospital treatment of asthma in the adult patient. Ann Emerg Med 1995; 26:469–473.
18. U.S. Department of Health and Human Services, Management of exacerbations of asthma: Guidelines for the Diagnosis and Management of Asthma, Bethesda, MD, 1991, pp. 89–115.
19. U.S. Department of Health and Human Services, Overview of approaches to asthma therapy: Guidelines for the Diagnosis and Management of Asthma, Bethesda, MD, 1991, pp. 35–43.
20. Uden DL, Goetz DR, Kohen DP, Fifield GC. Comparison of nebulized terbutaline and subcutaneous epinephrine in the treatment of acute asthma. Ann Emerg Med 1985; 14:229–232.
21. Elenbaas RM, Frost GL, Robinson WA, Collier RE, McNabney WK, Ryan JL, Singsank MJ. Subcutaneous epinephrine vs. Nebulized metaproterenol in acute asthma. Drug Intell Clin Pharm 1985; 19:7–8, 567–571.
22. Ruddy RM, Kolski G, Scarpa N, Wilmott R. Aerosolized metaproterenol compared to subcutaneous epinephrine in the emergency treatment of acute childhood asthma. Pediatr Pulmonol 1986; 2:230–236.
23. Turner JR, Corkery KJ, Eckman D, Gelb AM, Lipavsky A, Sheppard D. Equivalence of continuous flow nebulizer and metered-dose inhaler with reservoir bag for treatment of acute airflow obstruction. Chest 1988; 93:476–481.
24. Olshaker J, Jerrard D, Barish RA, Brandt G, Hooper F. The efficacy and safety of a continuous albuterol protocol for the treatment of acute adult asthma attacks. Am J Emerg Med 1993; 11:131–133.
25. Katz RW, Kelly HW, Crowley MR, Grad R, McWilliams BC, Murphy SJ. Safety of continuous nebulized albuterol for bronchospasm in infants and children. Pediatrics 1993; 92:666–669.
26. Rudnitsky GS, Eberlein RS, Schoffstall JM, Mazur JE, Spivey WH. Comparison of intermittent and continuously nebulized albuterol for treatment of asthma. Ann Emerg Med 1993; 22: 1842–1846.
27. Lin RY, Sauter D, Newman T, Sirleaf J, Walters J, Tavakol M. Continuous versus intermittent albuterol nebulization in the treatment of asthma. Ann Emerg Med 1993; 22:1847–1853.
28. Papo MC, Frank J, Thompson AE. A prospective, randomized study of continuous versus intermittent nebulized albuterol for severe status asthmaticus in children. Crit Care Med 1993; 21:1479–1486.
29. Emerman CL, Crafford WA, Vrobel TR. Ventricular arrhythmias during treatment for acute asthma. Ann Emerg Med 1986; 15:699–702.
30. Seider N, Abinader EG, Oliven A. Cardiac arrhythmias after inhaled bronchodilators in patients with COPD and ischemic heart disease. Chest 1993; 104:1070–1074.
31. Berenberg MJ, Baigelman W, Cupples LA, Pearce L. Comparison of metered-dose inhaler attached to an Aerochamber with an updraft nebulizer for the administration of metaproterenol in hospitalized patients. J Asthma 1985; 22:87–92.
32. Summer W, Elston R, Tharpe L, Nelson S, Haponik EF. Aerosol bronchodilator delivery methods. Relative impact on pulmonary function and cost of respiratory care. Arch Intern Med 1989; 149:618–623.
33. Gervais A, Begin P. Bronchodilation with a metered-dose inhaler plus an extension, using tidal breathing vs. jet nebulization. Chest 1987; 92:822–824.
34. Sly RM, Barbera JM, Middleton HB, Eby DM. Delivery of albuterol aerosol by aerochamber to young children. Ann Allergy 1988; 60:403–406.
35. Salzman GA, Steele MT, Pribble JP, Elenbaas RM, Pyszczynski DR. Aerosolized metaproterenol in the treatment of asthmatics with severe airflow obstruction: comparison of two delivery methods. Chest 1989; 95:1017–1020.
36. Idris AH, McDermott MF, Raucci JC, Morrabel A, McGorray S, Hendeles L. Emergency department treatment of severe asthma: metered-dose inhaler plus holding chamber is equivalent in effectiveness to nebulizer. Chest 1993; 103:665–672.

37. Colacone A, Afilado M, Wolkove N, Kreisman H. A comparison of albuterol administered by metered dose inhaler (and holding chamber) or wet nebulizer in acute asthma. Chest 1993; 104:835–841.
38. Kerem E, Levison H, Schuh S, O'Brodovich H, Reisman J, Bentur L, Canny GJ. Efficacy of albuterol administered by nebulizer versus spacer device in children with acute asthma. J Pediatr 1993; 123:313–317.
39. Chou KJ, Cunningham SJ, Crain EF. Metered-dose inhalers with spacers vs. nebulizers for pediatric asthma. Arch Ped Adol Med 1995; 149:201–205.
40. Parkin PC, Saunders NR, Diamond SA, Winders PM, MacArthur C. Randomized trial of spacer vs. nebulizer for acute asthma. Arch Dis Child 1995; 72:239–240.
41. Lin YZ, Hsieh KH. Metered dose inhaler and nebulizer in acute asthma. Arch Dis Child 1995; 72:214–218.
42. Levitt MA, Gambrioli EF, Fink JB. Comparative trial of continuous nebulization versus metered-dose inhaler in the treatment of acute bronchospasm. Ann Emerg Med 1995; 26:273–277.
43. Wilkinson JRW, Roberts JA, Bradding P, Holgate ST, Howarth PH. Paradoxical bronchoconstriction in asthmatic patients after salmeterol by metered dose inhaler. Br Med J 1992; 305: 931–932.
44. Wilson AF, Mukai DS, Ahdout JJ. Effect of canister temperature on performance of metered-dose inhalers. Am Rev Respir Dis 1991; 143:1034–1037.
45. Spiteri MA, Millar AB, Pavia D, Clarke SW. Subcutaneous adrenaline versus terbutaline in the treatment of acute severe asthma. Thorax 1988; 43:19–23.
46. Victoria MS, Battista CJ, Nangia BS. Comparison between epinephrine and terbutaline injections in the acute management of asthma. J Asthma 1989; 26:287–290.
47. Appel D, Karpel JP, Sherman M. Epinephrine improves expiratory flow rates in patients with asthma who do not respond to inhaled metaproterenol sulfate. J Allergy Clin Immunol 1989; 84:90–98.
48. Cydulka R, Davison R, Grammar L, Parker M, Mathews J. The use of epinephrine in the treatment of older adult asthmatics. Ann Emerg Med 1988; 17:322–326.
49. Fisher JD, Vinci RJ. Prehospital management of pediatric asthma requiring hospitalization. Pediatr Emerg Care 1995; 11:217–219.
50. Shrestha M, O'Brien T, Haddox R, Gourlay HS, Reed G. Decreased duration of emergency department treatment of chronic obstructive pulmonary disease exacerbations with the addition of ipratropium bromide to beta-agonist therapy. Ann Emerg Med 1991; 20:1206–1209.
51. Owens MW, George RB. Nebulized atropine sulfate in the treatment of acute asthma. Chest 1991; 99:1084–1087.
52. Abou-Shala N, MacIntyre N. Emergent management of acute asthma. Med Clin North Am 1996; 80:677–699.
53. Monserrat JM, Barbera JA, Viegas C, Roca J, Rodriguez-Roisin R. Gas exchange response to intravenous aminophylline in patients with severe exacerbation of asthma. Eur Respir J 1995; 8:28–33.
54. Littenberg B. Aminophylline treatment in severe, acute asthma: a meta-analysis. JAMA 1988; 259:1678–1684.
55. Fanta CH, Rossing TH, McFadden ER. Treatment of acute asthma: is combination therapy with sympathomimetics and methylxanthines indicated? Am J Med 1986; 80:5–10.
56. Murphy DG, McDermott MF, Rydman RJ, Sloan EP, Zalenski RJ. Aminophylline in the treatment of acute asthma when $beta_2$-adrenergics and steroids are provided. Arch Intern Med 1993; 153:1784–1788.
57. Rodrigo C, Rodrigo G. Treatment of acute asthma: lack of therapeutic benefit and increase of the toxicity from aminophylline given in addition to high doses of salbuterol delivered by metered-dose inhaler with a spacer. Chest 1994; 106:1071–1076.
58. Bittar G, Friedman HS. The arrhythmogenicity of theophylline: a multivariate analysis of clinical determinates. Chest 1991; 99:1415–1420.

59. Bahls FH, Ma KK, Bird TD. Theophylline-associated seizures with ''therapeutic'' or low toxic serum concentrations: risk factors for serious outcome in adults. Neurology 1991; 41:1309–1312.
60. Aitken ML, Martin TR. Life-threatening theophylline toxicity is not predictable by serum levels. Chest 1987; 91:10.
61. Stewart MF, Barclay J, Warburton R. Risk of giving intravenous aminophylline to acutely ill patients receiving maintenance treatment with theophylline. Br Med J 1984; 288:450.
62. Nopper M, Vanmaele L, Impens N, Schandevyl W. Bronchodilating effect of intravenous magnesium sulfate in acute severe bronchial asthma. Chest 1990; 97:373.
63. Skobeloff EM, Spivey WH, McNamara RM, Greenspon L. Intravenous magnesium sulfate for the treatment of acute asthma in the emergency department. JAMA 1989; 262:1210.
64. Okayama H, Aikawa T, Okyana M, Sasaki H, Mue S, Takishima T. Bronchodilating effect of intravenous magnesium sulfate in bronchial asthma. JAMA 1987; 257:1076–1078.
65. Green SM, Rothrock SG. Intravenous magnesium sulfate for acute asthma: failure to decrease emergency treatment or need for hospitalization. Ann Emerg Med 1992; 21:260–265.
66. Tiffany BR, Berk WA, Todd IK, White SR. Magnesium bolus or infusion fails to improve expiratory flow in acute asthma exacerbations. Chest 1993; 104:831–834.
67. Bloch H, Silverman R, Mancherje N, Grant S, Jagminas L, Scharf SM. Intravenous magnesium sulfate as an adjunct in the treatment of acute asthma. Chest 1995; 107:1576–1581.
68. Commey JO, Levison H. Physical signs in childhood asthma. Pediatrics 1976; 58:537–541.
69. Keens TG, Bryan AC, Levison H, Ianuzzo CD. Developmental pattern of muscle fiber types in human ventilatory muscles. J Appl Physiol 1978; 44:909–913.
70. Muller NL, Bryan AC. Chest wall mechanics and respiratory muscles in infants. Pediatr Clin North Am 1979; 26:503.
71. Robertson CF, Smith F, Beck R, Levison H. Response to low doses of salbutamol in acute asthma. J Pediatr 1985; 106:672–674.
72. Moler FW, Hurwitz ME, Custer JR. Improvement in clinical asthma score and $PaCO_2$ in children with severe asthma treated with continuously nebulized terbutaline. J Allergy Clin Immunol 1988; 81:1101–1109.
73. Bentur L, Canny GJ, Shields MD, Kerem E, Schuh S, Reisman JJ, Fakhoury K, Pedder L, Levison H. Controlled trial of nebulized albuterol in children younger than 2 years of age with acute asthma. Pediatrics 1992; 89:133–137.
74. Reisman J, Galdes-Sebalt M, Kazim F, Canny G, Levison H. Frequent administration by inhalation of salbutamol and ipratropium bromide in the initial management of severe acute asthma in children. J Allergy Clin Immunol 1988; 81:16–20.
75. Beck R. Use of ipratropium bromide by inhalation in the treatment of acute asthma in children. Clinical experience, Arch Pediatr 1995; 2(suppl2):145S–148S.
76. Milner A. Role of anticholinergic agents in acute bronchiolitis in infants. Arch Pediatr 1995; 2(suppl2):159S–162S.
77. Carter E, Cruz M, Chesrown S, Shieh G, Reilly K, Hendeles L. Efficacy of intravenously administered theophylline in children hospitalized with severe asthma. J Pediatr 1993; 122:470–476.
78. DiGiulio GA, Kercsmar CM, Krug SE, Alpert SE, Marx CM. Hospital treatment of asthma: lack of benefit from theophylline given in addition to nebulized albuterol and intravenously administered corticosteroid. J Pediatr 1993; 122:464–469.
79. Strauss RE, Wertheim DL, Bonagura VR, Valacer DJ. Aminophylline therapy does not improve outcome and increases adverse effects in children hospitalized with acute asthmatic exacerbations. Pediatrics 1994; 93:205–210.
80. Potter PC, Klein M, Weinberg EG. Hydration in severe acute asthma. Arch Dis Child 1991; 66:216–219.
81. Kass JE, Castriotta RJ. Heliox therapy in acute severe asthma. Chest 1995; 107:757–760.
82. Boorstein JM, Boorstein SM, Humphries GN, Johnston CC. Using helium-oxygen mixtures in the emergency management of acute upper airway obstruction. Ann Emerg Med 1989; 18:688–690.

30

The Severe Asthmatic: Intubated and Difficult to Ventilate

Paul Mayo
Albert Einstein College of Medicine, Bronx, and Beth Israel Medical Center, New York, New York

Michael Stavros Radeos
New York Medical College and Lincoln Medical and Mental Health Center, Bronx, New York

I. INTRODUCTION

As discussed elsewhere in this book, the decision to intubate the asthmatic requires careful clinical assessment. The intubation process has its own risks; once intubated, the patient presents formidable management problems, including the possibility of mortality and morbidity from the complex interaction between the patient and the ventilator. In a real sense, the ventilator is a potentially lethal weapon. This discussion will focus on safe use of the ventilator in these critically ill patients. The first section discusses the physiology of patient-ventilator interaction, and the second emphasizes specific clinical management issues.

In 1977, Petty et al. reported that *following* intubation, 39% of asthmatics died (1). Using newer management strategies, the risk of death is now reported as less than 1% (2–4). The use of permissive hypercapnia has evolved into standard medical intensive care unit (MICU) practice since it was first reported by Darioli et al. (2) in 1983, and subsequently refined in landmark articles by Tuxen et al. (5–7).

II. PHYSIOLOGY OF THE INTUBATED ASTHMATIC

The hallmark of severe asthma is expiratory air flow obstruction. Severe obstruction results in hyperinflation, which leads to very specific physiological effects:

1. Significant hyperinflation decreases respiratory system compliance. As the chest wall and lungs hyperinflate, they progressively resist further inflation by virtue of their elastic recoil characteristics. This is much like the way a rubber band

becomes progressively more difficult to stretch as it is stretched from its resting length.

2. As compliance decreases with hyperinflation, the inspiratory work of breathing increases. Simultaneously, passive recoil of the respiratory system increases, which may permit more rapid exhalation of tidal volume.
3. Significant hyperinflation increases the dead space fraction. Therefore, the proportion of each tidal volume (TV) that is wasted ventilation increases with increasing hyperinflation.
4. Hyperinflation *decreases* airway obstruction. Airway resistance is inversely related to the fourth power of the radius of the airway. At higher lung volumes, airway diameter increases due to radial traction by surrounding lung tissue. The clinician commonly views hyperinflation as deleterious, but in fact it may influence airflow obstruction favorably.

The challenge that faces the emergency physician is to defend the intubated patient against dangerous aspects of hyperinflation while recognizing that some degree of hyperinflation is acceptable—and perhaps desirable—because of its positive effect on airway resistance.

In the intubated asthmatic, hyperinflation exists when the respiratory system does not return to its normal resting volume (functional residual capacity, or FRC) before the next tidal breath. Rather, at the end of a passive exhalation, the next breath is initiated from an end-expiratory lung volume (EELV) that is above the individual's normal FRC (Figure 1). There are several ways that EELV might be elevated above FRC independent

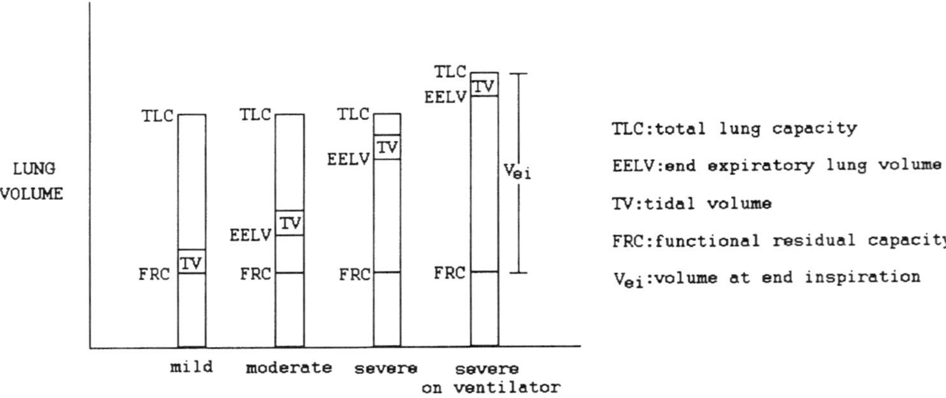

Figure 1 Lung volumes and capacities in asthma. As the patient develops more severe asthma, they hyperinflate. This results in a progressive increase in end-expiratory lung volume (EELV). During spontaneous breathing the degree of hyperinflation is limited by the reduction in system compliance that becomes maximal at total lung capacity (TLC), i.e., the patient cannot inspire above the TLC point, and EELV cannot be greater than TLC. If the patient is intubated with inappropriate settings (high rate, high TV), EELV may actually rise above normal TLC. The ventilator so over distends the respiratory system that TLC rises above that achievable during spontaneous effort.

of airflow obstruction. For example, very high respiratory rates in normal individuals, or the application of positive end-expiratory pressure, can result in an EELV elevated above FRC. In the asthmatic, hyperinflation results from slow emptying of the lungs due to airway obstruction. The degree of hyperinflation above FRC at the end of exhalation may be several liters of retained air, depending on ventilator settings and degree of airway obstruction (5).

Once the asthmatic patient is attached to the ventilator, a TV enters the patient's lungs. During exhalation, there is insufficient time for the TV to exit, and another TV is forced into the patient and so forth. This process, sometimes called breath stacking, may result in severe hyperinflation. Eventually, the patient reaches a steady state as the hyperinflation increases airway caliber and increases elastic recoil (see above) sufficiently for full TV exhalation to occur.

III. HYPERINFLATION AND AUTO-PEEP

In the intubated asthmatic, hyperinflation has other physiologic effects. Normally, end-expiratory alveolar pressure is atmospheric at the end of exhalation. Retained volume in the asthmatic results in positive alveolar pressure at end exhalation, called auto-PEEP (AP). Auto-PEEP is pressure that is associated with an EELV elevated above normal FRC. Depending on its severity, AP may cause severe cardiovascular dysfunction, just as high levels of applied PEEP may in intubated patients. PEEP and AP may reduce cardiac output to dangerous levels by impeding venous return to the heart. By elevating right ventricular (RV) afterload, they may also result in RV dilatation and ventricular septal movement that encroaches on left ventricular (LV) filling. This too may reduce cardiac output. Very high levels of auto-PEEP may result in shock from systemic hypoperfusion (8,9). The other major adverse effect of hyperinflation is barotrauma, such as pneumothorax (5). Recognizing, measuring, and controlling hyperinflation and AP in the intubated asthmatic is essential to good outcome.

IV. REDUCTION OF HYPERINFLATION AND AUTO-PEEP

Three strategies may be used to reduce hyperinflation and AP in the intubated asthmatic:

1. Reduction of respiratory rate (RR), permitting more complete exhalation before the next breath.
2. Reduction of TV, so that less volume must be exhaled before the next breath. This is effective only up to a certain point. If TV is reduced too far, dead space fraction will start to rise dramatically with consequent escalating disturbance of ventilatory function.
3. Shortening of inspiration to allow greater time for exhalation with each respiratory cycle. Each respiratory cycle may be subdivided into an inspiratory phase and an expiratory phase. Increasing inspiratory flow rate will decrease inspiratory time and increase expiratory time per breath cycle. This may be achieved by using high peak inspiratory flows with square wave pattern. Reduction in TV also shortens inspiratory time.

In selecting ventilator settings, changes in respiratory rate will have the greatest effect on auto-PEEP. Simple arithmetical principles explain this: Assume that a patient is on respiratory rate of 20/min with TV of 1.0 L with inspiratory flow of 1 L/sec (60 L/min) in square wave configuration. Inspiratory time is 1 sec and expiratory time is 2 sec, with a total breath cycle time of 3 seconds. These settings are completely inappropriate for an intubated asthmatic, and the operator wishes to correct the situation. The operator seeks to permit a far longer expiratory time per breath delivered in order to reduce auto-PEEP and hyperinflation. The operator may choose to reduce TV to 0.5 L and increase peak flow to 1.5 L/sec (90 L/min). The total cycle length remains 3 sec, but now inspiratory time is decreased to .33 sec and expiratory increases to 2.67 sec, a minimal change that is not likely to impact much on auto-PEEP risk. Alternatively, the operator may choose to reduce the respiratory rate to 10/min. Total breath cycle length increases to 6 sec, while inspiratory time remains at 1 sec. The patient now has 5 sec to exhale. Clearly, manipulation of the respiratory rate has a much greater effect than does shortening inspiratory time. In this example, tidal volume should be decreased, peak flow increased, and respiratory rate decreased in unison, of course, but the reduction in respiratory rate is proportionately more effective in reducing auto-PEEP and hyperinflation.

Modern ventilators permit the operator to select both peak inspiratory flow rate and flow configuration. In general, inspiratory flow of 60 L/min with decelerating wave form configuration is a reasonable initial setup for the intubated asthmatic. However, if reducing respiratory rate is insufficient to reduce auto-PEEP to acceptable levels due to unacceptable hypercapnia, the inspiratory time may be shortened to permit a proportionately longer time for exhalation per respiratory duty cycle. Reduction of tidal volume is appropriate but is limited by its progressive effect on dead space fraction. Both using a square wave flow pattern and increasing flow rate will shorten inspiratory time. High flow rates in square wave pattern will predictably result in high peak inspiratory pressures. This is not a dangerous situation. It will not increase the risk of barotrauma, and in fact will decrease it if auto-PEEP and hyperinflation are reduced as a result. Some clinicians fear that high pressures in this case may be dangerous to the patient. This is a false assumption. The entire concept that high peak pressures are directly injurious to the lung can be called into question (10,11). In addition, peak pressures are measured outside of the patient, and do not reflect alveolar pressures due to the elevated airway resistance, endotracheal tube resistance, and turbulent flow characteristics of the air entering the system at high flow rates. It is common for respiratory therapy personnel to express concern over the high peak pressures resulting from square wave high inspiratory flow rates that may be needed when ventilating the intubated asthmatic. It is important to be prepared to fully justify the physiological basis of their ventilator strategy to the respiratory therapy service in order to maintain the high level of cooperative effort needed to safely manage these difficult patients.

V. PERMISSIVE HYPERCAPNIA

Reduction in RR and TV may result in elevation of $Paco_2$. Asthmatics generally have an elevated deadspace fraction, which further predisposes them towards hypercapnia. In this case, the clinician permits hypercapnia in order to reduce deleterious hyperinflation. Hypercapnia is usually well tolerated and far more preferable to dangerous levels of hyperinflation (12). The only absolute contraindication to permissive hypercapnia is a coexisting disorder that causes elevation of intracranial pressure. Otherwise, hypercapnia and its resultant acidosis are well tolerated, especially in asthmatics who are generally without significant comorbid illness (12). The acceptable level of hypercapnia and acidosis differ among published guidelines, but, in general, $Paco_2$ of up to 80 mmHg and pH as low as 7.15 are considered acceptable (13). Administration of sodium bicarbonate remains an option should severe acidosis supervene, but the clinician must consider the complex metabolic effects of this therapy.

VI. MEASUREMENT OF HYPERINFLATION AND AUTO-PEEP

Since a goal of ventilator management is to avoid dangerous levels of hyperinflation and auto-PEEP, emergency physicians must be able to measure these endpoints accurately. In a research setting, hyperinflation may be assessed by respiratory inductance plethysmography, computer tomography (CT) scanning and gas dilution techniques. Tuxen et al. proposed a simple index of hyperinflation, the end-inspiratory volume, or V_{ei} (6). The passive intubated patient receives the set TV, and the ventilator is then shut off for a period of time. During this prolonged exhalation, the TV will be exhaled, followed by the additional volume of air accounted for by hyperinflation. V_{ei} is the total exhaled volume (TV plus the difference between EELV and FRC) (Fig. 1). In intubated asthmatics, the rate of complications increases with V_{ei} of > 1.4L (7). This measurement emphasizes the often dramatic difference between EELV and the FRC following prolonged exhalation. Modern ventilators are capable of measuring expiratory flow and volumes, although even those with advanced generation models may have limited ability to accurately assess V_{ei}, due to difficulties in measuring low flow rates following prolonged expiratory times. In that case, an additional expiratory flow-volume sensor is required, making this measurement impractical in a busy emergency department (ED). This, as well as concerns that the measurement has not been indexed to ideal body weight or to tubing expansion factors, suggest that V_{ei} measurement is not applicable in the ED environment.

The alternative to measuring hyperinflation volume above FRC is to measure AP directly. Auto-PEEP may be measured in several ways. Methods that require esophageal balloon insertion and placement of a flow sensor at the airway opening permit estimates of auto-PEEP by simultaneous examination of flow and pressure curves at the onset of inspiration. This approach is impractical for emergency medicine where this equipment is not available. A far simpler method is needed.

Unlike set-PEEP, which is determined by the physician and is readily visible on the manometer of the ventilator, auto-PEEP may be present but not evident by simple observation of the ventilator manometer. All ventilators in current use measure airway pressure continuously. Airway pressure, the designated pressure at airway opening (Pao), is measured outside of the patient, typically at the connection between the inspiratory and expiratory tubing, or even at the end of the expiratory tubing. In any case, it is measured well away from the alveolar compartment. During exhalation, Pao falls rapidly to 0 (unless set-PEEP is present) as Pao equilibrates rapidly with downstream atmospheric pressure upon the opening of the expiratory valve.

Auto-PEEP is not measurable by simple examination of the ventilator manometer. The manometer measures system pressure in the ventilator tubing outside of the patient, and not at the alveolar level. As soon as the expiratory valve opens, the tubing pressure rapidly falls to atmospheric (or to pre-set PEEP level) regardless of the alveolar pressure (Figure 2). Measurement of auto-PEEP requires closing of the expiratory valve or manual occlusion of the expiratory port in order that alveolar pressure may equilibrate with tubing pressure and the manometer sensor (Figures 2, 3A, and 3B). To measure end expiratory alveolar pressure, the operator must occlude the expiratory tubing at the end-expiratory point. This requires that the occlusion occurs instead of the next breath (Figures 2, 3A, and 3B). Either the ventilator rate must be temporarily turned down to a very low rate, or, if available, the ventilator may have design features that permit auto-PEEP measurement by microprocessor control. Advanced generation Puritan Bennett 7200 or Servo Ventilators have such auto-PEEP measurement capability. The clinician should not be discouraged if such a command is not available on their ventilator. Satisfactory auto-PEEP measurements can be easily performed by manually occluding the expiratory port at end-expiration (Figure 4), provided the occlusion is not interrupted by a subsequent breath and observing the buildup of pressure on the manometer (Figure 2). In measuring auto-PEEP it is essential to hold the occlusion for a sufficient time to permit equilibration of the Pao with alveolar pressure. In ventilator systems with nonhomogeneous time constants, it may take 20 sec or longer for the auto-PEEP occlusion maneuvers to reach steady state. The patient must be passive, otherwise respiratory effort will interrupt the measurement. Table 1 summarizes in detail how to measure auto-PEEP.

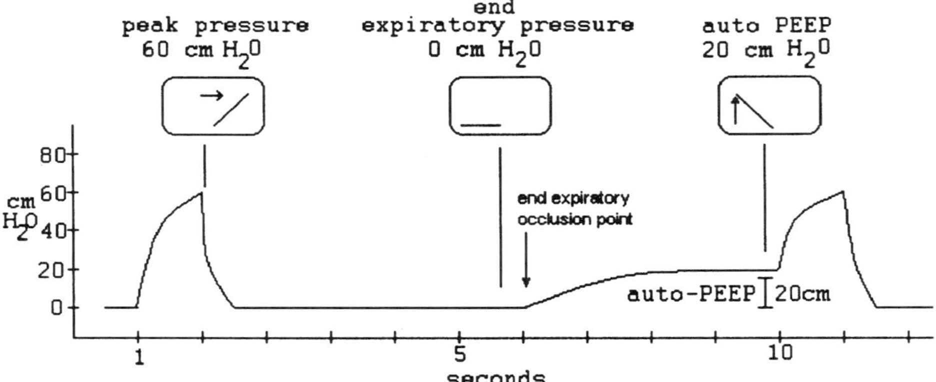

Figure 2 Airway pressure curve and manometer readings during measurement of auto-PEEP. The airway pressure curve graphically shows an auto-PEEP measurement. Ventilator settings are CMV at 10/min (respiratory cycle 6 sec), tidal volume 1.0 L, and inspiratory flow rate 60 L/min square wave. Instead of delivering the next breath as scheduled, the expiratory tubing is occluded for 5 sec. It is important to note that it takes several seconds for alveolar pressure to equilibrate with the manometer that is measuring system pressure outside of the patient. At the end of this technically acceptable auto-PEEP measurement, the machine cycles on to deliver the set tidal volume. It is evident that the patient must be passive, otherwise the end expiratory hold would be interrupted by the patient triggering the ventilator. In the absence of airway pressure graphics, the manometer readings can be used to give accurate measurement of auto-PEEP. From a management standpoint, the tidal volume should be immediately reduced in order to reduce auto-PEEP to acceptable levels.

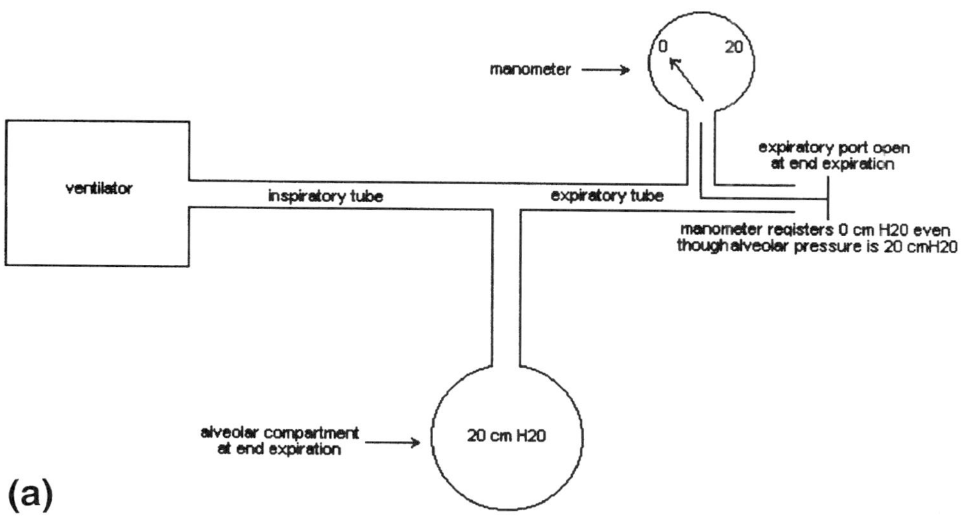

Figure 3a Schematic of ventilator circuit and manometer at end expiration without end-expiratory occlusion. In this example, the patient has an end-expiratory alveolar pressure of 20 cmH_2O. The manometer has equilibrated with atmospheric pressure due to its close proximity to the expiratory port of the ventilator. The manometer cannot detect the presence of auto-PEEP as long as the expiratory tubing is open to atmosphere. In order to measure auto-PEEP, the operator must occlude the expiratory port and allow equilibration of the alveolar compartment with the manometer. (See Figure 4b.)

Another way to assess hyperinflation and auto-PEEP in the passive intubated asthmatic is to follow plateau pressures (Ppl) (14). The Ppl is measured by blocking expiration immediately following TV injection. Ventilators in common use have an end-inspiratory plateau command available. The end-inspiratory Ppl is inversely related to respiratory system compliance and directly related to set-PEEP or auto-PEEP levels. Ppl of less than 30 cmH_20 is considered a reasonable target range, although literature does not validate this value as a therapeutic end point. Ppl is not an entirely satisfactory measurement of AP or hyperinflation, as factors other than AP may cause it to be high, e.g., acute respiratory distress syndrome (ARDS), pneumonia, chest wall disease, mainstem intubation, tension pneumothorax.

The authors favor repeated measurement of auto-PEEP level to track hyperinflation in intubated asthmatics. It is simple and safe to perform, reproducible, and easy to understand. This has major advantages in an ED situation. V_{ei} is less intuitively obvious as a concept and may not be easily measured on all ventilators. Unlike V_{ei}, there is no clear literature that defines a safe level of auto-PEEP. Auto-PEEP levels of 10–15 cmH_20 are generally well tolerated and do not carry risk of hemodynamic or barotrauma effect. Moreover, with severe asthma, it may not be possible or desirable to achieve lower levels even with high levels of permitted hypercapnia. In fact, some degree of hyperinflation may be beneficial due to its positive influence on airway resistance. Like V_{ei} and Ppl, auto-PEEP is not a perfect measurement. For example, it is quite likely that severely obstructed patients may have areas of air trapping and auto-PEEP that do not communicate with the

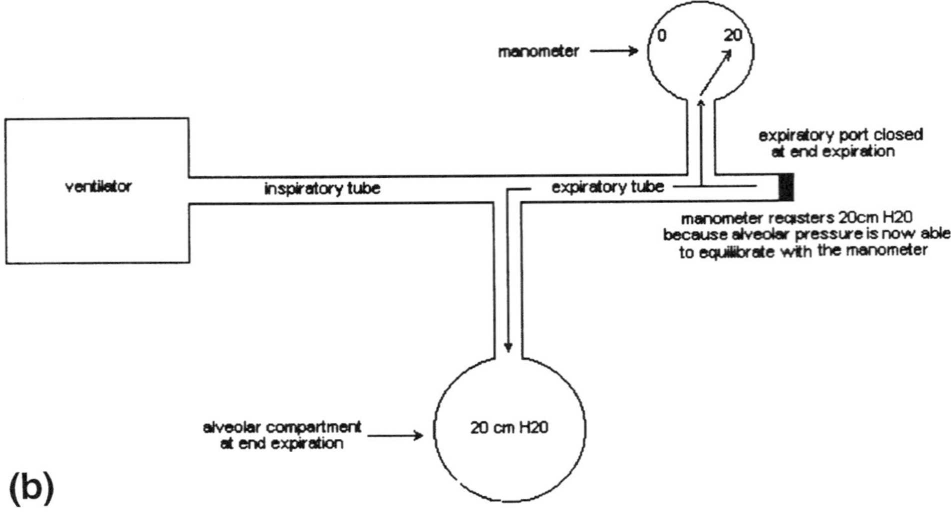

Figure 3b Schematic of ventilator circuit and manometer at end expiration with end-expiratory occlusion. In this example, the expiratory circuit has been occluded at end expiration. The alveolar pressure is 20 cmH_2O, and is readily detected by the manometer. Occlusion of the expiratory circuit permits equilibration of the alveolar compartment with the tubing circuit and manometer. Auto-PEEP is 20 cmH_2O.

central airway compartment (15). High levels of auto-PEEP in passive intubated asthmatics are of great concern. However, low or absent measured levels do not exclude the possibility of noncommunicating areas of auto-PEEP and hyperinflation that may hold danger for the patient.

VII. CLINICAL MANAGEMENT STRATEGY

Even in a busy ED, asthma that requires intubation is an uncommon event. When it happens, the complex physiological problems require a sophisticated management strategy. The emergency physician usually directs care for 30 min up to a few hours, and then turns responsibility over to the intensive care unit (ICU) team. The following discussion will therefore emphasize the pragmatic clinical challenge and pitfalls in the management of these difficult patients in the hours following intubation in the ED.

VIII. IMMEDIATE POSTINTUBATION PERIOD

The clinician must determine immediately whether the endotracheal tube (ET) is in proper position. Simple auscultation may not suffice, as the chest in the acute asthmatic may be silent due to reduced airflow; bilateral breath sounds may not audible even with correct ET tube placement. Expiratory return of condensate within the ET tube is a useful clue, as is palpation of the balloon in the suprasternal notch. For definitive check, an end tidal carbon dioxide detector is ideal. If available, an oximeter reading of 100% also supports successful intubation. A chest film should always be obtained to document appropriate depth of ET tube placement. The operator usually meets significant resistance in bagging the intubated patient with acute asthma due to high airway resistance. If not, proper inflation of the endotracheal tube balloon must be determined immediately by reinflation and cuff pressure check by palpation of the side arm balloon. Occasionally, the ET tube balloon may have been damaged by the patient's teeth, particularly if repeated attempts at intubation have been made. If the ET tube is correctly placed and the cuff balloon is properly inflated, absence of significant resistance to bagging suggests that the original diagnosis of asthma is incorrect and that intubation has bypassed an upper airway obstruction (e.g., functional stridor syndrome, tumor, foreign body) that is mimicking an acute asthma exacerbation.

The patient should always be bagged with 100% O_2 and pulse oximetry should be maintained. Saturation should be 100%. If not, the operator must immediately check that the bag is connected to a high flow O_2 source to assure high FIO_2.

IX. DESATURATION IN THE INTUBATED ASTHMATIC

Asthma alone cannot explain persistent oxygen desaturation if the patient is receiving a high FIO_2. The hypoxemia of asthma is due predominantly to V/Q mismatch physiology and, therefore, should respond readily to a high FIO_2. Right mainstem intubation and pneumothorax should be considered immediately. Because there is generally some delay in obtaining a chest film, rapid assessment of tube position may require fiberoptic exam to document that the ET tube is above the carina. As a fiberoptic scope is not available in most EDs, the clinician should make sure that the ET tube is placed at the *21 cm mark* on the incisors. This will generally exclude right mainstem bronchial intubation in adults but may be inaccurate in smaller persons.

Another cause of persistent oxygen desaturation may be pneumothorax. In the newly intubated asthmatic this diagnosis may be deceptive: the chest may be silent, the patient may be hypotensive due to auto-PEEP, visible chest wall hyperinflation is the rule in almost all the acute asthmatics, and the chest film is not usually immediately available. If the clinician is an experienced sonographer, immediate chest wall sonography may exclude pneumothorax (16). This resource is becoming more commonly available in the ED. Faced with this clinical situation, the emergency physician may be tempted to insert pleural drains, initially by accessing the pleural space with a small-diameter 16–18 g needle/cannula, followed by a chest tube. However, the clinician must always consider the possibility of massive auto-PEEP buildup due to severe airway obstruction with a resulting profound shock state. Unless there is unequivocal evidence of tension pneumothorax, i.e., unilateral chest wall expansion with obvious contralateral tracheal shift or subcutaneous emphysema, the first response should always be to stop ventilating the patient. If the silent chest and hypotension is due to auto-PEEP, permitting deflation of the system results in rapid improvement in blood pressure (8). Insertion of a pleural drain would have catastrophic consequence in a patient who did not have pneumothorax, since the visceral pleura of the hyperinflated lung would possibly be punctured, causing a pneumothorax. The operator may not realize that this has happened. Puncture of the lung will yield a release of air under pressure through the catheter just as would occur with relief of a tension pneumothorax. The resultant pneumothorax would likely be under tension,

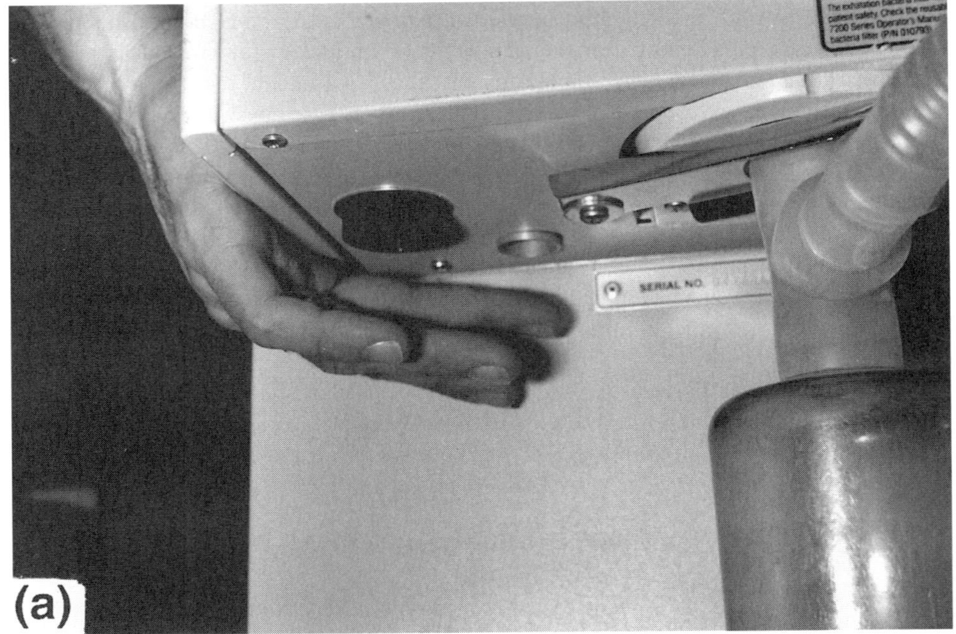
SERIAL NO.
(a)

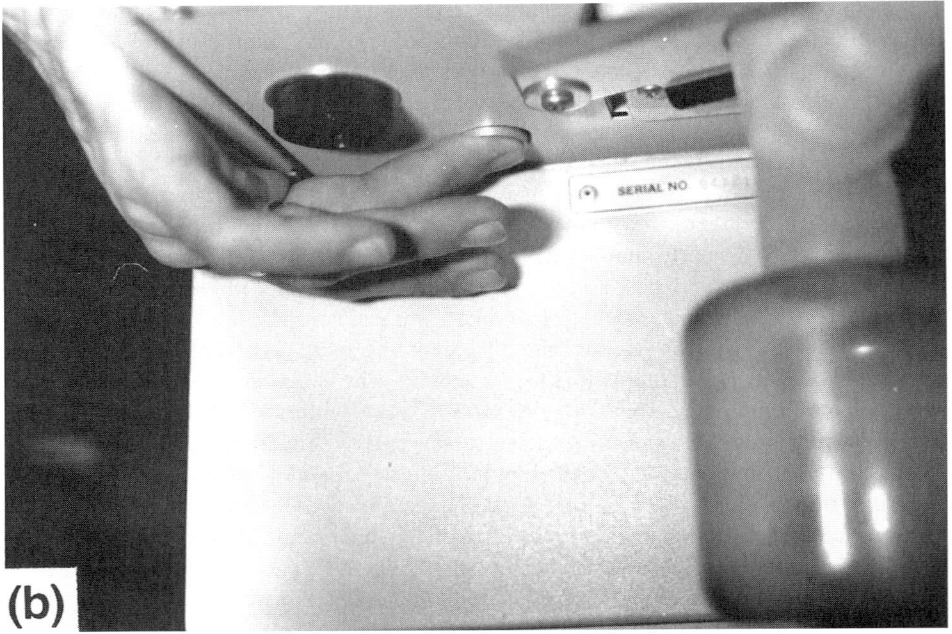
SERIAL NO.
(b)

as it would occur while on positive pressure ventilation with coexisting AP. Again, the most common cause of hypotension in the newly intubated asthmatic is AP effect (combined with sedatives used during recent intubation), *not* tension pneumothorax.

The clinician must instruct the person "bagging" the patient to use a very slow respiratory rate. Often the bagger, aware of preintubation hypercapnia, will attempt to hyperventilate the patient. This may also cause severe auto-PEEP with its untoward consequences. Bagging rates as low as 6–8/min are appropriate as long as the patient is adequately oxygenated and hypercapnia is not severe.

X. URGENT PLEURAL DRAINAGE OF AIR

If there is strong clinical or radiographic evidence of tension pneumothorax in the intubated asthmatic, pleural drainage may be life saving. A variety of rapid pleural access devices are commercially available, but immediate access may be provided by a simple device, such as a 16-gauge catheter with simple water seal for evacuation of pressure. The insertion should be in the second intercostal space in the midclavicular line. Two errors occur commonly (in the authors' experience):

1. The operator may inadvertently angle the insertion medially, with resulting catastrophic damage to mediastinal vascular structures. Great care needs to be exercised to insert the needle perpendicular to all axes of the chest wall.
2. The operator may tend to insert the needle catheter assembly too deeply, thereby penetrating both the parietal and visceral pleura with resultant placement of the catheter into lung tissue. The assembly is best passed slowly. With the first burst of air through the water seal attachment or into the air, no deeper insertion of the needle should occur, but rather advancement of the catheter should follow

---

Figure 4 Expiratory port occlusion on Puritan-Bennett 7200 ventilator in order to measure auto-PEEP. The expiratory port is located on the underside of the control panel. By watching the manometer on the machine, the operator can identify the appropriate moment to occlude the expiratory port, thereby permitting equilibration of end-expiratory alveolar pressure with the system manometer (see text). Individuals with small digits may not be able to fully occlude the orifice; an exam glove wrapped around the middle finger may permit a complete occlusion. Some modern ventilators have a command that permits auto-PEEP measurement by the ventilator. Many older models do not have this option, and so the clinician must be able to conveniently perform a manual end-expiratory auto-PEEP measurement. By way of example, the accompanying photographs demonstrate how to occlude the expiratory port on a PB 7200 ventilator. As a generic concept, all ventilators in common use have an end-expiratory port that can be briefly occluded at the end of expiration in order to measure auto-PEEP. Emergency physicians should be familiar with the ventilator design at their facility. The PB 7200 is in widespread clinical use and is therefore a suitable example. The same maneuver can be easily done on ventilators of a different design. (a) Manual occlusion of expiratory port of Bennett Puritan 7200 ventilator. Finger is off the expiratory port. (b) Manual occlusion of expiratory port. Finger has occluded the expiratory port as would occur during auto-PEEP measurement.

Table 1 How to Measure Auto-PEEP

1. Determine if the ventilator has a specific auto-PEEP or end-exhalation hold command. Advanced generation Puritan Bennett and Siemens ventilators may be so equipped. During machine controlled measurement, observe carefully to make sure that the auto-PEEP level reaches a sustained steady value, either on the manometer or with airway pressure graphics. If the patient actively fights the maneuver, the value may be inaccurate. If insufficient end expiratory hold time is used, there may not be full equilibration of the manometer with the alveolar space, and auto-PEEP will be underestimated.
2. If the ventilator does not have a specific auto-PEEP command, identify an appropriate point to manually block exhalation at the end of a breath cycle. Figure 4 identifies an appropriate site in a common ventilator, the Puritan Bennett 7200 series. As a generic concept, all ventilators have an expiratory port that can be occluded at an appropriate time.
3. Turn the ventilator rate to one breath per minute. Following the last breath, manually occlude the expiratory circuit at the time the next breath would be due. For example, at a set rate of 10/min, occlusion would be 6 sec following the onset of the previous breath. Because the machine rate is 1/min and the patient is not triggering, any auto-PEEP present will register on the machine manometer. Occlusion too early in exhalation will overestimate auto-PEEP. If the machine rate is not temporarily reduced, the auto-PEEP occlusion maneuver will be interrupted by a machine cycled breath.
4. It is important to maintain the occlusion for a sufficient period to permit equilibration of alveolar pressure with the patient's tubing. This may take many seconds to occur. If the occlusion is of insufficient duration, auto-PEEP will be underestimated. The presence of set-PEEP still permits an independent measurement of auto-PEEP.
5. During the manual auto-PEEP measurement, occlusion of the expiratory circuit must be complete and distal to the manometer connection to the ventilator tubing circuit. Individuals with small finger size may not be able to fully block the expiratory port of the Puritan Bennett ventilator. In that case, a rolled up examination glove may be used.
6. Always return ventilator rate to the previous value following the auto-PEEP measurements.

using the needle as a guide. Any simple needle catheter drainage system must always be quickly replaced by a more stable pleural drainage system.

XI. VENTILATOR MANAGEMENT

The next step in management involves attaching the patient to the ventilator. By this time, "peri-intubation" medication may be wearing off, and the patient may be combative and extremely uncomfortable due to the ET tube. The patient must be well sedated at the time of connection to the ventilator, or the patient runs the risk of accidental extubation, airway damage due to ET tube movement, and rapid accumulation of potentially lethal auto-PEEP as the patient triggers the ventilator at high respiratory frequency. If sedation is not sufficient to allow a passive "ventilator-patient" interaction, a brief period of paralysis with neuromuscular blocking agents (NMBs) may be required. The patient must be deeply sedated before use of NMBs to avoid the grave psychological stress of paralysis without adequate sedation. The only way to achieve permissive hypercapnia is to have a passive patient. An awake combative patient will resist this strategy by triggering the ventilator at high rates, coughing violently, and developing other dangerous elements of ventilator-patient dysynchrony. Heavy sedation reduces central respiratory drive, but transient neuromuscular blockade may still be necessary to ablate ventilator-patient dysynchrony. The duration of NMB use must be limited to avoid the debilitating muscle weakness syndrome of concomitant steroid and NMB use (17–19). This association between corticosteroid use, nondepolarizing NMBs, and prolonged muscle weakness appears to occur with all presently available NMBs: pancuronium, vecuronium, and atracurium have all been implicated. Following exposure, creatinine phosphokinase (CPK) levels rise, electromyograms (EMGs) reveal myopathy, and pathological study of affected muscles demonstrates muscle cell necrosis and disruption. The syndrome may yield profound muscle weakness, but, following a prolonged recovery phase, the patient generally recovers full function. The precise cause remains enigmatic. In some way, a prolonged neuromuscular blockade may dramatically accelerate steroid myopathic effect. A reasonable guideline is to avoid NMB of greater than 24-hr duration. Generally, deep sedation suffices past this point. An additional positive side effect of completely passive patient-ventilator interaction is that CO_2 production falls rendering the patient easier to ventilate.

XII. INITIAL VENTILATOR SETUP

Initial ventilator settings in the newly intubated adult asthmatic are summarized in Table 2. Following connection the ventilator will typically alarm immediately because the peak pressure limit is exceeded. Modern ventilators are designed to terminate TV injection when a preset peak pressure is reached. Due to high airway resistance, peak pressures may be very high in intubated asthmatics with resultant limitation of TV injection. In order to assure the patient receives the set TV, the operator may have to respond by increasing the peak pressure limit alarm, often to very high levels (e.g., 100 cmH_2O). Unless the peak pressure results from auto-PEEP, endotracheal tube kink or blockage, or other mechanical obstruction to inspiratory air flow, high peak pressures are predictable and completely acceptable in the intubated asthmatic. The clinician must then observe ventilator function to assure that TV is actually entering the patient. Once the peak pressure issue has been resolved, the operator should then rapidly assess for auto-PEEP, and, if appropriate, further reduce respiratory rate and TV while accepting hypercapnia. If the auto-PEEP is greater than 15 cm, the set respiratory rate should be turned down. Tidal volume may also be reduced. If this does not suffice to reduce auto-PEEP, the peak flow should be increased further to shorten inspiration. The initial target should be auto-PEEP between 10 and 15 cmH_2O if tolerated according to perfusion status. Until there is docu-

Table 2 Initial Ventilator Settings for the Intubated Asthmatic

1. Controlled mechanical ventilation at 10 breaths/min
2. TV at 5–8 cc/kg (ideal body weight)
3. Peak flow at 60 L/min with square wave
4. FIO_2 at 1.0

mentation of adequate O_2 saturation by ABG or oximetry, the initial FIO_2 should be 1.0. FIO_2 is then reduced as tolerated under continuous oximetry control. Characteristically, uncomplicated asthma does not require very high FIO_2 levels for adequate oxygenation function.

In the initial phase of management, frequent ABGs should be the rule. This is initially to document that oximetry is accurate, but subsequently to follow the $PaCO_2$. We favor a volume cycled ventilator (CMV) mode, as opposed to a pressure control mode (PC). Unless there is a strong institutional preference backed by extensive clinical expertise, pressure control is not appropriate for busy ED use. Although it is an effective ventilator strategy, its operation and troubleshooting is more complex than CMV. Also, the TV delivered with PC depends on airway resistance and respiratory system compliance, both of which may change rapidly in the intubated asthmatic. Volume cycled ventilator setup is intuitively obvious in its operation, and is therefore intrinsically safer and easier to use in the ED.

It may take up to 30 min for the patient's $PaCO_2$ to equilibrate at a steady state following machine connection or subsequent ventilator changes (PaO_2 will equilibrate much more rapidly). In the hours before MICU transfer, the clinician will be balancing auto-PEEP level, perfusion status, and $PaCO_2$ level, seeking an appropriate level of hypercapnia and tolerable hyperinflation. Continued passive ''ventilator-patient'' interaction is absolutely critical and requires ongoing sedation and possible paralysis to allow safe ventilator use with permissive hypercapnia.

A common clinical scenario results when a patient is inadequately sedated and triggering the ventilator at high rates, or when the ventilator strategy is targeted at achieving a normal $PaCO_2$. Massive hyperinflation and dangerous auto-PEEP levels may accumulate, and the clinician will be called to the bedside urgently due to profound hypotension. A silent chest is noted, and pneumothorax or other causes of shock considered. Before volume challenge, pressors, blind pleural invasion, or other responses to shock, the astute clinician may simply disconnect the ventilator for a period of time while closely following the pulse oximetry, and allow exhalation of retained volume and auto-PEEP. There will be a return of normal perfusion status, and the ventilator can be adjusted to more acceptable settings.

XIII. BARRIERS TO SAFE VENTILATOR MANAGEMENT

The emergency physician may have difficulty when using a strategy of permissive hypercapnia in a facility that does not have regular experience with the critically ill asthmatic. Medical, nursing, and respiratory therapy personnel are generally trained to run ventilators in order to achieve normal $PaCO_2$ levels. Respiratory therapists are trained to avoid high peak pressures when running ventilators, due to prevalent but erroneous belief that high peak pressure itself may cause barotrauma (10,11). The emergency physician must be vigilant in the hours before MICU transfer. Often, to reduce peak pressure, well-intentioned staff will place the patient on lower peak flows with decelerating wave form. This will lengthen inspiration, and cause further hyperinflation. Justification of the general approach of permissive hypercapnia and education of their colleagues, nurses, and respiratory therapy staff may be necessary.

XIV. MEDICAL TREATMENT OF THE INTUBATED ASTHMATIC

The challenge of the intubated asthmatic lies in the great danger of ventilator-induced injury. Once these issues have been addressed, the medical treatment of the patient is straightforward. Systemic corticosteroids are the mainstay of treatment. There has been ongoing controversy regarding dose. A definitive review of the literature suggests 40 mg Q 6 H of methylprednisolone or its equivalent is sufficient for the sickest asthmatic and higher doses are not more efficacious (20). Inhaled β-agonists are also indicated, their frequency and dose remaining an area of ongoing debate. Providing a well-designed reservoir system is used and sufficient puffs delivered, delivery of β-agonists via a metered dose inhaler (MDI) is as effective as nebulizers in intubated asthmatics, and is less expensive (21). Specific guidelines for MDI and nebulizer use in intubated patients are summarized in Tables 3 and 4 (21). It is extremely important to follow these guidelines, as bronchodilator deposition in the intubated patient is critically dependent on detailed technical issues. The optimal dose and frequency of bronchodilators for intubated asthmatics has yet to be determined. Four puffs of MDI-delivered albuterol appear to be maximally effective for at least 60 min in stable intubated patients with chronic obstructive pulmonary disease (COPD) (22). Patients with acute exacerbation of asthma who are intubated may benefit from higher doses. Eight sequential puffs would be a reasonable initial dose range with frequency determined by clinical response (21). Intravenous (IV) theophylline does not appear to improve outcome in hospitalized asthmatics (23), so its use in intubated patients is questionable.

The intubated asthmatic is often a high-profile patient in the ED and MICU. Young

Table 3 Technique for Using MDIs in Mechanically Ventilated Patients

1. Assure $V_T > 500$ mL (in adults) during assisted ventilation.
2. Aim for an inspiratory time (excluding the inspiratory pause) > 0.3 of total breath duration.
3. Ensure that the ventilator breath is synchronized with the patient's inspiration.
4. Shake the MDI vigorously.
5. Place the canister in actuator of a cylindrical spacer situated in inspiratory limb of the ventilator circuit.[a]
6. Actuate MDI to synchronize with precise onset of inspiration by the ventilator.[b]
7. Allow a breath hold at end inspiration for 3–5 sec[c]
8. Allow passive exhalation.
9. Repeat actuation after 20–30 sec until total dose is delivered.[d]

[a] With MDIs, it is preferable to use a spacer that remains in the ventilator circuit to avoid disconnecting the ventilator circuit for each treatment. Although bypassing the humidifier can increase aerosol delivery, it prolongs each treatment and requires disconnecting the ventilator circuit.

[b] In ambulatory patients with an MDI placed near the mouth, actuation is recommended briefly after initiation of inspiratory airflow. In mechanically ventilated patients using an MDI and spacer combination, actuation should be synchronized with the onset of inspiration.

[c] The effect of a postinspiratory breath hold has not been evaluated in mechanically ventilated patients.

[d] The manufacturer recommends repeating the dose after 1 min. However, MDI actuation within 20–30 sec after prior dose does not compromise drug delivery.

Source: Adapted from Ref. 21.

Table 4 Technique for Using Nebulizers in Mechanically Ventilated Patients

1. Place the drug solution in nebulizer, employing a fill volume (2–6 mL) that ensures greatest aerosol-generating efficacy.[a]
2. Place the nebulizer in inspiratory line at least 30 cm from the patient Y.[b]
3. Ensure airflow of 6–8 L/min through the nebulizer.[c]
4. Ensure adequate tidal volume (>500 mL in adults). Attempt to use duty cycle > 0.3 if possible.
5. Adjust minute volume to compensate for additional airflow through the nebulizer, if required.
6. Turn off flow-by or continuous-flow mode on ventilator.
7. Observe nebulizer for adequate aerosol generation throughout use
8. Disconnect nebulizer when all medication is nebulized or when no more aerosol is being produced.
9. Reconnect ventilator circuit and return to original ventilator settings.

[a] The volume of solution placed in the nebulizer, i.e., fill volume, that achieves maximal efficiency varies among nebulizers.
[b] Bypassing the humidifier has been suggested as a means of improving aerosol delivery in mechanically ventilated patients. However, administration of dry gas may lead to drying of the airway mucosa; therefore, administration with humidified gas is preferred for routine bronchodilatory therapy.
[c] The nebulizer may be operated continuously or only during inspiration; the latter method is more efficient. Some ventilators provide inspiratory gas flow to the nebulizer; alternatively, the nebulizer can be powered by continuous gas flow from an external source.
Source: Adapted from Ref. 21.

and otherwise healthy, they are appropriately considered highly salvageable patients. The staff may come under pressure to use modalities of treatment that are unnecessary. For example: systemic β-agonists do not appear more effective than inhaled β-agonists in very ill asthmatics (24), and their risks clearly are not worth their benefit once the patient has been intubated. Heliox has specific beneficial effects on airflow abnormality (25–27), and may have efficacy in avoiding an intubation decision. Once intubated, Heliox use has not been shown to improve clinical outcome. It is expensive and many ventilators are not designed with flow sensors calibrated for its use. Unless there is strong institutional preference and resource, its use should be discouraged once the patient is intubated.

General anesthesia has been advocated for patients who are intubated (12). Its use remains anecdotal and there are major logistical issues implicit in delivery. As it has not been shown to improve survival and is hazardous, its use should be limited to research based effort. Bronchoalveolar lavage has been advocated for severe asthma (28), in order to remove the mucous plugs so common in this condition. Its use remains unproven, and the procedure has substantial risks in the intubated asthmatic. Magnesium has been advocated for asthma, and although there is debate about its efficacy in severe asthmatics (29–31), its benefit in intubated asthmatics is unproven. Antibiotics are also not required for severe asthma (32), unless there is strong independent indication for their use (i.e., pneumonia).

Using a simple medical regimen and permissive hypercapnia ventilator strategy, acute asthmatics that have been intubated should have an excellent outcome. Additional techniques appear unnecessary, expensive, and occasionally hazardous.

The main responsibility of the emergency physician is to stabilize the intubated asthmatic until transfer to the MICU. This chapter will not discuss issues peculiar to treating these patients in an MICU environment, such as timing of extubation. However, occasionally an asthmatic has dramatic and rapid improvement of airflow obstruction following appropriate intubation. These patients often present with abrupt severe asthma that progresses to severe respiratory failure very rapidly without antecedent history of severe chronic asthma (33). The more standard patient typically presents with severe poorly controlled chronic disease and progressive unstable illness in the days before intubation. This patient requires a long period of treatment before extubation. The sudden onset asthmatic, on the other hand, may resolve airflow obstruction as rapidly as it commenced. It is possible that this subset of patients has pathophysiology related to anaphylaxis rather than progressive severe generalized bronchial inflammation with airway edema and mucous impaction. If the intubated asthmatic improves markedly while waiting for MICU transfer, the opportunity should be taken to extubate the patient. It is advisable to confirm physiological improvement sufficient to warrant extubation by measuring indices of airflow and airtrapping. Unfortunately, it is unusual for patients to clear their airflow obstruction so rapidly as to permit early extubation; nevertheless, this occasionally does occur.

The ED management of the critically ill asthmatic is crucial to good outcome, including, as it does, two very dangerous treatment processes: the intubation sequence and the initial ventilator setup. To summarize, the emergency physician is a key partner with the MICU in assuring excellent outcome for the intubated asthmatic. Steps to achieve this include:

1. Vigorous early use of sedation and paralysis (if needed) in order to achieve safe passive patient-ventilator interaction.
2. Ventilator setup with low respiratory rate, low tidal volume, and high inspiratory flow (i.e., short inspiratory time) with permissive hypercapnia, in order to avoid life threatening hyperinflation.
3. Targeting auto-PEEP level < 15, $V_{ei} < 1.4$ L or plateau < 30.
4. A simple medical regimen including systemic cortico- steroids and inhaled β-agonists.

REFERENCES

1. Scoggin CH, Sahn SA, Petty TL. Status asthmaticus: A nine year experience. JAMA 1977; 238:1158–1162.
2. Davioli R, Perret C. Mechanical controlled hypoventilation in status asthmaticus. Am Rev Respir Dis 1984; 129:385–387.
3. Braman SS, Kaemmeren JT. Intensive care of status asthmaticus: A ten year experience. JAMA 1990; 264:366–368.
4. Bellomo R, McLaughlin P, Tai E, Parkin G. Asthma requiring mechanical ventilation: a low morbidity approach. Chest 1994; 105:891–896.
5. Tuxen DV, Lane S. The effects of ventilatory pattern on hyperinflation, airway pressures, and circulation in mechanical ventilation of patients with severe air-flow obstruction. Am Rev Respir Dis 1987; 136:872–879.
6. Williams TJ, Tuxen DV, Scheinkestel CD, Czarny D, Bowes G. Risk factors for morbidity in mechanically ventilated patients with acute severe asthma. Am Rev Respir Dis 1992; 146: 607–615.
7. Tuxen DV, Williams TJ, Scheinkestel CD, Czarny D, Bowes G. Use of a measurement of

pulmonary hyperinflation to control the level of mechanical ventilation in patients with acute severe asthma. Am Rev Respir Dis 1992; 146:1136–1142.

8. Pepe EP, Marini JJ. Occult positive end-expiratory pressure in mechanically ventilated patients with airflow obstruction. Am Rev Respir Dis 1982; 126:166–170.
9. Wiener C. Ventilatory management of respiratory failure in asthma. JAMA 1993; 269:2128–2131.
10. Pierson DJ. Alveolar rupture during mechanical ventilation: role of PEEP, peak airway pressure, and distending volume. Respir Care 1988; 33:472–486.
11. Manning HL. Peak airway pressure: Why the fuss? Chest 1994; 105:242–247.
12. Tuxen DV. Permissive hypercapnic ventilation. Am J Respir Crit Care Med 1994; 150:870–874.
13. Feihl F, Perret C. Permissive hypercapnia. How permissive should we be? Am J Respir Crit Care Med 1994; 150:1722–1737.
14. Corbridge TC, Hall JB. The assessment and management of adults with status asthmaticus. Am J Respir Crit care Med 1995; 151:1296–1316.
15. Leatherman JW, Ravenscraft SA. Low measured auto-positive end-expiratory pressure during mechanical ventilation of patients with severe asthma: Hidden auto-positive end expiratory pressure. Crit Care Med 1996; 24:541–546.
16. Lichtenstein DA, Menu Y. A bedside ultrasound sign ruling out pneumothorax in the critically ill. Chest 1995; 108:1345–1348.
17. Douglass JA, Tuxen D, Horne M, Scheinkestel CD, Weinmann M, Czarny D, Bowes G. Myopathy in severe asthma. Am Rev Respir Dis 1992; 146:517–519.
18. Decramer M, Stas KJ. Corticosteroid-induced myopathy involving respiratory muscles in patients with chronic obstructive pulmonary disease or asthma. Am Rev Respir Dis 1992; 146: 800–802.
19. Griffin D, Fairman N, Coursin D, Rawsthorne L, Grossman JE. Acute myopathy during treatment of status asthmaticus with corticosteroids and steroid muscle relaxants. Chest 1992; 102: 510–514.
20. McFadden ER Jr. Dosages of corticosteroids in asthma. Am Rev Respir Dis 1993; 147:1306–1310.
21. Dhand R, Tobin MJ. Inhaled bronchodilator therapy in mechanically ventilated patients. Am J Respir Crit Care Med 1997; 156:3–10.
22. Dhand R, Duarte AG, Subran A, Senne SW, Fink JB, Fahey PJ, Tobin MJ. Dose response to bronchodilator delivered by metered-dose inhaler in ventilator-supported patients. Am J Respir Crit Care Med 1996; 154:388–393.
23. Murphy DG, McDermott MF, Rydman RJ, Sloan EP, Zalenski RJ. Aminophylline in the treatment of acute asthma when B_2-adrenergic and steroids are provided. Arch Intern Med 1993; 153:1784–1788.
24. Salmeron S, Brochard L, Mal H, Tenaillon A, Henry-Amar M, Renon D, Duroux P, Simonneau G. Nebulized versus intravenous albuterol in hypercapneic acute asthma: A multicenter, double blinded, randomized study. Am J Respir Crit Care Med 1994; 149:1466–1470.
25. Mauthous CA, Hall JB, Melmed A, Caputo MA, Walter J, Klocksieben JM, Schmidt GA, Wood LDM. Heliox improves pulsus paradoxus and peak flow in nonintubated patients with severe asthma. Am J Respir Crit Care Med 1995; 151:310–314.
26. Shive ST, Gluck EH. The use of helium-oxygen mixtures in the support of patients with status asthmaticus and respiratory acidosis. J Asthma 1989; 26:177–180.
27. Kass JE, Castriotta RJ. Heliox therapy in acute severe asthma. Chest 1995; 107:757–760.
28. Henke CA, Hertz M, Gustafson P. Combined bronchoscopy and mucolytic therapy for patients with severe refractory status asthmaticus on mechanical ventilation: A case report and review of the literature. Crit Care Med 1994; 22:1880–1883.
29. Green SM, Rothrock SG. Intravenous magnesium for acute asthma: Failure to decrease emergency room duration or need for hospitalization. Ann Emerg Med 1992; 21:260–265.

30. Tiffany BR, Berk WA, Todd IK, White SR. Magnesium bolus or infusion fails tc improve expiratory flow in acute asthma exacerbations. Chest 1993; 104:831–834.
31. Bloch H, Silverman R, Mancherje N. Intravenous magnesium sulfate as an adjunct in the treatment of acute asthma. Chest 1995; 107:1576–1581.
32. Graham VAL, Knowles GK, Milton AF, Davies RJ. Routine antibiotics in hospital management of acute asthma. Lancet 1982; 1:418–420.
33. McFadden ER Jr, Warren EL. Observations on asthma mortality. Ann Intern Med 1997; 127: 142–147.

31

The Acute Asthmatic in the Emergency Department

To Admit or Discharge?

Barry E. Brenner
The Brooklyn Hospital Center, member of New York–Presbyterian Hospitals, Weill Medical College of Cornell University, Brooklyn, New York

Kerry Alexander Powell
Johns Hopkins Bayview Medical Center, Baltimore, Maryland

The decision to admit or discharge a patient is a cornerstone of emergency medicine, and one we make many times each day, often with little data upon which to base our opinion. Fortunately, in most cases we are right or the nature of the disease allows the patient to return if they are not improving. However, asthma, like ischemic heart disease, has all the ingredients for a bad outcome if an incorrect decision is made. Acute asthma has the potential to be a life-threatening disease and a propensity for rapid deterioration. How can we best differentiate those patients that will do well from those that will not? In addition, can we select those patients that will need admission early to best use our resources?

The importance of these decisions is further underlined by an appreciation of the scale of the problem. In the United States, over 1 million adult emergency department (ED) visits are made each year for asthma (1). In addition for the last 20 years the incidence, morbidity, and mortality associated with asthma have continued to increase (see Chapters 5 and 17). The decision is made more difficult by the lack of clearly defined end points for the therapy of asthma in the ED, either clinical or spirometric.

I. CLINICAL PARAMETERS (Table 1)

Traditionally physicians have used patients' history to predict whether they will need admission. A previous history of frequent admissions (greater than two in the previous year), frequent ED visits (greater than three in the previous year), or previous intubation does increase the chances of admission (2,3). In addition, a patient with attacks of rapid development, changing from mild to severe bronchospasm in < 3 hr, is at greater risk of respiratory failure, lowering the threshold for admission to the hospital (4). In contrast, a patient with a slowly developing asthma attack over several days is also more likely to be admitted, partially because of the failure to respond to β-agonists that have already been heavily used at home (5). Although the presence of any one of these factors increases the chances of admission, none predicts the outcome for the individual patient.

The physical exam and vital signs have been used to define the severity of an asthma attack, and indeed the degree of dyspnea does generally correlate with the degree of bronchospasm (3,6). However, patients presenting without significant shortness of breath may still have severe airway obstruction and have an impairment in perceiving bronchospasm (see Chapter 13). Those asthmatics presenting with a pulse greater than 130 bpm generally having a higher incidence of in-hospital complications (7). The other, often quoted physical sign of severe airway obstruction is the presence of a pulsus paradoxus > 15 mmHg together with sternocleidomastoid retraction. Both of these findings result from the need to generate large negative intrapleural pressures to overcome the increased airway resistance. A pulsus paradoxus over 15 mmHg and sternocleidomastoid retraction are associated with $FEV_1 < 1$ L, suggesting the need for hospital admission (8–10). However, if a patient is breathing only small tidal volumes, then they may not generate a large negative intrapleural pressures, and these signs can be absent. In fact, in one study only 64% of patients with a peak expiratory flow rate (PEFR) < 100 L/min had pulsus paradoxus (11). Although if it is present, pulsus paradoxus does have some discriminating value. In the study of Rebuck and Reed, pulsus paradoxus was absent in all those whose FEV_1 was > 40% of predicted and elevated in all those whose $FEV_1$was < 20% of predicted (12). In summary the absence pulsus paradoxus does not exclude severe asthma. In fact, pulsus paradoxus may only regularly appear when the FEV_1 is < 20% of predicted. Many patients with severe bronchospasm may not develop pulsus paradoxus. Pulsus paradoxus is also notoriously difficult to measure accurately and a source of constant confusion as to how it is measured. Fortunately, accessory muscle use as explained above reflects the same pathophysiological process as pulsus paradoxus (e.g., high negative intrapleural pressures) and is much easier to evaluate and follow over time. Pulsus paradoxus and accessory muscle use may help in the assessment of the acute asthmatic when used together with other physical findings, particularly if the quality of spirometric data is in doubt. Marked tachycardia, pulsus paradoxus, or accessory muscle use, when present, suggest that a patient needs to be admitted to the hospital on presentation to the ED.

II. INDICATIONS FOR ADMISSION

Sometimes the decision to admit a patient can be fairly easy when there is an absolute indication (see Table 1). These are usually the occasional complications of asthma resulting from significant barotrauma, e.g., pneumothorax, pneumomediastinum, or pneumopericardium. Simple pneumonia in an acute asthmatic should also be considered a strong indication for admission. The presence of pneumonia acts as a continuing stimulus to bronchospasm and aggravates pre-existing hypoxia and ventilation/perfusion problems. Severe hypoxia (< 50 mmHg) is rarely present in acute asthma as an isolated finding, but, when present, suggests severe bronchospasm, profound ventilation/perfusion mismatch, and/or another coexistent pulmonary disease (e.g., multiple pulmonary emboli), which necessitate admission.

Salient psychiatric disturbances, poor access to medications, poor educability, drug abuse, fear of steroids, and evening discharges will predispose to relapse after discharge

Table 1 Admission Guidelines for Acute Asthma

Historical
Both abrupt and prolonged duration of symptoms
Frequent ED visits (> 3 per year)
Frequent hospitalizations (> 2 per year)
Endotracheal intubation
Physical
Pulse rate ≥ 130
Spirometric
See Table 4
Complications Indicating Admission
Barotrauma such as pneumothorax
Pneumonia
Hypoxia ≤ 50 mmHg rare in asthma, suggests other diagnoses, e.g., pneumonia, CHF, multiple pulmonary emboli
Other
Psychiatric illness
Poor educability
Fears of steroids
Discharge of patients during the evening
Chronic glucocorticoid use
Glucocorticoids stopped or tapered abruptly
Dysrhythmias

Source: Ref. 51.

from the ED (2,4,5) (see Chapters 34, 36, and 37). Lastly, patients on glucorticoids or those who have recently stopped taking glucocorticoids should be strongly considered for inpatient therapy.

III. PULSE OXIMETRY AND SPIROMETRY

A. Pulse Oximetry

In children, pulse oximetry has been useful to discern asthmatics that need admission to the hospital from those that can be safely discharged (see Chapters 32 and 34). In adults, however, pulse oximetry alone has not been shown to be helpful in predicting the course of acute asthma. In one study of 28 patients on a nonstandardized therapeutic regime, those that presented with an O_2 saturation ≤ 95% plus a change in PEFR ≤ 100 L/min either relapsed or required admission (13). The sensitivity was 73% and specificity was 88%.

B. Spirometry

Spirometry in the form of FEV_1 or PEFR has become the gold standards by which asthma is evaluated in the ED and outcome decisions are made. Before the utility of such measures was realized, patients were evaluated clinically and discharged when "wheeze free and asymptomatic." The history of this reliance on spirometry in the ED will be reviewed.

Kelsen et al. (14) studied 107 patients with acute asthma obtaining FEV_1 values at regular intervals and blinding the treating house officers in the ED from the results. Patients were treated and dispositions made on the usual clinical grounds of ''wheeze free and asymptomatic'' (14). They found that severe obstruction was present in 50% of asthmatics despite no accessory muscle use. Ten percent were discharged from the ED as sufficiently improved on a clinical basis, but these patients had no change in their FEV_1. In addition if the FEV_1 changed less than 400 mL, then 66% relapsed within 2 days. This study successfully demonstrated that clinical findings alone were unreliable in the decision to admit or discharge the acute asthmatic from the ED.

Shortly afterwards a study was published by Nowak et al. on the spirometric findings in 82 patients (15) during 85 ED visits. Again, the treating house officers were blind to the results and treated the patients according to the prevailing standards. The patients were followed up at 24–48 hr later in person or by telephone. Of these patients, 31% were admitted to the hospital, 26% were discharged and relapsed or had significant symptoms at follow up, and the remainder were discharged without problems. Thirty-five percent of the patients studied had an initial $FEV_1 < 0.6$ and a FEV_1 after treatment of < 1.6 L. Of these patients, 90% were admitted to the hospital or had a poor outpatient course, either relapsing or suffering significant symptoms. This study was the first to give spirometric criteria suggestive of poor outcome.

This was closely followed by a second study from the same group on a further 90 patients with over 109 ED encounters (16). Similar to the previous study, these patients were treated with a uniform treatment protocol for an average of 4.7 hr and then follow-up was performed at 48 hr. The treating physicians were not blind to the spirometric results that consisted of both FEV_1 and PEFR; however, the author notes that most of the physicians chose not to use the spirometric data in their decision making, since spirometric data were not yet accepted as valuable in decision making for patients with acute asthma. Those patients admitted to the hospital had an average predicted PEFR of 43% ± 19%. Those who were discharged and had a poor outcome, either relapse or continued symptoms, had an average predicted PEFR of 55% ± 21%. Those discharged with a successful outcome had an average predicted PEFR of 75% ± 25%. This study was the first to show clear differences in spirometry between those successfully discharged and those not. Thus spirometry could be used to help admission/discharge decisions for the acute asthmatic in the ED (see Table 2).

These findings were confirmed over the next decade by a variety of studies and clinical practice (15–20), so much so that they form the foundation for guidelines published by the World Health Organization (WHO) and the medical bodies of the United States (17), the United Kingdom (18), Canada, Australia/New Zealand, and South Africa (Table 3). All the guidelines are similar. All agree that spirometry should be the standard measure for the decision to discharge a patient from the ED. Sixty percent to 75% of the predicted value of the patient's PEFR or the patient's personal best are the desired values before discharge. All the published guidelines from the national bodies, however, add caveats to this dogma to allow flexibility for the treating physician. The guidelines from WHO are the strictest on this point, stating that the patient's PEFR should be >70% of predicted or personal best and sustained before discharge with no flexibility allowed. The Australian/New Zealand and U.K. guidelines also allow little flexibility. The Australian guidelines suggesting discharge only if the PEFR is > 60%. The U.K. guidelines also allow the discharge of patients whose PEFR is less than the recommended 75% of predicted but greater than 60% if this is unchanged after prolonged therapy; the nature or length of this prolonged therapy, however, is not clearly explained. The guidelines of South Africa, Canada, and the United States allow for the discharge of patients between

Table 2 Spirometric Criteria

Article	N	Spirometry	Outcome
Kelsen et al. (15)	107	FEV_1 < 400 mL improved during treatment	67% will relapse in 2 days
Banner et al. (16)	67	PEFR < 16% of predicted and improve < 16% of predicted with first treatment	All admitted or relapse
Nowak et al. (17)	82	FEV_1 < 0.6 initially and 1.6 L at end of therapy	90% relapse, poor home course or admitted to the ED
Nowak et al. (18)	90	PEFR < 45% of predicted	Admitted
		PEFR < 55% of predicted	Poor home course
		PEFR > 75% of predicted	Good home course
		Initial PEFR < 20–25% of predicted, receive parenteral β-agonists and PEFR still < 32–40% of predicted	85% admitted or poor outpatient course
		Initial PEFR < 20–25% of predicted and post-treatment < 70% of predicted	92% either admission or poor outpatient course
		If 300 L/min (approximately 70% of predicted PEFR in this study) is discharge criteria	14% will relapse
Fanta et al. (19)	102	Initial FEV_1 < 30% of predicted and < 40% after first hour	92% admitted or needed more than 4 hr to resolve
Fischl et al. (20)	112	Approximately 70% of predicted PEFR at time of discharge from ED	No relapses after discharge from ED
McFadden (23)	1084	PEFR < 20% of predicted and after 2 hr therapy PEFR < 40% predicted	Require admission with mean of 4.1 ± 0.2 days of inpatient care

Source: Ref. 51.

50–75%, 40–60%, and 50–70% of predicted or personal best, respectively, in the absence of risk factors. The nature of these risk factors are well-defined in both the Canadian and U.S. guidelines, are largely historical, and mirror many of the aforementioned comments. The Canadian guidelines include ''a previous near death episode,'' which is better defined in the U.S. guidelines as prior intubation or admission to an intensive care unit (ICU). Both include frequent hospitalizations or ED visits, sudden attacks, current or recent use of systemic steroids, unavoidable triggers, and poor compliance. The U.S. guidelines add low socioeconomic status, comorbid disease, psychiatric illness, and illicit drug use (see Tables 1 and 4).

This leads to the question of whether we can improve further upon spirometry and

Table 3 Discharge Criteria of Published Guidelines from Around the World

Guideline	Measure recommended	Percent predicted or personal best recommended for discharge
NHLBI/WHO Global Initiative (44)	PEFR or FEV_1	$>$ 70% of predicted and sustained
U.S./NHLBI	PEFR or FEV_1	$\geq$ 70% or $>$ 50% but $<$ 70% without risk factors
Canada (45)	PEFR or FEV_1	$>$ 60% or $>$ 40% but $<$ 60% without risk factors
Australia/New Zealand (46)	PEFR or FEV_1	$>$ 60% "generally discharged"; 40–60% generally admitted
United Kingdom	PEFR	$>$ 75% or $>$ 60% after more treatment
South Africa (47)	PEFR or FEV_1	$>$ 75% or $>$ 50% but $<$ 75% without risk factors

determine even earlier those patients who are going to do badly, and thus spare them a 3–4 hr stay in the ED before determining their outcome. This problem has been addressed in a number of studies. One of the earliest of these was by Fanta et al. (19). In this study 102 patients were treated on a fixed protocol. They found that if the initial FEV_1 was less than 30% of predicted initially and failed to improve after the first hour to better than 40% of predicted, these asthmatics had a 92% chance of admission or required more than the standard 4 hr to resolve. They noted that the greatest rate of improvement occurred in the first hour.

Table 4 Risk Factors Quoted in U.S. and Canadian Guidelines

United States	Canada
Past history of sudden severe exacerbation	Previous near death episode
Prior intubation for asthma	Recent ED visits
Prior admission to an intensive care unit	Frequent hospitalizations
Two or more hospitalizations in last year	Steroid dependent or recent use
Three or more emergency care visits in the past year	Sudden attacks
Hospitalization or an emergency care visit for asthma in last month	Allergic/anaphylactic triggers
Current use or recent withdrawal from steroids	Prolonged duration of attack
Difficulty perceiving airflow obstruction or severity	Poor compliance/understanding
Comorbidity, as from cardiovascular disease or COPD	Returning to same environment
Serious psychiatric disease or psychosocial problems	Asthma triggers
Low socioeconomic status and urban residence	
Illicit drug use	
Sensitivity to *Alternaria*	

Further attempts were made to refine this and better predict those patients that will need admission earlier in the course of ED treatment. Notably, Fischl et al. (20) developed a multifactorial index that had a sensitivity of 0.97 and a specificity of 0.95 for predicting relapse or admission to the hospital using data obtained at the time of presentation of the patient to the ED. In this study the patients were placed on a specific protocol of epinephrine, isoetharine, and intravenous (IV) aminophylline with a time limit of 8–12 hr in the ED. This study also confirmed the previous findings of Nowak that a PEFR of 70% of predicted or more at the time of discharge from the ED was associated with a low relapse rate (16). However, no steroids were given at the time of discharge from the ED. Repeated attempts were made to validate this predictive index (21,22) without success, but these studies failed to follow the same rigid protocol for the treatment of the patients. Therefore, indices such as those of Fischl may be beneficial, but only if the exact protocol used is followed, and perhaps may not be generalized to other EDs due to differences in the patient population and ED resources. The study did inadvertently support the findings of Nowak that patients discharged with a PEFR of greater than 70% of predicted had a low rate of relapse.

The largest study looking at spirometric criteria was by McFadden et al. (23), who studied a total of 1084 acute asthmatics in the ED. Patients that presented with an initial peak flow of less than 20% of predicted and failed to improve to better than 40% of predicted within 2 hr, despite intensive therapy (steroids, aminophylline, and inhaled β-agonists every 20 min), were unlikely to improve within 24 hr and on average required 4 days of inpatient therapy (23).

Similarly, an index has been developed in Uruguay by Rodrigo and Rodrigo predicting the need for hospitalization 30 min after initial β-agonist therapy (24). In this study, physicians were blinded from the PEFR values and admission/discharge decisions were made within 6 hr of the initial ED presentation based on clinical findings. A patient would be discharged from the ED if they were asymptomatic with minimal wheezing, absence of accessory muscle use at rest, and ability to walk 60 feet without exacerbation of bronchospasm. ED therapy consisted of albuterol by metered dose inhaler (MDI) and spacer (2.5 mg/hr), 500 mg hydrocortisone intravenously, and, at discharge from the ED, 40 mg prednisone for 5 days. There were 184 adults in the study. The patients that were discharged from the ED compared to those admitted had a better PEFR (expressed as percent predicted) at the time of initial ED presentation (32 vs. 25%, $p < 0.01$), after 30 min (50 vs. 28%, $p < 0.001$), and at the end of ED therapy (58 vs. 31%). Similar results have been reported by others (3,16,19,23), where the patients that are eventually hospitalized with acute asthma had a lower PEFR on presentation to the ED and at every time point during ED therapy, responding most vigorously within the first 30 min to 2 hr of initial therapy. Using discriminant analysis and stepwise addition of variables, an index was developed based on the percent predicted PEFR at 30 min, change in the PEFR from baseline at 30 min, and subjective impression of accessory muscle use (Table 5). They found that a index score of 4 or more had a sensitivity of 0.86, specificity of 0.96, positive predictive value of 0.75, and negative predictive value of 0.75. The validation and applicability of this index to other institutions awaits further study. The study population was unusual in that 40% had not used β-agonist inhalants before the ED visit and their relapse rate at two weeks was only 10% as compared to 17% in the U.S.-based Multicenter Asthma Research Collaboration (MARC) (personal communication C. Camargo Jr., principal investigator, MARC, March 1998).

In summary, spirometry supplements clinical judgment in assessing the acute asth-

Table 5 Predictive Index Scoring System

Variable	Score 0	Score 1	Score 2
	Score		
PEFR variation at 30 min (L/min)	> 50	50–20	< 20
PEFR at 30 min (%predicted)	> 45	45–35	< 35
Accessory muscle use at 30 min[a]	0–1	2	3

[a] 0 = no accessory muscle use; 1 = mild accessory muscle use; 2 = moderate accessory muscle use; 3 = severe accessory muscle use with retraction or depression.
Source: Ref. 24.

matic. The likelihood of relapse or severe continued symptoms is much less if the patient has a PEFR or $FEV_1 > 70\%$ at the time of discharge. If the patient presents with a PEFR 20–30% and fails to improve to > 40% in the first 1–2 hr, then they are unlikely to resolve in less than 24 hr (see Table 2 and the ''Perspective'' section later in this chapter).

IV. ADMISSION TO THE INTENSIVE CARE UNIT

We have been discussing the indicators for admission to the hospital and those criteria that suggest a poor outpatient course and high likelihood of relapse. In patients that are admitted, what are the indicators of severe illness and can we predict those acute asthmatics that may deteriorate further leading to respiratory failure? That is, what are the selection criteria for admission to the intensive care unit? In this situation spirometry is of little value, because the patient is usually unable to perform spirometric tests and clinical factors are of the utmost importance.

If the patient was found in or near respiratory arrest and arrives intubated, the decision to admit the patient to the ICU is straightforward. In addition, a pco_2 greater than 45 mmHg, profuse sweating, recumbence, decreased muscle tone, or a desire to lie down (25), as well as any mental status changes, such as somnolence, suggest hypercapnea and impending respiratory arrest. Other signs, not as catastrophic as some of those above but still indicators of severe disease, include the classic ''silent'' chest that occurs as fatigue develops and tidal volume falls leading to decreased air movement, until there is insufficient air movement to generate a ''wheeze.'' The same process is occurring when the patient is unable to speak in that they are unable to generate sufficient airflow across the vocal cords to speak. Thus, unless these signs can be quickly reversed, the patient should be considered for admission to an ICU (see Chapter 26).

A few asthmatics, usually when there is accompanying heart disease, may also develop dysrhythmias secondary to methylxanthines or β-agonists self-administered, administered by EMS during transport, or given in the ED. Admission to the ICU would be required where adequate monitoring can be provided (Table 6).

V. GLUCOCORTICOIDS: DO THEY ALTER THE ADMISSION/DISCHARGE DECISION?

Glucocorticoids undoubtedly play a pivotal role in the management of asthma; however, the delay in the onset of action is the limiting factor on their impact in the management

Table 6 Admission Guidelines to the Intensive Care Unit

1. Respiratory arrest
2. $P_{CO_2} > 45$ mmHg
3. Signs of near respiratory arrest
   - Diaphoresis with recumbency
   - Somnolence
   - Staring facies
   - Bradypnea
4. Dysrhythmias (multifocal PVCs, tachyarrhythmias)

The patient needs admission to the hospital even with dramatic improvement if he or she presents or develops any of the above during the ED stay.
Source: Ref. 51.

and decision to admit an acute asthmatic. Essentially, should we keep an asthmatic in the ED awaiting the effect of steroids and will that delay avoid some admissions? The rapid resolution of an acute asthmatic in 1–2 hr does not require steroids nor do steroids increase the rate of improvement (26,27). In another important study by Fanta et al., hydrocortisone was administered intravenously (2 mg/kg bolus then 0.5 mg/kg/hr infusion) in a double-blind fashion to 20 patients following 8 hr of unsuccessful conventional bronchodilator therapy (28). The treated group had a 118 ± 25% change in FEV_1 and the placebo group had only a 35 ± 22% change. The difference was statistically significant. The difference between the groups was initially noticed at 6 hr when the first FEV_1 was measured. Therefore an earlier effect cannot be excluded. Stein and Cole countered this with a study on 91 patients given a fixed therapeutic protocol and 125 mg methylprednisolone (29). They failed to detect any significant effect in their patients; however, the asthmatics were only followed for 6.5 hr, which probably was insufficient time to see an effect. The average PEFR of the study patients upon presentation was 250 L/min, suggesting the degree of bronchospasm was not particularly severe and also possibly explaining the lack of a detectable response. In a meta-analysis of the 30 studies performed on the subject of whether steroids have a role in the treatment of acute asthma, Rowe et al. concluded that steroids are effective agents within 6 hr (30). In general, between 6 and 12 hr are needed for steroids to have an effect and relieve acute bronchospasm, with 160 mg of methylprednisolone per day being the optimum dose (28,31–34) (see Chapter 22). From the earlier data of McFadden et al. (23), we can conclude that some of the factors that determine whether steroids will have an impact on the ED course are dependent on the initial severity of illness. If the patient fails to respond to initial bronchodilator therapy and the PEFR remains below 40% of predicted after 2 hr of therapy, then the patient is unlikely to respond, because on average the exacerbation of acute asthma would take 4 days to resolve due to the much slower resolution of airway inflammation. Therefore, waiting for the onset of action of glucocorticoids would be fruitless. If the patients PEFR is greater than 40% of predicted after 2 hr of therapy, then it is reasonable to wait for the onset of the action of steroids depending on ED resources. If the patient has already been given steroids on arrival in the ED, then time is saved.

VI. DURATION OF THERAPY

We have discussed criteria by which it is possible to decide whether to discharge a patient with acute asthma from the ED. However, a patient whose PEFR is 50% of predicted after 4 hr of therapy may reach 70% of predicted after 12 hr of continued therapy, particularly with the delayed onset of action of steroids. So how long should a patient stay in the ED before a decision is made to admit or discharge? There is no definite answer to this question, because the answer will depend primarily on the resources available in the ED as well as inpatient and intensive care services of the hospital. Frequently people cite cost as a reason to prolong ED stay and avoid admission. Although cost is legitimately a factor, it does not always favor a prolonged stay in the ED or observational ward because the additional cost of a prolonged stay may not be reimbursed (see Chapter 33). Thus the usual length of stay of patients varies widely between EDs. Therefore, when applying the spirometric criteria for admission, the rate of improvement must be considered and whether the usual length of stay will allow time for sufficient improvement. Some of these problems can be ameliorated by the presence of a holding or observation unit for patients with acute asthma in which a 12 hr stay is allowed, which can avoid up to 60% of admissions (35). However, outcome may be affected adversely by having patients languish without timely treatments in an ED without such a specialized observation unit. For example, if adequate staffing dedicated to the unit is not provided, the patient may be neglected at times while the ED staff undertake other duties, and the benefits of the observation unit is lost.

VII. PREVENTION OF RELAPSE

In assessing admission and discharge of patients from the ED, relapse has come to be the outcome measure reflecting an inappropriate or unsuccessful discharge from the ED. Relapse is often viewed as return visits to the ED, unscheduled visits to the private medical doctor for bronchospasm, or increase in medications since discharge (see Chapter 34). But the patient who does none of the above but is highly symptomatic at home, cannot sleep or exercise, or misses days from work or school represents an unsuccessful discharge from the ED. This standard was used in the studies by Nowak et al. (15,16). On the other hand, a patient who returns to the ED after discharge may return for reasons other than a relapse with acute bronchospasm. The patient may not have acquired the necessary medications, and uses the ED for all forms of therapy. The patient may be ''relapsing'' to acquire inhalant canisters as adjuncts for their drug use. If relapse is to be related to the index ED visit, then the relapse should soon follow the ED visit. In most studies, relapse within two to three weeks of the ED visit has been considered a ''true'' relapse. This presumption, however, has not been verified.

In the discussion of the spirometric criteria for admission or discharge from the ED, the incidence of relapse was an important component. Relapse may be partially regarded as the emergency physician's failure either to recognize or treat the disease on the initial presentation, but as mentioned earlier the reasons for the relapse may be multifactorial. Most would agree that an asthmatic returning to the ED two or three times within a week, each time with significant airway obstruction, reflects relapse and requires admission. However, the study of relapse is greatly complicated by a lack of a consistent definition of what constitutes relapse. How many visits in a week should be allowed? A return to the ED within 72 hr for recurrent asthma would undoubtedly be considered relapse. The importance of relapse lies in it being an indicator of serious disease and poor outcome. Studies of relapse show that 60–83% of patients that relapse are admitted to the hospital (20,36) and of patients admitted to the ICU 30–50% had been treated in the ED within the preceding days or weeks, i.e., before they relapsed (37). Relapse rates vary between 16 and 24% in the first 2–10 days after treatment in the ED (14,16,23,38). Seventy-five percent of these relapses occur within the first 4 days and represent early relapse (20,36,38). A risk factor for frequent relapse is previous relapse (39,40). Excluding the use of correct criteria for discharge from the ED, two interventions have been shown to reduce the incidence of relapse: steroids and providing adequate patient education and follow-up.

A. Steroids

A short outpatient course of steroids was studied by Fiel et al. (41) in patients discharged from the ED following treatment for acute asthma. The patients were treated in a double-blind placebo controlled fashion with a 8-day tapering course of methylprednisolone, starting with a dose of 32 mg twice a day or placebo. They were then followed up at 7–10 days later to assess their degree of symptomatology. The results revealed a dramatic decrease in the relapse rate: 5.9% in the treated group and 15.6% in the placebo group. The results were similarly marked in the degree of symptomatology reported at follow-up, with 21% having significant pulmonary symptomatology in the treated group as compared to 36.4% in the placebo group. The number of side effects reported was the same in both the treated and placebo groups. These dramatic results were successfully repeated and expanded upon by Chapman et al., who gave a short course of prednisone in a double-blind placebo controlled fashion at discharge from the ED (38). They stratified the patients on their percentage predicted PEFR achieved at discharge. The results were similar to those above with a relapse rate of 6% in those treated and 24% in those given placebo. In those whose PEFR was less than 70% at the time of discharge from the ED, the relapse rate was 13% if given steroids and 50% if given placebo. Thus there appears to be a greater difference giving steroids to those given whose PEFR is less at the time of discharge, reflecting the predominately inflammatory process in the more severe asthmatics.

B. Patient Education

A short course of steroids reduces the risk of relapse to only 6%. However, any discharged patient remains at risk of relapse and appropriate education and follow-up can potentially prevent a return to the ED. From the Multicenter Asthma Research Collaboration, 40% of adults with an episode of acute asthma did not see a primary care provider (PCP) in the previous year and the ED serves as their primary source of asthma therapy and education (42). A time of crisis is often when a patient is their most receptive to education. The effectiveness of such patient education programs was demonstrated by Mayo et al. (43). This study took 47 of 104 moderately severe asthmatics—all frequent visitors to the ED—and randomized them to receive (n = 47) or not receive (n = 67) an intensive program on the correct use of inhaler spacers and inhaled steroids and taught self-management techniques that included the self-administration of 3-day courses of prednisone 40 mg for exacerbation. They then followed the patient for a year and found a threefold reduction in readmission rate and shorter hospital stays when admitted for the group receiving education.

The patient does not just need only education, but also the provision of follow-up care. Emerman and Cydulka reported that 79% of their 10-day relapses occurred within the first 4 days, with almost half of the patients relapsing before the scheduled appointment (see Chapters 34 and 35). Importantly, they found that relapse was reduced if the outpatient appointment was scheduled at the time of discharge from the ED rather than giving the patient the responsibility. Clearly the follow-up appointment should occur soon after the ED visit to adjust the patient's asthma medications when the risk for relapse is the highest.

VIII. PERSPECTIVES ON ADMISSION CRITERIA

In this chapter, the utility of spirometric criteria to assist in admission and discharge decisions of the asthmatic from the ED has been emphasized. It is clear that the most commonly used test, peak flow, is fraught with problems. The peak flow nomogram varies with the race/ethnic group. The equipment is not calibrated, occasionally the dial ''sticks,'' and ideally we should use the patient's personal best and not a nomogram to determine the patient's predicted values (see Chapter 14). Nevertheless, this hand-held peak flow meter is the best spirometric equipment that we have in common use.

From the results of Nowak et al. (17,18) and Fischl et al. (20), those acute asthmatics with PEFR values over 70% of predicted are less likely to relapse or have an unsuccessful discharge from the ED. However, others have stated that there was too much overlap in the spirometric data on admitted vs. discharged asthmatics for these criteria to be useful clinically. One such study evaluated 2-day relapse and blinded the physicians to the spirometric results (48). They tried to develop spirometric predictors of relapse based on the response to the first ED treatment with a β-agonist. The applicability of this study to current recommendations concerning admit/discharge of the asthmatic is difficult, since their protocol gave inadequate β-agonist therapy over the 6 hr ED protocol and did not assess the final spirometric values in the ED before discharge, and the admission rate to the hospital was only 10% as compared to 22%, which is our national ED admission rate for acute asthma (personal communication C. Camargo Jr, personal communication, March 1998).

In a similar study, Worthington and Ahuja looked at spirometric criteria to predict relapse as defined as the need for further medical attention or increase in asthma medications within 5 days of the ED visit (49). The physicians were blinded to the spirometric values. The spirometric values in this study were unable to differentiate admitted, discharged, or relapsed patients except that those patients with an FEV_1 over 2.4 L had only a 10% incidence of relapse. However, the length of time that the patient could be treated in the ED was at the physician's discretion. Obviously, the longer a physician treats an acute asthmatic in the ED, the higher the discharge FEV_1 may be. Also in this study there was only a 10% admission rate; therefore, as mentioned earlier, the applicability of these results to 1998 is questionable.

More recent studies have used a 3–5 hr protocol for ED treatment of acute asthma. In evaluating relapse at 3 days, no differences in post-treatment spirometric values between those that relapsed and those that did not were noted (39). In this study, however, the physicians were not blinded to the spirometric values and may have been using the results for admission/discharge decision making.

In summary, although Rodrigo and Rodrigo, as noted earlier, have developed a predictive index for admission after initial response to treatment in the ED, this index awaits further validation by other emergency departments (24). Prospective studies are needed to determine if discharging patients after a fixed therapeutic protocol with a PEFR of greater than 70% will reduce relapse and unsuccessful discharges from the ED.

Changes in pulmonary function within the time frame of a stay in the ED will affect whether the patient will be admitted or discharged from the ED. If the length of time that the asthmatic is allowed to be treated within the ED is increased, more time is allowed for the patient to demonstrate that their bronchospasm and pulmonary function is reversible; therefore, fewer patients would need admission to the hospital (35). Likewise, if a new therapy is highly effective in acute asthma, e.g., inhaled corticosteroids, rapidly reducing bronchospasm during the allowed time period in the ED, then there would be a quicker improvement in the spirometric tests and more acute asthmatics would reach the "cutoff" values for admission/discharge from the ED (50). Therefore, even if validated, spirometric criteria will never be static in time or universally applicable to all EDs. They will depend on institutional policies such as the length of time the asthmatic can remain in the ED, the presence of an observation unit, and the development of more effective therapeutic modalities that would reduce bronchospasm more rapidly than previously.

REFERENCES

1. Weiss KB, Gergen PJ, Hodgson TA. An economic evaluation of asthma in United States. New Engl J Med 1992; 326:862–866.
2. Williams MH. Increasing severity of asthma from 1960–1987. N Engl J Med 1989; 320:1015–1016.
3. Rodrigo G, Rodrigo C. Assessment of the patient with acute asthma in the emergency department: A factor analytic study. Chest 1993; 104:1325–1328.
4. Kallenbach JM, Frankel AH, Lapinsky SE, et al. Determinants of near fatality in acute severe asthma. Am J Med 1993; 95:265–272.
5. Appel DA, Karpel JP, Sherman M. Epinephrine improves expiratory flow rates in patients with asthma who do not respond to inhaled metaproterenol sulphate. J Allergy Clin Immunol 1989; 84:90–98.
6. Bailey WC, Higgins DM, Richards BM, et al. Asthma Severity: A factor analytic investigation. Am J Med 1992; 263–269.
7. Cooke NJ, Crompton GK, Grant IWB. Observations on the management of acute bronchial asthma. Br J Dis Chest 1979; 73:157–163.
8. Knowles GK, Clark TJH. Pulsus paradoxus as valuable sign indicating severity of asthma. Lancet 1973; 2:1356–1358.
9. Rebuck AS, Read J. Assessment and management of severe asthma. Am J Med 1971; 51: 788–798.
10. McFadden ER Jr, Kiser R, DeGroot WJ. Acute bronchial asthma: Relations between clinical and physiological manifestations. N Engl J Med 1973; 288:221–225.
11. Pearson MG, et al. Value of pulsus paradoxus in assessing acute severe asthma. Brit Med J 1993; 307:659.
12. Rebuck AS, Read J. Patterns of ventilatory response to carbon dioxide during recovery from severe asthma. Clin Sci 1971; 41:13–21.
13. Hedges JR, Amsterdam JT, Cionni DJ, Embry S. Oxygen saturation as a marker for admission of relapse with acute bronchospasm. Am J Emerg Med 1987; 5:196–200.
14. Kelsen SG, Kelsen DP, Fleeger BF, et al. Emergency room assessment and treatment of patientswith acute asthma: Adequacy of conventional approach. Am J Med 1978; 64:622–628.
15. Nowak RM, Gordan KR, Wroblewski DA, et al. Spirometric evaluation of acute bronchial asthma. J Am Coll Emerg Phys 1979; 8:9–12.
16. Nowak RM, Pensier MI, Sarker DD, et al. Comparison of peak expiratory flow and FEV_1 admission criteria for acute bronchial asthma. Ann Emerg Med 1982; 11:64–69.

17. NHLBI. National Asthma Education Program, Expert Panel Report. Guidelines for the diagnosis and management of asthma. J Allergy Clin Immunology 1991; 88:425–534.
18. British Thoracic Society, Research Unit of the Royal College of Physicians of London, King's Fund Centre, National Asthma Campaign. Guidelines for the management of asthma in adults: II. Acute severe asthma. Br Med J 1990; 301:797–801.
19. Fanta CH, Rossing TH, McFadden ER Jr. Emergency room treatment of acute asthma: Relationships among therapeutic combinations, severity of obstruction, and time course of response. Am J Med 1982; 72:416–422.
20. Fischl MA, Pitchenik A, Gardener LB. An index predicting relapse and need for hospitalization in patients with acute bronchial asthma. N Engl J Med 1981; 305:783–789.
21. Centor RM, Yarbrough BY, Wood JP. Inability to predict relapse in acute asthma. N Engl J Med 1984; 310:577–580.
22. Rose CC, Murphy JG, Schwartz JS. Performance of an index predicting the response of patients with acute asthma to intensive emergency department treatment. N Engl J Med 1984; 310:573–577.
23. McFadden ER Jr, Elsanadi N, Dixon L, et al. Protocol therapy for asthma: therapeutic benefits and cost savings. Am J Med 1995; 99:651–661.
24. Rodrigo G, Rodrigo C. A new index for early prediciton of hospitalization in patients with acute asthma. Am J Emerg Med 1997; 15:8–13.
25. Brenner BE, Abraham E, Simon R. Position and diaphoresis in acute asthma. Am J Med 1983; 74:1005–1009.
26. McFadden ER Jr, Kiser R, deGroot WJ, Holmes B, Kilker R, Viser G. A controlled study of the effects of single doses of hydrocortisone on the resolution of acute attacks of asthma. Am J Med 1976; 60:52–59.
27. Kattan M, Gurwitz D, Levison H. Corticosteroids in status asthmaticus. J Pediatr 1980; 96: 596–599.
28. Fanta CH, Rossing TH, McFadden ER Jr. Glucocorticoids in acute asthma. A critical controlled trial. Am J Med 1983; 74:845–851.
29. Stein LM, Cole RP. Early administration of corticosteroids in emergency room treatment of acute asthma. Ann Intern Med 1990; 112:822–827.
30. Rowe BH, Keller JL, Orman AD. Effectivenes of steroid therapy in acute exacerbations of asthma: a meta-analysis. Am J Emerg Med 1993; 22:1829–1835.
31. McFadden ER Jr. Dosages of corticosteroids in asthma. Am Rev Respir Dis 1993; 147:1306–1310.
32. Pierson WE, Bierman CW, Kelley VC. A double-blind trail of corticosteroid therapy in status asthmaticus. Pediatrics 1974; 54:282–288.
33. Collins JV, Clark TJH, Brown D, Townsend J. The use of corticosteroid in the treatment of acute asthma. Quart J Med 1975; 174:259–273.
34. Haskell RJ, Wong BM, Hansen JE. A double-blind, randomized clinical trail of methylprednisolone in status asthmaticus. Arch Intern Med 1983; 143:1324–1327.
35. McDermott MF, Murphy DG, Zalenski RJ, et al. Comparison between emergency diagnostic and treatment unit and inpatient care in the treatment of asthma. Arch Intern Med 1997; 157: 2055–2062.
36. Newcomb RW, Akhter J. Outcomes of emergency room visits for asthma. J Allergy Clin Immunol 1986; 77:309–314.
37. Westerman DE, Benatar Sr, Potgieter PD, et al. Identification of the high-risk asthmatic patient. Experience with 39 patients undergoing ventilation for status asthmaticus. Am J Med 1979; 66:566–572.
38. Chapman KR, Verbeek R, White JG, Rebuck AS. Effect of a short course of prednisone in the prevention of early relapse after the emergency room treatment of acute asthma. New Engl J Med 1991; 324:788–794.

39. Emerman CH, Cydulka RK. Factors associated with relapse after emergency department treatment for acute asthma. Ann Emerg Med 1995; 26:6–11.
40. Ducharme FM, Kramer MS. Relapse following emergency treatment for acute asthma: Can it be predicted or prevented? J Clin Epidemiol 1993; 46:1395–1402.
41. Fiel SB, Swartz MA, Glanz K, et al. Efficacy of short-term corticosteroid therapy in outpatient treatment of acute bronchial asthma. Am J Med 1983; 75:259–262.
42. Woodruff PG, Singk AK, Camargo CA Jr. Role of the emergency department in chronic asthma care. Am J Respir Crit Care Med 1998; 157(3, Part 2):A161.
43. Mayo PH, Richman J, Harris HW. Results of a program to reduce admissions for adult asthma. Ann Intern Med 1990; 112:864–871.
44. National Institutes of Health: Global Strategy For Asthma Management and Prevention NHLBI/WHO Workshop Report, National Heart, Lung, and Blood Institute, Bethesda, MD, 1995, NIH Publication No. 95-3659.
45. Beveridge RC, Grunfeld AF, Hodder RV, et al. for the CAEP/CTS Asthma Advisory Committee, Guidelines for the Emergency Department management of asthma in adults, Can Med Assoc J 1996; 155:25–37.
46. Woolcock A, Rubenfeld AR, Seale JP, et al. Asthma management plan, Med J Aust 1989; 151:650–653.
47. Statement by a Working Group of the South African Pulmonology Society, Guidelines for the management of asthma in adults in South Africa. Part II. Acute asthma, South Afr Med J 1994; 84:332–338.
48. Martin TG, Elenbaas RM, Pingleton SH, et al. Failure of peak expiratory flow rate to predict hospital admission in acute asthma. Ann Emerg Med 1982; 11:466–470.
49. Worthington JR, Ahuja J. The value of pulmonary function tests in the management of acute asthma. Can Med Assoc J 1989; 140:153–156.
50. Rodrigo G, Rodrigo C. Inhaled flunisolide for acute severe asthma. Am J Respir Crit Care Med 1998; 157:698–703.

32

The Acute Asthmatic in the Pediatric Emergency Department
To Admit or Discharge?

Jill M. Baren
University of Pennsylvania School of Medicine, Philadelphia, Pennsylvania

I. INTRODUCTION

Asthma is the most prevalent chronic disease in childhood with 2.7 million under the age of 18 affected (1). It is a frequent cause of emergency department (ED) visits that often result in hospitalizations. It is estimated that there are 200,000 hospitalizations per year for asthma in the pediatric population (1). In the last few decades, hospitalization rates from asthma among children have increased from 112 per 100,000 in the early 1970s to 279 per 100,000 in the 1980s (2). Children under 4 years of age are disproportionately affected, with an average increase in hospitalization of 5.0% per year compared to 4.5% for all children age 0–17 years (3). Mortality from asthma in children under age 15 years has doubled over the same time period from an all-time low of 54 deaths in 1977 to 125 deaths in 1985 (3). These increases have occurred despite advancements in the understanding of disease pathophysiology and in the number of therapeutic modalities available (4–7). The reasons for these increases are still unclear (6–9). In addition to increasing hospitalization rates, relapse or return unscheduled visits by pediatric asthma patients to the ED or other health care facilities have been reported to be as high as 30% (2). From the third Multicenter Asthma Research Collaboration (MARC3), nationally representative rates for admission for approximately 750 asthmatic children from 30 states in 1997 for children ages 2–17 are 22% [20–25 confidence interval (CI)] with relapse rates of 17% in two weeks for acute asthma that presented to the ED. Neither admission nor relapse rates varied significantly with age (personal communication, C. Camargo, principal investigator for MARC3, May 1998).

Assessing the severity of an acute asthma exacerbation in a child and accurately predicting the outcome (admit vs. discharge) of the exacerbation remains one of the most challenging problems in emergency medicine. Acutely ill children are more difficult to assess than adults due to a variety of physiological and behavioral characteristics. This is especially true for younger, preverbal children. Routine methods for estimating the severity of acute asthma in adults, adolescents, and older children often cannot be applied in younger children. The lack of available objective methods to assess asthma severity in children and the lack of ''gold standard'' criteria for admission may contribute to both excessive hospitalization rates and high relapse rates.

II. PEDIATRIC VS. ADULT ASTHMA PATIENTS

A. Definition of Disease

Making the definitive diagnosis of asthma in the pediatric population is complex, requires multiple observations over time, and is often fraught with disagreement amongst clinicians (1). Pediatricians are reluctant to label young children with the diagnosis of asthma until a clear pattern of reversible bronchospastic episodes can be demonstrated. Nomenclature is often confusing because a number of poorly defined terms are in existence, such as ''reactive airways disease,'' ''wheezing associated respiratory infection,'' and ''wheezy bronchitis'' (1).

Different patterns of disease progression are also characteristic of childhood wheezing or asthma. Many will manifest wheezing with an episode of infectious bronchiolitis before age 1 or 2 years and may remain wheeze-free until later in life. Some begin an episodic pattern of wheezing shortly after an episode of bronchiolitis. Treatment regimens effective for asthma are not necessarily proven to be effective for bronchiolitis. Thus, emergency physicians are left with a confusing diagnostic and therapeutic dilemma.

B. Physiological Differences

Infants and children are more prone to respiratory failure than their adult counterparts. They have less functional reserve due to increased airway resistance, decreased elastic recoil properties, early airway closure, unstable rib cage structure, weaker diaphragmatic muscles, small caliber airways, and a more immature immune system (1,10). Therefore, ED treatment may need to be more aggressive with a lower threshold for admission. A wide range of normal respiratory rates, heart rates, and blood pressure exist for children of different age groups. Without this knowledge, assessment of asthma severity in children will be impaired. Specific clinical signs of respiratory distress may be more prominent and useful in children than adults; for example, retractions are a very visible sign of respiratory distress in children due to a thin and compliant chest wall.

C. Behavioral/Developmental Differences

Infants and young children rely on parents and guardians to administer medications, to access the health care system, and to provide historical information during an acute episode of asthma. Young infants and children cannot verbalize subjective feelings of dyspnea or respiratory distress. The emergency physician must rely on caretakers' impressions of disease severity, which may not be accurate or reliable, and on direct observation without the patient's input. Children also have limited ability to perceive their degree of airway obstruction (11).

Older children and adolescents are often permitted and encouraged to self-administer asthma medications. This particular group of patients is also at high risk for noncompliance due to a variety of psychosocial factors such as denial of asthma and its severity (12). Delay in seeking medical care and minimization of symptoms is not unusual and may also increase the difficulty of the ED evaluation and disposition decision. The cognitive and social development of children must be taken into account when devising management and treatment plans (11).

III. TOOLS AVAILABLE TO ASSESS ASTHMA SEVERITY IN PEDIATRIC PATIENTS

A. Estimation of Severity of the Exacerbation

The emergency physician has several types of information available to estimate asthma severity in a pediatric patient that will provide the basis for a disposition decision: (1) historical information about baseline disease status, medication usage and compliance, and events leading up to the ED visit; (2) clinical parameters assessed during the ED visit, upon presentation, and after treatment; and (3) objective measurements taken during the ED visit, upon presentation, and after treatment. The decision to discharge or admit the patient is usually based on a combination of factors, and there is tremendous variability among practitioners. To date, no single factor or combination of factors has been shown to be satisfactorily predictive of who will require hospitalization and who can be safely discharged without fear of relapse. However, since the assessment of airway obstruction in children is clinically difficult, objective measures are exceedingly important in making a correct assessment and in monitoring the response to treatment.

B. Historical Information

Emergency physicians should identify risk factors that are known to be associated with a more severe episode of asthma and possibly the need for hospitalization. These include: (1) frequency of previous asthma exacerbations; (2) recent visit to the ED for asthma; (3) recent hospitalization and duration of hospitalization; (4) prior admission to an intensive care unit; (5) previous near fatal asthma or long delay in seeking medical care; and (6) current use of systemic steroids to control asthma symptoms (13). Although the identification of these risk factors may be helpful in determining disposition, it is important to realize that they may be confounded by institutional practice and policy and by socioeconomic factors (13).

C. Assessment of Severity by Physical Examination and Clinical Scoring Methods

Typical physical findings present during an asthma exacerbation are tachypnea, accessory muscle use, wheezing or other abnormal breath sounds, and color change. Studies have shown that several of these signs will correlate somewhat with pulmonary function measurements (14–19). When examined as predictors of outcome of an acute exacerbation, physical exam findings lack the sensitivity and specificity necessary to become useful clinical tools (20). In addition, interobserver correlation, when it has been measured, is poor (13). For example, respiratory rate in children is state dependent: more rapid when the child is awake and crying as compared to being asleep. Unless the child's measurements are taken in identical states at all times, results are not likely to be reproducible (13).

Many investigators have combined physical findings with other clinical parameters such as pulmonary function measurements and have designed multivariate clinical scoring systems for acute asthma. These scoring systems are primarily subjective, and few have been systematically evaluated (13). Attempts to validate clinical scores have also been disappointing (13). It is still worthwhile to review the subject of clinical scoring systems especially in the context of pediatric asthma, since routine assessment of airway obstruction by measurement of peak expiratory flow (PEF) or spirometric indices is not an option in younger patients (14).

Clinical scores have been devised for several purposes: (1) to assess the severity of asthma at a single point in time; (2) to predict the need for hospitalization, or the likelihood of relapse after discharge; and (3) to evaluate changes in the severity of asthma over time, usually in response to therapy (14). A clear and thorough review of multivariate clinical scores for preschool children (ages 0–5 years) is presented by van Der Windt et al. (14). The authors found 16 scores that appeared in the literature as of 1994. The scores were evaluated based on a predefined set of criteria that included purpose of the score, description of the score, suitability for use in children, interobserver agreement, and validity (14).

To summarize, Van der Windt et al. found that interobserver agreement of scores was not often tested or reported despite that fact that clinical signs in the scores like cyanosis and retractions required subjective judgment. They also found that the ability of the asthma scores to predict the outcome of an acute episode of asthma was limited due to different treatment responses measured. The authors noted several pitfalls with asthma scores in children such as the state-dependent nature of certain variables and the difficulty with certain measurements like pulsus paradoxus. Most of the scores did include accessory muscle use or retractions, dyspnea, and wheezing, and the authors commented that these items showed a better correlation with pulmonary function than other clinical signs (14,21). Although several clinical asthma scores have been used in research settings, none have made their way into routine clinical practice and none have sufficient validity to be used as a decision rule for admission versus discharge (14).

D. Objective Measurements That Assess Severity

1. *Pulmonary Function Tests*

Pulmonary function tests (PFTs) are integral in defining the presence and baseline degree of airway obstruction in asthmatic patients. Airway responsiveness (bronchial challenge) maneuvers and other PFTs such as absolute lung volumes and airways resistance can only be obtained by large, expensive equipment, clearly unsuitable in the ED setting (22). Spirometric measures usually include forced expiratory volume in 1 sec (FEV_1), forced vital capacity (FVC), forced expiratory flow between 25% and 75% of FVC (FEF_{25-75}), and the ratio of FEV_1/FVC. These are relatively easy to perform, the equipment is available at a reasonable cost, and test interpretation is standardized (22). Ambulatory monitoring of airway obstruction can be performed with hand-held inexpensive spirometers and with PEF meters, which are widely available and therefore amenable for use in the ED (22).

PFTs are the best measurement of the degree of airway obstruction and should be measured whenever possible (23). Failure to perform routine spirometry in children results in underdiagnosis of airflow obstruction and may even result in failure to optimize therapy (24). Adult studies have shown that physicians tend to underestimate the degree of airway obstruction in acute asthma, especially when a patient is initially assessed, and that knowing the results of PFT may change management in a significant number of patients (25). Inaccurate assessment of asthma severity of patients by parents can be a major reason to delay seeking care and is linked to increased morbidity and mortality (26).

The National Asthma Education and Prevention Program (NAEPP) Guidelines developed by an expert panel recommends the routine use of objective measures of pulmonary function in the ED management of acute asthma for both children and adults (23). For a variety of reasons, it may be more difficult for emergency physicians to comply with this standard in the case of children. As discussed, clinical assessment is more difficult because of a wide variation in verbal and developmental skills. In the case of PEF, the breathing maneuver is strenuous and often requires effort that cannot be mounted during an acute period of dyspnea (22). Submaximal efforts may create falsely low readings and there may be wide variability between readings (22). For both spirometry and PEF measurements, younger children may not be able to perform the maneuver in a coordinated fashion without intensive prior training. The utility of teaching the maneuver in the ED under circumstances of increased anxiety and breathlessness is questionable. Despite these obstacles, emergency physicians should attempt to perform objective measures of lung function on all children greater than the age of 5 who present with acute asthma and on younger children who have been trained in the maneuver or who seem sophisticated and amenable to performing the tests. In general PFTs can be performed reliably by most children by 5 or 6 years of age (27).

The most valuable of all PFT for assessing severity, response to treatment, and for formulating patient dispositions are FEV_1, PEF, and FEF_{25-75} (28). FEV_1 is the most reproducible airway function parameter. It varies inversely with airflow obstruction and is more sensitive than examination of the lungs, symptoms felt by the patient, or clinical signs noted by health care workers (22). Similar to FEV_1, PEF reflects changes in the degree of upper, larger airways obstruction and is the most common form of ambulatory monitoring available due to low cost, which makes it ideal for use in the ED (22). Disadvantages of using PEF to assess acute asthmatics is that it is effort dependent. Results may show high variability, but it is helpful in most cases when making therapeutic decisions.

Normal FEV_1 and PEF values do not always indicate that all other PFTs are normal (26,29–31). Results from several recent investigations in children with asthma have shown that FEF_{25-75} is the most sensitive and specific measure of airway obstruction (26,31). FEF_{25-75} reflects the function of both large and small airways. In some patients reduction in FEF_{25-75} occurred when PEF and FEV_1 were still within normal range and the patients were experiencing symptoms of acute asthma (26). In the future, devices that measure FEF_{25-75} may be more readily available for routine use in the ED.

ED personnel should follow the NAEPP Guidelines for the Diagnosis and Management of Asthma regarding the use of objective lung function measurements. For acute exacerbations, PEF should be measured on all patients greater than 5 years of age initially upon presentation or after initial bronchodilator treatment to gauge response, and before discharge from the ED. Patients should be questioned about prior training and home use of PEF monitors to ascertain their ''personal best.'' If personal best is not known, percent predicted PEF for age, height, and race may be obtained from charts like the one illustrated in Table 1. General guidelines for PEF values are: PEF $\geq$ 70% predicted, disease is stable

Table 1 Predicted Peak Expiratory Flow Rates (L/min) in Children Based on Sex and Height

Height (cm)	Female	Male
110	145	145
115	157	160
120	170	175
125	184	191
130	199	208
135	216	226
140	234	247
145	253	269
150	274	293
155	296	319
160	321	348
165	347	379
170	376	414
175	407	451
180	441	491

Source: Adapted from Ref. 45.

with good response to bronchodilator; PEF $\geq$ 50% but $<$ 70% predicted, incomplete response to bronchodilator, consider hospitalization; and PEF $<$ 50% predicted, poor response to bronchodilator, hospitalization required, consider intensive care setting (23).

2. *Pulse Oximetry*

Due to its ease of use and noninvasive properties, pulse oximetry for measurement of arterial oxygen saturation (O_2sat) is routinely used in many EDs to help evaluate the severity of an asthma exacerbation (32,33). Several studies have examined the usefulness of pulse oximetry as a predictor of outcome. Geelhoed et al. found that the initial O_2sat was highly predictive of outcome in 52 asthmatic patients ages 2–14. O_2sat $<$ 91% was associated with an unfavorable outcome defined as admission or need for re-presentation to the ED (34). In a similar study of 100 pediatric asthma patients in an ED, Bishop and Nolan showed that pretreatment O_2sat of $<$ 91% had a sensitivity of only 36% and specificity of 57% for an unfavorable outcome (35). The sensitivity and specificity improved to 42% and 78%, respectively, when measured after bronchodilator treatment; however, the positive and negative predictive values calculated for admission were only 75% and 46%, respectively. The authors emphasize that a high negative predictive value is desirable to minimize the risk of discharging patients inappropriately from the ED. They conclude, however, that pulse oximetry is still a useful diagnostic tool due to its high specificity and should be used in conjunction with other diagnostic tests that have high sensitivity (35).

Geelhoed et al. in a later study examined how O_2sat compared with PEF as an indicator of asthma severity and a predictor of relapse after ED treatment (36). O_2sat and PEF were measured in 110 children on arrival by the investigators, while independent disposition decisions were made by treating physicians who only had access to PEF values.

Seventy-nine children were discharged home and 15 of those subsequently needed more medical care. Thirty-one children were hospitalized. O_2sat and PEF were lower in admitted patients. There was no statistical difference in the PEF between those who were discharged and subsequently required more care versus those who were simply discharged; however, initial O_2sat was found to be lower in children who were discharged and required more care. The authors concluded that PEF was less discriminating than O_2sat and that O_2sat had a greater potential to predict outcome in those not admitted (36).

Geelhoed et al. hypothesized that O_2sat may be superior to PEF for several reasons: hypoxia may impair a child's ability to perform a PEF; O_2sat has a normal range of values that applies to all ages whereas PEF is variable; and O_2sat may be a more accurate reflection of the multiple pathologic processes that occur in asthma resulting in ventilation-perfusion inequality, while PEF predominantly reflects only major airway obstruction (36).

Despite the advantages of providing continuous, noninvasive monitoring of arterial oxygen saturation, limitations of pulse oximetry must be recognized by ED personnel. Pulse oximetry provides no information about the adequacy of ventilation and may not be accurate when the oxygen carrying capacity of blood is decreased or during hyperventilation when O_2sat is increased by a shift in the hemoglobin-oxygen dissociation curve to the left. In addition, low perfusion states such as shock will not allow detection of the pulse signal and therefore will not provide accurate readings (10).

3. Pulsus Paradoxus

In adult asthmatics, pulsus paradoxus (PP), or an exaggeration of the normal fall in systolic blood pressure during inspiration, is thought to relate to the severity of the attack, and it has been recommended that the measurement be routinely sought (37,38). Since large swings in intrathoracic pressure are thought to be responsible for PP, investigators have noted that some severely ill patients may not be able to generate these pressures and may not demonstrate a PP (39). Pearson et al. in a study of 766 adult asthmatics reported only a weak association between worsening airflow obstruction and PP. One-third of patients with PEF less than 200 L/min did not manifest the sign (39). They concluded that PP is a poor guide to asthma severity in individual patients and noted that in a busy ED it is not easy to perform and interpret the maneuver (39).

Measuring PP in children is difficult and also shows a weak association with airflow obstruction and asthma severity. In one study of 40 asthmatic children, those with PP of greater than 25 mmHg tended to have higher $Paco_2$ values, but this association did not reach statistical significance (40). In another study of 111 asthmatic children, only 63–76% of children were able to be assessed for PP, and the authors state that the maneuver was distressing to young children and even interfered with further assessment and treatment (33). In routine ED practice, PP is not often attempted in children and does not often contribute to management decisions.

4. Arterial Blood Gases

Routine measurement of arterial blood gases (ABGs) in all asthmatic children who present to an ED with an exacerbation is not necessary. The test is invasive and painful. In the majority of cases of mild to moderate exacerbations, clinical assessment, PFT, and oximetry are sufficient to determine severity, although there is at least one study indicating that ABG was the only satisfactory method for assessing severity in asthmatic children with all but the "slightest" attacks (40).

ABGs are often performed in children who fail to respond to therapy in the ED or develop signs of increased work of breathing, impending respiratory failure, or decreasing PEF. The most common pattern seen on the ABG is hypoxemia, hypocapnia, and respiratory alkalosis (37). Normal or elevated $Paco_2$ indicates progression to respiratory failure. There is some evidence that children are more prone to develop failure at a lower $Paco_2$ value as the transition from alveolar hyperventilation to hypoventilation occurs at a slightly lower value than in adults (37 vs. 40 torr) (41). Since a decision to intubate an asthmatic child should always be made on clinical grounds, ABGs are often unnecessary and only provide superfluous information.

5. *Chest Radiograph*

A chest X-ray is seldom helpful in either the assessment of severity of an acute exacerbation or in determining outcome. Therefore, a chest X-ray should be reserved for those patients who do not improve as expected with treatment or in whom complications such as pneumothorax, other barotrauma, or bacterial pneumonia are suspected.

IV. DISPOSITION FROM THE ED

There are no absolute criteria dictating which pediatric asthma patients require hospitalization for continued treatment and which patients may be safely treated at home without the risk of relapse. However, there are a number of suggested guidelines that can assist emergency physicians in making sound disposition decisions, limiting the number of inappropriate hospitalizations and discharges.

The NAEPP Guidelines for the Diagnosis and Management of Asthma suggest initial assessment of severity in a child and initial treatment with nebulized albuterol (23). Depending on the response to this treatment a number of pathways may be followed (Figure 1). The treatment algorithm depends heavily on serial assessment of clinical parameters and repeated measurements of PEF and O_2sat. Supplemental oxygen is given to keep $O_2\text{sat} \geq 90\%$. Steroid therapy is initiated for all patients except those with the mildest exacerbations who have an excellent response to the initial inhaled bronchodilator or for those that recently took systemic steroids at home (23). A poor response is defined by a $\text{PEF} < 50\%$ of predicted along with other worrisome clinical parameters and is grounds for an immediate decision to admit (23).

These are sound guidelines developed by an expert panel. They are evidenced based, where possible, and should be followed whenever possible. Other countries with high asthma prevalence and high hospitalization rates have developed similar guidelines (42). The NAEPP Guidelines are probably the most well known and frequently used guidelines for ED treatment and decision making although they are still not used in all EDs for a variety of reasons (43). Clinical judgment, not objective measurements, is the basis for a large number of disposition decisions in younger children; in these instances the guidelines are often not used. In addition, there may be regional, local, or institutional variations in admission practice that will result in various interpretations of the guidelines.

Many authors have offered suggested criteria for hospitalization of a pediatric asthma patient, although not necessarily linked to a treatment-response algorithm like that found in the NAEPP Guidelines (11,44–46). These criteria are listed in Table 2. All or some of these factors may be useful to emergency physicians for decision making and will be individually applied to patients in different situations. With the increasing number of asthma short-stay observation units being created, these criteria will have to undergo

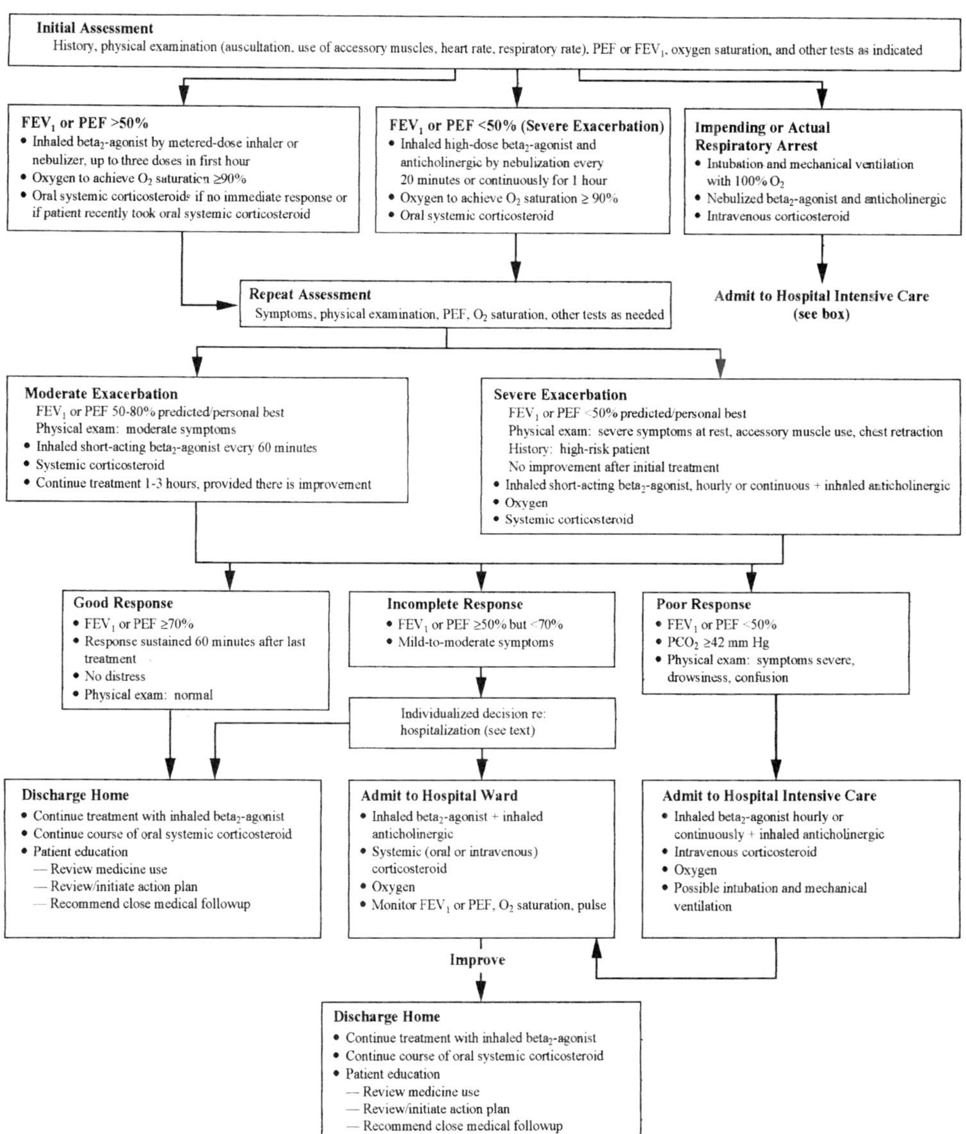

Figure 1 Algorithm for ED management of acute asthma exacerbations. (From Expert panel report 2, Guidelines for the diagnosis and management of asthma 1997. Clinical practice guidelines. NIH publication #4051. U.S. Department of Health and Human Services, NHLBI, National Asthma Education and Prevention Program, Bethesda, MD; Ref. 23.)

Table 2 Suggested Criteria for Hospitalization of a Pediatric Asthma Patient

Respiratory failure (Pa_{O_2}, 60 mmHg in 40% oxygen, $Pa_{CO_2} > 40$ mmHg)[a]
Severe respiratory distress with impending respiratory failure[a]
Alteration in consciousness[a]
Severe retractions
Hypotension[a]
Poor social situation
Prior hospitalization for respiratory failure
Past history of life-threatening asthma or near fatal asthma
Significant complications of asthma
Pneumothorax
Pneumonia
Extrapleural air
Theophylline toxicity
Cardiac arrhythmia
Previous ED treatment within last 24 hr
Inability to tolerate oral medications
Significant other diseases
Congenital heart disease
Bronchopulmonary dysplasia
Cystic fibrosis
Immunosuppression
Psychiatric disease

[a] Should be strongly considered for admission to an intensive care unit.

further refinement to accommodate a new subset of patients who can benefit safely from shorter inpatient treatment.

V. RELAPSE FROM THE ED

A. Predictors of Relapse

Studies have indicated that between 4 and 30% of children with an acute asthma exacerbation treated in an acute care setting will return for an unscheduled medical visit within 10 days following this treatment (5,44). These relapse visits may be viewed as treatment or disposition ''failures'' and there are often multiple factors that influence the rate of relapse in any given institution or geographical area. As previously discussed in this chapter, attempts to predict the outcome of a visit for acute asthma by assessing or scoring asthma severity have been unsuccessful to date.

Some investigators have tried to improve the prediction of relapse by looking at historical or sociodemographic variables in addition to variables present at the time of the exacerbation. Ducharme and Kramer in a prospective study of 314 acutely ill asthmatic children discharged from an ED collected information on multiple variables and found that a number were significantly associated with relapse (5). Relapse was defined as a second ED visit for asthma within 10 days of the first (5). The two most significant predictors of relapse that emerged were the number of ED visits for acute asthma in the past year, which seemed to have a dose-response effect, and the use of short-acting theophylline as part of the ED treatment regimen, although the latter was done at the discretion of the treating physician and should be interpreted with caution (5).

This study also found that the severity of the attack and the response to treatment were not important determinants of relapse (5). The authors concluded that a child's past medical history may be more important than the severity of the attack or the response to treatment and suggest that the frequency of ED visits be used as a stratifying variable in future studies of relapse (5). It may be prudent to explore these variables in the ED setting as well when evaluating young children since objective measures of severity are not always obtainable.

B. Follow-Up and Patient Education

Other suggested methods for reducing relapse after ED care are timely and coordinated referral for follow-up and simplification of asthma management plans. Emergency physicians should strive to view the exacerbation as part of the patient's overall management and facilitate communication between themselves, the patient, and their primary care providers (47). Many patients, particularly those who are economically disadvantaged, may depend on the ED as a routine source of asthma care. Efforts should be made to do some asthma management education in the ED and to make the follow-up process as simple as possible (47). Although referral to the primary care pediatrician is indicated in most instances, some authors have demonstrated that facilitated referral to an asthma specialist at the time of an exacerbation reduces relapses and return ED visits (48).

C. Corticosteroids and Relapse

Scarfone et al. have demonstrated that the administration of oral corticosteroids to children in the ED reduces the need for subsequent hospitalization when assessed within 4 hr of treatment (4). It is possible that oral corticosteroids are the most useful intervention by the ED physician in terms of preventing relapse, but this has not been conclusively proven. Chapman et al. followed 93 adults with acute asthma randomized to receive either prednisone or placebo at discharge from the ED and for 8 days afterwards to determine relapse within 21 days. The risk of relapse was significantly lower in the placebo group especially within the first half of the follow-up interval (49).

Shapiro et al. demonstrated rapid improvement in children with acute asthma after ED administration of steroids versus a group who had been treated with placebo. No relapses occurred in either the treatment or placebo group, indicating that study subjects may have had fairly mild disease exacerbations (50). A few additional studies in children have demonstrated protection against relapse by treatment with short courses of corticosteroids (51). One study compared intravenous methylprednisolone to placebo and showed a protective benefit of treatment in reducing relapse over the next 4-week period (52). Additional well-controlled studies are needed in the pediatric population to delineate the true effect of steroids on preventing relapse and to define the optimal dose, route, frequency, and duration of corticosteroid therapy.

REFERENCES

1. Brugman SM, Larsen GL. Asthma in infants and small children. Clin Chest Med 1995; 16(4): 637–656.
2. Bloomberg GR, Strunk RC. Crisis in asthma care. Pediatr Clin N Am 1992; 39(6):1225–1241.

3. Gergen PJ, Weiss KB. Changing patterns in asthma hospitalization among children: 1979 to 1987. JAMA 1990; 264(13):1688–1692.
4. Scarfone RJ, Fuchs SM, Nager AL, et al. Controlled trial of oral prednisone I in the emergency department treatment of children with acute asthma. Pediatrics 1993; 92:513–518.
5. Ducharme EM, Kramer MS. Relapse following emergency treatment for acute asthma: Can it be predicted or prevented? J Clin Epidemiol 1993; 46(12):1395–1402.
6. Infante-Rivard C, Sukia SE, Roberge D, et al. The changing frequency of childhood asthma. J Asthma 1987; 24(5):283–288.
7. Mitchell EA, Burr D. Comparison of the characteristics of children with multiple admissions to hospital for asthma with those with a single admission. N Z Med J Med 1987; 100:736–738.
8. Mitchell EA, Dawson KP. Why are hospital admissions of children with acute asthma increasing? Eur Respir J 1989; 2:470–472.
9. Bishop J, Carlin J, Nolan T. Evaluation of the properties and reliability of a clinical severity scale for acute asthma in children. J Clin Epidemiol 1992; 45(1):71–76.
10. Baren JM, Seidel JS. Emergency management of respiratory distress and failure, In: RM Barkin, ed., Pediatric Emergency Medicine Concepts and Clinical Practice, 1997, 95–105.
11. Gern JE, Scroth MK, Lemanske RF. Childhood asthma in older children and adolescents. Clin Chest Med 1995; 16(4):657–670.
12. Martin AJ, Campbell DA, Gluyas PA, et al. Characteristics of near-fatal asthma in childhood. Pediatr Pulmonol 1995; 20:1–8.
13. de Blic J, Thomson A. Short-term clinical measurement: acute severe episodes. Eur Respir J 1996; 9(521):4s–7s.
14. van der Windt DAWM, Nagelkerke AF, Bouter LM, et al. Clinical scores for acute asthma in pre-school children: A review of the literature. J Clin Epidemiol 1994; 47(6):635–646.
15. Kesten S, Maleki-Yazdi R, Sanders BR, et al. Respiratory rate during acute asthma. Chest 1990; 97:58–62.
16. Tanaka T, Shimazaki T, Kusakawa I, et al. Analysis of breathing pattern in children with asthma. Acta Paediatr Jpn 1990; 32:365–372.
17. Baughman RP, Loudon RG. Quantitation of wheezing in acute asthma. Chest 1984; 86:718–722.
18. Commey JO, Levison H. Physical signs in childhood asthma. Pediatrics 1976; 58:537–541.
19. Galant SP, Groncy CE, Shaw KC. The value of pulsus paradoxus in assessing the child with status asthmaticus. Pediatrics 1978; 61:46–51.
20. O'Connor GT, Weiss ST. Clinical symptom measures. Am J Respir Crit Care Med 1994; 149: S21–S28.
21. Kerem E, Canny G, Tibshirani R, et al. Clinical physiologic correlations in acute asthma of childhood. Pediatrics 1991; 87:481–486.
22. Enright PL, Lebowitz MD, Cockroft DW. Physiologic measures: pulmonary function tests. Asthma outcome. Am J Respir Crit Care Med 1994; 149:S9–S18.
23. Expert Panel Report 2: Guidelines for the diagnosis and management of asthma, Clinical practice guidelines, NIH publication #4051, U.S. Department of Health and Human Services, NHLBI, National Asthma Education and Prevention Program, Bethesda, MD, 1997.
24. Bye MR, Kerstein D, Barsh E. The importance of spirometry in the assessment of childhood asthma. Am J Dis Child 1992; 146:977–978.
25. Emerman CD, Cydulka RK. Effect of pulmonary function testing on the management of acute asthma. Arch Intern Med 1995; 155:2255–2228.
26. Klein RB, Fritz GK, Young A, et al. Spirometric patterns in childhood asthma: peak flow compared with other indices. Pediatr Pulmonol 1995; 20:372–379.
27. Mueller GA, Eigen H. Pediatric pulmonary function testing in asthma. Pediatr Clin N Am 1992; 39:(6)1243–1258.
28. Pederson S, Management of acute asthma in children, In: Byrne PO and Thomson NC, eds., Manual of Asthma Management, 1995, 511–541.

29. Sly PD, Cahill P, Willet K, et al. Accuracy of mini peak flow meters in indicating changes in lung function in children with asthma. Br Med J 1994; 308:572–574.
30. Perin PV, Weldon D, McGeady SJ. Respiratory pathophysiologic responses. Objective indicators of severity of asthma. J Allergy Clin Immunol 1994; 94:517–522.
31. Lebecque P, Kiakulanda P, Coates AL. Spirometry in the asthmatic child: Is FEF_{25-75} a more sensitive test than FEV_1/FVC. Pediatr Pulmonol 1993; 16:19–22.
32. Yamamoto LG, Wiebe RA, Anaya C, et al. Pulse oximetry and peak flow as indicators of wheezing severity in children and improvement following bronchodilator treatments. Am J Emerg Med 1992; 10:519–524.
33. Connett GJ, Lenney W. Use of pulse oximetry in the hospital management of acute asthma in childhood. Pediatr Pulmonol 1993; 15:345–349.
34. Geelhoed GC, Landau LI, LeSouef PN. Predictive value of oxygen saturation in emergency evaluation of asthmatic children. Br Med J 1988; 297(6645):395–396.
35. Bishop J, Nolan T. Pulse oximetry in acute asthma. Arch Dis Child 1991; 66(6):724–725.
36. Geelhoed GC, Landau LI, LeSouef PN. Oximetry and peak expiratory flow in assessment of acute childhood asthma. J Pediatr 1990; 117(16):907–909.
37. McFadden ER. Management of patients with acute asthma: What do we know? What do we need to know? Ann Allergy 1994; 72:385–388.
38. Mountain RD, Sahn SA. Clinical features and outcome in patients with acute asthma presenting with hypercapnia. Am Rev Respir Dis 1988; 138:535–539.
39. Pearson MG, Spence DP, Ryland I, et al. Value of pulsus paradoxus in assessing acute severe asthma. Br Med J 1993; 307(6905):659.
40. McKenzie SA, Edmunds AT, Godfrey S. Status asthmaticus in children. Arch Dis Child 1979; 54:581–586.
41. Moler FW, Hurwitz ME, Custer JR. Improvement in clinical asthma score and $Paco_2$ in children with severe asthma treated with continuously nebulized terbutaline. J Allergy Clin Immunol 1988; 81:1101–1109.
42. International consensus report on diagnosis and treatment of asthma, National Institute of Health, NIH publication #92-3091, U.S. Department of Health and Human Services, Bethesda, MD, 1992.
43. Crain EF, Weiss KB, Fagan MJ. Pediatric asthma care in US emergency departments: Clinical practice in the context of the National Institute of Health Guidelines. Arch Pediatr Adcl Med 1995; 149(8):893–901.
44. McWilliams B, Kelly HW, Murphy S. Management of acute severe asthma. Pediatr Ann 1989; 18(12):774–783.
45. Letourneau MA, Schuh S, Gausche M. Respiratory disorders, In: Barkin RM, ed., Pediatric Emergency Medicine Concepts and Clinical Practice, 1997; 1078–1088.
46. Kulick RK, Ruddy RM. Allergic emergencies, In: Fleisher GR and Ludwig S, eds., Textbook of Pediatric Emergency Medicine, 3rd Ed., Fleisher GR, Ludwig S, eds., 1993; 858–867.
47. Garrett J. Hospital practice, In: Byrne PO and Thomson NC, eds., Manual of Asthma Management, 1995; 791–804.
48. Zeiger RS, Heller S, Mellon MH, et al. Facilitated referral to asthma specialist reduces relapses in asthma emergency room visits. J Allergy Clin Immunol 1991; 87:1160–1168.
49. Chapman KR, Verbeek PR, White JG, et al. Effect of a short course of prednisone in the prevention of early relapse after the emergency room treatment of acute asthma. New Engl J Med 1991; 324:788–794.
50. Shapiro GG, Furukawa CT, Pierson WE, et al. Double-blind evaluation of methylprednisolone versus placebo for acute asthma episodes. Pediatrics 1983; 71:510–514.
51. Engel T, Heinig JH. Glucocorticosteroid therapy in acute severe asthma—a critical review. Eur Respir J 1991; 4:881–889.
52. Younger RE, Gerber PS, Herrod HG, et al. Intravenous methylprednisolone efficacy in status asthmaticus of childhood. Pediatrics 1987; 80:225–230.

33

Asthma and Emergency Department Observation Units

Eric S. Nadel
Harvard Medical School and Brigham and Women's Hospital, Boston, Massachusetts

Louis G. Graff
University of Connecticut School of Medicine, Farmington, Connecticut

Michael F. McDermott
Cook County Hospital, Chicago, Illinois

I. THERAPY OF EMERGENT CONDITIONS IN THE EMERGENCY DEPARTMENT

Emergency departments (EDs) provide treatment to patients with emergent conditions such as asthma. Traditionally, 60–80% of asthma patients can be successfully treated in the first 3–4 hr (1–4). When initial therapy does not successfully resolve the asthma exacerbation, the patient is admitted to the hospital. With the use of an observation unit, the treatment regimen initiated in the ED can be extended. With an additional 8 hr of treatment the physician can avoid hospitalization in 80% of patients who would otherwise need hospitalization (5,6). Presently 53% of funds used for the care of asthmatic patients is for hospitalization during acute attacks. A more robust outpatient approach to the treatment of the asthmatic patient with the use of observation units can dramatically lower the overall true cost of services for this common serious condition.

II. OBSERVATION UNITS AND DECISIONS TO ADMIT

Patients are admitted to the acute care hospital from the ED when the patients' needs cannot be met by the ED visit. Most medical patients come to the ED for the evaluation of a critical diagnostic syndrome: chest pain, abdominal pain, syncope. They are admitted to the hospital when a serious disease is identified: acute myocardial infarction in patients with chest pain, appendicitis in patients with abdominal pain. Other patients come to the

ED for treatment of an emergent condition: asthma, congestive heart failure, hyperglycemia. They are admitted if they have not been sufficiently treated during their 2- to 3-hr ED stay.

There is a certain inexactness to the decision process on hospitalization. Often the physician makes a decision to admit a patient based on clinical suspicion of serious disease or projection that treatment may be extensive. ''Cookbook'' lists of criteria for hospital admission have been promulgated by payers to limit their need to pay for inpatient services but can not be relied upon by the clinician. They have only 60–80% sensitivity, and 80–90% specificity for identifying serious disease (7).

Observation units enlarge the time window the emergency physician has for evaluation and treatment of patients. For patients being evaluated for a diagnostic syndrome, this allows the emergency physician added time to more fully evaluate the patient and avoid failing to diagnose patients with an atypical presentation of a serious disease. In chest pain evaluation the period of observation nearly eliminates the usual 5% miss rate of acute myocardial infarction (CHEPER study) (8). In addition, many patients with symptoms that are worrisome to the physician can avoid a hospital admission with a period of observation. Twenty-five percent of patients with chest pain who would otherwise have needed hospital admission can be safely released home without hospital admission with reassurance that they have been rigorously and fully evaluated (8). In patients being treated for emergent conditions, this allows the emergency physician added time to further treat the patient's condition and avoid having to admit many patients who need 6–12 hr of additional treatment. As will be discussed below, one-third of asthma patients are not successfully treated in a 3- to 4-hr ED visit and are admitted to the hospital. With an observation unit, ED treatment is continued and 80% of patients who would otherwise have needed hospitalization can be discharged (5,6). The goal is to provide patient service based on what is ideal given the pathophysiology of the patient's disease and not based on what is required to meet the financial architecture, physician comfort, or even patient expectations.

III. OBSERVATION UNIT SERVICES

Many emergency physician groups around the world have developed observation units. In the United States, the American College of Emergency Physicians (ACEP) developed standards on ''Management of Observation Units'' in 1988 and a revision of those standards in 1995 (9). Three textbooks are available from ACEP to aid emergency physicians in providing these services: *Observation Medicine* (10) evaluates the scientific basis for the provision of observation services, *Observation Units: Implementation and Management Strategies* (11) describes how to develop and manage an observation unit, and *Emergency Department Design* (12) reviews how to design an observation unit. EDs providing observation services require a physical facility, staff to provide the services, management to organize and administer the services, protocols and continuous quality improvement to ensure the value of the service, and a billing structure to fund the service.

The design of the physical facility for the observation unit depends upon the quantity and types of services. Some observation units only offer nonmonitored services, such as treatment of asthma and evaluation of patients with abdominal pain. Other observation units have electrocardiographic monitors and off-monitored services such as treatment of patients with congestive heart failure and evaluation of patients with chest pain. A rough estimate, based on expert opinions, of the number of beds is 1–2 beds per 10,000 visits per year for monitored services and 1–2 beds per 10,000 visits per year for nonmonitored services (11). Thus an ED with 40,000 visits per year would need an observation unit with between 8 and 16 beds if it offered all types of services that are appropriate for an observation unit.

Adequate staff must be available to ensure appropriate services are provided. The average observation patient requires 2.5 times the amount of services that are required by the average ED patient (13). The amount of nursing services tends to follow the level of intensity of services provided. Nonmonitored services (asthma treatment, abdominal pain evaluation) require a 1:8 or 1:12 nurse-to-patient ratio, similar to services provided on hospital floors. Monitored services (chest pain evaluation, congestive heart failure treatment) require a 1:4 nurse-to-patient ratio, similar to services provided on a telemetry floor. Most ED observation units utilize emergency nurses, and the observation unit could be one of many possible assignments for the nurses each shift. Cross-training and flexibility is the key to observation services as in all aspects of emergency medicine.

Management must be selected to organize and administer the services. The observation unit brings a new level of complexity to the ED, the hospital, and the organization of the local health care system. Properly managed, the creation of this third disposition pathway enables the ED to function as the hub of the health system. Not properly managed, the observation unit becomes a ''dumping ground'' where decisions and treatments are delayed, and the health care system fails to effectively and efficiently provide high-quality services. Documentation requirements increase as the complexity of interactions increase between different health care professionals.

Mandatory for the structuring of any observation unit's functioning is the delineation of the ''line of authority.'' It needs to be clear at all times for all patients which physician is responsible for the patient's care. Multiple physicians may be involved in the care of a patient, e.g., an asthmatic patient with an emergency physician, a private internist, a resident physician, and a pulmonary physician. Yet one physician must be clearly identified for each patient as the one responsible. That physician is responsible that services are provided appropriately and that a correct disposition is made in a timely manner.

The development and implementation of clinical protocols and a continuous quality improvement process are essential. There needs to be clear inclusion and exclusion criteria for which patient is appropriate for services in the observation unit. The health care institution comes to a consensus on standards for how those services should be provided. A continuous quality improvement (CQI) model is used for surveillance and intervention as needed. If high utilization of steroids in asthma patients is the best practice and the CQI monitoring shows less than ideal utilization, then the CQI team/committee works to identify the roadblocks to ideal care. If the standard is that 80% of asthmatic patients treated in an observation unit can be discharged home and the department's own monitoring shows 40% of observation unit asthmatic patients are being admitted to the hospital, then the CQI team/committee works to identify the problem. This is similar to the management of an ED but with added complexity given the increased length of stay and the increased number of personnel involved in the care of each patient.

A billing structure for the observation unit is necessary to fund the services provided in the observation unit. A facility fee is charged for the observation unit service. This is usually proportional to the level of services provided (monitored vs. nonmonitored service). A physician fee is charged for the physician service. There are two sets of CPT 4 codes for physician services to observation patients (11). Which set of codes the physician uses depends on whether the observation services are provided all on the same date or provided over two different dates. In some parts of the country the provider negotiates with the payer contractors to provide the service based on per diem, on case rates, or on capitated contract. The true costs are lower than providing these services on an inpatient basis, so the payer can negotiate lower expenses than if the service was provided as an inpatient while the provider can still remain financially viable.

IV. STUDIES ON THE USE OF OBSERVATION UNITS FOR ASTHMATIC PATIENTS

Although observation units are commonly used to treat patients with asthma, there is limited literature that describes the medical and cost effectiveness of this approach. In an era focused on cost containment, emergency physicians are challenged to reduce hospital admission rates while maintaining quality of care. One method that may reduce costs without sacrificing quality of care is the development of ED observation units. Asthmatic patients are transferred to these units when they are not appropriate for ED discharge and a brief course of continued therapy might avoid inpatient admission.

At the University of North Carolina, Zwicke et al. (1) performed a retrospective analysis of 46 asthmatics treated in the ED over a 4-month period. Patients were either treated and released, admitted to the observation unit, or admitted to the inpatient service. Initial disposition and final disposition were determined, including rate of relapse. Clinical variables (demographic, historical, physiological, treatment) were assessed in order to evaluate appropriate candidates for ED discharge, observation unit admission, and inpatient admission. Marked overlap was seen when these clinical variables were evaluated. Analyses of these variables could not predict which observation unit patients would require admission and which observation unit patients would be stable for discharge.

The authors suggest that observation units might prevent admission of patients to an inpatient unit. These patients would be admitted if an observation unit were unavailable. They also recognize that there is a group of patients who might have been discharged from the ED if an observation unit were unavailable, and that these patients may have done well at home. The effect on hospitalization rates cannot be determined from the data. However, relapse rates within 10 days were determined and found to be 41% relapse among patients initially discharged, while the relapse rate from the observation unit was only 4%. This high relapse rate is likely statistical variance from a small sample size. The authors appropriately raise the question of whether overutilization of an observation unit is preferred over ED relapse.

Brillman and Tandberg (14) evaluated the impact of the opening of an observation unit (OU) on admission rates and charges in asthmatic patients. The retrospective comparative cohort study evaluated 834 asthmatic patients seen in the 14 months prior to opening an observation unit and 390 asthmatic patients treated after the opening of the OU. The decision to admit a patient to the observation unit was at the discretion of the attending physician and the house staff and based on the following general criteria: the patient was likely to require 3–18 hr of additional care; the patient had received a thorough ED evaluation and trial of therapy usually including steroids and nebulized β-agonists; and the need for vital sign measurement was no more than every 2 hr. There were no strict entrance criteria into the OU [i.e., peak expiratory flow rate (PEFR)]. Outcome measures were admission and discharge rates from the ED and OU, and measurement of charges of the admitted patients in both groups.

There were 47 patients admitted to the OU during the postobservation period. As a result of an alternative site for disposition, direct admissions of all asthmatics to the inpatient service decreased 5.3% ($p = 0.01$), and discharges directly from the ED decreased 6.7% ($p = 0.005$). Of the 47 patients admitted to the OU, 10 patients (21%) were later admitted to the inpatient service. The decline in the total admission rate of 16.1% in the preobservation group to 13.4% in the postobservation group was not statistically significant. Charges were measured only for admitted patients in the preobservation and postobservation groups and were not significantly different.

There were several limitations of the study. The study does not compare overall charges of the preobservation group to the postobservation group. Comparison of only admitted patients has limited value in determining potential cost savings of an observation unit. Data on measurement of severity, ED length of stay, and overall length of stay in both groups were not available. Patients seen in the ED prior to the opening of the observation unit may have had prolonged length of stay prior to disposition. Follow up data including relapse rates were unavailable. However, the study raises legitimate concerns about whether some patients are admitted to an observation unit who might otherwise have been safely discharged if an observation unit were not available.

The most comprehensive study thus far on the utility of ED observation units in the treatment of asthma has been published by McDermott et al. (5). A study at Cook County Hospital and the University of Illinois Hospital enrolled 222 asthmatic patients unable to be discharged from the ED. Patients were randomized to an emergency diagnostic and treatment unit (EDTU) or inpatient admission on the medical service. The objective of the study was the evaluation of the medical and cost effectiveness, assessment of patient satisfaction, and quality of life in an EDTU compared to an inpatient facility. Patients aged 18–55 were enrolled in the study if they were unable to be discharged after 3 hr of ED evaluation and treatment. In the first 3 hr in the ED, patients received oral or intravenous steroids within the first hour and 3 or more treatments of nebulized albuterol. After 3 hr patients were discharged if the expected PEFR was 50% of predicted. High-risk patients were discharged if the PEFR was 60% of predicted. High-risk patients were defined as patients with a short-term relapse, ICU admission, endotracheal intubation, hospitalization in the past year, three or more ED visits within 6 months, or use of oral steroids for more than half of the prior year. Exclusion criteria included $Paco_2 > 45$ mmHg, $Pao_2 < 55$ mmHg, PEFR of 80 L/min after one treatment, 10 pack-years smoking history, pregnancy, pneumonia, or history of congestive heart failure or restrictive lung disease.

Eligible patients were randomized to the EDTU or to the inpatient medical service. Patients were discharged from the EDTU when the above-mentioned discharge criteria were met. At the end of a 9-hr EDTU course, if patients were not able to be discharged based on PEFR criteria, patients would be admitted to the medical service. For all patients admitted to the medical service, patient discharge was at the discretion of the medical service and based on national guidelines (15).

Patients had medical follow-up appointments at 1 and 8 weeks. Patients had telephone follow-up at 3, 5, and 7 weeks. Follow-up encounters measured symptoms of cough, wheezing, dyspnea, nocturnal awakenings, lifestyle limiting events, and unscheduled visits for asthma treatment. Outcome measures included discharge rate from the EDTU, total length of hospital stay, relapse rates, days missed form work or school, days incapacitated, symptom free days and nights, nocturnal awakenings, patient satisfaction, and quality of life.

Of those patients admitted to the EDTU, 59% were discharged to home with an average length of stay of 8.8 hr. Among the inpatient group average length of stay was 59 hr. Of interest is that 41% of patients required admission, and these patients had an average length of stay of 77 hr. There was no difference in the relapse rates between the EDTU and inpatient groups over 8 weeks, and no deaths were reported. There was no significant difference between the EDTU and inpatient groups when comparing nocturnal awakening, rates of missing work or school, days incapacitated, or frequency of mild symptoms.

Analysis of cost difference between the two groups revealed a mean cost per patient of $1,202 for the EDTU group, which includes discharges and subsequent admission, vs. $2,247 for the inpatient group. Assessment of quality of life and patient satisfaction at 1 week follow-up revealed significantly better outcomes in the EDTU group.

McDermott et al. conclude that the majority of patients admitted to an EDTU are able to be discharged and avoid inpatient admission. Observation unit patients had no increase in relapse rates and no increase in morbidity. The use of a system that includes an observation unit can reduce overall cost and improve patient satisfaction and quality of life.

V. PEDIATRIC OBSERVATION UNITS

Three studies have been published on the use of observation units for pediatric patients with asthma. The findings are consistent with the studies in the adult population. The use of observation units avoids the need to admit many patients to the acute care hospital.

O'Brien et al. (2) performed an uncontrolled study with 434 pediatric patients seen in the ED at Children's Hospital National Medical Center. Seventy-six percent (328) of the patients were sent home after initial treatment. The remaining 106 patients received further treatment in the holding unit. Sixty-seven percent of the patients treated in the holding unit were discharged. The recurrence rate at one week of these discharged patients was 7% with hospital admission required for four out of five relapses. The overall hospital admission rate was 8%. Additional cost would have been incurred had the patients that were successfully treated in the holding unit been admitted to an inpatient facility instead.

Subsequently, Willert et al. (3) conducted a randomized trial at the Children's Memorial Hospital in Chicago. Patients included in the study were > 1 year old and had an asthma score < 5 (16). After a standardized treatment regimen, eligible patients for further therapy were randomized to a holding unit or an inpatient facility. Therapy using aminophylline and isoetharine was standardized for both inpatient and holding unit groups. Steroids and other β-agonists were given at the discretion of the physician. Multiple clinical variables were assessed. Seventy percent of patients were able to be discharged after initial treatment. Of the patients randomized to the holding unit, 67% were discharged and 33% required admission after 18–24 hr. Of the randomized inpatients, only 31% were discharged after 1 day of treatment. Relapse rates of both groups, measured at 7 days and 1 month, were not statistically different. Patients randomized to the holding unit had fewer hospital days and lower hospital therapy and room costs.

More recently, Gouin et al. (17) evaluated the effect of opening an ED observation unit on the admission and relapse rates of asthmatic children. The authors conducted a retrospective review of patients aged 1–18 seen in the ED during a 1-year period before the opening of an observation unit, and during a 1-year period after the opening of an observation unit. There were 1,979 patients in the preobservation group and 2,248 patients in the postobservation group. General criteria for admission to the observation unit included respiratory distress after 2 hr of treatment with systemic steroids and inhaled bronchodilators, some signs of improvement, and not expected to need more than 12 hr of treatment. Patients expected to require more than 12 hr of continuous care were admitted to the inpatient service. Patients were able to be discharged from the observation unit if the respiratory status was stable, the patients used inhaled bronchodilator every 4 hr, and the social circumstances were stable. In the preobservation unit group, patients were admitted to the inpatient service if there was persistent respiratory distress after 4 hr of treatment in the ED with steroids and inhaled bronchodilators.

Randomized samples of both groups ($n = 702$) were compared. There were no significant differences in baseline characteristics of the groups. In the preobservation unit group, 31% of children were admitted, while in the postobservation unit group 24% required admission ($p < 0.01$). In the postobservation group, 15% were admitted directly from the ED and 9% were admitted from the observation unit. The relapse rate within 72 hr, measured by a computerized list of ED discharge diagnoses, was 3.2% in the preobservation unit groups and 5.0% in the postobservation unit group ($p < 0.01$) This represents the largest of the pediatric observation unit studies, and includes current treatment regimens. The authors conclude that there was a reduction in the rate of hospitalization, but an increase in ED relapse rates when an observation unit was introduced in a pediatric ED.

VI. CONCLUSION

Asthma is a common condition managed in the ED. Well-structured and -managed protocols are effective in managing asthmatic patients on an outpatient basis. Observation units are a tool for rational restructuring of emergent treatment providing high-quality, cost-effective services.

REFERENCES

1. Zwicke DL, Donohue JF, Wagner EH. Use of the emergency department observation unit in the treatment of acute asthma. Ann Emerg Med 1982; 11:77–83.
2. O'Brien SR, Hein EW, Sly RM. Treatment of acute asthmatic attacks in a holding unit of a pediatric emergency room. Ann Allergy 1980; 45:159–162.
3. Willert C, Davis AT, Herman JJ, Holson, BB, Zieserl E. Short-term holding room treatment of asthmatic children. J Pediatr 1985; 106:707–711.
4. Camargo CA Jr on behalf of the MARC Investigators. Management of acute asthma in US emergency departments: The Multicenter Asthma Research Collaboration (abstr). Am J Respir Crit Care Med 1998; 157(3, Part 2):A623.
5. McDermott MF, Murhpy DG, Zalenski RJ, et al. A comparison between emergency department diagnostic and treatment unit and inpatient care in the management of acute asthma. Arch Intern Med 1997; 157:2055–2062.
6. Murphy DG, Zalenski RJ, Raucci JC, et al. The utility of extended emergency department

treatment of asthma: An analysis of improvement in peak expiratory flow rate as a function of time (abstr). Ann Emerg Med 1989; 18:467.

7. Graff L, Mucci D, Radford M. Decision to admit: Objective DRG criteria vs. clinical judgment. Ann Emerg Med 1988; 18:943–952.
8. Graff LG, Dallara J, Ross MA, et al. Impact on the care of the emergency department chest pain patient from the chest pain evaluation registry (CHEPER) study. Amer J Cardiol 1997; 80:563–568.
9. Brillman J, Graff LG, L Dunbar, et al. American College of Emergency Physicians section of observation services. Management of observation units. Ann Emerg Med 1995; 25;823–830.
10. Graff L, ed. Observation medicine. Boston, MA: Butterworth Heineman, 1993.
11. Graff LG, ed. Observation units: Implementation and management strategies, Dallas, TX: American College of Emergency Physicians, 1998.
12. Riggs L, ed. Emergency department design, Dallas, TX: American College of Emergency Physicians, 1994.
13. Graff L, Wolf S, Dinwoodie R, Buono D, Mucci D. Emergency physician workload: A time study. Ann Emerg Med 1993; 22:1156–1163.
14. Brillman JC, Tandberg D. Observation unit impact on emergency department admission for asthma. Am J Emerg Med 1994; 12:11–14.
15. National Heart, Lung, and Blood Institute. Guidelines for the diagnosis and management of asthma: National asthma education program expert panel report. Publication No. 91-3042 Bethesda, MD: National Institutes of Health, 1991.
16. Wood DW, Downes JJ, Lecks HI. A clinical system for the diagnosis of respiratory failure. Preliminary report on childhood status asthmaticus. Am J Dis Child 1972; 123:227–228.
17. Gouin S, Macarthur C, Parkin PC, Schuh S. Effect of a pediatric observation unit on the rate of hospitalization for asthma. Ann Emerg Med 1997; 29:218–222.

34

Follow-Up and Prevention of Relapse in Adults After Disposition from the ED

Rita Kay Cydulka
MetroHealth Medical Center/Case Western Reserve University, Cleveland, Ohio
Mona Shah
Oregon Health Sciences University, Portland, Oregon

I. INTRODUCTION

The term *relapse* is an inexact one. In fact, little agreement as to its definition exists within the asthma literature (1–3). McNamara defined relapse as return to ED within 7 days after discharge (1) whereas Chapman defined it as return to the emergency department (ED) within 3 weeks of the index visit (2,4). McFadden regards relapse as symptomatic episodes of asthma that occur within 2 days of an ED visit (3).

The definition of relapse is directly tied to discharge criteria, which are, at best, loosely defined (5). In fact, the entire study of relapse after acute exacerbation raises more questions than it answers. Does relapse represent incomplete resolution of a prior exacerbation or does it represent a new exacerbation? Is relapse related to compliance with medication regimen, avoidance of environmental triggers, poorly understood pathophysiology, or all of these factors?

Most clinical research directed at ED disposition and prevention of relapse was conducted in the era before steroids were routinely administered in the ED for acute asthma exacerbation. Currently, The National Asthma Education and Prevention Program strongly advocates the routine use of oral steroids after ED treatment (4). However, further, larger, prospective clinical trials to establish the impact of steroid use in long-term prevention of relapse are needed because few studies exist that determine the impact of steroid use in prevention of relapse (2,7).

II. EMERGENCY DEPARTMENT DISPOSITION

Disposition decisions about the asthmatic patient treated in the ED currently take in to account a combination of subjective parameters, such as resolution of wheezing, improvement in air exchange as assessed by auscultation and patient opinion, and objective measures, such as normalization of pulmonary function tests (PFTs) or peak expiratory flow rate (PEFR) measurements (4,5,8). In the 1970s and '80s, relapse rates in patients treated and discharged from the ED remained as high as 26–30% (10,11), necessitating further ED care or hospitalization. In 1979, Nowak et al. reported that 92% of patients with a pretreatment PEFR < 100 L/min and a posttreatment value of < 300 L/min required admission (9). Furthermore, they found that 27% of patients discharged from the ED later relapsed and required admission. Kelsen et al. identified a relapse rate of 26%, with 6% of patients initially discharged requiring hospitalization on repeat visit (10). Fischl et al. documented a relapse rate of 25%, with 83% of patients in the relapsed group requiring admission. The high rate of relapse prompted them to develop an index to predict relapse and need for hospitalization. The index combined subjective criteria, such as dyspnea, wheezing, and accessory muscle use with objective criteria, such as pulse rate > 120/min, respiratory rate > 30/min, pulsus paradoxus > 18 mmHg, and PEFR < 120 L/min. On a scoring system of 0–7, with higher scores reflecting increasing severity of symptoms, an index score of 4 correlated accurately in predicting risk of relapse and need for hospitalization (11). Unfortunately prospective studies by Centor et al. (6) and Rose et al. (12) failed to confirm utility and validity of this index, which was developed retrospectively. Asthma was later recognized largely as an inflammatory disease and these data reflect reality in the era before steroid use in asthmatics was commonplace.

In the 1980s asthma exacerbation was clearly recognized as a biphasic disease. The early phase is comprised of bronchoconstriction, followed by mucous secretion and airway edema. The late phase is characterized by airway inflammation, bronchial hyperresponsiveness, and persistent airflow obstruction. Individuals with late-phase response during acute exacerbation account for most admissions to the hospital (13–16). Those that are well enough to be discharged from the ED also have a high incidence of relapse (10,13), suggesting that all phases of asthma exacerbation may not be completely resolved at the time of discharge from the ED. Clearly, some degree of residual airflow obstruction, airway lability, and inflammation always persists (10,13).

Unfortunately no single treatment program can be recommended for all patients discharged home from the ED following treatment of an asthma exacerbation. A short course of oral steroids in addition to the use of β_2-agonist bronchodilators reduces relapse amongst asthma patients considered well enough for ED discharge (3,7). Probably the single most common omission leading to severe asthma attacks is the failure to begin oral corticosteroids during the early phases of a serious attack (17). McNamara reported a significantly lower relapse rate in patients receiving intramuscular (IM) prednisolone (6.7%), compared to the patients receiving placebo (31%), during ED treatment for asthma exacerbations. In this study, 50% of all patients with relapse within 7 days subsequently required admission (1). Although some investigators have compared steroids with placebo tablets and found a decrease in the incidence of relapse (2), others have demonstrated a high relapse rate despite the routine use of steroids (4). Emerman and Cydulka (4) noted a relapse rate of over 25% within 3 weeks of discharge. Almost two-thirds of the relapses occurred while the patients were still on oral steroid therapy. They reported that patients with a history of previous ED visits and hospitalization were at highest risk of relapse regardless of ED management. In addition, incidence of relapse within 3 days was greater in patients with eosinophilia. McFadden et al. determined that they could discharge 77% of asthmatics presenting to the ED and decrease relapse rate within 1 week of ED treatment to 7% by enforcing a strict ED treatment protocol that dictated timing and dose of β-agonist therapy, administration of steroids and aminophylline, and timing of PEFR and arterial blood gas measurements. These figures represented a significant improvement from the preprotocol period (18).

The NAEPP has developed general guidelines to determine hospitalization/discharge criteria based on response to aggressive ED treatment (5). A good response to treatment is demonstrated by complete resolution of symptoms and a PEFR or $FEV_1 >$ 70% predicted. Such individuals can be safely discharged home without concerns of relapse (see Chapter 31). Patients with a poor response to treatment are defined as those with persistent symptoms and FEV_1 or PEFR $< 40\%$ predicted or less. Such patients are likely to have persistent wheezing and dyspnea at rest despite intense treatment in the ED. They are at risk for developing hypercapnic respiratory failure, necessitating intubation and mechanical ventilation (17). The NAEPP proposes immediate admission for these patients to monitor for respiratory failure. An incomplete response to treatment—the midground—is defined as some persistence of symptoms, and a PEFR or $FEV_1 < 70\%$ and $> 40\%$ of predicted. A large percentage of the asthmatic patients treated in an ED fall in this category. Current knowledge does not permit rapid and reliable identification of patients within this intermediate category of response or deterioration who should be hospitalized because of the likelihood of deterioration following ED discharge (5).

In addition, patients with complications of their asthma, such as pneumonia, pneumothorax, and atelectasis, should be seriously considered for hospitalization.

The role of steroids in long-term prevention of relapse is yet to be identified. However, current recommendations by the NAEPP suggest that all patients with an FEV_1 or PEFR $< 70\%$ of baseline after aggressive ED treatment should receive at least a course of oral steroids (5).

Follow-up medical care must be arranged following an acute asthma exacerbation to assure resolution of exacerbation, and to review the long-term medication plan for chronic management of asthma (5). The high relapse rate, despite routine use of steroids, strongly suggests the need for follow-up within days of the ED visit. Making an appointment for patients may help them get timely care more easily. Fitzgerald and Hargreave reported that patients with acute asthma who have direct access to medical care have lower rates of illness and death than patients who need to contact their primary care physician in order to receive approval to obtain urgent medical care (19). All patients with asthma *must* have an appropriate plan of action that deals with an acute worsening of symptoms.

Finally, patient education delivered during patient disposition from the ED has been demonstrated to reduce the frequency of subsequent ED visits and therefore must become an integral part of ED care (19). The ED physician should provide basic education on asthma and help link the patient with a primary care provider while providing discharge instructions. Review of the patient's discharge medications, technique of inhaler use, and the use of peak flow monitoring, are just some of the issues the ED physician can teach and emphasize. Hopefully, this will increase disease awareness as well as better compliance among patients.

III. SUMMARY

The decision to discharge an asthma patient from the ED depends on both subjective and objective criteria. Although pre- and posttreatment pulmonary function have been useful in guiding disposition decisions, posttreatment pulmonary function has failed to identify all patients at risk for relapse. The benefit of steroids in the prevention of relapse has been demonstrated by some investigators but the full impact of steroids in prevention of relapse remains uncertain. Further investigation is needed to elucidate this. Nevertheless, most current literature suggests that oral steroids should be administered to patients in the ED when PEFR is $< 70\%$ predicted prior to discharge (4).

Besides aggressive pharmacological management, one of the most important roles of the emergency physician is to educate asthmatics about their disease, thereby facilitating patient understanding and compliance. Finally, the high relapse rate currently seen after ED discharge mandates close medical follow-up, especially in patients with history of previous ED visits and hospitalization for asthma exacerbation.

REFERENCES

1. McNamara RM, Rubin JM. Intramuscular methylprednisolone acetate for the prevention of relapse in acute asthma. Ann Emerg Med 1993; 22:1829–1835.
2. Chapman KR, Verbeek PR, White JG, Rebuck AS. Effect of a short course of prednisone in the prevention of early relapse after the emergency room treatment of acute asthma. N Engl J Med 1991; 324:788–794.
3. McFadden ER. Management of patients with acute asthma: What do we know? What do we need to know? Ann Allergy 1994; 72:385–389.
4. Emerman CL, Cydulka RK. Factors associated with relapse after ED treatment for acute asthma. Ann Emerg Med 1995; 26:6–11.
5. National Asthma Education Program, Expert Panel Report II. Executive Summary: Guidelines for the diagnosis and management of asthma, DHHS Publication/NIH Publication No. 97-4051, 1997.
6. Centor RM, Yarborough B, Wood JP. Inability to predict relapse in acute asthma. N Engl J Med 1984; 310:577–580.
7. Fiel SB, Swartz MA, Glanz K, Francis ME. Efficacy of short-term corticosteroid therapy in out-patient treatment of acute bronchial asthma. Am J Med 1983; 73:845–851.
8. Nowak RM, Gordon KP, Wroblewski DA, et al. Spirometric evaluation of acute bronchial asthma. JACEP 1979; 8:9–12.
9. Nowak RM, Penslar MI, Sarkar DD, et al. Comparison of peak expiratory flow and FEV_1 admission criteria for acute bronchial asthma. Ann Emerg Med 1982; 11:64–69.
10. Kelsen SG, Kelsen DP, Fleegler BF. Emergency room assessment and treatment of patients with acute asthma: adequacy of the conventional approach. Am J Med 1978; 64:622–628.
11. Fischl MA, Pitchenik A, Gardner LB. An index predicting relapse and need for hospitalization in patients with acute asthma. N Engl J Med 1981; 305:783–789.
12. Rose CC, Murphy JG, Schwartz JS. Performance of an index predicting the response of patients with acute bronchial asthma to intensive ED treatment. N Engl J Med 1983; 310:573–577.
13. McFadden ER. Clinical physiologic correlates in asthma. J Allergy Clin Immunol 1986; 77: 1–5.
14. McFadden ER, Kiser R, deGroot W. Acute bronchial asthma: Relations between clinical and physiologic manifestations. N Engl J Med 1973; 288:221–225.

15. Fanta CH, Rossing TH, McFadden ER. Emergency room treatment of asthma. Relationships among therapeutic combinations, severity of obstruction, and time course of response. Am J Med 1982; 72:416–422.
16. Fanta CH, Rossing TH, McFadden ER. Glucocorticoids in acute asthma. A critical controlled trial. Am J Med 1983; 74:845–851.
17. Fanta CH. Acute asthma, In: Weiss EB and Stein M, eds., Bronchial asthma: Mechanisms and therapeutics, 3rd Ed., Boston, MA: Little, Brown, and Co., 1993.
18. McFadden E, Jr, Elsanadi N, Dixon L, et al. Protocol therapy for acute asthma: Therapeutic benefits and cost savings. Am J Med 1995; 99:651–661.
19. Fitzgerald JM, Hargreave FE. Acute asthma: ED management and prospective evaluation of outcome. Can Med Assoc J 1990; 142:991–995.
20. Maiman LA, Green LW, Gibson G. Education for self-treatment by adult asthmatics. JAMA 1979; 241:1919–1922.

35

Follow-Up and Prevention of Relapse in Children After Disposition from the ED

Ellen F. Crain
Albert Einstein College of Medicine and Jacobi Medical Center, Bronx, New York

Prevention of relapse to the emergency department (ED) begins with appropriate determination regarding the patient's readiness for discharge. ED physicians are most familiar with physiological and physical examination criteria for discharge. These have been reviewed in detail in Chapter 13 on clinical manifestations and differential diagnosis. Early studies suggested that physiological parameters were paramount in determining which patients were likely to relapse to the ED following treatment for an asthma exacerbation. Fischl et al. (1) found that an index using a combination of presenting factors—pulse rate $\geq$ 120/min, respiratory rate > 30/min, pulsus paradoxus > 18 mmHg, peak expiratory flow rate (PEFR) < 120 L/min, moderate to severe dyspnea, accessory muscle use, and wheezing—predicted relapse in adults with 95% accuracy if it was 4 or higher. Later, however, Baker (2) showed that pretreatment scores on a similar index, the Wood-Downes-Lecks score, were not related to ongoing disability after discharge, including relapse.

It makes intuitive sense that physiological criteria alone would not predict relapse. At the minimum, the patient requires an adequate treatment plan, access to medications and devices required for medication delivery, a caretaker able to give the medications and assess the child's response, and a home environment where triggers can be avoided or minimized. Thus, in addition to the more familiar physiological criteria, prior to deciding that the child can be discharged home the physician should review three additional areas for risk factors for relapse (Table 1).

Steps recommended to prevent relapse are summarized in the Guidelines for the Diagnosis and Management of Asthma (3), the Global Initiative for Asthma (4), and the 1997 Expert Panel Report II (5). They include five actions to be taken at the time of discharge from the ED: (1) identify and avoid the trigger factor that precipitated the exacerbation; (2) instruct the patient (parent) to contact the child's health provider or asthma specialist within 24 hr of discharge and make a follow-up appointment within a few days

Table 1 Risk Factors for Relapse due to Asthma

Physiological factors at time of ED discharge
Respiratory rate
Retractions
Quality of speech
Peak expiratory flow rate
Degree of wheeze
Family factors
Condifence of caregiver to assess and monitor child's condition
Ability of caregiver to assess and monitor child's condition
Caregiver's understanding of medication plan and use of adjunctive devices
Environmental factors
Presence of smokers in the home
Presence of other/new triggers for child's asthma
Access factors
Availability of medications and adjunctive devices
Distance from the ED
Availability of transportation
Availability of a telephone

of discharge to assure that lung function has improved prior to stepping down therapy; (3) prescribe a 5-day course of short-acting β-agonist therapy and (in most cases) 5 days of oral prednisone; (4) review the patients inhaler technique and use of peak flow meter to monitor therapy at home; and (5) review and, if necessary, modify the action plan to ensure that the parent can recognize signs of worsening asthma, start treatment early, and reach medical care. With regard to referring the patient to follow-up, the February 1997 Expert Panel Report II has specifically added that the emergency physician should notify the patient's health care professional that the patient was in the ED for an exacerbation, and, whenever possible, schedule the follow-up appointment prior to the patient's discharge from the ED. The new guidelines also recommend that the emergency physician consider issuing a peak flow meter and provide patient education on how to measure and record daily PEF rates.

Although many of these recommendations are the product of expert opinion, in the remainder of this chapter we will review existing data that support and modify these recommendations as well as how they apply to children

In children, identification of the trigger factor is often difficult. For many children, an asthma exacerbation is precipitated by an upper respiratory infection (URI), although smoking, pets, cockroaches, and dust mites are common in the homes of children with asthma. One treatment modality that has been shown to reduce ED visits by children is to give oral prednisone at the first sign of a URI (6). However, in the setting of the ED, it is often difficult to get parents to adapt such an aggressive management plan. The physician should determine if possible whether there have been any recent changes in the home or other environment such as a new babysitter who smokes or the acquisition of a new pet that may have triggered the attack. If the child can be removed from exposure to the trigger, even for a few days, it may reduce the likelihood of relapse.

Instructing the parent to contact the child's health care provider within 24 hr of discharge from the ED and to make a follow-up appointment within a few days of discharge is important for documenting whether the child has returned to baseline or requires further aggressive therapy with anti-inflammatory medications. Although this is probably a critical step for avoiding relapse, many parents do not contact their child's provider or make an appointment to have the child evaluated. They frequently do not appreciate the chronic nature of asthma and assume that as symptoms resolve the asthma is "going away" so their child does not need a follow-up visit. Helping parents to understand that asthma is persistent and chronic and explaining to them what the provider will do to determine whether the child has returned to baseline may help to increase adherence to the follow-up visit. The new 1997 guidelines include a list of items to be reviewed and questions to be asked at follow-up visits, and reviewing them with parents prior to discharge from the ED may be helpful (Table 2). Although data on this subject are sparse, reports from over 300 parents of inner-city children with asthma enrolled in the National Cooperative Inner-City Asthma Study who were interviewed approximately four weeks after an ED visit for asthma suggest that only 60% of families who receive a follow-up appointment at the time of discharge from the ED or who are told to make an appointment actually keep it. The biggest barrier to keeping an appointment is the belief that the child is better and so does not need a follow-up visit with the health care provider (7).

Table 2 Examples of Topics to Review with Parents Prior to Discharge from the Emergency Department

Monitoring signs and symptoms at home
Coughing/wheezing
Shortness of breath/chest tightness
Waking up at night
Symptoms with play or exercise
Monitoring pulmonary function (if child uses a peak flow meter)
Highest and lowest peak flow since ED visit
Whether child's peak flow has dropped below ____ L/min (80% of personal best or expected) since ED visit
What parent did when this occured
Need to bring peak flow meter to follow-up visit and show health care provider how parent (and child) measure the peak flow rate
Monitoring functional status
Days of school missed due to asthma
Need to tell provider about this ED visit and any other recent unscheduled asthma visists
Monitoring the environment
Changes in home/school/other environment where child spends time (smokers, pets)
Monitoring pharmacotherapy
Ability to adhere to/problems with medication plan
Other medicines or remedies tried
Side effects
Review inhaler technique (with or without a spacer device)
Take inhaler and spacer to follow-up visit and review use with the health care provider

Source: Adapted from Ref. 5.

While the impact on relapse of providing early follow-up after treatment of an asthma exacerbation in the ED has not been studied, the 1991 and 1997 Guidelines for the Evaluation and Management of Asthma as well as the Global Initiative for Asthma recommend early follow-up. Improvement in rates of follow-up appointment keeping will require effort on the part of physicians and administrative staff providing care in the ED as well as in the primary care setting. A survey by Butz et al. (8) of 136 children ages 7–12 years treated for an acute asthma exacerbation in the pediatric ED of an inner-city teaching hospital found a 26% relapse rate over the 8 weeks that the study continued. Only 26% had a scheduled follow-up visit over the course of the study period. Barnett and Oberklaid studied the medical records of 422 children with asthma seen in the ED of a pediatric teaching hospital in Australia over a 1-year period (9). For more than one-third, no documentation of follow-up arrangements was made. Another study by Mak et al. (10) found that almost half of inner-city children who were seen in the ED for asthma care reported that the ED was their only source of asthma care.

From the perspective of ED practice, there is little literature on follow-up patterns for asthma care for adults or children following an ED visit. A recent survey of ED directors from 376 hospitals representing U.S. children's, public, and community hospitals found that only 20% of ED directors reported knowing how long it took children with asthma to obtain follow-up (11). Those ED directors reported that only 61% of children obtained follow-up within 2–3 days and only 74% obtained any follow-up at all. Appointments for follow-up could be made only during daytime hours in 71% of the EDs.

In the same survey, only 3.3% of ED directors reported that their ED confirms whether a child seen in the ED for an asthma exacerbation and scheduled for follow-up actually obtains follow-up. Although it may not be the ED's job to track whether patients actually obtain follow-up, as more patients with asthma are enrolled in managed care, case management is likely to become more important and tracking of patients to follow-up is likely to become more common (12,13).

Even if a process is developed to track patients to follow-up, how likely is it that families will take advantage of opportunities for a follow-up visit? We have touched on some of the reasons why they might not with respect to lack of understanding of the chronic nature of asthma. Other issues related to enhancing patient follow-up come from studies on enhancing return to the ED. Although we cannot extrapolate from this body of data directly to the topic of enhancing follow-up for asthma, there are some lessons to be learned. Data from a study by Chande et al. (14) suggest that a one-time educational intervention in the ED does not alter ED utilization habits. Parents of 130 patients seen in the pediatric ED for minor illnesses were randomized to receive education about use of their primary care provider and provided information about common pediatric illnesses, while the control group received usual discharge instructions. There were no differences between the groups in total number of return visits to the pediatric ED or return visits for minor illnesses. The authors suggest that more extensive education and greater availability of primary care providers may be needed to decrease use of the ED for minor illnesses. The authors also note that for minor illnesses, there was no need for a follow-up visit with the primary care provider, perhaps diluting the impact of the educational intervention. In addition, families who seek care in the ED for minor illnesses may not have had a strong relationship with their primary care provider and so may have been less amenable to the intervention.

Asthma is not a minor complaint and most experts consider a follow-up visit to be essential for reducing the likelihood of relapse. However, the lack of impact of a one-time intervention in reducing use of the ED suggests that it may be difficult to change parental behavior when the recommendation to obtain follow-up is initiated by the ED staff alone. There are many reasons to suspect that it will be difficult to change parental behavior regarding use of the ED for their child's asthma management. Wasilewski et al. (15) interviewed the parents of children who received care for their asthma in the ED to identify psychosocial and behavioral factors that correlated with ED use for childhood asthma. Parents receiving Medicaid brought their children more frequently to the ED than parents not receiving Medicaid. Younger children were taken to the ED more frequently than older children with asthma. Other factors associated with increased utilization of the ED for asthma care included more days with asthma symptoms; more asthma medications prescribed; a prior hospitalization for asthma; a lower level of parental confidence in the efficacy of asthma medications; and not using a specific standard, such as that the child's breathing slowed after treatment, for deciding to continue treating the asthma at home.

Changing parental behavior regarding the need for follow-up visits for asthma may require a coordinated effort by ED and primary care provider staff. Although children with asthma were not specifically enrolled in the trial, data from Nelson et al. (16) suggest that providing post-ED visit support from a nurse practitioner can improve the use of follow-up care. In 86% of the cases, the nurse practitioner intervention consisted of only a single telephone call, and in the majority of cases the call lasted less than 5 min. Parents in the intervention group were significantly more likely to comply with follow-up instructions including keeping appointments that had been scheduled. Although unnecessary revisits to the ED were unusual in both the intervention and control groups, they occurred with equal frequency. The intervention was much more effective in encouraging appropriate follow-up visits than in preventing revisits to the ED; if this type of intervention were applied to patients with asthma exacerbations, in combination with appropriate use of anti-inflammatory medications, which will be discussed below, it might have a substantial impact on early revisits to the ED.

Wissow et al. (13) noted a 50% drop in acute care visits for asthma by children whose families were enrolled in a case-management program in which a nurse discussed proper medication use and home management, gave the parent a phone number for 24-hr consultation, and reviewed the child's medical care with the primary physician. Also using a pre-/post-design, Greineder et al. (12) reported that an outreach program involving an allergy nurse, a nurse-practitioner, and an allergist was able to reduce ED visits by 79% among children with asthma who were patients in a staff-model health maintenance organization. Although the impact of the program on relapse was not specifically reported, the asthma outreach nurse performed all of the tasks recommended by the guidelines to prevent relapse, including a review of asthma triggers, warning signs, and medications; review of peak flow meter use; monitoring compliance with visits to the pediatrician; provision and review of a written medication plan; and, where necessary, environmental avoidance instructions.

One of the most important steps for preventing relapse is to properly identify which children need a course of oral steroids following discharge from the ED. There are two-main categories of patients who should be discharged with steroids. The first is the group of children who required more than one nebulized β-agonist treatment to return to baseline or to reach discharge values for respiratory rate, oxygen saturation, peak expiratory flow rate, and other parameters, which have been discussed in Chapter 22. Although use of oral steroids for this situation is clearly described in the guidelines, it is often not done in many EDs. In the survey of ED directors by Crain et al. (11), only 45% of ED directors

Table 3 Risk Factors for Death from Asthma

Past history of sudden severe exacerbation
Prior intubation for asthma
Prior admission to an intensive care unit
Two or more hospitalizations for asthma in the past year
Three or more ED visits for asthma in the past year
Hospitalization or an emergency visit for asthma within the past month
Use of > 2 canisters per month of inhaled short-acting β-agonists
Current use of sytemic corticosteroids or recent withdrawal from systemic corticosteroids
Difficulty perceiving airflow obstructions or its severity
Comorbidity, as from cardiovascular disease or other serious pulmonary condition
Serious psychiatric disease or psychosocial problems
Low socioeconomic status and urban residence
Illicit drug use
Sensitivity to *Alternaria*

Source: Ref. 5.

reported that steroids were used after the first treatment if there is poor or no response to β-agonists.

The other important category of indications for steroid prescription at discharge includes children who have an asthma exacerbation after recently taking steroids or have had symptoms such as nighttime wakening, chest tightness, or coughing for several days prior to presenting to the ED. In the survey of ED directors, only 57% of directors reported that steroids were used as a routine part of the initial treatment of children who experience an asthma attack while they are taking steroids. The low use of steroids in the ED was documented despite recent emphasis on the inflammatory nature of asthma (17,18) and the apparent benefits of steroids in reducing the need for hospitalization (19).

Most physicians in the ED regularly assess their patient's asthma activity by asking about hospitalizations, intensive care unit admissions, and intubation, as well as frequency of attacks and time of the last attack. Although this is important to help determine the patient's risk for life-threatening asthma (Table 3), many children with severe inflammation and risk for further episodes will be missed unless the emergency physician also asks about the recent impact of asthma on their daily activities (Table 4). Many children who have not had an overt exacerbation in months to years will be found to have significant restriction in their daily activities or regular nighttime wakening and should be sent home to take a course of oral steroids.

Table 4 Areas of Quality of Life to Be Assessed in the ED

Missed school due to asthma
Reduction in usual activities (play, exercise, athletics, work, school)
Disturbances in sleep (nighttime wakening due to asthma)
Changes in caretaker's sleep/activites due to child's asthma

Source: Adapted from Ref. 5.

Although most experts believe that prescribing steroids when appropriate is essential to preventing relapse, there are few data from ED studies to document this. In the study by Butz et al. (8), two-thirds of the children were prescribed medication for 2 weeks and then as needed, while one-third were prescribed continuous medications and/or steroids. Relapse rates over the 8 weeks following an ED visit were similar in the two groups. In this study, relapse was associated with maternal smoking, female gender, prior hospitalization for asthma, cough, and medication use during the last two weeks of the study period.

Less than a decade ago, theophylline was the mainstay of the discharge medication plan for pediatric patients with asthma (20). Theophylline and β-agonists were given by the oral route. Now, most adolescents as well as many children with asthma are sent home to take β-agonists by the inhaled route. Most adolescents and many school aged children are now prescribed β-agonists by metered dose inhaler (MDI). According to the Guidelines and Global Initiative for Asthma, an important step to help reduce the likelihood of relapse is to review the medication plan and the patient's inhaler technique. When the ED physician reviews the discharge medication plan, it is essential not only to ask whether the patient has an adequate supply of medication at home but also to inquire about how the patient takes the medications. All children and adolescents should be using inhaled β-agonists. School-aged children and adolescents should be asked to demonstrate their use of the inhaler prior to discharge. Although there are few data to document the adequacy of use of MDIs by children, one indication of inappropriate use may be relapse to the ED despite what appears to be proper adherence to an adequate medication plan. The Expert Panel Report II includes an educational intervention and recommendations for proper use of an MDI that can be provided to patients as part of the discharge teaching, as reproduced here.

Please demonstrate inhaler technique at every visit:

1. Remove the cap and hold inhaler upright.
2. Shake the inhaler.
3. Tilt your head back slightly and breathe out slowly.
4. Position the inhaler in one of the following ways (see Figure 1: (a) or (b) is optimal, but (c) is acceptable for those who have difficulty with (a) or (b); (c) is required for breath-activated inhalers).
5. Press down on the inhaler to release medication as you start to breathe in slowly.
6. Breathe in slowly (3–5 sec).
7. Hold your breath for 10 sec to allow the medicine to reach deeply into your lungs.
8. Repeat puff as directed. Waiting 1 min between puffs may permit second puff to penetrate your lungs better.
9. Spacers/holding chambers are useful for all patients. They are particularly recommended for young children and older adults and for use with inhaled steroids.

Avoid inhaler mistakes. Follow these inhaler tips:

1. Breathe out *before* pressing your inhaler.
2. Inhale *slowly*.
3. Breathe in through your mouth, not your nose.
4. Press down on your inhaler at the *start* of inhalation (or within the first second of inhalation).

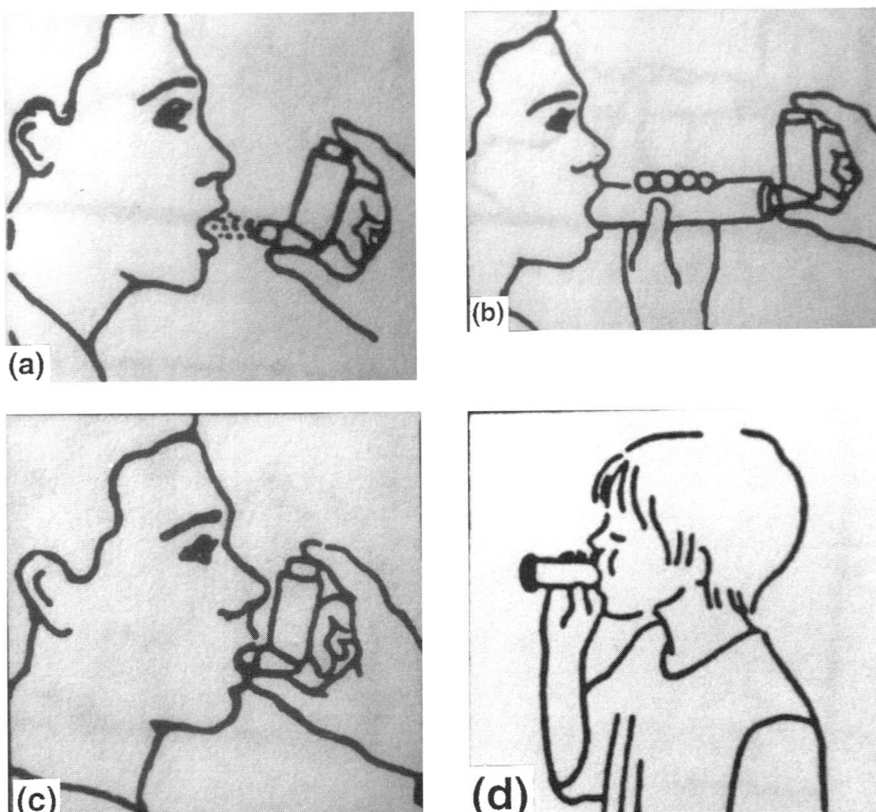

Figure 1 Inhaler use. (a) Open mouth with inhaler 1 to 2 in. away. (b) Use spacer/holding chamber (that is recommended especially for young children and for people using corticosteroids). (c) In the mouth—do not use for corticosteroids. (d) Inhaled dry powder capsules require a different inhalation technique. To use a dry powder inhaler, it is important to close the mouth tightly around the mouthpiece of the inhaler and to inhale rapidly.

5. Keep inhaling as you press down on inhaler.
6. Press your inhaler only *once* while you are inhaling (one breath for each puff).
7. Make sure you breathe in evenly and deeply.

It may be best to assume that most children cannot use an MDI properly. In one multicenter study of childhood asthma, over 80% of children under the age of 12 with asthma who had been prescribed an inhaler device could not use it correctly when tested on a nine-item scale (21). Because inhaled medications are essential to successful asthma management, emergency physicians may want to incorporate more formal evaluation of inhaler technique in their discharge planning (Table 5). Certainly, all health care providers in the ED should review the technique and be certain that they are all teaching the same, correct method. Several studies have evaluated MDIs with spacer devices compared to usual therapy for children both in the ED as well as at home. Studies comparing MDI

Table 5 Bailey Test of MDI Use

Desirable behavior	Yes	No
1. Patient shakes canister for 5 sec	1	2
2. Patient attaches spacer correctly	1	2
3. Patient positions finger on the top of the medication canister and provides support	1	2
4. Patient places the spacer tube or mouthpiece into the mouth between the teeth	1	2
5. Patient closes lips around the spacer tube or mouthpiece	1	2
6. Patient exhales normally	1	2
7. Patietn correctly presses down the top of the medication canister to release the medication	1	2
8. Patient inhales medication deeply and slowly	1	2
9. Patient holds the medication inside lungs a minimum of 10 sec before exhaling	1	2

and spacer use vs. nebulizers for β-agonist therapy for the treatment of acute asthma in hospitalized patients or in the ED have found no differences between the methods (22–24). A study by Cunningham and Crain (25) compared asthma symptoms, school attendance, and unscheduled medical visits among children receiving β-agonist therapy at the time of discharge from the ED via MDI with a spacer compared to a group receiving standard inhaled or oral β-agonists. Those receiving the MDI with spacer had substantial improvement in clinical outcomes (25). Cunningham's study was particularly important because it showed that, contrary to popular opinion, a device that was thought to require time-consuming education and reinforcement could be introduced in a busy ED and lead to improvement in symptoms.

Simply prescribing a spacer device is not adequate, however. Proper use of the MDI with the spacer must be reviewed with the patient and the caretaker prior to discharge from the ED. It may be harder for patients to use a spacer if one is simply prescribed rather than given to the patient. Asthma disproportionately affects inner-city poor children who may be uninsured or insured by Medicaid. The cost of the spacer device may be prohibitive, and in some states, such as New York, Medicaid will pay for one spacer device every 2 years. The prescription for the spacer device requires prior approval from an office that is only open during the daytime hours. Unfortunately, many asthmatic children present to the ED for care during the evenings and on weekends, making it impossible to obtain the prior approval number. This policy provides a substantial barrier to providing inhaled medications to children and illustrates the need for the ED physician to be familiar with reimbursement policies that affect their prescribing behaviors (26).

In summary, prevention of relapse requires attention to far more than physiological or physical examination parameters at the time of presentation or discharge from the ED. It includes ensuring that the patient has an appropriate medication plan and access to the medications and adjunctive devices required for their use. The family's ability to implement the plan as well as assess the child's response to treatment must also be evaluated. In the best of circumstances, the patient and caretaker should leave the ED with a follow-up appointment already scheduled and an understanding of what they should be ready to discuss with their child's regular physician at the time of the follow-up visit.

REFERENCES

1. Fischl MA, Pitchenik A, Gardner LB. An index predicting relapse and need for hospitalization in patients with acute bronchial asthma. N Engl J Med 1988; 305:783–789.
2. Baker D. Pitfalls in the use of clinical asthma scoring. Am J Dis Child 1988; 142:183–185.
3. National Institutes of Health, National Heart, Lung, and Blood Institute. Guidelines for the Diagnosis and Management of Asthma, Publication No. 91-3042, Bethesda, MD: U.S. Department of Health and Human Services, 1991.
4. National Institutes of Health, National Heart, Lung, and Blood Institute. Global Initiative for Asthma: Global strategy for asthma management and prevention. NHLBI/WHO workshop report, March 1993, Publication No. 95-3659, Bethesda, MD: U.S. Public Health Service, January 1995, p. 106.
5. National Asthma Education and Prevention Program, National Hearth, Lung, and Blood Institute, Expert Panel Report II: Guidelines for the Diagnosis and Management of Asthma, NIH Publication No. 97-4051 February 1997 (http://www.nhlbi.nih.gov/nhlbi.htm).
6. Brunette MG, Lands L, and Thibodeau LP. Childhood asthma: Prevention of attacks with short-term corticosteroid treatment of upper respiratory tract infection. Pediatrics 1988; 81: 624–628.
7. Leickly FE, Wade SL, Crain EF, Kruszon-Moran D, Wright L, Evans R. Self-reported adherence, management behavior, and barriers to care after an ED visit by inner city children with asthma. Pediatrics 1998; 101: electronic pages (http://www.pediatrics.org).
8. Butz AM, Eggleston P, Alexander C, Rosenstein BJ. Outcomes of emergency room treatment of children with asthma. J Asthma 1991; 18:255–264.
9. Barnett PJ, Oberklaid F. Acute asthma in children: Evaluation of management in a hospital emergency department. Med J Aust 1991; 154:729–733.
10. Mak H, Johnston P, Abbey H, Talamo RC. Prevalence of asthma and health service utilization of asthmatic children in an inner city. J Allergy Clin Immunol 1982; 70:367–372.
11. Crain EF, Weiss KB, Fagan MJ. Pediatric asthma care in U.S. emergency departments. Arch Pediatr Adolesc Med 1995; 149:893–901.
12. Greineder DK, Loane KC, Parks P. Reduction in resource utilization by an asthma outreach program. Arch Pediatr Adolesc Med 1995; 149:415–420.
13. Wissow LS, Warshow M, Box J, Baker D. Case management and quality assurance to improve care of inner-city children with asthma. Am J Dis Child 1988; 42:748–752.
14. Chande VT, Wyss N, Exum V. Educational interventions to alter pediatric emergency department utilization patterns. Arch Pediatr Adolesc Med 1996; 150:525–528.
15. Wasilewski Y, Clark NM, Evans D, Levison MJ, Levin B, Mellins RB. Factors associated with emergency department visits by children with asthma: Implications for health education. Am J Publ Health 1996; 86:1410–1415.
16. Nelson EW, Van Cleve S, Swartz MK, Kessen W, McCarthy PL. Improving the use of early follow-up care after emergency department visits. Am J Dis Child 1991; 45:440–445.
17. Fraenkel DJ, Bardin PG, Sanderson G, Lampe F, et al. Lower airway inflammation during rhinovirus colds in normal and asthmatic children. Am J Respir Crit Care Med 1995; 151: 879–886.
18. Sampson AP, Castling DP, Green CP, Price JF. Persistent increase in plasma and urinary leukotrienes after acute asthma. Arch Dis Child 1995; 73:221–225.
19. Scarfone JF, Fuchs SM, Nagar AL, Shane SA. Controlled trial of oral prednisone in the emergency department treatment of children with acute asthma. Pediatrics 1993; 92:513–518.
20. Fleisher GR, Surpure JS, Rosenberg NM, and Kulick R. Management of asthma. Pediatr Emerg Care 1992; 8:167–170.
21. Unpublished data, National Cooperative Inner-City Asthma Study, NIH/NIAID, 1991–1996.
22. Chou KJ, Cunningham SJ, Crain EF. Metered dose inhalers with spacers vs. nebulizers for pediatric asthma. Arch Pediatr Adolesc Med 1995; 149:201–205.

23. Karem E, Levison H, Schuh S, O'Brodovich H, Reisman J, et al. Efficacy of albuterol administered by nebulizer versus spacer device in children with acute asthma. J Pediatr 1993; 123: 313–317.
24. Benton G, Thomas RC, Nickerson BG, McQuitty JC, Okikawa J. Experience with a metered dose inhaler with a spacer in the pediatric emergency department. Am J Dis Child 1989; 143: 678–681.
25. Cunningham SJ Crain EF. Reduction of morbidity in asthmatic children given a spacer device. Chest 1994; 106:753–757.
26. National Asthma Education and Prevention Program Task Force Report on the Cost Effectiveness, Quality of Care, and Financing of Asthma Care, Supplement, Am J Respir Crit Care Med 1996; 154:S81–S130.

36

Compliance Issues in Acute Asthma

Paul Mayo
Albert Einstein College of Medicine, Bronx, and Beth Israel Medical Center, New York, New York

I. INTRODUCTION

Asthma exacerbation is a common cause for emergency department (ED) visits. This is no more evident than in inner-city areas where there may exist an unfortunate congruence of socioeconomic, cultural, and environmental factors in populations that are immunogenetically predisposed to asthma. These reasons have resulted in small geographic areas that have extremely high hospital utilizations and death rates from the disease (1–3). Any emergency physician (EP) who has worked in a busy inner-city area knows only too well the frequent occurrences of severe asthma exacerbation. This pattern of ED visit for asthma is a paradox. The disease is easily treated on an outpatient basis with a variety of highly effective medicines, and guidelines for therapy (4) have been widely disseminated to the medical profession. Despite this, poorly treated asthma remains a common cause for ED visits. The reasons for this are multiple, but chief among them must be listed problems with compliance. This chapter will discuss compliance as it relates to the ED treatment of acute asthma.

II. GENERAL ISSUES RELATED TO COMPLIANCE

Noncompliance with medical treatment is a very common occurrence in clinical practice. It is estimated that 50% of patients do not comply with their physician's instruction in a typical outpatient setting (5). Noncompliance—and its less pejorative synonym, nonadherence—appears to be independent of patient age, gender, race, ethnicity, and socioeconomic and educational level (5). As a corollary, physicians may have difficulty in predicting to what extent a given patient will adhere to a medical regimen (5). Certain patient groups are especially likely to be noncompliant with medical treatment: patients with severe mental illness such as schizophrenia and major depression, adolescents, substance abusers, and patients with overwhelming psychosocial dysfunction.

Outpatient physicians face an especially daunting task in treating chronic ailments such as diabetes, hypertension, atherosclerotic heart disease, and asthma. The physician must convince the patient of the need to take medicines on a long-term basis. Asthma increases the challenge, as it requires constant readjustment of medication levels in response to varying disease activity levels.

Powerful forces are arrayed against clinicians in their quest for adherence. For example, fear of side effects from medicines is ubiquitous in outpatient practice. This is a reasonable fear, and it provides a strong internal logic to the patient that favors noncompliance. Economic forces may favor noncompliance. The cost of medicines may simply prohibit their use by the patient. The asthma patient who lacks adequate prescription plan coverage may pay $50 per metered dose inhaler (MDI) at a typical retail pharmacy in New York City. These patients are often the working poor who face a simple decision: compliance with their inhaled corticosteroids or food on the table for their children. Cultural forces may favor noncompliance. Cultural beliefs concerning a disease process and its treatment may result in dissonance between treatment plan and the patient's acceptance of it. Mistrust of the care provider, be it for personal or cultural reasons, is also a potential cause for noncompliance. Unless the patient and physician have a trusting therapeutic alliance, nonadherence to even the simplest medical treatment plan may occur.

Any discussion of adherence tends to be patient oriented, but another form of nonadherence plagues outpatient treatment of asthma. Physicians themselves may be guilty of nonadherence to widely available standard treatment guidelines for asthma. Patients who are treated incorrectly by their physicians may be labeled as being noncompliant with acceptable treatment methods, when in fact the blame rests squarely on their care provider, who has mistreated the patient. The noncompliant patient is often judged to have made a conscious willful decision not to follow a doctor's care plan. Nothing could be further from the truth. A complex cascade of events results in noncompliance. Rather than blaming the patient, the physician should always focus on improvement of the process that results in compliance.

III. GENERAL ISSUES RELATED TO COMPLIANCE AND ASTHMA

The current outpatient treatment of asthma is straightforward: as-needed β-agonists, an appropriate dose of twice-daily inhaled corticosteroids (ICS) delivered via spacer, and a well-structured self management plan that includes a supply of oral corticosteroids for self administration for severe exacerbations should suffice to treat the vast majority of outpatient asthmatics. The well-treated asthmatic should seldom need to visit the ED. The challenge to the clinician is not so much of regimen design, but rather of patient compliance. The two powerful tools available to the clinician are a strong therapeutic alliance combined with an appropriate medical regimen. A strong therapeutic alliance requires time, effort, and commitment. The successful outpatient physician who treats the socioeconomically deprived inner-city asthmatic must be sensitive to the challenging ethnic, cultural, economic, and personal psychodynamic issues required to develop a relationship of mutual trust between the patient and care provider. It is beyond the scope of this chapter to discuss the nuances of this important relationship. Suffice it to say that the emergency physician treats the outpatient physicians' failure on a regular basis. However, a strong therapeutic alliance will not benefit the asthmatic unless combined with an appropriate medical regimen. The regimen must be developed and negotiated within the context of the therapeutic partnership. To improve the probability of adherence, the medical regimen should be safe, effective, and simple. Simplicity is critical, and includes choosing a regimen of asthma medications that uses the fewest medicines as infrequently as possible. Asthma regimens are often unnecessarily complex. The clinician is not realistic if he prescribes multiple medications multiple times per day. Patients do not adhere to complex chronic asthma regimens. For example, dosing of ICS in chronic asthma has been studied using microprocessor-equipped metered dose inhalers capable of measuring time and number of actuations over weeks of study time (6). Compliance with QID dosing is lower compared to BID schedules (7). Disease activity does not modulate compliance with ICS either (8). In another study, patients assigned to QID inhaled ipratropium had marked noncompliance, including some patients who claimed good compliance supported by diary and MDI weight but who were detected to use hundreds of actuations just prior to seeing their physician, i.e., they were ''dumping'' the medicine in order to appear compliant (9). The clinician who prescribes ICS on a QID basis and inhaled β-agonists on a set schedule fosters noncompliance. Simplification of the asthma medical regimen remains a cornerstone of improving compliance.

Metered dose inhalers represent a challenge to the outpatient asthma clinician. These devices are essential to outpatient asthma treatment. Unfortunately, patients have great difficulty in using them properly (10,11). This form of nonadherence is self-perpetuating. Reasonably, the patient may become nonadherent with the MDI if the device is ineffective due to poor technique. If the MDI does not work, why use it? This form of noncompliance is generally judged to be patient related, i.e., the patient is blamed for not being able to use the device. This blame may be misplaced. Care providers, who are themselves responsible for training patients in proper use of the MDI, may themselves be ignorant of its correct use (12,13). This extends not only to use of the MDI itself, but also to spacer use (14). Clearly, adherence to MDI technique on the patient's part requires a clinician who is skilled in their use to train the patient.

Other issues related to compliance with MDI and spacer derive from the cost of the devices. This is especially relevant to the uninsured working poor, as previously mentioned. Medicaid patients may receive the MDI free of charge; on the other hand, spacers are not so easy for them to actually obtain. Regarded by administrative decision as being a durable medical device, spacers require a complex preapproval process before being obtained by the patient. This particular barrier must be considered as a culprit in fostering noncompliance with spacer use in Medicaid populations. Outpatient clinic operations may improve adherence with spacers by allocating resources to obtain an on-site supply of MDI and spacers for patients who require them.

The research effort targeted at identifying methods to improve compliance with outpatient asthma treatment falls into two general categories. One approach to research has been to develop highly specific interventions, such as written brochures, videotapes, classes for patients, and educational efforts directed at care providers, and to then measure compliance with treatment plan following the intervention. An alternative approach has been to design global treatment strategies using multiple simultaneous interventions that may improve adherence and search for outcome improvement. Typically, outcome measurements include reduction in ED usage, hospitalizations, and overall cost. Any improvement is considered to result from improvement in patient adherence to medical treatment plan. Although the precise improvement that has greatest effect cannot be specifically identified, this global improvement strategy has the merit of yielding pragmatic clinical benefit to the treated patient population.

Several studies have demonstrated that specialized asthma programs may have positive effects on asthma activity (15). Severe asthmatics enrolled in these programs have reduced disease activity and lower exacerbation rates requiring ED visit and hospitalization than do patients treated by the usual means. The designs of these successful programs have similar characteristics. They combine simple and safe medical regimens with an intensive personalized education strategy. Most programs rely on the care provider to provide both medical treatment and education on a one-to-one basis. The details of clinic design emphasize elements that foster close therapeutic alliance between patient and care provider. For example, short wait times, extended hours, long visits, and open-ended interview and discussion techniques are common features of clinic operation. In addition to effective medication treatment that emphasizes inhaled corticosteroids and β-agonists, patients are generally trained in aggressive self-management strategy to control exacerbations that would ordinarily result in ED visit.

The emergency physician is unlikely to treat a patient with acute asthma from a well-organized asthma specialty clinic. More typically, they see patients who have ready access to medical care but of the wrong kind. Confusing and ineffective medicines; physicians who are harried, uncommunicative, or incompetent; and clinic systems that dissuade attendance due to long waiting times and inconvenient hours are the more common lot of the inner-city asthmatic. These factors combine with ethnic, cultural, language, and socioeconomic issues to result in a final common pathway of nonadherence that is not the patient's fault. The system itself guarantees a pattern of noncompliance. The patient may become trapped in a vicious cycle of relapsing asthma. The patient is discharged from the ED or hospital and cared for by a system that encourages a passive patient response to asthma exacerbation. The uneducated patient has no self-management strategy available and an inflexible clinic system to contend with. With no recourse, disability and relapse finally lead to ED visit, and the cycle prevails.

Tactics used in specialized asthma clinics, so successful in treating populations of severe asthmatics, may have application for the EP. In the following sections, many management suggestions will be derived from the methods used commonly in such a clinic operation (16).

IV. COMPLIANCE WITH ASTHMA TREATMENT IN THE ED PREHOSPITAL PHASE

The emergency physician cannot influence compliance with asthma treatment in the period before the patient arrives in the ED. The patient's need for treatment may derive from nonadherence to medical treatment. However, the pattern of noncompliance may be useful in predicting the patient's course in the ED. Patients who seek ED treatment for asthma exacerbation due to the simple fact that they ran out of β-agonists (for example, due to lack of money or doctor's prescription) generally respond to treatment in the ED and are likely not to require hospitalization. On the other hand, if the patient has been taking some asthma medications and presents with exacerbation, the attack will commonly result in hospitalization (17).

The emergency physician should be alert for patients who are likely to be highly noncompliant in the period leading up to the ED visit. Patients in these categories may require special treatment in the postdischarge period. For example, patients with mental illness may be highly noncompliant with medical treatment as their asthma exacerbation progresses. Schizophrenic patients may have such severe thought disorder as to seriously impair their ability to take medicines (18,19), e.g., hallucinations, paranoid ideation, and delusional thoughts. Likewise, patients with severe depression may be unable to comply with medical treatment for asthma. Depression has been reported as a risk factor for severe exacerbation and potentially fatal asthma (20–22). Noncompliance in the face of severe asthma may be a manifestation of suicidal ideation and lead to death. Others have speculated on a more direct causal relationship between depression and asthma activity (23). In any case, the EP should be alert to the dangerous combination of mental illness and asthma exacerbation. Their coexistence might encourage early hospitalization decision.

Adolescent patients also present a special challenge to the EP. They face the turmoil of teenage years and may neglect compliance with asthma treatment in testing the limits of self-expression and independence (24). Asthma exacerbation in the adolescent should always alert the EP to high risk for noncompliance and the need for urgent outpatient follow-up following ED discharge.

A particularly difficult type of patient requires mention: the patient with overwhelming psychosocial problems that result in nonadherence with appropriate outpatient asthma treatment. This patient may not have any definable mental illness or intellectual deficit. They are often cared for by highly organized inner-city clinics and have access to free medication by virtue of Medicaid coverage. Despite the best efforts of well-intentioned care providers, the patient relapses repeatedly and is often a well-known figure in the inner-city ED. The life problems of the patient are so overwhelming as to render the patient incapable of compliance with a medical regimen designed to treat their asthma. In a sense, the will of the patient is paralyzed by the pervasive psychosocial failure. The problem is compounded by the fact that the hospital may be the only safe and supportive haven for the patient. There at least they are cared for by an attentive staff, and life's problems are temporarily at bay. Careful appraisal of the patient's psychosocial structure reveals a familiar pattern. In this author's experience, risk factors include middle age, physical abuse by spouse, drug abuse by spouse, abandonment by spouse, severe poverty, chronic unemployment, living in decaying housing stock, and ongoing threat of personal injury due to high levels of neighborhood criminal activity. There is often a lack of supportive extended family, and in particular the children of the patient may have suffered early death by infections such as AIDS, criminal action, or drug abuse. Living children may imprisoned. The EP needs to be alert to this type of patient, as standard methods to improve compliance are not likely to benefit the patient.

Finally, substance abuse and asthma may unite to yield high rates of noncompliance. The reasons for this are obvious: drug-seeking behavior takes precedence over compliance with medical regimen. This general pattern of noncompliance is amplified by specific pharmacological effects of substance abuse. For example, inhalation of cocaine may directly result in asthma exacerbation (25,26). An equally dangerous but more subtle effect occurs with narcotic use. The patient with worsening asthma may derive subjective benefit from narcotic use as the narcotic suppresses his sense of dyspnea. The addict may delay presentation to the ED until they are in extremis by using narcotics instead of asthma medications to attenuate symptoms. There is a strong association between death from asthma and substance abuse (27). This relates ultimately to the noncompliance of these patients with asthma treatment. The EP may need to modify discharge treatment for these patients as discussed below.

Substance abusers may manifest another pattern of behavior that results in noncompliance. In order to fund their recreational drug use, this author is aware of diversion of appropriately prescribed asthma medications for resale back to unscrupulous pharmacy operations. Alternatively, β-agonists may be resold by the patient on the street to cocaine abusers, as there is a prevalent but unproven belief amongst cocaine users that prebronchodilation with β-agonists will improve the uptake of crack cocaine. In addition, the beta-sympathomimetic effect of the inhaled β-agonists may mimic the peripheral adrenergic effects of cocaine, giving the abuser a sense of synergy in using both the MDI and cocaine. In any case, the EP may be placed in the uncomfortable position of wishing to prescribe an MDI, while being aware that it is not likely to be used, or worse, that it will be diverted for patient profit.

In summary, regarding non-adherence before ED visit, the EP may be a passive observer of the results of non-compliance with asthma treatment plan. However, the information that is derived by careful history and assessment of the psychologic state of the patient may allow the EP to develop a strategy that will improve post discharge treatment and compliance.

V. COMPLIANCE ISSUES IN THE PERIOD POSTDISCHARGE FROM THE ED

The patient who is treated in the ED for asthma exacerbation will either be hospitalized or, if improved, discharged from the ED. The ED treatment may be perfect and the discharge decision appropriate, but if relapse occurs, some blame may rest with the EP. Just as nonadherence may result in the initial ED visit, nonadherence with postdischarge medical plan must necessarily be a major factor in many relapses requiring retreatment in the ED. For this reason, the EP must make every effort to ensure compliance with treatment plan until such time as the patient comes under treatment by his assigned outpatient care provider. It is critical to develop an effective strategy to bridge the patient to outpatient follow-up during this period, understanding that many patients will not follow-up with a primary care provider (28).

Successful clinics that target asthmatics have had considerable success in reducing asthma activity in populations of severe asthmatics form inner-city areas, as discussed earlier. The techniques used in these clinic operations may have application in improving adherence to medical treatment in the ED postdischarge period. There is little literature examining specific ED-based interventions on compliance with asthma treatment in the postdischarge period (29). What follows is a pragmatic approach based on experience with clinic operations targeted at severe adult asthmatics.

VI. SPECIFIC SUGGESTIONS THAT MAY IMPROVE COMPLIANCE IN THE POSTDISCHARGE PERIOD

1. The patient should be seen very soon postdischarge by a competent outpatient care provider. The ideal system would require the patient to be seen the following day

or even the same day. The author's experience is that follow-up visits from the ED of 1 or 2 weeks yield negligible show rates. On the other hand, early follow-up appointments have been very difficult to achieve in urban clinics due to heavy scheduling and the lack of ability to make a clinic appointment at the time of the discharge from the ED. This remains a vexing problem. In arranging early clinic visit, the EP must be confident in the quality of the follow-up. It does the patient little good to be treated by an incompetent outpatient service. It is essential that the EP find a source of high-quality asthma care for referral of their difficult patients, especially in areas of high asthma prevalence in the inner city. This represents formidable organizational challenges. Additionally, a managed care environment may restrict the EP's ability to select a particular clinician. To improve quality and access to high-quality care may require a major cooperative effort that involves the ED and outpatient medical providers. This is difficult to achieve given the limited resources available to the inner-city ED and outpatient areas. As an alternative, individual ED physicians might attempt to develop a close working relationship with an outpatient clinician with expertise in asthma. Sadly, the most prevalent outpatient follow-up given to the high risk of an inner-city asthmatic may simply be a telephone number of a clinic to contact for follow-up postdischarge. It is known that this approach yields low levels of compliance with outpatient follow-up following ED treatment (28). Every effort should be made to give the patient an actual scheduled appointment. Obviously, patients with private medical follow-up are in a favorable position, but this does not hold for indigent patients. Traditionally, the ED and their outpatient colleagues have not cooperated and coordinated with each other in the effort against asthma. The seamless pass, transfer, and capture by a high-quality outpatient clinic requires the EP to have a close working relationship with the outpatient asthma care providers who will be seeing the patient in early follow-up. The importance of early follow-up cannot be overemphasized. In one study, 91% of patients who required ED revisit for relapse had not seen their primary care physician before having to return to the ED (30).

2. The postdischarge medical regimen should be very simple, well tolerated, and effective. The ED clinician has a very specific goal in the postdischarge period: to prevent relapse and reduce disability from asthma until the patient comes under early outpatient control. Unless the patient has had a very mild exacerbation, the discharge regimen will usually include a course of systemic steroids to suppress disease activity until the patient visits the outpatient care provider, as well as β-agonists to control symptoms. Obedient to the concept of simplicity, the corticosteroid dose should be given as a single daily dose. More frequent dosing, or dosing that requires precise timing will greatly increase risk of noncompliance. Patients are knowledgeable regarding the side effects of oral corticosteroids, and the clinician must be prepared to discuss these issues exhaustively. If these concerns are not met, the patient will simply not take the medicine. Nonadherence has a strong internal logic when the patient fears the medicine. The clinician will foster nonadherence unless the fears of the patient are addressed. Specific issues that may reassure the patient include a frank discussion of the very real dangers of corticosteroids, their clinical effectiveness, as well as the need to use them for only a short period of time. If outpatient follow-up will be delayed, the patient is often placed on a tapering oral regimen, thereby increasing the complexity of the regimen and greatly increasing the probability of nonadherence if the patient is fearful of the medication or develops side effects. The EP may elect to start high dose ICS in order to permit rapid taper of oral corticosteroids. This being the case, the patient must be educated as to their use. More concentrated formulations of ICS are now available. Using these, the clinician may reduce the number of

puffs required and so increase likelihood of adherence. Likewise, all ICS are effective BID, another factor fostering compliance.

Inhaled β-agonists are the second mainstay of treatment. There is a tendency to prescribe them on a standing-order basis. This fosters nonadherence as such regimens are simply not taken by patients. Instead, the clinician should encourage compliance by assigning them on an as-needed basis which is equally efficacious (see Chapter 19 on β-agonists). The patient may be warned that excessive need indicates that the asthma may be recurring in a dangerous pattern.

One issue that concerns patients relates to the safety of inhaled β-agonists. This author notes a common fear among asthma patients that β-agonists may cause cardiac damage and may be ''addicting.'' To increase compliance, both of these issues must be addressed in an understanding way. The author, when faced with a patient expressing concern regarding safety of the β-agonist, often inhales six puffs in a row of albuterol in front of the patient. This is valuable as a teaching method for MDI use, as well as to assuage patients' fear related to toxicity. Seeing a physician using the medication reassures the patient of its safety. Unless the patient's fears are sufficiently allayed, the patient will not take the medication. It is essential that the clinician address these fears in a supportive and convincing manner.

In keeping with the need for simplicity, the institution of methyl xanthines, long-acting β-agonists, mast cell stabilizer, and leukotriene inhibitors should be reserved for the outpatient physician. Their use needlessly complicates the task of the EP and greatly increases the probability of nonadherence by the patient. All effort should be focused on assuring compliance with the oral corticosteroids (with ICS if needed) and β-agonists during the critical period between ED discharge and outpatient clinic visit. For economic reasons as well as practical ones, patients may not be able to obtain prescriptions following discharge from the ED. This form of noncompliance may result in an early ED revisit. A simple solution to this problem is to provide selected patients with sufficient medicines to last until outpatient follow-up upon discharge from the ED. This resource allocation may be justified if it reduces early relapse rates. A medicine is only effective if the patient actually has it to take.

3. The patient should be given specific training in MDI use. Unless this is done, the clinician may be fostering a form of physician-induced noncompliance. If the patient does not use the MDI correctly, they are innocently nonadherent. The medication will have no clinical effect, and the clinician is to blame. Giving an MDI, especially to a new-onset asthmatic, without specific training is akin to giving the diabetic patient insulin and syringes without training the patient in their use. MDI technique is difficult to master, and every EP must be completely proficient in MDI use before they can attempt to train the patient. In training the patient, both the trainer and patient must have an MDI at hand. Simple verbal instruction may be ineffective. Training requires hands-on demonstration, repetition, and multiple re-checks (31). If the ED has sufficient resources, I would strongly recommend the distribution of spacers to acute asthmatics, as they guarantee intrabronchial delivery of medication. Limited ED resource may not absolutely justify this type of resource allocation, especially if the patient will be seen promptly by a skilled outpatient provider. Certainly, spacers are an essential part of management once the patient is under regular outpatient treatment.

4. Specific teaching techniques should be used to improve postdischarge adherence. The worst case scenario can be seen in any busy ED. The patient is improved and

ready for discharge. A quick sign out occurs, and the patient is given a phone number to call for follow-up. This chain of events guarantees a high rate of noncompliance with the medical plan.

On the other hand, it is unrealistic for the ED to provide the patient with a full-service outpatient visit. Given the intrinsic limitations of a busy ED, I would suggest the following basic requirements for educating asthmatic patients before discharge.

a. The discharge instruction must be given in a quiet area not subject to interruption with both patient and clinician seated comfortably.

b. The discussion must be unhurried, detailed, and repetitive. The treatment regimen should be simple, i.e., not with an excessive number of separate instructions (32).

c. The patient must be able to clearly explain in his own words the discharge medications and when, where, and with whom he will be obtaining early outpatient follow-up.

d. The session must include clear demonstration by the care provider of MDI use, and the patient must personally demonstrate adequate technique before discharge.

e. The instructor should specifically discuss all patient questions related to medication effect and toxicity.

f. The culture, language, and socioeconomic background of the patient need to be considered. If possible, all instruction should be in the native language of the patient. Family members may be key players in the instruction phase. Written instruction should be regarded as supplementing rather than replacing verbal communication. The training session can typically be accomplished in about 10–15 min. This allocation of valuable time resource is counterbalanced by the major potential benefit of reduced relapse rate. The care provider assigned the task of discharge training does not need to be a medical doctor. Nurses practitioners (33) and respiratory therapists are highly effective in training asthma patients.

Turning now to those patients who are very likely to be highly noncompliant with any medical treatment plan, the EP faces the difficult challenge of the mentally ill asthmatic, the adolescent, the psychosocial failure, and the substance abuser. The adolescent patient, highly vulnerable to relapse due to noncompliance, is obviously a high priority. Every family resource must be mobilized to assure immediate follow-up by a highly competent adolescent medicine expert. Regarding the other three categories, there is a high probability that they will not take a course of oral corticosteroids or inhaled medications, and they will not visit their outpatient provider. Although transiently improved by ED treatment, their nonadherence greatly increases the probability of early ED revisit. Death from asthma is not out of the question. What should the emergency clinician do?

A large dose of depot long-acting corticosteroids is a therapeutic option in these patients who will not otherwise take oral or inhaled medication. Several studies demonstrate that intramuscular (IM) depot triamcinolone can have prolonged antiasthma effect (34,35). By using a long-acting injectable preparation, the clinician insures compliance with an effective asthma medication.

This approach has the obvious drawback that the patient is exposed to the usual side effects of long-duration systemic corticosteroids. The patient may also receive additional doses if he or she visits multiple EDs. For this reason, the use of this medication by ED staff should be restricted to those patients who will obviously not comply with a conventional bridging regimen to outpatient follow-up visit. Most patients are appropriately treated with a brief course of oral corticosteroids and inhaled medication in order to prevent relapse between ED discharge and early outpatient follow-up. IM triamcinolone, while effective, should be reserved for those patients at very high risk for noncompliance.

VII. SUMMARY

Noncompliance with asthma treatment is a major contributor to ED visit for asthma exacerbation. Using straightforward techniques, the EP may impact favorably on compliance rates in the critical period between ED discharge and outpatient follow-up. Certain patient groups have very high rates of noncompliance, and represent difficult challenges to the emergency physician.

REFERENCES

1. Carr W, Zeitel L, Weiss K. Variations in asthma hospitalizations and deaths in New York City. Am J Public Health 1992; 82:59–65.
2. DePalo VA, Mayo PM, Friedman P, Rosen MJ. Demographic influences on asthma admission rates in New York City. Chest 1994; 106:447–451.
3. Gottlieb DJ, Beiser AS, O'Connor GT. Poverty, race, and medication use are correlates of asthma hospitalization rates. A small area analysis in Boston. Chest 1995; 108:28–35.
4. Guidelines for the diagnosis and management of asthma. NIH Publication No. 97-4051A, 1997.
5. Mellins RB, Evans D, Zimmerman B, Clark NM. Patient compliance: Are we wasting our time and don't know it? Am Rev Respir Dis 1992; 146:1376–1377.
6. Spector SL, Kinsman R, Mawhinney H, Siegel SC, Rachelefsky GS, Katz RM, Rohr AS. Compliance of patients with asthma with an experimental aerosolized medication: implications for controlled clinical trials. J Allergy Clin Immunol 1986; 77:65–70.
7. Mann M, Eliasson O, Kaushik P, ZuWallack RL. A comparison of the effects of bid and qid dosing on compliance with inhaled flunisolide. Chest 1992; 101:496–499.
8. Mann M, Eliasson O, Kaushik P, ZuWallack RL. An evaluation of severity-modulated compliance with qid dosing of inhaled beclomethasone. Chest 1992; 102:1342–1346.
9. Rand CS, Wise RA, Nides M, Simmons MS, Bleecker ER, Kusek JW, Li VC, Tashkin DP. Metered dose inhaler adherence in a clinical trial. Am Rev Respir Dis 1992; 146:1559–1564.
10. Shim C, Williams MH Jr. The adequacy of inhalation of aerosol from canister nebulizers. Am J Med 1980; 69:891–894.
11. Oprehek J, Gayard P, Grimaud C, Chapin J. Patient error in use of bronchodilator metered aerosols. Br Med J 1976; 1:76.
12. Kelling JS, Strohl KP, Smith RL, Altose MD. Physician knowledge in the use of canister nebulizers. Chest 1983; 83:612–614.
13. Guidry GG, Brown WD, Stogner SW, George RB. Incorrect use of metered dose inhalers by medical personnel. Chest 1992; 101:31–33.
14. Hanania NA, Wittman R, Kesten S, Chapman R. Medical personnel's knowledge of and ability to use inhaling devices, metered dose inhalers, spacing chambers, and breath actuated dry powder inhalers. Chest 1994; 105:111–116.
15. Bartter T, Pratter MR. Asthma: Better outcome at lower cost? The role of the expert in the care system. Chest 1996; 110:1589–1596.
16. Mayo PM, Richman J, Harris WH. Results of a program to reduce admissions for adult asthma. Ann Intern Med 1990; 112:864–871.

17. Brenner BE, Leber M, Kohn MS, Camargo C. ED visits for acute asthma by patients who recently ran out of their beta-agonist inhaler. Ann Emerg Med 1997; 30(abstr):427.
18. Patterson R. Greenberger PA, Patterson DR. Potentially fatal asthma: the problem of non-compliance. Ann Allergy 1991; 67:138–142.
19. Sonin L, Patterson R. Corticosteroid-dependent asthma and schizophrenia. Arch Intern Med 1984; 144:554–556.
20. Picado C, Montserrat JM, dePablo J, Plaza V, Agusti-Vidal A. Predisposing factors to death after recovery from a life threatening asthmatic attack. J Asthma 1989; 26:231–236.
21. Strunk RC, Mrazek DA, Wolfson GS, LaBreque JF. Physiologic and psychological characteristics associated with deaths due to asthma in childhood: a case study. JAMA 1985; 254:1193–1198.
22. Bosley CM, Fosbury JA, Cochrane GM. The psychological factors associated with poor compliance with treatment in asthma. Eur Respir J 1995; 8:899–904.
23. Miller BD. Depression and asthma: a potentially lethal mix. J Allergy Clin Immunol 1987; 80:481–486.
24. Lewiston NJ, Rubinstein S. The young Damocles. The adolescent at high risk for serious or fatal status asthmaticus. Clin Rev Allergy 1987; 5:273–284.
25. Rebhun J. Association of asthma and freebase smoking. Ann Allergy 1988; 60:339–342.
26. Rubin RB, Neugarten J. Cocaine-associated asthma. Am J Med 1990; 88:438–439.
27. Levenson T, Greenberger PA, Donoghue ER, Lifschultz BD. Asthma deaths confounded by substance abuse: An assessment of fatal asthma. Chest 1996; 110:604–610.
28. Thomas EJ, Burstin HR, O'Neil AC, Orav ES, Brennan TA. Patient non-compliance with medical advice after the emergency department visit. Ann Emerg Med 1996; 27:49–55.
29. Maiman LA, Green LW, Gibson G, MacKensie EJ. Education for self-treatment by adult asthmatics. JAMA 1979; 241:1919–1922.
30. Emerman CL, Cydulka RK. Factors associated with relapse after emergency department treatment for acute asthma. Ann Emerg Med 1995: 26:6–11.
31. Resnick DJ, Gold RL, Lee-Wong M, Feldman BR, Rajasekar R, Davis WJ. Physicians metered dose inhaler technique after a single teaching session. Ann Allergy Asthma Immunol 1996; 76:145–148.
32. Guishard K, Rogove V, Chudian F, Griffith E, Seally A, Pomeranz H. A study of physician communication and patient retention of discharge instructions. Acad Emerg Med 1997; 4:473.
33. Mayo PM, Weinberg JW, Kramer BH, Richman J, Seibert-Choi OS, Rosen MJ. Results of a program to improve the process of inpatient care of adult asthmatics. Chest 1996; 110:48–52.
34. Ogirala RG, Aldrich TK, Prezant DJ. High-dose intramuscular triamcinolone in severe chronic life threatening asthma. N Engl J Med 1991; 324:585–589.
35. Ogirala RG, Sturm TM, Aldrich TK, Miller FF, Pacia EB, Keane AM, Finkel RI. Single high-dose intramuscular triamcinolone acetonide versus weekly oral methotrexate in life threatening asthma: A double-blind study. Am J Respir Crit Care Med 1995; 152:1461–1466.

37

Access, the Emergency Department, and Asthma

Lynne D. Richardson
Mount Sinai School of Medicine, New York, New York

The reported increases in morbidity and mortality from asthma over the past two decades, particularly in poor communities of color, have not been adequately explained (1–3). Lack of access to primary health care has been hypothesized to contribute to the increased risk of asthma morbidity and mortality (4,5). This chapter will explore the relationships between emergency department (ED) visits and access to primary care and the complex interactions of these two phenomenon in patients with asthma.

I. ACCESS

Access to care is an issue that has been widely discussed in the health services and public health literature. In recent work, the distinction between potential access and realized access has been emphasized. Access is best defined as the actual use of personal health services and everything that facilitates or impedes the use of personal health services (6, 7). To examine this issue, the clinician's usual focus on individual patient characteristics must be expanded. Understanding the complex individual and interactive effects of myriad personal, medical, environmental, psychosocial, organizational, and institutional factors on service utilization is necessary to understanding the issue of access (8,9) (see Table 1).

Effective measures of access must incorporate patient level, provider level, and systems level characteristics (6,7). Since access to health services that are inadequate or deleterious are of no value, measures of access also assess issues of quality. Disease-specific access is an emerging concept that is particularly relevant to patients with asthma. Clearly, many patients with asthma have unmet needs; they underuse necessary services and fail to achieve optimal control of their disease (10–12). This situation may well be exacerbated

Table 1 Factors That Influence Access to Medical Care

Patient Factors	Provider Factors
Financial barriers	medical knowledge
unemployment	communication skills
lack of insurance	clinical competence
low income	cultural competence
Personal/psychosocial barriers	discrimination
health status	Systems Factors
functional status	hours of operation
literacy	waiting time
education	structural barriers
ability to negotiate complex bureaucracies	payment policies
personal preference/choice	number of providers
discrimination	location of services
social support	type of providers
Cultural barriers	characteristics of providers
cultural values	appointment availability
health beliefs	preauthorization
language	institutional racism
traditional customs	
alternative health remedies	
Environmental barriers	
housing	
occupation	
community disadvantage	
violence	
travel times	

by competitive pressures on health care providers under managed care and future changes in Medicaid, Medicare, and public health expenditures (13,14).

Certain barriers are disproportionately encountered by specific socioeconomic or racial groups (15). Many of these are of particular relevance to the populations experiencing the highest rates of morbidity and mortality from asthma (16,17). The poor of all races face more intractable financial barriers than those with higher incomes. Racial minorities report that they experience more delays in seeking needed care, and are twice as likely as whites to report that getting specialty care is a major problem (18). Both poverty and race may limit access due to cultural and institutional barriers (19–21).

Understanding the barriers to appropriate access to care for patients with asthma is essential to the design of effective interventions to reduce asthma morbidity and mortality. The ED offers a unique and important perspective from which to study factors that limit access to other sources of care and the effect of limited access on patient outcomes. It has been reported that individuals without primary care physicians, those without insurance, and those with public insurance disproportionately utilize EDs to obtain care (22,23).

II. THE EMERGENCY DEPARTMENT

ED utilization is a multifaceted reflection of the many forces impacting on the health care delivery system. The development of new therapeutic modalities and the improvements in diagnostic technology that have accompanied the establishment of emergency medicine as a specialty have raised the public's expectations regarding acceptable levels of care and created a widespread demand for services that did not exist 30 years ago. The ED is a unique practice setting in two respects. The first is its capacity to deliver a full range of medical services to acutely ill or injured patients, regardless of the nature of the presenting complaint. Second, the complete accessibility of the ED is assured not only by the professional and ethical standards of emergency physicians but by federal, and in many cases, state law. Either or both of these two defining characteristics may influence a patient's decision to use the ED.

Patients with an unarguable need for emergency care may have a serious illness or injury resulting from a catastrophic event that could not have been predicted or prevented by even the most astute and experienced primary physician, or resulting from an unmanaged disease process due to the lack of appropriate primary care. On the other hand, complaints that could be competently managed outside of the ED may be brought by patients without access to other settings (who may or may not appreciate the lack of urgency of their problem), or by patients who prefer the more sophisticated resources and immediate availability of the ED, despite their access to alternative sources of care that could competently manage their condition (24,25).

The ED is thus many things to many people: the provider of choice for some, a provider of convenience for others, and the provider of last resort for many. A useful framework to analyze ED utilization must link the patient's previous experience with primary health care to the nature of the presenting complaint (see Figure 1). Current patterns of ED utilization have undesirable consequences for both the patient and the system. The ED visit addresses the immediate clinical issues but it is not an acceptable substitute for regular medical attention. Care rendered in the ED lacks the continuity of information and the attention to health maintenance issues that are necessary for high-quality primary care. ED care is also more costly. Although of comparable cost to a primary care visit,

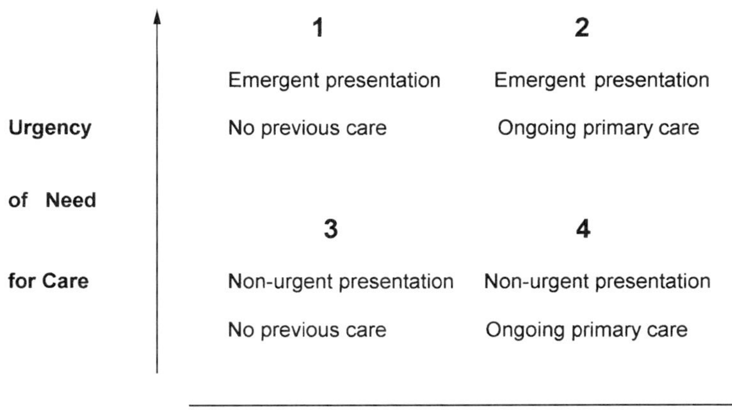

Figure 1 Emergency department visits. ED utilization must be analyzed as a function of: (1) the nature, acuity, and severity of the presenting complaint; and (2) the patient's experience with other health care settings prior to the ED visit.

it has been estimated to be as much as five times the average charge for a clinic or physician's office in the same community (26,27).

The relatively high charges for emergency care have caused a great deal of attention to be focused on the occurrence of what are called (inappropriately, I believe) ''inappropriate emergency department visits'' (28–31). The characterization and quantification of these ''inappropriate emergency visits'' have been hampered by widespread confusion between retrospective and prospective judgments on whether or not evaluation and treatment on an emergency basis were warranted. Since the patient's decision to seek emergency care is made based on the presenting symptoms without knowledge of the findings of the as yet to be performed ED evaluation, the appropriateness of an ED visit cannot be determined retrospectively based on ED diagnosis. However attractive this method may be to cost-conscious payors, it is useless to either describe or modify the behavior of patients.

It is true that a significant portion of the care rendered to patients in EDs could be competently delivered in other practice settings if such settings were similarly equipped and staffed and were immediately available at all hours. Unfortunately, it is unlikely that total costs to the system would be reduced by creating 24 hours per day walk-in capacity in primary care centers. In the presence of existing financial, temporal, and institutional barriers to appropriate primary care, the decision by a patient to forgo an ED visit for a nonurgent problem (Figure 1, quadrant 3) may lead to the later occurrence of a life-threatening problem that necessitates an emergent ED visit (Figure 1, quadrant 1). From the perspective of an individual with limited resources, an ED visit may be the only available source of health care; and such a visit may be far more appropriate than seeking no care at all. From the perspective of the health care delivery system, access to adequate primary care would not only result in a decrease of ED visits for nonurgent problems as patients received care for these in primary care settings, but also a decrease in ED visits for urgent and emergent problems as serious episodes of illness and injury are avoided or prevented by effective primary care. This is likely to be particularly true of patients with asthma. Current efforts to erect barriers to ED access are ill advised and in the interests of neither the patients nor the health care system.

III. ASTHMA

The number of ED visits made by a patient with asthma has long been regarded as a marker for serious disease (32,33). Regardless of the surrounding circumstances or underlying cause, a visit to the ED for an acute asthmatic attack represents a clinical failure to control the disease. This may occur despite appropriate management as the result of an unavoidable physiological, environmental, or psychosocial insult that precipitates the attack, or it may occur as the result of inadequate medical management.

Visits to the ED for asthma therefore represent an easily measurable variable that is related both to the severity of illness and the quality of the previous clinical management received by the individual (34). In fact, patients with asthma can be found in all four quadrants of Figure 1. ED visits for asthma are very common, as high as 10% in many urban EDs. Patients with asthma who are well managed and on optimal therapy may occasionally present in respiratory failure (Figure 1, quadrant 2); patients who are not receiving adequate primary care are even more likely to present with serious respiratory compromise (Figure 1, quadrant 1). Patients who lack primary care may visit the ED with minimal symptoms but needing prescription refills (Figure 1, quadrant 3). Patients with excellent access to primary care but little insight into their symptomatology may present to the ED rather than complying with their self-management regimen (Figure 1, quadrant 4).

The relationship between hospitalization for asthma and the availability of primary care providers has been extensively studied (36–38). It has been demonstrated using small area analysis that the frequency of asthma hospitalization is inversely proportional to the level of primary care in a given area; this has led to the description of asthma as a ''primary care sensitive condition.'' Primary care sensitive conditions (also called ''ambulatory care sensitive conditions'') are diagnoses for which hospitalization can usually be avoided by appropriate treatment in the outpatient setting. When there are delays in seeking care, manifestations or complications of these primary care sensitive conditions that were initially preventable or treatable result in clinical deterioration requiring hospitalization.

It is reasonable to extrapolate from hospitalizations to ED visits. Since virtually all admissions of patients without a regular source of primary care are made through the ED, ED visits would be expected to increase to the same extent as hospitalizations in areas with decreased primary care. In fact it is likely that ED visits are increased to a greater extent than hospitalizations because there are undoubtedly occasions when ED management is sufficient to treat the acute problem and the patient is not hospitalized. ED visits for asthma may be an even more ''primary care sensitive'' indicator than hospitalizations.

It is also true that the kind of partnership between the patient and the primary care provider espoused by the National Heart, Lung and Blood Institute (NHLBI) National Asthma Education and Prevention Program would decrease visits for asthma in all quadrants of Figure 1. The NHBLI's Second Expert Panel on the Management of Asthma describes successful asthma management as requiring patients and families to effectively carry out complex pharmacological regimens, institute environmental control strategies, detect and self-treat most asthma exacerbations, and communicate appropriately with health care providers (40). Their report also emphasizes the importance of assessing and responding to cultural or ethnic beliefs or practices that may influence patients. The report urges that educational messages and discussions of clinical care plans be provided in the patients primary language by an individual who is knowledgeable about medical terms and fluent in both English and the patient's primary language (41).

The recommendations contained in NHBLI's Second Expert Panel Report (EPR-2) require a significant commitment from both patients and primary care providers in their approach to asthma management. Unfortunately, the guidelines contained in EPR-2 constitute a vision of what asthma care should encompass, not a description of prevailing practices. The fact is that many patients with asthma, particularly those who are poor or African-American or both, do not now have access to such primary care (34,35). Widespread changes in clinical practice may ultimately result from dissemination and implementation of the NHLBI guidelines, but such changes will not occur quickly.

In the meantime, the challenge presented to emergency physicians is threefold: (1) to prevent the creation of barriers to ED access; (2) to deliver high-quality medical care to all patients who present to the ED; and (3) to recognize that the ED visit may be a teachable moment when important educational messages about the patient's disease and the patient's use of appropriate health care services can be delivered. Identifying providers who are delivering effective primary care for asthma and creating linkages with these providers for ED patients may have as important an effect on patient outcomes as our performance of critical medical interventions.

REFERENCES

1. National Institutes of Health, National Heart, Lung and Blood Institute, Global Strategy for Asthma Management and Prevention, Publication No. 95-3659, 1995.
2. Centers for Disease Control, Asthma—United States, 1982–1990. MMWR 1995; 43(51–52): 95.
3. Gergen PJ, Mullally DI, Evans, R III. National survey of prevalence of asthma among children in the United States, 1976–1980. Pediatrics 1988; 81:1–7.
4. Weiss KB, Gergen PJ, Crain EF. Inner city asthma: The epidemiology of an emerging US public health concern. Chest 1992; 101:362S–367S.
5. Findley SE, McLean DE, Stevens K. Interactive effects of race and poverty on asthma. Am J Respir Dis Crit Care 1996; PA429(abstr).
6. Anderson R. Revisiting the behavioral model and access to medical care: Does it matter? J Health Soc Behav 1995; 36:1–10.
7. Anderson R, Newman J. Societal and individual determinants of medical care utilization in the United States. Milbank Mem Fund Q Health Soc 1973; 54:95–124.
8. Giblin P, Poland M, Ager J. Effects of social supports on attitudes, health behaviors and obtaining prenatal care. J Community Health 1990; 15:357–368.
9. Lillie-Blanton M, Laveist T. Race/ethnicity, the social environment, and health. Soc Sci Med 1996; 43:83–91.
10. Fossett J, Perloff J. The ''New'' Health Reform and Access to Care: The Problem of the Inner City, Washington, DC: The Kaiser Commission on the Future of Medicaid, 1995.
11. Kelley M, Perloff J, Morris N, Liu W. The role of perceived barriers in the use of a comprehensive prenatal care program. In: Nellie P Tate, ed., Health Care for the Poor & Uninsured: Strategies That Work, Hawthorne Press, 1992.
12. Austin R. Asthma and the unmet needs of minorities. In: Bernstein E and Bernstein J, eds., Case Studies in Emergency Medicine and the Health of the Public, Sudbury, MA: Jones and Bartlett Publishers, 1996, 152–157.
13. Hurley R, Freund D, Taylor D. Emergency room use of primary care case management: Evidence from four Medicaid demonstration programs. Am J Publ Health 1989; 79:843–846.
14. Rowland D, Rosenbaum S, Simon L, Chait E. Medicaid and managed care: Lessons from the literature, A Report of the Kaiser Commission on the future of Medicaid, The Henry J. Kaiser Family Foundation, CA, 1995.
15. Nickens HW. The role of race/ethnicity and social class in minority health status, Health Serv Res 1995; 30:151–162.
16. Weiss KB, Wagener DK. Changing patterns of asthma mortality; identifying target populations at risk. JAMA 1990; 264:1683–1687.
17. Weiss KB, Wagener DK. Geographic variation in US asthma mortality: Small area analyses of excess mortality, 1981–1985. Am J Epidemiol 1990; 132:S107–S115.
18. National Comparative Survey of Minority Health Care, New York: The Commonwealth Fund, 1995.
19. Krieger N, Rowley DL, Herman AA, et al. Racism, sexism and social class: Implications for the studies of health, disease, and well-being. Am J Prev Med 1993; 9:82–122.
20. Schulman KA, Rubinstein LE, Chesley FD, Eisenberg JM. The roles of race and socioeconomic factors in health services research. Health Serv Res 1995; 30:179–195.
21. Scott CJ. Ethnicity, culture, and the delivery of health-care services. In: Bernstein E and Bernstein J, eds., Case Studies in Emergency Medicine and the Health of the Public, Sudbury, MA: Jones and Bartlett Publishers, 1996, 139–151.
22. General Accounting Office, Emergency Departments: Unevenly Affected by Growth and Change in Patient Use, Washington, D.C., Publication No. B-251319, 1993.
23. Richardson LD, Ford JG. Use of the emergency department by patients with asthma in an indigent urban African-American community, presented at the 10th Annual Meeting of the Association for Health Services Research; Washington, DC, June 1993.

24. Lowe RA, et al. Indigent health care in emergency medicine: an academic perspective. Ann Emerg Med 1991; 20:790–794.
25. Allison EJ, DeHart KL. The ultimate safety net. Ann Emerg Med 1991; 20:820–821.
26. U.S. Department of Health and Human Services, Office of the Inspector General, Use of Emergency Rooms by Medicaid Recipients, 1992.
27. Blumenthal D, Mort E, Edwards J. The efficacy of primary care for vulnerable population groups. Health Serv Res 1995; 30:253–273.
28. Guterman JJ, et al. Inappropriate emergency department visits. Ann Emerg Med 1985; 14: 1191–1196.
29. Pane GA, Farner MC, Salness KA. Health care access problems of medically indigent emergency department walk-in patients. Ann Emerg Med 1991; 20:730–733.
30. Shesser R, et al. An analysis of emergency department use by patients with minor illness. Ann Emerg Med 1991; 20:743–748.
31. Buesching DP, et al. Inappropriate emergency department visits. Ann Emerg Med 1985; 14: 672–676.
32. National Institutes of Health, National Heart, Lung and Blood Institute, National Asthma Education Program; Expert Panel Report. Guidelines for the Diagnosis and Management of Asthma, Publication No. 91-3042, 1991.
33. Richardson LD, Jagoda A. Management of life-threatening asthma in the emergency department. Mount Sinai J Med 1997; 64:275–282.
34. Richardson LD, McLean DE, Ford JG, et al. Factors associated with frequent ED use for asthma. (abstr.) Acad Emerg Med 1996; 3:A123.
35. Richardson LD, McLean DE, Ford JG, Findley SE, Zhang W. Reducing emergency asthma care in Harlem: primary care access is not enough (abstr). New York: American Public Health Association, 1996.
36. Gergen PJ, Weiss KG. Changing patterns of asthma hospitalization among children: 1979–1987. JAMA 1990; 264:1688–1692.
37. Billings J, Zeitel L, Lukomnik J, et al. Impact of socioeconomic status on hospital use in New York City. Health Aff Millwood 1993; 12:162–173.
38. Billings J, Anderson G, Newman L. Recent findings on preventable hospitalizations. Health Aff Millwood 1996; 14:239–249.
39. Bindman A, Grumbach K, Osmond D, Komaromy M, Vranizan K, Lurie N, Billings J, Stewart A. Preventable hospitalizations and access to health care. JAMA 1995; 274:305–311.
40. National Institutes of Health, National Heart, Lung, and Blood Institute, Expert Panel report 2: Guidelines for the Diagnosis and Management of Asthma, Publication No. 97-4051, 1997.
41. Woloshin S, Bickell NA, Schwartz LM, Gany F, Welch HG. Language barriers in medicine in the U.S. JAMA 1995; 273:724–728.

Index

Page references followed by f *and* t *denote figures and tables, respectively.*

About the Editor

BARRY E. BRENNER is Vice-Chairman and Research Director of the Department of Emergency Medicine, Director of the Brooklyn Acute Asthma Center, and Director of the Physician Research Associate Program, at The Brooklyn Hospital Center, a member of New York–Presbyterian Hospitals, an academic affiliate of Weill Medical College of Cornell University. The Brooklyn Hospital Center receives over 4000 adult and pediatric visits for acute asthma each year. A nationally recognized authority on acute asthma and the author or coauthor of over 70 research articles, academic books, and book chapters, he has been a Fellow of the American College of Emergency Physicians, the American College of Physicians, the American College of Chest Physicians, the New York Academy of Medicine, and a member of the New York Academy of Sciences. Dr. Brenner received the B.A. degree (1971) from Bard College, Annandale-on-Hudson, New York, and the M.D. (1974) and Ph.D. (1976) degrees from the Medical College of Virginia, Richmond.

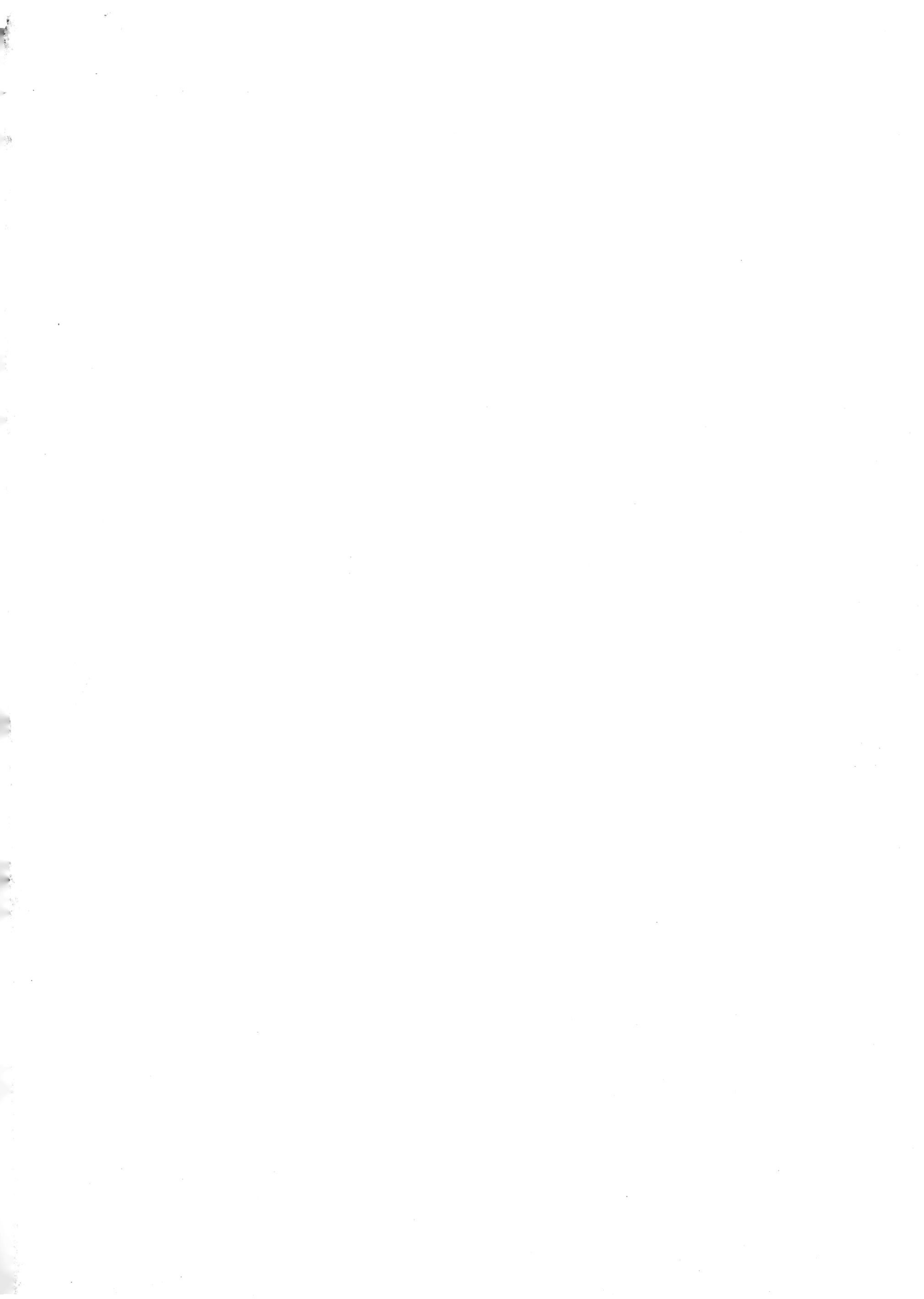